Psychiatric Care in Severe Obesity

Sanjeev Sockalingam • Raed Hawa
Editors

Psychiatric Care in Severe Obesity

An Interdisciplinary Guide to Integrated Care

Springer

Editors
Sanjeev Sockalingam
Toronto Western Hospital Bariatric Surgery Program
Centre for Mental Health
University Health Network
Toronto, ON, Canada

Department of Psychiatry
University of Toronto
Toronto, ON, Canada

Raed Hawa
Toronto Western Hospital Bariatric Surgery Program
University Health Network
Toronto, ON, Canada

Department of Psychiatry
University of Toronto
Toronto, ON, Canada

ISBN 978-3-319-42534-4 ISBN 978-3-319-42536-8 (eBook)
DOI 10.1007/978-3-319-42536-8

Library of Congress Control Number: 2016959007

Printed on acid-free paper

This Springer imprint is published by Springer Nature
The registered company is Springer International Publishing AG
The registered company address is: Gewerbestrasse 11, 6330 Cham, Switzerland

Contents

Contributors

Giovanni Amodeo, M.D. Department of Psychiatry, Department of Molecular Medicine and Development, University of Siena School of Medicine, Siena, Italy

Molly Atwood Department of Psychology, Ryerson University, Toronto, ON, Canada

Kathleen S. Bingham University Health Network, Toronto, ON, Canada

Stephanie E. Cassin, Ph.D., C.Psych. Department of Psychology, Ryerson University, Toronto, ON, Canada

Department of Psychiatry, University of Toronto, Toronto, ON, Canada

Centre for Mental Health, University Health Network, Toronto, ON, Canada

Satya Dash, Ph.D., M.B.B.S., M.R.C.P(U.K.), F.R.C.P.C. Division of Endocrinology, Department of Medicine, Toronto General Hospital, University Health Network, Toronto, ON, Canada

Lauren David Department of Psychology, Ryerson University, Toronto, ON, Canada

Karen Davison, Ph.D., M.Sc., B.A.Sc., R.D. Faculty of Health and Faculty of Science and Horticulture, Kwantlen Polytechnic University, Surrey, BC, Canada

Chau Du Toronto Western Hospital Bariatric Surgery Program, University Health Network, Toronto, ON, Canada

Markus Duncan School of Kinesiology, University of British Columbia, Vancouver, BC, Canada

Guy Faulkner School of Kinesiology, University of British Columbia, Vancouver, BC, Canada

Alexis M. Fertig, M.D., M.P.H. Department of Psychiatry, Western Psychiatric Institute and Clinic, University of Pittsburgh Medical Center, Pittsburgh, PA, USA

Aliza Friedman, M.A. Department of Psychology, Ryerson University, Toronto, ON, Canada

Weronika Gondek, M.D. Department of Psychiatry and Behavioral Sciences, Johns Hopkins University School of Medicine, Baltimore, MD, USA

Lorraine Gougeon, R.D. Toronto Western Hospital Bariatric Surgery Program, University Health Network, Toronto, ON, Canada

Raed Hawa Toronto Western Hospital Bariatric Surgery Program, University Health Network, Toronto, ON, Canada

Department of Psychiatry, University of Toronto, Toronto, ON, Canada

Roger C.M. Ho, M.B.B.S(H.K.), D.P.M(Ire), M.R.C.Psych(U.K.), F.R.C.P.C. Department of Psychological Medicine, National University of Singapore, Singapore, Singapore

J.J. Hunter, M.D. F.R.C.P.C. Division of Consultation-Liaison Psychiatry, Department of Psychiatry, Mount Sinai Hospital, University of Toronto, Toronto, ON, Canada

Timothy Jackson, B.Sc., M.D., M.P.H., F.R.C.S., F.A.C.S. Minimally Invasive and Bariatric Surgery, Division of General Surgery, Department of Surgery and Institute of Health Policy, Management and Evaluation Faculty of Medicine, University Health Network, Toronto Western Hospital, University of Toronto, Toronto, ON, Canada

Patti Kastanias, M.Sc.(A.), N.P. Toronto Western Hospital Bariatric Surgery Program, University Health Network, Toronto, ON, Canada

Catherine Laird Toronto Western Hospital Bariatric Surgery Program, University Health Network, Toronto, ON, Canada

Tho Lan Le, Ph.D. Candidate Institute of Medical Science, University of Toronto, Toronto, ON, Canada

Elliott Kyung Lee, M.D., F.R.C.P.(C.), D. A.B.S.N. Department of Psychiatry and Institute for Mental Health Research (IMHR), Royal Ottawa Mental Health Center (ROMHC), University of Ottawa, Ottawa, ON, Canada

Wynne Lundblad, M.D. Department of Psychiatry, Western Psychiatric Institute and Clinic, University of Pittsburgh Medical Center, Pittsburgh, PA, USA

Karyn Mackenzie Toronto Western Hospital Bariatric Surgery Program, University Health Network, Toronto, ON, Canada

Rodrigo B. Mansur, M.D. Mood Disorders Psychopharmacology Unit, University Health Network, Toronto, ON, Canada

R.G. Maunder Division of Consultation-Liaison Psychiatry, Department of Psychiatry, Mount Sinai Hospital, University of Toronto, Toronto, ON, Canada

Roger S. McIntyre, M.D., F.R.C.P.C. Mood Disorders Psychopharmacology Unit, University Health Network, Toronto, ON, Canada

Department of Psychiatry and Pharmacology, University of Toronto, Toronto, ON, Canada

Brain and Cognition, Discovery Foundation (BCDF), University of Toronto, Toronto, ON, Canada

Kristel Lobo Prabhu, M.D., F.R.C.S.C. University of Toronto, Toronto, ON, Canada

Minimally Invasive and Bariatric Surgery, Division of General Surgery, Department of Surgery and Institute of Health Policy, Management and Evaluation Faculty of Medicine, University Health Network, Toronto Western Hospital, University of Toronto, Toronto, ON, Canada

Gary Remington, M.D., Ph.D., F.R.C.P.C. Schizophrenia Division, Centre for Addiction and Mental Health, Toronto, ON, Canada

Sandra Robinson, M.N., N.P. Toronto Western Hospital Bariatric Surgery Program, University Health Network, Toronto, ON, Canada

Becky Smith School of Continuing Studies, University of Toronto, Toronto, ON, Canada

Sanjeev Sockalingam Toronto Western Hospital Bariatric Surgery Program, Centre for Mental Health, University Health Network, Toronto, ON, Canada

Department of Psychiatry, University of Toronto, Toronto, ON, Canada

Mehala Subramaniapillai, H.B.Sc., M.Sc. Mood Disorders Psychopharmacology Unit, University Health Network, Toronto, ON, Canada

Marlene Taube-Schiff, Ph.D., C.Psych. Department of Psychiatry, Sunnybrook Health Sciences Centre, Toronto, ON, Canada

Department of Psychiatry, University of Toronto, Toronto, ON, Canada

Lynn Tremblay, M.S.W., R.S.W. Toronto Western Hospital Bariatric Surgery Program, University Health Network, Toronto, ON, Canada

Jessica Van Exan, Ph.D., C.Psych. Toronto Western Hospital Bariatric Surgery Program, University Health Network, Toronto, ON, Canada

Anna Wallwork, M.A., M.S.W. Toronto Western Hospital Bariatric Surgery Program, University Health Network, Toronto, ON, Canada

Wei Wang Toronto Western Hospital Bariatric Surgery Program, University Health Network, Toronto, ON, Canada

Katie Warwick, R.D. Toronto Western Hospital Bariatric Surgery Program, University Health Network, Toronto, ON, Canada

Susan Wnuk, B.A., M.A., Ph.D. Toronto Western Hospital Bariatric Surgery Program, University Health Network, Toronto, ON, Canada

Richard Yanofsky Toronto Western Hospital Bariatric Surgery Program, University Health Network, Toronto, ON, Canada

Department of Psychiatry, University of Toronto, Toronto, ON, Canada

Shira Yufe, B.A. Department of Psychology, York University, Toronto, ON, Canada

Melvyn W.B. Zhang, M.B.B.S., D.C.P., M.R.C.Psych. Biomedical Institute for Global Health Research & Technology (BIGHEART), National University of Singapore, Singapore, Singapore

Carrol Zhou, M.D. Department of Psychiatry, University of Toronto, Toronto, ON, Canada

Part I

Introduction

1 Introduction to Severe Obesity for Psychiatrists

Raed Hawa and Sanjeev Sockalingam

The obesity epidemic is a well-recognized phenomenon in North America and has led to the recognition of obesity as a disease by the American Medical Association. Moreover, this rapid increase in the prevalence of obesity has been a driver for the increased focus on treatments for severe obesity, specifically weight loss surgery. As a result of the complex psychiatric co-morbidities in severely obese patient populations, mental health needs have been recognized as a critical component to caring for obese patients in clinicians' practice.

With the increase in the number of bariatric surgeries performed over the last 15 years and evidence for its efficacy in treating severe obesity, more healthcare providers are now involved in pre- and post-surgery patient care, including the assessment and management of psychiatric issues. Despite the growing evidence on the relationship between mental health issues and severe obesity management, and the emergence of evidence-based treatments for weight loss in severe obesity, there are a limited number of mental health resources to assist clinicians and interprofessional teams in a comprehensive approach to severe obesity care and bariatric surgery.

The proposed textbook is designed to present a comprehensive and state-of the-art approach to assessing and managing bariatric surgery psychosocial care. This textbook will provide clinicians with a biopsychosocial understanding of patients' obesity journey and psychosocial factors contributing to their obesity and its management. The textbook is divided into three sections based on guideline-based care: understanding obesity and its management, assessment of psychosocial issues in severe obesity, and psychological and pharmacological treatments of mental illness in severe obesity.

Initial chapters will focus on obesity prevalence and its relationship to psychiatric illness and social factors. Genetic, neurohormonal pathways and developmental factors for obesity, including childhood adversity, will be discussed and will inform subsequent chapters focused on medical and surgical treatments of obesity. The second section of the textbook will focus on evidence and strategies for assessing a range of common psychiatric issues in severe obesity. The

R. Hawa (✉)
Toronto Western Hospital Bariatric Surgery Program, University Health Network, 399 Bathurst Street, Toronto, ON, Canada M5T 2S8

Department of Psychiatry, University of Toronto, Toronto, ON, Canada
e-mail: Raed.Hawa@uhn.ca

S. Sockalingam
Toronto Western Hospital Bariatric Surgery Program, Centre for Mental Health, University Health Network, 200 Elizabeth Street, Toronto, ON, Canada M5G 2C4

Department of Psychiatry, University of Toronto, Toronto, ON, Canada
e-mail: sanjeev.sockalingam@uhn.ca

S. Sockalingam, R. Hawa (eds.), *Psychiatric Care in Severe Obesity*,
DOI 10.1007/978-3-319-42536-8_1

authors will review common psychiatric presentations, their impact on bariatric surgery and key assessment features for weight loss. In the last section of the textbook, chapters will focus on evidence-based psychosocial and pharmacological treatments for supporting patients' mental health during weight loss and bariatric surgery. Experts on non-pharmacological interventions such as mindfulness, cognitive-behavioral therapy, and nutrition education will describe treatment approaches in each modality.

This comprehensive resource will address established gaps in not just the assessment of psychosocial concerns in severe obesity, but also its management. The unique components of this textbook include its patient-centered approach, specifically patient narratives introducing mental health concerns in severe obesity care. In addition, this textbook provides an interprofessional approach to severe obesity management and bariatric surgery care, which is a salient feature to managing psychiatric concerns in obesity management programs. Each chapter provides clinical pearls and is supplemented with illustrative cases and/or clinical tools to facilitate translation of chapter content into clinical practice. We feel that these unique and clinically relevant features will support clinicians in managing mental health concerns emerging during the care of patients with severe obesity.

A textbook of this magnitude and design would not be possible without the help and mentorship of several people. First, we would like to thank our co-authors who devoted extensive time and creativity in each of their chapters. We would also like to thank Patrick Carr and the team at Springer for their support in developing this textbook. We would also like to thank our families who provided us with ongoing support to pursue our passion in creating this textbook. Finally, we would like to thank our patients who provided us with inspiration each day to create a resource that would improve the mental health care for all patients being treated for severe obesity. We hope that this textbook will be a resource for the thousands of clinicians caring for patients with severe obesity and considering treatments, including bariatric surgery, for their obesity.

2 Severe Obesity: A Patient's Perspective

Becky Smith and Catherine Laird

2.1 Patient Story #1

Becky Smith

I was not born obese. Not many people are! My parents actually report that there was concern that I was not quite hefty enough. My birth-weight was 6 lb and 7 ounces (2.9 kg). Almost 43 years later, I hit a peak of 320 lb (145.1 kg). In other words, for someone of my height (5′10″ or 178 cm), I was severely obese. My journey towards severe obesity was not a gradual slope, but more of an undulating one. The same could be said of my journey towards bariatric surgery, which I had 7 months ago.

Throughout my early childhood, my weight was normal. I was actually something of a fussy eater and recall frequently being made to sit at the table until my plate was empty. I was a tall girl from a young age and one of the first in my class to hit puberty. I have thick bones—thick ankles and thick wrists. My feet are very large for a female and since my teens I've had to buy shoes in specialist shoe stores. I distinctly remember family and friends saying what a "big girl" I was. In my head, I interpreted this as fat, but now, when I look back at photographs of that period, I see myself as a perfectly normal, if shapely, young woman. My female friends were less shapely and, on the whole, thinner and more petite than I was. In comparison I felt somewhat oafish. My friends seemed more elegant in their movement and were generally better at sports than I was. Sports that involved running were physically hard for me and I hated them. I was constantly out of breath and red-faced. I didn't hate all sports, just those that involved running. Swimming and skiing were my preferred sports and I both enjoyed and excelled at those in my youth. However, I grew to detest sport at school because most activities involved running and I was often the last to be picked for teams.

2.1.1 Weight Gain Journey

I left home aged 18 and went off travelling the world for a year with a friend before going to university. Having always had home-cooked and fairly balanced meals, the freedom to eat and drink what I wanted in quantities of my choice meant that my diet was less healthy than it had been. Convenience foods and alcohol also played

B. Smith (✉)
School of Continuing Studies, University of Toronto, 252 Bloor Street West, Room 4-160, Toronto, ON, Canada M5S 1V6
e-mail: b.smith@utoronto.ca

C. Laird
Toronto Western Hospital Bariatric Surgery Program, University Health Network, Toronto, ON, Canada
e-mail: catherinelaird1042@yahoo.ca

S. Sockalingam, R. Hawa (eds.), *Psychiatric Care in Severe Obesity*,
DOI 10.1007/978-3-319-42536-8_2

their part during my student days. My weight started to creep up and, at the age of 22, I was diagnosed with high blood pressure. I made various attempts to diet on the recommendation of health practitioners, but my weight seemed to "yo-yo" up and down.

In my mid-twenties, I had to have surgery to remove a pilonidal sinus. There were no major complications, but thereafter I experienced acid indigestion on a regular basis. Not long after that surgery, I moved overseas for a period of 2 years and, when the acid indigestion arose, I suppressed it by eating. Returning home to the UK at the age of 27, my weight had increased to 252 lb (114.3 kg). I now shopped exclusively in plus-size stores and didn't feel quite as young and trendy anymore. A year later, with my housemate's support and frequent company, I joined a slimming club and began going to the gym, swimming, and doing yoga regularly. Over the next couple of years, I was successful at losing 50 lb (22.8 kg), proudly gaining a certificate in the process. By the time my 30th birthday came around, I remember feeling toned and comfortable with my size. People commented on how fit I looked.

My thirties was a period of highs and lows where I feel I spent a lot of time searching for myself. My heart was broken twice (for which I sought therapy), I completed a Masters degree, I developed my career, I bought a new house, and I moved countries a few more times. Prior to immigrating to Canada at the age of 37, I spent a year living and working in the Netherlands. There, I was very lonely and unhappy. I lacked social interaction and felt very isolated. On reflection, I probably should have sought treatment for depression. Instead, I ate my feelings. I became lethargic and, although I cycled to and from work, spent almost every evening lying on the couch watching TV.

I left the Netherlands at the end of my 1-year contract and just as my Canadian residency came through. Part of the immigration process required a medical exam and it was then that the examining doctor found blood in my urine. On my return to the UK, prior to my move to Canada, a 'leaky' kidney was diagnosed with protein in my urine.

2.1.2 Pre-Surgical Weight Loss Efforts

Moving to Canada was a positive step and I began to feel my old self again. Initially, I was confident in my decision, challenged in my new job and engaged with my new environment making friends and exploring new places. Again, I joined a slimming club and lost some weight. However, about 6 months after I arrived, I changed jobs and spent the next 9 months quite uncomfortable at work. I was bullied by a colleague and the thought of going to office became a dread. Again, I began to eat my feelings. My new family doctor decided to investigate my 'leaky' kidney issue, referring me to a nephrologist, and also recommended I see a doctor who specialised in weight management. All the doctors were concerned about my weight, my blood pressure, and my kidneys.

At the time, I would say when asked that I felt generally healthy and looking in the mirror saw myself as curvy but not obese. I don't think I really recognised that having to lie on the couch every night after work with your ankles up high because they were swollen, lacking in energy, over-reacting emotionally, and sleeping poorly were indicators that my body was not functioning well.

My nephrologist encouraged me to lose weight and I started seeing the weight-management doctor on a regular basis. I did not have a particularly easy relationship with the latter, but kept going as I recognised that despite our disconnection personality-wise, he was trying to get to the root of my weight issue. For the first time in dealing with health practitioners, I felt I was actually being offered structured support rather than just simply being told I needed to lose weight. Although not a psychiatrist, he had a special interest in nutritional orders and had collaborated with a psychologist on a number of papers linking Attention Deficit Hyperactivity Disorder (ADHD) and weight management. He diagnosed me with ADHD and I was put on atomoxetine, which I feel has helped me with my ability to maintain focus and be less impulsive. I was also sent for a sleep study where it was determined that although I did not have sleep apnea, I was a very light sleeper, easily disturbed by noise. We talked about my seasonal mood changes and he suggested I purchase a seasonal affective disorder (SAD) light therapy lamp and use it every day, which I did. He arranged for me to have a 24-h blood pressure monitoring test and also increased my blood pressure medication to include hydrochlorothiazide and, later, amlodipine. My doctor also encouraged me to go to mindfulness classes, which I hated, but lead to me finding an alternative plus-size yoga class, which I loved and, apart from the occasional swim, hike, cross-country ski, or annual 10 km walk for charity, was pretty much all the physical activity I did apart from everyday walking. He encouraged me to be more aware of my health and self-care by, for example, going for regular massages, getting enough vitamin D and omega-3, and not waiting to sort out minor health niggles. He put me on a very low calorie powdered diet, which I used for two meals a day supplemented with a regular meal and was actually quite successful for a while. I lost about 25 lb (11.4 kg) over the year I was on it; I found it quite easy not having to cook. At one point, I was also tried on topiramate (and later naltrexone) to see if that might help stave off food cravings and encourage weight loss. He sent me to see a psychologist who I saw for about three sessions before the psychologist and I agreed it wasn't really that beneficial for me at that point. I wasn't feeling particularly emotionally distressed or troubled and felt that we had had talked through my feelings regarding my weight issues in the sessions. The main driver in seeing the psychologist was really my weight management doctor. I think I went ahead with it because I was keen to try anything to resolve my weight issue, but, at the same time, I don't think I really felt a strong intrinsic motivation to talk through my feelings compared to the previous times I had undergone psychological therapy. From quite early on in our consultative sessions, my weight-management doctor raised the prospect of bariatric surgery, but I was totally resistant to the idea.

My view was that my weight was something that I should be able to control and that surgery was too risky and dramatic. I am generally a very capable person who succeeds when I apply myself and so, in my mind, I felt I should be able to lose weight without resorting to surgery. I was also conflicted in that I felt, and still feel, that someone's aesthetic should not influence how they are perceived but, deep down, I know I felt it did. I have experienced people's judgements and criticisms about my physical being on a number of occasions. It hurts, even if they mean well in terms of their concern for your health. It also presses my 'rebel' buttons and I begin to dig my heels in further. Take me as I am or get out of my life! However, at the same time, I recognised I was (feeling) less attractive and had lost interest in relationships and my appearance. Shopping for clothes, for example, was no longer fun and dating was non-existent.

I think I tried to pretend I was body-confident externally, but really I wasn't. I no longer felt good about my body in terms of its attractiveness. I even tried to boost my confidence by taking part in a nude photo shoot as part of a public art project. I didn't tell anyone about this because I was embarrassed!

During the process of trying various weight-loss strategies under the guidance of the weight-management doctor, I independently met two people who had had bariatric surgery. Speaking to them and hearing about their experiences really helped me start to revaluate the prospect of surgery. I heard first-hand that they felt it was beneficial, what the surgical process was like, what the post-surgery eating situation was like for people who tend to socialise around food-based events and enjoy food, and how they dealt with the excess skin they now had. I got the 'warts and all' version but the overwhelming sentiment was that it was a positive experience. One of them, who knew me professionally as well as personally, also made the point that I was a smart and capable woman, and that having a weight-problem that I could not control did not make me a failure in life—this struck a chord. I bought some books on weight-loss surgery and started to read articles and blogs as well as visit bariatric chat rooms. I began to educate myself on the surgical process from a medical and psychological perspective. Eventually, I agreed to being referred to the local bariatric program.

2.1.3 Pre-Surgical Support

I went along to an introductory information session at the hospital, which outlined the various procedure and requirements for surgery, the risks and benefits as well as post-operative lifestyle and eating changes. I took copious notes. Later, I again connected with one of my friends who had had surgery and quizzed her and her partner about their experiences, contextualizing all that I had learnt. By this point, I was fairly confident that surgery was something I was going to do. A few months later, my first appointments at the hospital came around and I met with a social worker, a nurse practitioner, and a psychologist. I asked the questions I needed to, and by the end of this stage, was determined that surgery was the right thing for me. The psychologist encouraged me to go along to the bi-weekly bariatric support group at the hospital where she suggested I ask my outstanding questions regarding my intended surgery.

I was somewhat reluctant to go to the support group meeting as I was guarded about sharing my emotions and feelings with strangers. However, by the end of the meeting I felt very much more positive about it. I valued the companionship of others going through or having been through the process. I recognised the variety of individuals who for one reason or another had become obese. I had learnt some useful tips. My query had been listened to and I had had constructive suggestions made and real examples provided. I felt the group was a safe space to express my concerns. I have continued going to the group, which alternates between an open forum and lecture-style learning sessions, on a regular basis and feel it is very beneficial.

Following my first support group experience, I decided that I would limit the people I told about my planned surgery to a small group: my parents (in the UK), my doctors, my immediate boss who is also a friend, and a few other trusted close friends here in Canada that I felt would be supportive, non-judgemental and would, to be honest, suspect that I was dealing with a health issue. I didn't want them to worry I was seriously ill and knew I would need their practical support given the distance from my family. I decided to keep it at that. I think the support group gave me the confidence to focus on my own preferences and stop worrying what others would think. I felt strong enough to say to myself that there are people in my life for whom it really is none of their business what I choose to do with my body and they don't need to know everything about me to still belong in my social circle. This was empowering in many ways; I felt I was in the driving seat about the decisions.

My parents, who are both also overweight, were supportive of my decision when I told them of the proposed surgery, but had questions regarding surgical risks. They offered to fly over during the period of surgery and recovery, but I indicated I did not feel this was necessary. My friends were outwardly very accepting and supportive, although wanted to be sure the main reason I was doing it was for health rather than aesthetic reasons. They also wanted to know how it might affect my ability to socialise. I asked one of my friends to be my support person in terms of helping me home and staying with me for a few days as advised by the hospital. She agreed. My doctors and boss were totally positive and supportive.

My next round of appointments came through and I saw the nurse practitioner and had a very helpful nutritional lesson presented by the dietician providing guidance on pre- and post-surgery nutrition.

Things became very real when I was given a surgical date after my surgical consult and I actually felt quite excited about the prospect of what lay ahead in terms of being able to see a solution to my weight problem.

2.1.4 Pre-Surgery

The final appointment was to do various pre-surgery examinations (blood, cardiac, etc.) and I met with a pharmacist to go over my medications and an anaesthetist who went over my surgical risks. I also saw another team member that day. She asked me about my support person and we started chatting about my parents and when I would next see them (6 months post-surgery). She then said: "Oh, how wonderful! You'll be all skinny and beautiful when you next see them!" Her comment really upset me, but I didn't say anything at the time. I don't think she meant to be anything but positive, but the implications of the words she chose, as I 'heard' them was (a) you are not beautiful now and (b) skinny = beautiful. It still bothers me.

As my surgery date came closer I felt comfortable in my decision, but, as I think many people feel pre-surgery, there were still the concerns that something might go wrong. I rewrote my will; perhaps telling in terms of some of my underlying fears.

Prior to my surgery, I began the process of preparing for surgery by "shrinking" my liver and went on the same powdered very low calorie diet I'd been on previously, but, this time, with no regular food intake at the same time. There was a period of about a week before starting this diet when I binged on my favourite food and drinks as a kind of farewell to old friends. In my mind, I would never eat these things again so wanted one last sentimental taste. These items included pizza, handmade cannelloni, Chinese take-out, Portuguese custard tarts, a gin and tonic, a pint of beer, and mango ice cream.

For the next 3 weeks, I was just on the powdered drinks and allowed other low calorie drinks, but no actual food. In my case, my drinks of choice were water and diet soda. I was quite anxious about this diet as the first few days of being on it coincided with attending a work-related conference involving a number of social events and receptions. Despite my fears, it was actually OK. The first couple of days were the hardest and I felt as if all my senses were heightened in the awareness of food smells and tempting food. Restaurants seemed to jump out at me! However, I navigated my way through and had no real hunger after day 3. I actually quite enjoyed my shakes and the feeling that my journey towards better health had commenced.

2.1.5 Hospital Stay

On the day of my surgery, I called the hospital to check everything was still OK and they asked if I could come in a bit earlier as they were running ahead of schedule. I walked to the hospital with my little suitcase and was warmly greeted by the receptionist who made me feel very positive by telling me his sister was 6 months post-bariatric surgery and how she was very happy with her progress and felt it had been a good decision. Next, the surgeon (whom I had not met before) came in and he was very friendly. I was a bit taken aback though when he lifted my gown and signed my stomach as I was completely naked underneath—we'd hardly said hello! He then, kindly, asked for the number of my support person so he could call her after the surgery was over.

Next, I was taken to sit in a comfy chair with my feet up and a nicely warmed blanket was placed over me. The anaesthetist came and prepped me. It all moved very quickly and the next thing I knew I was being walked down to the operating theatre. This was very strange for me as, based on my previous experience of surgery, I had been expecting to be wheeled down. I was led into the theatre, where the radio was playing, and introduced to the staff in the room. They asked me to get on the table, I was strapped down and then sleep ensued as the anaesthetic took effect.

I woke up in the recovery room and the first thing I noticed was that my back hurt. I had been advised this might be the case, due to the gases used in keyhole surgery. My surgeon was at the end of my bed and told me he'd already called my friend and that everything with the surgery had gone well. He also advised me that the operation had taken longer than anticipated as they found I had a hiatus hernia when they went in so he had to fix that prior to doing the Roux-en-Y gastric bypass. Thankfully, all issues with acid indigestion have now been completely resolved with no reoccurrence post-surgery.

I was still a bit sleepy when I was wheeled up to the ward and was given my liquids, some medicine cups, and instructed on how often I had to drink. A few hours later, one of the nurses encouraged me to go for a walk around the corridors. He kindly stayed behind me as I pushed the intravenous drip trolley since I was worried I might fall because I felt very light-headed. I did a circuit and then had the confidence to unplug myself from the monitors and do a few rounds every few hours.

My first night in hospital was not great. I was very tired but couldn't sleep. I was told I had to stay sitting up and couldn't lie down flat. Every time I was about to drop off to sleep an alarm would go off. My breathing kept slowing and set the alarms off. I felt really bad as I must have kept the lady in the bed next to me awake half the night as well.

The next day was better and I managed to doze a bit between drinking from the little cups, sipping broth and eating some gelatine pudding. I felt very nauseous at one point and had to have some intravenous anti-nausea medication. My support person visited and one of the nurses told me that my other friend, who had previously had bariatric surgery, had been calling every hour the night before to check on my well-being. In the late morning, a different surgeon came with some students to check on me and was very pleased I was sitting in a chair and had been walking and using the bathroom.

The second night I slept better and the next morning I was seen by a resident and some other students. The resident agreed I could go home.

2.1.6 Recovery at Home

Almost 48 h after my surgery, I was on my way home via taxi with my support person assisting me. I felt tired and weak as I hadn't eaten much at all for 3 days, but was happy to be home. My support person stayed at my place for two nights. I slept a lot but we went for a short walk each day. I also started the liquid diet stage, which I now refer to as the 'white' diet because all the food I ate seemed to be white—yogurt, sieved mushroom soup, sieved chicken soup with protein powder in. By the end of the 2 weeks, I was so bored of the 'white' food that the pureed stage was a delight! Two weeks is nothing in the scale of things, but when I could finally have crunchy food again in the form of saltine crackers I was so excited.

I was very touched and appreciative when I received a call from the tele-health support nurse at the hospital on day 2 after being discharged. She just wanted to check in on how I was doing. On the third day after getting out of hospital, I went to see my family doctor. We discussed how I was doing and looked at my medications. We agreed on a phased reduction in my blood pressure medication and she asked me to check my blood pressure daily. She also helped me get new prescriptions so that all the medications I was on, including some prescribed by the hospital to take for the first few weeks post-surgery, were small enough in size that I could digest them. I was advised to never take anything bigger than an M&M post-surgery.

One disconcerting thing to arise immediately following my surgery was that my body odour changed. It felt almost as if someone else was inhabiting my body and I didn't like the change in smell at all. I was quite anxious about this, but spoke to others who had surgery and at least two people said they had had the same thing. It lasted a few days and possibly was due to the surgical gases leaving my body, but it was a bit discombobulating.

The first few weeks were quite exciting in terms of seeing the effect the surgery had had. I checked the scale daily and could see the weight coming off. However, at my first support group meeting post-surgery, the issue of checking the scale obsessively was raised by another member and I resolved to then only weigh myself once a week. I have stuck to this and track my weight weekly on a smartphone app.

I ended up being off work for 4 of the anticipated 6 weeks recovery period. It actually did me a lot of good to rest, relax, and build up my strength with my daily walks. I also think it helped me adjust to my new eating and vitamin regime. I was able to focus on my health and my new routine with no other distractions. This was important since I no longer felt hunger and initially kept forgetting to eat so had to get used to eating my meals according to the clock in order not to get 'hangry'. The days actually went by very quickly and the weather was good, so my daily walks were a pleasure.

The first week back at work was fine and I took my snacks and lunch in every day. The only real issues I had around this time were that I got dizzy if I stood for longer than a couple of minutes and that I felt very nauseous about an hour after taking my morning vitamins, which were taken 30 min after my breakfast as per the dietician's instructions. I either had to lie down or have some protein drink to suppress the nausea.

At 8 weeks post-surgery, I went on a vacation by myself. I took a lightweight suitcase and booked accommodation without meals so I could figure out in my own way what I wanted to eat and when. I had been anxious about this and made sure I took plenty of protein bars with me, but it was actually fine. I was pleasantly surprised to discover that I could usually find something suitable on offer in restaurants or the supermarket. I also started drinking coffee again after 6 years. The reason for this was I found it difficult to go to a café and only have water. I don't really like tea that much and soda of any kind is no longer an option. The biggest issue I had was asking wait staff to bring me smaller portions. I explained I had a medical issue that meant I couldn't eat much, but they would bring exactly the same size served to others even though I had asked for a small portion. I hate wasting food and as I couldn't store food anywhere, I couldn't easily take any leftovers away with me to have later. The wait staff would always look shocked at how much was left on the plate and I felt guilty about the wasted food. A few months on, I've got used to this a bit more now, but am very appreciative of friends who are willing to share food dishes. When eating out now, I usually opt for an appetizer instead of a main meal.

2.1.7 New Habits

I didn't lift anything heavy for 3 months and abstained from any exercise other than walking until my 3-month check up, as advised by the hospital staff. At 3 months, I started swimming and went back to my yoga class, having let my yoga instructor know my situation. I also changed my job and started a secondment that meant I would not be travelling overseas for work. I saw this as a good move in that I could stick to my eating routine and not have to deal with airline, hotel, and restaurant meals quite as much. My new job also meant that I could start cycling to and from work (15 min each way) on a daily basis. I did this until the cold weather started. My swimming routine has not really stuck, but I am still going to yoga regularly and am generally out and about walking more than pre-surgery. I know I should do more 'proper' sport though.

Around this time, people who didn't know I'd had surgery started to comment on how great I was looking. Very few people made any comment about the fact I had lost weight. I found this interesting and, even now, 7 months on and approaching 100 lbs (45.4 kg) less in weight, very few people actually make note of the fact I have lost weight. They do, however, say I'm looking very well.

Initially, it was only by standing on the scale and because my clothes were looser that I noticed the weight coming off. Personally, I didn't see a visual change for a few months. Eventually though, I noticed my double chin had disappeared and that my face was becoming more defined. Next, I saw it at the top of my shoulders and then around my bust. The weight seemed to be coming off my top half first, but I'm not sure if it was just easier to see the significant change in my upper body at first.

My clothes were getting really too big and they either looked billowy or simply fell off my hips. I had a purge of my wardrobe and also began to learn how to sew by taking classes. I really enjoy my new hobby and the fact I can now alter my clothes to fit has been both satisfying and cost-saving during this transitional period. I was able to donate most of my discarded clothes to my plus-sized yoga classmates and to a local charity.

I started to get interested in shopping for clothes again around this time and had a couple of splurge trips where I bought new clothes. I was, however, conscious that I needed to exercise caution due to the risk of transferring my food addiction to becoming a shopping addiction. I asked friends to keep a watchful eye on my clothes spending. Although I have bought a few new items, this splurging has settled down.

Around the 4-month post-surgery mark, I began to notice chunks of my hair coming out when I brushed it. I had been warned by the dieticians that this could happen due to post-surgical shock and protein absorption, but it still made me anxious as my hair is quite fine and thin anyway. On the dietician's advice, I started to take a zinc supplement and, following my own research, also began using a keratin-based shampoo and hair oil spray in an attempt to reduce breakage. I was advised not to take the zinc for more than 2 months, but during this time the hair loss slowed, so, despite my initial anxiety, I felt comfortable stopping the zinc at 2 months. My hair is now back to normal in terms of both growth and shedding.

My new eating and vitamin regime had also begun to feel normal. I now take two multivitamins and have six calcium citrate chews spread throughout the day with a B12 tablet every other day; although I'm not always as compliant as I should be with the B12 as I don't like taking this due to the chalky residue it leaves. I also try to ensure I am getting enough protein in and still rely on ready-made protein shakes or bars to supplement my diet. Through trial and error, I've noticed the shakes tend to cause what can be quite uncomfortable constipation so I am shifting to the bars instead.

Apart from 3 episodes in the first 3 months, I have not had any ill effects due to overeating, eating too quickly, or eating foods that are difficult to digest. The first time I vomited was after having eaten a piece of toast for the first time post-surgery. It did not sit comfortably for about 45 min and I felt very queasy. Eventually, it came back up as regurgitation. I had a similar experience two other times when I think I ate my breakfast too quickly. I seem to have learned what is the right pace for eating now and chew my food very thoroughly. I have tried bread since when eating out and it's been OK in small quantities. I have not yet tried rice or pasta, and don't really plan to. Most other foods are fine, but I seem to have trouble digesting tough, dry chicken or meat and find I just have to stop after a few bites. I now try to avoid meat grilled on a barbecue or re-heated in a microwave.

2.1.8 Noticing Shifts

My 6-month check up went very well and I was told, by the dietician and nurse practitioner, that I had lost 53 % of my excess weight and 15 cm from my waist. I had also recently come off all blood pressure medication, although I was still taking the atomoxetine. The hospital staff seemed pleased with my progress.

Shortly thereafter, I went on vacation with my parents. Interestingly, they did not really make a big deal of my weight loss when they saw me, although my mum did comment on my bust having shrunk and that I looked almost as I had done around the age of 17. I think initially they were a bit uncertain about how to deal with my new eating habits, but, after a few days, I think they got used to it and saw it as advantageous to share meals with me in terms of managing their own consumption and also from a financial point of view. This was also the first time I had really spent time around people drinking alcohol socially. I have been surprised at how little I have actually missed drinking alcohol. It really is not something I have craved, even when socialising. I did try alcohol over the holiday period having a glass of wine on one occasion and a gin and tonic on two other occasions. I noticed that I felt the effects more quickly and to a stronger degree than previously.

During this vacation, we took part in a few adventurous activities and I really noticed how much fitter I felt. I no longer was out of breath, red, and sweaty on climbing to the top of a hill. This felt good and I could actually feel my health, as well as my body-size, had shifted.

Looking at photographs of this trip, I can see that I am looking thinner all over. My legs are really starting to look slimmer. I am more comfortable in clothes as I am aware my tummy, my upper arms, and inner thighs are quite saggy in terms of the excess skin. I feel it looks a bit like an old woman's skin—as if the fat has been sucked out. However, it doesn't bother me too much and didn't inhibit me from wearing beach clothes on vacation. I am hopeful that with time and exercise, it will tone up as I have quite good skin generally. I have noticed that it seems to be much drier though and I need to moisturise a lot more to reduce itching.

I also recently looked at some photographs of myself pre-surgery and the contrast is very marked. What struck me most though was that I could now see how overweight I looked. At the time, I don't think I could see it in the same way I can now. It's as if I didn't see it as distinctly previously and that some sort of visual distortion was occurring when I looked in the mirror or at photographs. I saw what I was wearing and whether I was smiling or not, but not my size and shape. Now, I see what I think is my true self in both the 'before' photographs and in the mirror. Someone said to me at support group that prior to surgery they only focused on their face when looking in the mirror and now they focus primarily on their body. I wonder if a similar type of behaviour is at play with me.

2.1.9 Conclusion

I recognise I am, in many ways, still in the early stages of post-operative life and that I am still adjusting. I don't know yet where my weight loss journey will end, or if it ever will, but I do know that, as of today, I am very pleased that I made the leap to have the surgery. I am glad it took me a long time to actually get there in terms of making the decision to have surgery as I feel I needed that time to really explore the options and get my head around the psychological side of it. I am also immensely grateful for the support I have received from all the healthcare professionals, the bariatric program, my support group, colleagues, friends, and family. I feel that I was truly ready, supported, and prepared to make the lifestyle shift, and although it's still a work in progress, the real physical benefits I am seeing and feeling now provide me with incentive to continue working towards better health.

2.2 Patient Story #2

Catherine Laird

2.2.1 My Story

It has been a long 6 years since my weight loss surgery. Along with many continued health issues, I have also been dealing with mental health problems, mainly depression and anxiety. However, I have been receiving medical help and guidance. As they say, "I have come a long way baby!".

The path is still not clear, nor have the problems fully gone away, but I am much further now than I have ever been. Presently, I am on duloxetine for the anxiety and depression and lisdexampfetamine for my attention deficit hyperactivity disorder (ADHD). The diagnosis of ADHD was definitely an eye-opener—I will explain more in detail later on.

So here is my story… I began life as a very skinny, "wirey", very active child. I always needed to be busy. I constantly struggled with school and keeping things in order (hence the ADHD). I battled with dyslexia, but did not find out until I was in Grade 7, at which time the school I was attending suggested to my parents that I be put into a vocational school (schooling that was based on performance and not academic ability). It was such a wonderful time for me, going from grades of 40s and 50s to 80s and 90s. It was certainly a great self-esteem builder, while I was there. However, when I made academic mistakes, it was not the school that pointed it out, but rather by my mother and my siblings. Their comments got to the point where I would simply not say a thing when we were out as a family. There really was no point—defending myself was like talking to a wall. No one cared, or even heard me. I was constantly hearing the messages; "little girls should be seen and not heard", or "if you can't do anything right, don't do it at all".

The ADHD put a damper on my ability to be careful as I was always running into things and getting physically injured, "an accident waiting to happen" my grandmother would often say. I was also unable to complete projects or focus on what

I felt were simple tasks. I was not only surprised, but thankful that my bariatric psychiatrist was able to diagnose me with this problem and help me manage it. I still have my issues, such as my ongoing tendency to be what I call a *perfectionist-procrastinator* (someone who is afraid to start something new for fear of not doing it right). I am not too sure what is worse, being degraded for not being an academic success, or not being able to start or complete things I have started. Even writing this story has been a very big ordeal for me, despite the encouragement I received from my supports. Forgetfulness has been one of my strongest characteristics. The ADHD medication works wonders for me and keeps me focused and on top of things when I need it. I am sure it was great for my doctor to finally make some sense of what I was saying, instead of me going off in 20-different directions.

Now, I turn to the part in the story focused on how I came to the decision of having a Roux-en-Y Gastric By-Pass. As I mentioned in the beginning I was a very skinny, active child and my weight was not something my mother or family worried about early on. All the way up to age 12 years old, I had no issues with my weight gain even though sugar and sweets, and fast food, were not as prevalent as they are these days. Home desserts were a part of my life growing up and my Scottish descent also meant using a decent amount of butter. With the onset of puberty, came all the problems. I started gaining a significant amount of weight around the age of 15, a time when a teen needs more understanding and security. I was told often that "you have such a pretty face", a comment that comes with a hidden meaning. It was not a very good time to be feeling insecure and vulnerable. It was a time to be social, not socially awkward, the latter being the reality for me. The harder it was to keep the weight off, the more reclusive I became. Hiding in my room, I would keep a secret stash of "goodies" and eat my McDonald's fries. If it was forbidden to eat, I snuck it into my room, or simply wolfed it down my throat.

I was not the only one dealing with problems. My mother and grandmother dealt with weight issues all of their lives. At first my Grandmother would tell me, "We are all "big boned". The translation of these comments was "you'll always be fat not matter how much you lose". As a result, when my mother went on a diet, I was expected to do the same, and of course the diets worked— for a short time, but really, how long can one sustain eating grapefruits or bananas for every meal? After weeks of eating little to nothing and losing the weight, 1–2 months would pass and the weight would return with just that little bit extra. So we played the "merry-go-round" or as I like to call it the "diet-losing-gain it back" game together: go on a diet and lose weight; then have fun and feel good briefly; continue poorly managed eating habits with the hope that you will correct them later; followed by gaining back the weight and often gaining more. After each "diet-losing-gain it back" attempt, I would start all over again. It was exhausting and depressing.

I felt hope as the pounds melted away and I began to receive compliments as my figure improved, but this was soon followed by the feeling of failure, the judgments, and the comments made as the weight returned. It made me feel less of a person. Was I someone who is incapable of accomplishing a simple task? I used to repeat to myself "lose weight and keep it off—others do it so why can't I?".

Over many years of failing diets and my learning disability, I could feel my self-esteem slipping further and further into a hole. When I was in my 20s, it was the first time I had realised I had some mental health struggles. I did not seek help and these feelings built up to the point where I could not take it anymore, so I took some pills in an overdose. Fortunately, for me they weren't all that strong; but I was taken to the hospital and was referred to a psychologist. What I found out in this treatment was something I already knew. I wouldn't be happy, until I could get a job, lose some weight, and find someone to love. Wow! I thought to my self, "what an insight - I can finally move on!" (sarcasm). I quickly lost faith in seeking anymore professional help and as a result, and, I stopped the treatment.

I eventually found work lost weight, and found love, and did this several times.

At the age of 28, I decided once again to participate in a diet program, and once again I was successful. During this time, I was a slim, blonde, and singer for a band. This is when I met my husband now, and soon after was pregnant. Pregnancy was one of the few times that I was not judged for what I was eating or my weight. During pregnancy, I gave myself permission to eat my favourite foods and again, no one thought it was an issue. They assured me, that I would lose most of it once the baby was born, and the rest would come off later. So I continued to enjoy myself.

After three children, many more ineffective diets, more weight gain and lost jobs, I finally gave up and succumbed to my weight issues. I remember thinking, "I am fat, I am always going to be fat and that is all there is to it!". I confined myself to my home and found it hard to do things that others in my life could do. I didn't care anymore. No more diets, no more fighting to look like everyone else. I was done. Then one day at church, a girl who was obese started losing a massive amount of weight. I asked her what she was doing and she told me about a gastric bypass procedure. Curious, I immediately started looking into this. It took me 3 years to make the decision to see someone about it. My family doctor was initially against this procedure, and it wasn't until I received my first appointment for a bariatric surgery orientation that I told my family about my plan to pursue bariatric surgery. To my surprise, I did not get the reaction I thought I was going to get.

I thought they would be happy to know that I found something that could help me lose the weight I was carrying around, especially after their years of focusing on my weight gain. Instead, I felt overwhelmed by my family telling me not to do this surgery. I have to admit, I started to feel unsure again, but I also knew that I had right up until the time of the seeing the surgeon to change me my mind. In the end, I did not change my mind, but things did not go as I had planned. I began to think my family was right again. I came very close to death following a leak after surgery and I fell into a major depression that took me close to 5 months to reach a point of stability as I bounced in and out of hospital after my surgical complication.

My problems didn't end there, that depression hung around, and problem after problem did not help my recovery. I was told I was the rare patient with recurring problems after surgery, but it did not help how I was feeling. Each time I became physically ill, I was sent back to the hospital to see my surgeon, and each time I entered that hospital, I had a feeling that I would not come out alive. I want to be clear that there was never a feeling of ending my life. I loved my kids too much to do that to them, but I didn't know what to do. I was at my bottoms-end and things were not looking good. Just when I thought I couldn't take another procedure or problem, I had my first after surgery check up with the bariatric surgery program, check up. Things were going to change.

Six months from the time I had the surgery, got sent home for good, and managed to eat food without being sick, I was able to re-connect with my bariatric surgery clinical team. While in the clinic, I was seen alone by the nurse who saw me curled up on the table in the fetal position. The nurse asked me what was going on. I told her I had not eaten in the last 3 days and that everytime I ate I was throwing up "black stuff" and feeling pain. I then had to tell three other people and each time I begged them not to send me back to the hospital where I had had my surgery. Their response was all the same, "I needed to be taken care of by the doctor that performed the surgery".

Finally after reaching my dietitian, whom I had been keeping in contact with over these last few months, she advocated for me and to this day, I see her as a "guardian angel". She gathered my team outside my examination room and told them that no matter what, I was not to go back to that hospital. When the dietitian returned to the room to let me know what was going to happen in terms support, I felt more relieved. My fears were slowly going away.

After undergoing an endoscopy, the clinical team discovered an ulcer. I was given two new doctors and I began treatment for my depression under the great care of the bariatric clinic psychiatrist. Among these three people, I started a journey of several illness, surgeries, and procedures, followed by many ups and downs. Yet, I was now comforted by knowing that I was being cared for by this bariatric team.

From a psychological perspective, I was taught how to work through my feelings, using procedures such as a cognitive behavioural therapy. I was even taught how to use a "scale of intensity" to label my feelings. Besides started going to support groups, I said "yes" to whatever was available to keep myself involved in the clinics psychosocial programs and I remained engaged with treating the many health issues over time. Attending the support groups was the only way I felt I could keep myself going some days.

I have undergone this procedure and continue to have challenges with eating and my mood, but I am managing. I continue to attend the support group and have worked with my bariatric team to manage my diet and emotion during this journey. I continue to receive psychiatric support and am now in individual psychotherapy to gain a deeper understanding of my emotions and self-image.

Despite these efforts, I was faced with yet another challenge impacting my physical and mental health. I would like to share my reflections during this critical time in my weight loss journey. I was struggling with just having yet another endoscopy done and the surgeon indicated that I needed to have a surgical revision in order to fix some ongoing issues related to strictures, ulcers, a hernia, and other problems. I was nervous, as I was also dealing with problems with my body image at this point after surgery. I had heard similar challenges with body image discussed by other members in the support group. Given these challenges, I wrote this poem. It was a response to a friend's question about how I saw myself after my weight loss and surgery in the context of these challenges.

The Person that I See, Is not the Person that is Me

Things have changed, I know that know. What once was me has changed…
but how?
I'm still the person deep inside. I've only changed my shape and size.
Can it be? I say, "No way, not me."
The person that I see is not the person that is me
Hold on, there's something wrong
As I stare from foot to head—I long…for it to be true in what I see
This person's different; it's just not me
Can it be? I say "No way, not me."
The person that I see is not the person that is me
I'm big and ugly and don't fit the norm. My body shames me in its form
I'm different from the rest of you. I have no meaning. My life's askew.
I fought a battle to win a race. To lost the pounds so I could face,
discussed looks of my demise. Yet soon I'm back to staring eyes.
So I gave up, said "What's the Use" I'm fat and ugly; I'll be recluse
The cries unanswered "Please set me free!" To a person who can truly see
It's ME I say, No way, can't be
The person that I see is not the person that is me
I shamed away from society, of years with my obesity.
I hid my food for no one else. An empty life of doubt in self
So when I look how can it be?
The person that I see is not the person that is me
Suppose it's me.
Not sure as yet, the eyes and brain cannot detect…
That person standing here in front, is different than what I confront
I hear myself, I've tried to change. To make my eyes and brain arrange
Believe in who you are—what you've become. The work was hard to now succumb.
But yet to hear me say!
It's Me you see! No way, can't be
The person that I see is not the person that is me
I could not listen anymore. And so I opened one more door
And Praise to God
He gave me more
So the Mantra of my new life must be
This person that I see,
Really IS—The person that is Me

At the current time, I have lost a total of 243 lb; I still struggle with the excess skin and this holds me back from feeling good about my appearance.

I am still under the care of my bariatric team. I make regular visits to my psychiatrist and attend regular support groups. I also get involved with any additional programs being offered, which help me keep focused. I still have contact with my dietitian and any other care providers on an as needed basis. My weight is still something I worry about, but not quite as much. I am presently under the care of a psychotherapist to look deeper into why I do certain things and hopefully find the answer to my "WHY's".

The day will come, when I will no longer be able to receive help from the program due to the "program 5-year graduation", as they make room for future patients. It will not be easy for me to let go, but I know it will be yet another leap of faith in my journey.

I don't know where mental health will be in the future, with advances in future of technology and researchers pushing the horizon of knowledge. I do hope that those going through similar things as I did will hopefully not have to suffer quite as much as I did early in life.

In summary, as I reflect on my journey, I do want to thank a few people in my life. To my Husband, who was initially against me having this operation, yet took (and still takes) excellent care of me whenever needed based on my health status. To my sister who diligently came to my rescue, on many occasions when I needed it. To my sons, whom I probably have scared to death several times during my journey and who remained patient with me whenever I struggled. Last but not the least, the bariatric team at Toronto Western Hospital, University Health Network, without whom I would not have survived.

Part II

Causes and Treatment of Obesity: From Genes to Integrated Care Models

3 Causes of Severe Obesity: Genes to Environment

Satya Dash

3.1 Introduction

Obesity is a growing public health concern, both in the developed and developing world. It is associated with a number of complications including type 2 diabetes, dyslipidemia, hypertension, cardiovascular disease, nonalcoholic fatty liver disease, obstructive sleep apnea, and malignancy [1]. This causes considerable morbidity and increased mortality. Further, lifestyle changes such as diet and exercise and/or treatment with medications do not usually result in sustained weight loss [2, 3]. Bariatric surgery is the only treatment that results in sustained weight loss with resolution/improvement in obesity-associated complications [4]. Understanding the regulation of food intake and energy expenditure and ultimately body weight regulation is therefore of paramount importance and may ultimately need to better treatments of obesity and its complications. In this chapter, we will review the regulation of food intake and energy expenditure by genetic and environmental factors and how this pertains to the etiology of severe obesity.

S. Dash, Ph.D., M.B.B.S., M.R.C.P(U.K.), F.R.C.P.C. (✉)
Division of Endocrinology, Department of Medicine, Toronto General Hospital, University Health Network, 12EN-213, 200 Elizabeth Street, Toronto, ON, Canada M5C 2C4
e-mail: satya.dash@uhn.ca

3.2 Definitions

Obesity is defined as a body mass index (BMI) (weight in kilograms divided by height in meters squared) of greater than 30 in adults or greater than the 95th percentile in the pediatric population. Morbid obesity is defined as either a body mass index of greater than 35 with more than one obesity-associated comorbidity or a BMI of greater than 40. Many use the same criteria to define severe obesity. In the pediatric population, a BMI of greater than 120 % of the 95th percentile has been suggested as a definition of severe obesity with a BMI>140 % of the 95th centile representing more severe obesity [5, 6].

Case Vignettes

Here we highlight two clinical cases of severe obesity, followed by a discussion of the etiology of severe obesity. We will return to the cases toward the end of the chapter.

Case 1: KM is a 24-year-old Caucasian female. She was born at 40 weeks. She weighed 2.7 kg (third centile). She achieved all her developmental milestones on time. Her BMI was on the 75th centile at the age of 10. She started to gain weight afterward and was on the 95th centile by age 12 and 2 standard

(continued)

S. Sockalingam, R. Hawa (eds.), *Psychiatric Care in Severe Obesity*,
DOI 10.1007/978-3-319-42536-8_3

(continued)

deviations (SDS) above the 95th centile at age 15. Her current BMI is 42 kg/m^2. Her menarche was at age 11. Her cycles were irregular occurring every 30–45 days and now occur every 2–3 months. Both parents have had issues with their weight throughout their adult life. She eats a cereal bar for breakfast, pizza for lunch, and pasta for dinner. She has a can of soda with her lunch and dinner. She snacks frequently, especially in the evening. She typically snacks on chips, cookies, and chocolate. She watches 3–4 h of TV in the evening. She has difficulty falling asleep and often wakes up at night and has a snack. She has 3–4 beers every Friday night. She is not very active but has recently started to go for a 10 min walk twice a week as she is worried about her weight. On examination, she has acanthosis nigricans in her neck and axillae with centripetal adiposity. Her BP is 140/86 mm Hg. Her blood tests show impaired fasting glucose, mild hypertriglyceridemia, low HDL, and mild transaminitis.

Case 2: WM is an 11-year-old Caucasian male. He was born at 40 weeks and weighed 3.6 kg (50th centile). His mother noted that he had a voracious appetite. By the age of 4 he had a height of 1.1 m and weight of 25 kg, BMI of 20.7 kg/m^2 (3 SDS above mean for gender). He was >95th centile for height. He continued to gain weight throughout childhood despite efforts to reduce his food intake including a strict dietary regime. He would often steal food from the refrigerator. He is always hungry. He did not have a history of developmental delay. He currently weighs 120 kg with a height of 1.65 m and a BMI of 44 kg/m^2 (3 SDS). His father has had weight issues since his childhood, as have two of his siblings and father. His mother is reported to be in good health. On examination, he has acanthosis nigricans in his neck and axillae with centripetal adiposity. His BP is 110/68 mm Hg. His blood tests show normal fasting glucose, mild hypertriglyceridemia, and mild transaminitis.

3.3 Regulation of Food Intake and Energy Expenditure

Obesity ultimately results from chronic energy surplus with dietary caloric intake exceeding energy expenditure. Our knowledge of factors regulating appetite and energy expenditure has improved tremendously with discoveries from rodent studies and monogenic causes of human obesity [7]. A detailed overview of this topic is beyond the scope of this review and hence a brief overview is provided.

3.3.1 Regulation of Food Intake

The central nervous system (CNS), in particular, the hypothalamus and brain stem, are critical regulators of energy homeostasis (Fig. 3.1). The hypothalamus integrates signals from the periphery which ultimately regulate food intake. These signals include hormones secreted by the gastrointestinal tract, pancreas, adipocytes, thyroid, and adrenal glands [7, 8] as well as circulating nutrients such as glucose, amino acids, and lipids [9]. In the fasted state, circulating concentration of nutrients and anorexigenic hormones (see later) are low while ghrelin, a hormone secreted by the stomach, is increased. This promotes food intake. Postingestion, increased concentration of anorexigenic hormones (such as glucagon-like peptide 1 and peptide YY, secreted by L cells in the gut in response to food intake), pancreas (insulin), and adipocytes (leptin) suppresses appetite. In addition, afferent neural connections between the gut and NTS (nucleus tractus solitaris) in the brainstem suppress food intake [7–9]. The arcuate nucleus in the hypothalamus is a critical region which responds to circulating signals from the periphery. It comprises anorexigenic POMC (Pro-Opio-Melanocortin) and CART (Cocaine and Amphetamine Regulated Transcript) neurons and orexigenic AGRP (Agouti related peptide) neurons, both of which connect with other hypothalamic regions such as the ventral medial hypothalamus and lateral hypothalamus as well as the brainstem to regulate food intake [8]. These neural pathways have

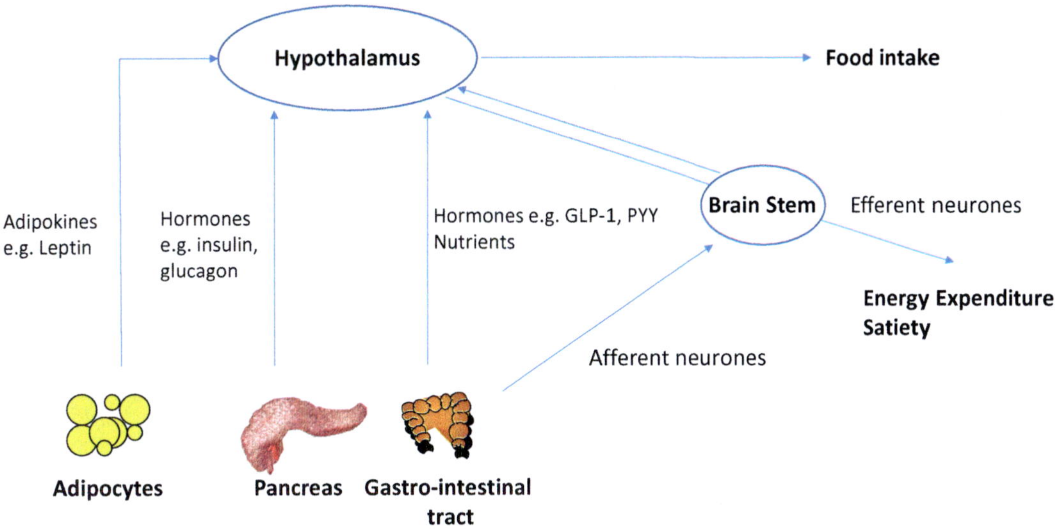

Fig. 3.1 Basic schemata of the regulation of satiety and energy expenditure. The arcuate nucleus in the hypothalamus receives and integrates nutritional and endocrine signals from the peripheral tissues including the gastrointestinal tract, pancreas, and adipocytes. It can then activate or inhibit second-order neurons to other hypothalamic nuclei or the brain stem in response to these signals to regulate food intake and satiety. The brainstem also receives peripheral signals including those from afferent neurons which also regulate satiety, either directly or via communication with the hypothalamus. The hypothalamus and brainstem can also regulate energy expenditure in response to peripheral signals by modulating autonomic outflow to tissues such as brown and beige adipocytes. In addition to these circuits, sensory signals such as sight and smell as well as endocrine inputs such as leptin and ghrelin can regulate cortical and limbic regions which influence the rewarding/hedonic aspects of food intake. *GLP-1* glucagon-like peptide 1, *PYY* peptide YY

been most extensively studied in response to leptin. Leptin activates POMC neurons and suppresses AGRP neurons. POMC neurons secrete αMSH (Melanocyte stimulating hormone), a posttranslational cleavage product of POMC which activates MC4R (Melanocortin 4 receptor) in second-order neurons to suppress appetite [7, 8]. Conversely, activation of AGRP neurones by Neuropeptide Y/AGRP suppresses POMC neurones to stimulate appetite [7, 8]. Circulating leptin, in addition to being modulated by fasting and feeding as described earlier is also directly proportional to fat mass which may serve as a long-term control of food intake. The available evidence would suggest that in common forms of obesity, high leptin concentration fails to suppress appetite suggestive of leptin resistance [8]. In addition to the hypothalamus, cortical regions engaged in executive function as well as striatal regions are important in processing the rewarding value of food and the hedonic (i.e., the 'liking' and 'wanting' of food) drive to eat [7, 8]. These can respond to stimuli such as sight and smell. In recent years it has also been shown that anorexigenic hormone such as leptin, glucagon-like peptide 1, and Peptide YY regulate striatal regions in the brain to reduce the rewarding properties of food and thus the hedonic drive to eat [10–12]. Conversely, ghrelin increases the rewarding property of food [13]. Whether this is a direct effect of these hormones in these regions or mediated via other CNS regions is unknown. In addition to the hypothalamus, the brainstem (regions such as the nucleus tractus solitaris and dorsal vagal complex) is important in regulating food intake. Afferent neurons from the gut can communicate to the brain stem in response to food intake to suppress appetite. It may also respond to signals from the hypothalamus or directly to circulating hormones. In addition, it can relay afferent signals from the periphery to the hypothalamus [9].

In summary, the central nervous system receives and integrates numerous endocrine, nutritional, and neural stimuli to regulate appetite. In addition, cortical and limbic structures can also respond to peripheral stimuli to regulate the hedonic aspects of food ingestion.

3.3.2 Regulation of Energy Expenditure

Energy expenditure is determined by physical activity as well as resting metabolic rate. A major determinant of resting metabolic rate is lean mass in particular skeletal muscle [14, 15]. The neural pathways affecting appetite can also influence energy expenditure. The brainstem, either directly in response to endocrine and neural inputs or indirectly via hypothalamic inputs, can regulate energy expenditure by regulating autonomic outflow [16]. This is achieved, at least in part, by regulation of brown and beige adipose tissue. Unlike white adipose tissue which stores energy in the form of triglyceride, brown adipose is capable of expending energy from substrates such as glucose and triglyceride, in the form of heat in response to a cold stimulus [17]. In addition, humans have 'beige adipocytes,' which are white adipocytes that are capable of becoming more "brown like" to generate heat and expend energy [17]. In addition to cold stimuli, brown and beige adipocytes can be activated by the sympathetic nervous system, which in turn can be regulated by many factors including the leptin–melanocortin system, thyroid hormones, glucagon, and fibroblastic growth factor 21 [18–20]. Exercise may also regulate beige adipocytes, at least in rodents, by promoting secretion of hormones termed myokines from skeletal muscle in response to exercise [18, 19]. These findings need to be confirmed in human studies. The presence of brown/beige adipocytes is inversely related to BMI in humans although causality has not been established. In addition to physical activity and resting metabolic rate, diet-induced thermogenesis (increase in energy expenditure in response to food ingestion) may influence energy balance [21], although its contribution to energy balance in humans has not been established. The underlying regulators of this process have not been firmly established but it may be regulated by brown/beige adipocytes.

Although brown/beige adipocytes can be activated by acute cold exposure, whether this strategy translates into long-term weight loss is not known. Similarly, pharmacological administration of β3 receptor agonists has also been shown to acutely activate brown adipose tissue (BAT) and increase energy expenditure but its long-term effects are not known. Short-term unwanted effects include tachycardia and hypertension [22]. Notably many obese patients lack detectable BAT/beige adipocytes and therefore these agents and/or future agents targeting these adipocytes may not have therapeutic benefits. As highlighted later, thus far the available evidence from genetic causes of obesity and lifestyle interventions suggests that increased food intake is likely the major contributor to obesity in most obese individuals.

In summary, energy expenditure is dependent on physical activity and resting energy expenditure. The latter is regulated by lean mass and potentially brown/beige adipocytes. Many of the CNS regions involved in appetite regulation may also modulate energy expenditure, in response to peripheral stimuli, by modulating sympathetic outflow to brown/beige adipocytes.

3.4 Etiology of Severe Obesity

In this section, we will focus on the etiology of obesity secondary to rare mono/oligogenic causes, 'common' obesity, and obesity secondary to other medical conditions.

3.4.1 Mono/Oligogenic Causes of Obesity

These disorders are caused by mutations in single genes or by structural rearrangements affecting a few genes and have helped further our understanding of human biology as patients harboring these mutations are 'human knockouts.' A major reason for highlighting these cases is that they illuminate the functional significance of pathways regulating energy balance discussed in the previous section. Unlike common cases of obesity, these genetic changes are invariably associated with severe obesity. Although rare, an awareness of these conditions is important as it may have ramifications for the patient and their management. For example, these patients may have additional complications beyond that seen with common obesity. Further, due to the nature of the condition, screening of relatives may be indicated. In some instances, it may be possible to offer effective management, which differs from standard management of obesity. An intricate knowledge of the details of these various genetic disorders is not expected for a nonspecialist. A more pertinent question for a general physician seeing a severely obese patient is: when should one consider these rare monogenic causes of obesity and refer to a specialist physician? Onset of extreme obesity in early childhood (BMI>3 standard deviations from the mean) is typically seen in these patients. Parental consanguinity may be present. Additional clinical features beyond obesity, particularly developmental delay, are also suggestive [7]. A detailed review of every genetic disorder is beyond the scope of this chapter but we have discussed conditions that are relatively common and/or that inform us of pathways regulating human energy balance and those that may have management implications.

3.4.1.1 The Leptin–Melanocortin Pathway

Leptin (*LEP*) and Leptin Receptor (*LEPR*) Mutations

Leptin was first identified in mice as a hormone secreted by adipocytes and suppressed appetite. Ob/Ob mice which lack leptin are obese as are db/db mice which lack its receptor [23, 24]. The importance of leptin in human body weight regulation was confirmed by the identification of humans with congenital leptin deficiency [25]. These cases are usually due to homozygous loss-of-function (usually truncation) mutations in the *LEP* gene and were initially reported in a consanguineous family. Hyperphagia was a prominent feature in these children with marked weight gain (BMI >3 standard deviations from age and gender-matched mean). In addition to obesity, they had impaired immune function and hypogonadotropic hypogonadism. Importantly, treatment with leptin significantly reduced appetite with significant weight loss. Although there was no effect on energy expenditure corrected for lean mass, it is worth noting that energy expenditure usually decreases with weight loss. Associated immune dysfunction and hypogonadotropic hypogonadism also resolved [26]. More recently, cases of severe early onset obesity and similar clinical features to congenital leptin deficiency, but with detectable leptin level, were found to have a homozygous missense mutation in leptin [27, 28]. Treatment with leptin led to reduction in body weight and associated phenotypes. Homozygous and compound heterozygous mutations in the long isoform of the leptin receptor (*LEPR*) are also associated with similar phenotype, but this does not respond to leptin treatment [29].

SH2B1 Deficiency

Sarc Homology 2 B adapter protein 1 (SH2B1) is an adapter protein important in tyrosine kinase signaling in response to a variety of ligands including leptin, insulin, growth hormone, and nerve growth factor. Humans with heterozygous loss-of-function mutations have been identified with hyperphagia, severe early onset obesity, developmental delay and maladaptive behavior, short stature and disproportionate insulin resistance likely reflecting impaired leptin, nerve growth factor, growth hormone, and insulin signaling, respectively [30]. In addition, large, rare chromosomal deletions in chromosome 16 have been identified in children with severe obesity. These deletions encompass a number of genes including SH2B1. Those with larger deletions encompassing a locus previously implicated in autism and cognitive impairment, also had mild developmental delay [31, 32].

POMC Deficiency and PC1/3 Deficiency

POMC (pro-opiomelanocortin) neurons are anorexigenic and direct targets of leptin. They secrete POMC which undergoes posttranslational cleavage by prohormone convertase 1/3 (PC1/3) to yield αMSH and βMSH which are MC4R receptor agonists. Rare loss-of-function mutations in POMC result in obesity with other phenotypes including ACTH (a cleavage product of POMC) and cortisol deficiency and red hair in Caucasians [33]. PC1/3 deficiency, due to mutations in the *PCSK1* gene which encodes PC1/3, also results in severe early onset obesity and ACTH deficiency with additional features such as reactive hypoglycemia, hypogonadotropic hypogonadism and diarrhea likely due to impaired processing of other prohormones including pro-GNRH, proinsulin, and proglucagon peptides (which yield glucagon-like peptides 1 and 2 from enteroendocrine cells) [34].

Melanocortin 4 Receptor (MC4R) Mutations

This is the commonest monogenic cause of severe obesity with mutations reported in up to 1 % of obese patients and 5 % of severely obese patients in some cohorts. Most cases are heterozygous and caused by loss-of-function mutations in the gene encoding the MC4R, a G protein-coupled receptor [35, 36]. This receptor is activated by αMSH and βMSH, peptides generated by cleavage of POMC protein expressed by neurons in the hypothalamus. These POMC-expressing neurons are activated by signals from the periphery in particular leptin. In addition to early onset obesity, increased linear growth is often seen. MC4R signaling is an important mediator of sympathetic outflow which may explain why these patients often do not develop hypertension despite being obese [37]. MC4R agonists are being evaluated as treatment for obesity and have been shown to increase energy expenditure acutely potentially by increasing sympathetic outflow [38]. Its long-term effects have not been evaluated.

SIM1 Deficiency

Single-minded 1 (SIM1) is a basic helix-loop-helix transcription factor, which based on murine models, implicated in development of the paraventricular nucleus of the hypothalamus [39]. Loss-of-function mutations in SIM1 in humans are associated with hyperphagia, early onset obesity, increased linear growth, and impaired autonomic function which are features also seen with MC4R mutations [40]. In mice, MC4R agonist reduces food intake and body weight in wild-type mice but not SIM-1 heterozygous knockout mice suggesting it acts downstream of MC4R [39].

BDNF and TrkB

Brain-derived neurotrophic factor (BDNF) is a neuronal growth factor which binds to a tyrosine kinase receptor TrKB to initiate downstream signaling pathways such as MAP Kinase which is important for cell growth and proliferation. Genetic loss of *BDNF* is associated with obesity in rodent models highlighting the role of neurotrophic factors in obesity [41]. In addition, *BDNF* administration rescues the hyperphagia in *Mc4r* knockout mice suggesting that it acts downstream of the leptin–melanocortin pathway [42]. It also highlights the plasticity in neuronal circuits which are thus potentially amenable to treatment. In humans, a mutation in *TrKB* which resulted in loss of function was associated with early onset obesity, developmental delay, and reduced nociception [43]. A patient with severe hyperphagia, obesity, hyperactivity, and developmental delay was noted to have an inversion in one copy of chromosome 13 which involved the *BDNF* gene and resulted in loss of expression of the gene [44].

KSR2

Kinase suppressor of Ras 2 (KSR2) is a scaffolding protein that regulates multiple pathways including the MAP kinase growth pathway and interacts with AMP kinase, a cellular energy sensor. Consistent with the phenotype of mice with targeted deletion of *KSR2*, humans with loss-of-function mutations in KSR2 which impair MAP kinase signaling and interaction with AMPK, have hyperphagia, obesity, severe insulin resistance, and impaired fatty acid and glucose oxidation [45]. Treatment with metformin, an AMPK activator, improved glucose and fatty acid oxidation in vitro. Notably, unlike most monogenic causes of obesity, mutations in *KSR2* are also associated with reduced energy expenditure which very likely contributes to obesity [45]. Thus far, this is the only monogenic cause of obesity associated with reduced energy expenditure.

Prader–Willi Syndrome

This autosomal dominant condition has a prevalence of 1:10,000–1:30,000 and is caused by absent expression of the paternally derived chromosome 15q11.2–15q13 locus resulting in loss of expression of several genes [46]. This may be seen either due to a deletion in the paternal chromosome or complete absence of the paternal chromosome with two maternally derived copies of chromosome 15. As many of the genes in this locus from the maternal chromosome are usually silent, due to the phenomenon of imprinting, loss of paternally derived genes in this locus leads to complete absence of expression of these genes [46]. These genes encode multiple small nucleolar RNA, which when deleted in humans reproduces features of Prader–Willi syndrome [47]. Clinical features include poor feeding and hypotonia initially followed by the onset of severe hyperphagia and weight gain with morbid obesity thereafter. Elevated ghrelin levels have been reported and likely contribute to the hyperphagia and obesity [48]. Dysmorphic features and hypopigmentation are common. Cognitive impairment and behavioral problems such as temper tantrums and obsessive compulsive disorder are also a feature. Short stature due to growth hormone deficiency along with hypogonadotropic hypogonadism, central hypothyroidism, and adrenal insufficiency is frequently seen. Growth hormone replacement can help improve height, body composition, and reduce body weight [49].

Bardet–Biedl Syndrome

This is a complex syndrome associated with obesity, hypogonadism, retinitis pigmentosa, developmental delay, polydactyly, and renal malformations. Mutations in multiple genes affecting primary ciliary formation have been identified [50].

Albright Hereditary Osteodystrophy

This condition is associated with short stature, skeletal abnormalities, shortened metacarpals, and obesity. Loss-of-function mutations in the *GNAS* gene, which encodes the Gsα subunit of G proteins, have been identified. If the mutation is seen in the maternal allele, additional features including resistance to the action of hormones acting via G protein-coupled receptors such as PTH (pseudohypoparathyroidism 1a), thryoid stimulating hormone (TSH), and gonadotropin-releasing hormone (GNRH) are seen. This is because the paternal allele of this gene is usually silenced and hence loss of the maternal allele leads to complete loss of function [51].

In summary, mono/oligogenic causes of obesity usually cause severe childhood onset obesity, often with the presence of additional clinical features including developmental delay. They are invariably associated with hyperphagia which predisposes toward severe obesity.

3.4.2 Etiology of Common Obesity

3.4.2.1 Genetic Factors

Bodyweight is a highly heritable trait. Studies in families including monozygotic and dizygotic twins raised together or apart have suggested that the heritability of bodyweight is between 40 and 70 % [52–54]. The heritability appears to be higher at a younger age suggesting that environmental influences become more important with time. At a population level, bodyweight has a normal distribution. It has been previously posited that individuals at the extreme ends of this distribution, particularly those in whom the phenotype manifests at a younger age, are more likely to have a monogenic cause for the phenotype. This has been validated in numerous studies that have identified highly penetrant monogenic disorders causing severe obesity in children as highlighted earlier [7]. In most individuals however, numerous genetic variants with small affect sizes contribute to the heritability of bodyweight. These variants interact with environmental influences to influence the individual's phenotype.

These findings have been confirmed in recent genome-wide association studies that have identified more than 100 single nucleotide polymorphisms (SNPs) associated with bodyweight [55]. It is worth highlighting that these variants explain less than 15 % of the heritability of bodyweight. These genetic variants have small affect sizes with odds ratios ranging between 1 and 1.5. The variant with the largest effect size is an intronic variant near the FTO gene. Individuals that are homozygous for the risk variant are an average, 3 kg heavier than those without the risk variant. Heterozygotes have an intermediate bodyweight [56]. The basic premise of genome-wide associated studies (GWAS) is that multiple common variants underlie the heritability of complex traits. In view of the unexplained heritability of traits such as obesity, it is possible that rarer variants with larger effect sizes may also contribute to complex traits. A further limitation of genome-wide association studies is that they do not establish causality but merely association between these variants and obesity. Further, many of these variants are in noncoding regions of the genome. Therefore, traditionally the nearest gene has been assigned as the named gene of interest [57]. In some cases, the nearest gene encodes a protein that is known to affect bodyweight based on rodent and/or human monogenic disorders—two examples being SNPs near the genes encoding *MC4R* and *BDNF* [55]. However, in many cases the nearest gene's biological function has not been established. There is growing evidence that these noncoding variants can influence the expression of genes, both in close proximity and beyond, involved in the biology of bodyweight regulation. For example, the variant in FTO has been found to influence the expression of several genes in its vicinity [58]. More recent endeavors such as the ENCODE project will help disentangle the effects of noncoding variants on expression of relevant genes and pathways implicated in complex phenotypes including obesity [59].

As alluded to earlier, elucidating the functional effects of genetic variants identified by GWAS and how they influence bodyweight has been challenging. This is further compounded by the small affect sizes of the variants in question. The FTO variant, which has the largest effect size with an odds ratio of ~1.5, has been studied in some detail. Initial studies have suggested that individuals carrying the risk variant have increased caloric intake compared to noncarriers [60]. In one study, circulating concentrations of the orexigenic hormone ghrelin were found to be higher in these individuals and thought to underlie their phenotype. This study also reported that the risk variant of FTO influenced Ghrelin mRNA expression in leukocytes [61]. The contribution of leukocytes to circulating ghrelin, which predominantly originates from the stomach, is unknown. A more recent study has suggested that the FTO risk variant causes obesity by reducing energy expenditure. It has been suggested that it does so by increasing the expression of two nearby genes *IRX5* and *IRX3*, which in turn prevent the conversion of white adipocytes, which store energy as fat, into beige adipocytes which increase fat oxidation to generate energy in the form of heat [58]. A major limitation of this study is that these effects were seen in vitro and ex vivo. There is currently no evidence that carriers of the FTO risk variant have reduced energy expenditure, thermogenesis, or beige adipocytes depots [62].

An important point to note is that the common genetic variants found in GWAS studies have been associated with BMI and associated measures either in healthy controls or obese individuals. The majority of the studies did not include individuals with severe obesity. A pertinent question, therefore, is whether these variants contribute to severe obesity. A recent study assessed the contribution of 32 GWAS loci, previously implicated in obesity, in approximately 1000 severely obese patients referred for bariatric surgery compared to healthy controls [63]. They found that two loci were significantly associated with severe obesity: a common variant in *FTO* as well as a previously described SNP in *NEGR1*. They found that a cumulative weighted genetic risk score was associated with severe obesity but did not predict the variance in BMI within the extreme obesity cohort [63]. This would suggest that additional, as yet unidentified, genetic factors may play a role in severe obesity. This is consistent with the finding of Wheeler et al. who performed genome-wide association studies in children with severe early onset childhood obesity [64]. They found nine common variants associated with severe obesity. These included previously described variants in *FTO*, *MC4R*, *TMEM18*, and *NEGR1*. They also found four novel loci including variants in the leptin receptor (*LEPR*) and genes previously not known to be involved in energy and hemostasis including *PRKCH*, *PACS 1*, and *RMST*. In addition, they found rare copy number variants (large regions of deleted DNA or multiple copies of a region of DNA encompassing multiple genes) associated with severe childhood obesity [64]. Whether severe obesity in adults shares the same or similar underlying genetic architecture as severe early onset childhood obesity is unknown.

In summary, multiple genetic variants with small effect sizes have been found to be associated with obesity. The underlying mechanistic link between these variants and obesity has not been established. In addition, these variants explain a minority of the heritability of obesity suggesting that as yet unidentified genetic variants may underlie the heritability void.

3.4.2.2 Environmental and Diet Factors

As mentioned in the previous section, heritability of obesity and bodyweight measures are estimated to be between 40 and 70 % depending on age. Environmental factors very likely explain the remainder. In this section, we will discuss some of these environmental factors.

Diet

Obesity results from chronic energy surplus. Dietary energy intake is likely the major determinant of overall energy balance. This is based on the finding from human trials that reduction in caloric intake can result in substantial weight loss in the short term irrespective of macronutrient composition [65]. The recent obesity epidemic has paralleled the recent increase in caloric intake with the availability of highly processed calorically dense food, usually high in refined carbohydrates and fat [66]. The recent increase in portion sizes has also contributed to increased caloric intake. In a prospective study assessing three cohorts totaling more than 100,000 individuals, intake of potatoes and potato chips, unprocessed red meat, processed meat, and sugar sweetened beverages was directly associated with weight gain whereas the consumption of unprocessed food including vegetables, fruit, nuts, and yogurt were inversely related to weight gain [67].

Eating Patterns

In addition to dietary composition, the pattern of eating also likely contributes to bodyweight. These factors include restrained eating, binge eating, and night eating. Restrained eating, that is the conscious limitation of food intake is often seen in normal weight individuals suggesting that a lack of inhibition likely contributes to weight gain [68]. An extreme form of lack of inhibition is seen with binge eating disorder (BED) in which individuals have uncontrolled periods of significantly increased, usually rapid caloric intake (binges) [69]. This persists beyond the state of satiety despite physical discomfort and is associated with subsequent feelings of guilt. This may in some cases be associated with subsequent purging. In some reports, between 23 and 46 % of individuals seeking treatment for obesity have binge eating disorder [70]. It is worth noting however that not all individuals with binge eating disorder are obese [70]. It has also been suggested that some obese individuals, especially those with BED, may have 'food addiction' akin to drug addiction and as a consequence crave and seek out food. Questionnaires such as the Yale Food Addiction score have been developed to identify these symptoms. In some studies, obese individuals have been found to have blunted striatal dopamine response (indicating reduced reward) to food due to reduced dopamine D2 receptor expression, similar to the reduced striatal dopamine response to drugs in drug addicts. It has been suggested that as a consequence these individuals have to eat larger amounts of food to compensate for the lack of hedonic value to the food, analogous to the reward deficiency hypothesis of drug addiction [71]. However, although the neurobiology of drug addiction and obesity, particularly in patients with BED, has similarities there are important differences. There are no convincing symptoms of withdrawal or tolerance seen with food. Further, studies have shown increased, decreased, and normal striatal dopamine responses to food [71].

Night eating, that is the consumption of at least 25 % of daily caloric intake between the evening meal and breakfast is associated with increased bodyweight [69, 72]. In a recent study, reduction in night time food intake and as a consequence prolonging the overnight fast resulted in weight loss and improved metabolic parameters despite no attempt to reduce caloric intake [73].

Physical Activity

The recent obesity epidemic has also coincided with a time period in which sedentary behavior has increased which has very likely contributed to the epidemic [74, 75]. Based on available data from interventional trials, exercise causes modest additional weight loss when added to dietary changes suggesting that dietary factors are the primary environmental drivers of obesity. Exercise, however, helps maintain weight loss in the longer term and has metabolic benefits beyond weight loss and is therefore an important aspect of the management of obesity [3, 76].

Television Watching

Epidemiological studies have found a link between time spent watching television and obesity [77]. In addition, reducing television viewing time has been shown to result in weight loss [78]. It has been suggested that watching television promotes sedentary behavior, increases food intake especially of fast food, and possibly disrupts sleep [79].

Socioeconomic Factors

Rates of obesity are disproportionately higher in low social economic groups. This is likely to be secondary to some of the environmental factors listed earlier. This includes poor nutritional education, increased consumption of processed foods which are cheaper, and lack of access to sidewalks and playgrounds [80].

In Utero Environment

Longitudinal studies have shown that maternal undernutrition and overnutrition as well as maternal hyperglycemia can adversely affect the offspring's bodyweight [81, 82]. The Dutch famine study demonstrated that in for uterine growth retardation and small for gestational age babies are at risk for increased weight gain and metabolic disease later on in life when faced with surplus nutrients [83]. Studies in rodents suggest that this may be due to epigenetic changes that affect the expression of metabolically relevant genes [81].

Medications

A number of medications are implicated in weight gain. These include atypical antipsychotic medications (e.g., olanzapine and clozapine), lithium, anticonvulsants (valproate and carbamazepine), insulin, and glucocorticoids [84, 85]. Medications acting via the central nervous system such as antipsychotic agents, lithium, and anticonvulsants likely have direct effects on food intake. Insulin has known anabolic actions and may promote food intake and weight gain secondary to glucose lowering as suggested by the presence of weight gain with intensive glycemic control [86]. Glucocorticoids are known to stimulate adipogenesis and food intake [87, 88].

Physiological Changes

Weight gain often occurs with certain physiological changes such as puberty, pregnancy, menopause, and aging [89–91]. Although modest, this can predispose toward obesity.

Gut Microbiota

Obesity is associated with alterations in the gut microbial population, which has been postulated to contribute to obesity [92]. Antibiotic use in early life has been associated with obesity in animal models but this has not been confirmed in humans [93]. Changes in microbiota have also been reported after diet-induced weight loss and bariatric surgery. In rodents, these changes in microbiota have been causally linked to obesity in experiments in which microbiota from obese mice are transferred to lean nude mice lacking gut microbes and vice versa [92]. A definitive causal relationship between altered microbiota and obesity in humans has not been established. Transfer of microbiota from insulin-sensitive to insulin-resistant individuals has been associated with improvement in insulin sensitivity suggesting that microbiota may influence human metabolism [94].

In summary, numerous environmental factors including caloric intake, macronutrient composition, pattern and timing of food intake, reduced physical activity, and medications may predispose to weight gain. Rodent models suggest that novel factors such as alterations in gut microbiota may also be causally linked to obesity.

3.4.2.3 Gene–Environment Interaction

There is growing evidence of interactions between genetic and environmental factors. One of the limiting factors in studying gene–environment interaction is that detailed data about environmental risk factors, such as those outlined earlier, may not be available [95]. Further, due to the small effect sizes of the common genetic variants associated with obesity, large sample sizes are needed in order to detect an interaction [96, 97]. Two approaches to circumvent these issues are to assess the interaction between a variant with a relatively large effect size and a predefined environmental factor or to calculate a cumulative genetic risk score based on the weighted effects of each risk variant and assess the interaction between the risk score and an environmental variable. A caveat with using a risk score is that it is not possible to ascertain which individual gene–environment interactions are biologically significant. An example of gene environment interaction for a single genetic variant comes from the studies of food intake and the *FTO* risk variant, which has the largest effect size, among common genetic variants associated with obesity. Cecil et al. found that this genetic variant was associated with increased consumption of energy-rich foods [60]. Interestingly, it was also reported to be associated with increased physical activity. Although an initial study suggested that individuals with the FTO risk variant had decreased odds of being obese if they were physically active [98], these findings were not always reproducible until a large meta-analysis of 45 studies eventually confirmed this finding, underpinning the need for adequately powered studies to assess gene–environment interactions [99]. An example of a study assessing gene–environment interaction with weighted genetic risk scores is a report by Qi et al. [100]. They found that an increasing genetic risk score was associated with higher BMI but this was further modulated by intake of sugar sweetened beverages. For each increase in ten risk alleles, the increase in BMI was 1.0 for those consuming <1 serving per month vs. 1.78 for those consuming >1 serving per day, i.e., a relative increase of 78 % [100]. The same group reported similar interactions between fried food consumption and genetic risk score [101].

In summary, genetic and environmental factors can interact to modulate the risk of obesity in an individual. Due to the small effect sizes of common genetic variants, large sample sizes are typically needed to establish these interactions. Future studies in large population cohorts with well-documented environmental influences are needed to assess these interactions further.

3.4.2.4 Obesity Secondary to Other Medical Conditions

Increased weight gain can be seen secondary to other medical conditions including hypothyroidism, Cushing's syndrome, and hypothalamic lesions particularly after treatment.

Primary Hypothyroidism

Primary hypothyroidism, characterized by elevated TSH (thyroid stimulating hormone) and low thyroid hormones (free T4 and T3), is associated with weight gain. Other features including fatigue, low mood, cold intolerance, edema, menorrhagia, bradycardia, myalgia, and dyslipidemia may be seen. It can be due to autoimmune disease or treatments such as radioactive iodine and surgical thyroidectomy [102].

Cushing's Syndrome

This is characterized by glucocorticoid excess either due to endogenous or exogenous glucocorticoid. Endogenous sources of glucocorticoids include benign and malignant adrenal cortical lesions and pituitary adenomas. In addition to weight gain, altered fat distribution (centripetal, dorsocervical, supraclavicular, and facial), thin skin, easy bruising, striae, proximal myopathy, hypertension, glucose intolerance, facial plethora, osteopenia/osteoporosis, and fragility fractures may be seen. Very high ACTH and cortisol secretion may be seen secondary to malignancy such as small cell carcinoma of the lung but due to the rapid onset of disease and poor prognosis, hypertension and hypokalemia due to mineralocorticoid action of cortisol and increased pigmentation are more prominent than weight gain [103].

Hypothalamic Lesions

Hypothalamic lesions, in particular craniopharyngiomas, may present with weight gain, although this tends to be more pronounced post-surgery and radiotherapy with reported rates of increase in obesity of 50 %. As stated earlier the hypothalamus is an important regulator of energy balance. Both increased food intake and reduced activity have been reported in patients with treated craniopharyngioma [104, 105].

3.5 Review of Case Histories

Case 1

The patient in this case has had a gradual increase in weight since puberty. She has a family history of obesity but does not have early childhood onset severe obesity. A number of environmental factors are contributing to her increased body weight including consumption of processed food and beverages high in saturated fat and sugar, night time eating, television watching, and a sedentary lifestyle. Her history and physical examination suggest she may have a number of obesity-related complications including insulin resistance, polycystic ovarian syndrome, and fatty liver disease based on the presence of acanthosis nigricans, irregular menses, and transaminitis. She also has hypertension and dyslipidemia. Her obesity is likely caused by a combination of polygenic factors interacting with numerous environmental contributors.

Case 2

The patient in this case clearly has early childhood onset severe obesity secondary to hyperphagia which is suggestive of a monogenic cause. In addition, there appears to be a family history of early onset obesity. There is no developmental delay. He has signs of insulin resistance (acanthosis nigricans) and dyslipidemia but is normotensive. A mutation in the MC4R gene, the commonest monogenic cause of childhood obesity, could account for his obesity and his normal blood pressure.

Conclusion

Obesity results from chronic energy surplus. In most individuals, a combination of multiple genetic and environmental factors interacts to predispose toward obesity. The majority of the genetic component of obesity as well as its interaction with the environment has not been established. Discovering these genetic variants and how they interact with the environment will undoubtedly improve our understanding of obesity and may potentially translate to better treatments.

References

1. Malnick SD, Knobler H. The medical complications of obesity. QJM. 2006;99:565–79.
2. Douketis JD, Macie C, Thabane L, Williamson DF. Systematic review of long-term weight loss studies in obese adults: clinical significance and applicability to clinical practice. Int J Obes (Lond). 2005;29:1153–67.
3. Look ARG, Wing RR, Bolin P, et al. Cardiovascular effects of intensive lifestyle intervention in type 2 diabetes. N Engl J Med. 2013;369:145–54.
4. Puzziferri N, Roshek 3rd TB, Mayo HG, Gallagher R, Belle SH, Livingston EH. Long-term follow-up after bariatric surgery: a systematic review. JAMA. 2014;312:934–42.
5. Jensen MD, Ryan DH, Apovian CM, et al. 2013 AHA/ACC/TOS guideline for the management of overweight and obesity in adults: a report of the American College of Cardiology/American Heart Association Task Force on Practice Guidelines

and the Obesity Society. Circulation. 2014;129: S102–38.
6. Skinner AC, Skelton JA. Prevalence and trends in obesity and severe obesity among children in the United States, 1999–2012. JAMA Pediatr. 2014;168: 561–6.
7. van der Klaauw AA, Farooqi IS. The hunger genes: pathways to obesity. Cell. 2015;161:119–32.
8. Coll AP, Farooqi IS, O'Rahilly S. The hormonal control of food intake. Cell. 2007;129:251–62.
9. Schwartz GJ, Zeltser LM. Functional organization of neuronal and humoral signals regulating feeding behavior. Annu Rev Nutr. 2013;33:1–21.
10. De Silva A, Salem V, Long CJ, et al. The gut hormones PYY 3–36 and GLP-1 7–36 amide reduce food intake and modulate brain activity in appetite centers in humans. Cell Metab. 2011;14:700–6.
11. Farooqi IS, Bullmore E, Keogh J, Gillard J, O'Rahilly S, Fletcher PC. Leptin regulates striatal regions and human eating behavior. Science. 2007; 317:1355.
12. Rosenbaum M, Sy M, Pavlovich K, Leibel RL, Hirsch J. Leptin reverses weight loss-induced changes in regional neural activity responses to visual food stimuli. J Clin Invest. 2008;118: 2583–91.
13. Malik S, McGlone F, Bedrossian D, Dagher A. Ghrelin modulates brain activity in areas that control appetitive behavior. Cell Metab. 2008;7:400–9.
14. Speakman JR, Selman C. Physical activity and resting metabolic rate. Proc Nutr Soc. 2003;62:621–34.
15. Zurlo F, Larson K, Bogardus C, Ravussin E. Skeletal muscle metabolism is a major determinant of resting energy expenditure. J Clin Invest. 1990;86:1423–7.
16. Schneeberger M, Gomis R, Claret M. Hypothalamic and brainstem neuronal circuits controlling homeostatic energy balance. J Endocrinol. 2014;220: T25–46.
17. Kajimura S, Spiegelman BM, Seale P. Brown and beige fat: physiological roles beyond heat generation. Cell Metab. 2015;22:546–59.
18. Cohen P, Spiegelman BM. Brown and beige fat: molecular parts of a thermogenic machine. Diabetes. 2015;64:2346–51.
19. Lee P, Greenfield JR. Non-pharmacological and pharmacological strategies of brown adipose tissue recruitment in humans. Mol Cell Endocrinol. 2015;418(Pt 2):184–90.
20. Richard D, Carpentier AC, Dore G, Ouellet V, Picard F. Determinants of brown adipocyte development and thermogenesis. Int J Obes (Lond). 2010;34 Suppl 2:S59–66.
21. Kozak LP. Brown fat and the myth of diet-induced thermogenesis. Cell Metab. 2010;11:263–7.
22. Cypess AM, Weiner LS, Roberts-Toler C, et al. Activation of human brown adipose tissue by a beta3-adrenergic receptor agonist. Cell Metab. 2015;21:33–8.
23. Friedman JM. Leptin, leptin receptors, and the control of body weight. Nutr Rev. 1998;56:s38–46. discussion s54–75.
24. Friedman JM, Halaas JL. Leptin and the regulation of body weight in mammals. Nature. 1998;395: 763–70.
25. Montague CT, Farooqi IS, Whitehead JP, et al. Congenital leptin deficiency is associated with severe early-onset obesity in humans. Nature. 1997;387:903–8.
26. Farooqi IS, Matarese G, Lord GM, et al. Beneficial effects of leptin on obesity, T cell hyporesponsiveness, and neuroendocrine/metabolic dysfunction of human congenital leptin deficiency. J Clin Invest. 2002;110:1093–103.
27. Wabitsch M, Funcke JB, Lennerz B, et al. Biologically inactive leptin and early-onset extreme obesity. N Engl J Med. 2015;372:48–54.
28. Wabitsch M, Funcke JB, von Schnurbein J, et al. Severe early-onset obesity due to bioinactive leptin caused by a p.N103K mutation in the leptin gene. J Clin Endocrinol Metab. 2015;100:3227–30.
29. Farooqi IS, Wangensteen T, Collins S, et al. Clinical and molecular genetic spectrum of congenital deficiency of the leptin receptor. N Engl J Med. 2007;356:237–47.
30. Doche ME, Bochukova EG, Su HW, et al. Human SH2B1 mutations are associated with maladaptive behaviors and obesity. J Clin Invest. 2012;122:l 4732–6.
31. Bochukova EG, Huang N, Keogh J, et al. Large, rare chromosomal deletions associated with severe early-onset obesity. Nature. 2010;463:666–70.
32. Walters RG, Jacquemont S, Valsesia A, et al. A new highly penetrant form of obesity due to deletions on chromosome 16p11.2. Nature. 2010;463:671–5.
33. Krude H, Biebermann H, Luck W, Horn R, Brabant G, Gruters A. Severe early-onset obesity, adrenal insufficiency and red hair pigmentation caused by POMC mutations in humans. Nat Genet. 1998;19: 155–7.
34. Jackson RS, Creemers JW, Farooqi IS, et al. Small-intestinal dysfunction accompanies the complex endocrinopathy of human proprotein convertase 1 deficiency. J Clin Invest. 2003;112:1550–60.
35. Farooqi IS, Yeo GS, Keogh JM, et al. Dominant and recessive inheritance of morbid obesity associated with melanocortin 4 receptor deficiency. J Clin Invest. 2000;106:271–9.
36. Vaisse C, Clement K, Durand E, Hercberg S, Guy-Grand B, Froguel P. Melanocortin-4 receptor mutations are a frequent and heterogeneous cause of morbid obesity. J Clin Invest. 2000;106:253–62.
37. Greenfield JR, Miller JW, Keogh JM, et al. Modulation of blood pressure by central melanocortinergic pathways. N Engl J Med. 2009;360:44–52.
38. Chen KY, Muniyappa R, Abel BS, et al. RM-493, a melanocortin-4 receptor (MC4R) agonist, increases

resting energy expenditure in obese individuals. J Clin Endocrinol Metab. 2015;100:1639–45.
39. Kublaoui BM, Holder Jr JL, Gemelli T, Zinn AR. Sim1 haploinsufficiency impairs melanocortin-mediated anorexia and activation of paraventricular nucleus neurons. Mol Endocrinol. 2006;20:2483–92.
40. Ramachandrappa S, Raimondo A, Cali AM, et al. Rare variants in single-minded 1 (SIM1) are associated with severe obesity. J Clin Invest. 2013; 123:3042–50.
41. Kernie SG, Liebl DJ, Parada LF. BDNF regulates eating behavior and locomotor activity in mice. EMBO J. 2000;19:1290–300.
42. Xu B, Goulding EH, Zang K, et al. Brain-derived neurotrophic factor regulates energy balance downstream of melanocortin-4 receptor. Nat Neurosci. 2003;6:736–42.
43. Yeo GS, Connie Hung CC, Rochford J, et al. A de novo mutation affecting human TrkB associated with severe obesity and developmental delay. Nat Neurosci. 2004;7:1187–9.
44. Gray J, Yeo GS, Cox JJ, et al. Hyperphagia, severe obesity, impaired cognitive function, and hyperactivity associated with functional loss of one copy of the brain-derived neurotrophic factor (BDNF) gene. Diabetes. 2006;55:3366–71.
45. Pearce LR, Atanassova N, Banton MC, et al. KSR2 mutations are associated with obesity, insulin resistance, and impaired cellular fuel oxidation. Cell. 2013;155:765–77.
46. Kalsner L, Chamberlain SJ. Prader-Willi, Angelman, and 15q11-q13 duplication syndromes. Pediatr Clin North Am. 2015;62:587–606.
47. de Smith AJ, Purmann C, Walters RG, et al. A deletion of the HBII-85 class of small nucleolar RNAs (snoRNAs) is associated with hyperphagia, obesity and hypogonadism. Hum Mol Genet. 2009;18: 3257–65.
48. Haqq AM, Farooqi IS, O'Rahilly S, et al. Serum ghrelin levels are inversely correlated with body mass index, age, and insulin concentrations in normal children and are markedly increased in Prader-Willi syndrome. J Clin Endocrinol Metab. 2003;88: 174–8.
49. Haqq AM, Stadler DD, Jackson RH, Rosenfeld RG, Purnell JQ, LaFranchi SH. Effects of growth hormone on pulmonary function, sleep quality, behavior, cognition, growth velocity, body composition, and resting energy expenditure in Prader-Willi syndrome. J Clin Endocrinol Metab. 2003;88:2206–12.
50. Badano JL, Mitsuma N, Beales PL, Katsanis N. The ciliopathies: an emerging class of human genetic disorders. Annu Rev Genomics Hum Genet. 2006;7: 125–48.
51. Weinstein LS, Chen M, Liu J. Gs(alpha) mutations and imprinting defects in human disease. Ann N Y Acad Sci. 2002;968:173–97.
52. Maes HH, Neale MC, Eaves LJ. Genetic and environmental factors in relative body weight and human adiposity. Behav Genet. 1997;27:325–51.
53. Stunkard AJ, Harris JR, Pedersen NL, McClearn GE. The body-mass index of twins who have been reared apart. N Engl J Med. 1990;322:1483–7.
54. Wardle J, Carnell S, Haworth CM, Plomin R. Evidence for a strong genetic influence on childhood adiposity despite the force of the obesogenic environment. Am J Clin Nutr. 2008;87:398–404.
55. Locke AE, Kahali B, Berndt SI, et al. Genetic studies of body mass index yield new insights for obesity biology. Nature. 2015;518:197–206.
56. Frayling TM, Timpson NJ, Weedon MN, et al. A common variant in the FTO gene is associated with body mass index and predisposes to childhood and adult obesity. Science. 2007;316:889–94.
57. Visscher PM, Brown MA, McCarthy MI, Yang J. Five years of GWAS discovery. Am J Hum Genet. 2012;90:7–24.
58. Claussnitzer M, Dankel SN, Kim KH, et al. FTO obesity variant circuitry and adipocyte browning in humans. N Engl J Med. 2015;373:895–907.
59. Maher B. ENCODE: the human encyclopaedia. Nature. 2012;489:46–8.
60. Cecil JE, Tavendale R, Watt P, Hetherington MM, Palmer CN. An obesity-associated FTO gene variant and increased energy intake in children. N Engl J Med. 2008;359:2558–66.
61. Karra E, O'Daly OG, Choudhury AI, et al. A link between FTO, ghrelin, and impaired brain food-cue responsivity. J Clin Invest. 2013;123:3539–51.
62. O'Rahilly S, Coll AP, Yeo GS. FTO obesity variant and adipocyte browning in humans. N Engl J Med. 2016;374:191.
63. Magi R, Manning S, Yousseif A, et al. Contribution of 32 GWAS-identified common variants to severe obesity in European adults referred for bariatric surgery. PLoS One. 2013;8:e70735.
64. Wheeler E, Huang N, Bochukova EG, et al. Genome-wide SNP and CNV analysis identifies common and low-frequency variants associated with severe early-onset obesity. Nat Genet. 2013;45:513–7.
65. Johnston BC, Kanters S, Bandayrel K, et al. Comparison of weight loss among named diet programs in overweight and obese adults: a meta-analysis. JAMA. 2014;312:923–33.
66. Swinburn BA, Sacks G, Hall KD, et al. The global obesity pandemic: shaped by global drivers and local environments. Lancet. 2011;378:804–14.
67. Mozaffarian D, Hao T, Rimm EB, Willett WC, Hu FB. Changes in diet and lifestyle and long-term weight gain in women and men. N Engl J Med. 2011;364:2392–404.
68. Konttinen H, Haukkala A, Sarlio-Lahteenkorva S, Silventoinen K, Jousilahti P. Eating styles, self-control and obesity indicators. The moderating role of obesity status and dieting history on restrained eating. Appetite. 2009;53:131–4.
69. Allison KC, Grilo CM, Masheb RM, Stunkard AJ. Binge eating disorder and night eating syndrome: a comparative study of disordered eating. J Consult Clin Psychol. 2005;73:1107–15.

70. de Zwaan M, Mitchell JE. Binge eating in the obese. Ann Med. 1992;24:303–8.
71. Ziauddeen H, Farooqi IS, Fletcher PC. Obesity and the brain: how convincing is the addiction model? Nat Rev Neurosci. 2012;13:279–86.
72. Mostad IL, Langaas M, Grill V. Central obesity is associated with lower intake of whole-grain bread and less frequent breakfast and lunch: results from the HUNT study, an adult all-population survey. Appl Physiol Nutr Metab. 2014;39:819–28.
73. Gill S, Panda S. A smartphone App reveals erratic diurnal eating patterns in humans that can be modulated for health benefits. Cell Metab. 2015;22:789–98.
74. Church TS, Thomas DM, Tudor-Locke C, et al. Trends over 5 decades in U.S. occupation-related physical activity and their associations with obesity. PLoS One. 2011;6:e19657.
75. Maher CA, Mire E, Harrington DM, Staiano AE, Katzmarzyk PT. The independent and combined associations of physical activity and sedentary behavior with obesity in adults: NHANES 2003-06. Obesity (Silver Spring). 2013;21:E730–7.
76. Gerstein HC. Do lifestyle changes reduce serious outcomes in diabetes? N Engl J Med. 2013;369:189–90.
77. Dietz Jr WH, Gortmaker SL. Do we fatten our children at the television set? Obesity and television viewing in children and adolescents. Pediatrics. 1985;75:807–12.
78. Robinson TN. Reducing children's television viewing to prevent obesity: a randomized controlled trial. JAMA. 1999;282:1561–7.
79. Council on Communications and Media, Strasburger VC. Children, adolescents, obesity, and the media. Pediatrics. 2011;128:201–8.
80. Drewnowski A. The economics of food choice behavior: why poverty and obesity are linked. Nestle Nutr Inst Workshop Ser. 2012;73:95–112.
81. Ozanne SE. Epigenetic signatures of obesity. N Engl J Med. 2015;372:973–4.
82. Baptiste-Roberts K, Nicholson WK, Wang NY, Brancati FL. Gestational diabetes and subsequent growth patterns of offspring: the National Collaborative Perinatal Project. Matern Child Health J. 2012;16:125–32.
83. Ravelli AC, van Der Meulen JH, Osmond C, Barker DJ, Bleker OP. Obesity at the age of 50 y in men and women exposed to famine prenatally. Am J Clin Nutr. 1999;70:811–6.
84. Leslie WS, Hankey CR, Lean ME. Weight gain as an adverse effect of some commonly prescribed drugs: a systematic review. QJM. 2007;100:395–404.
85. Bray GA, Ryan DH. Medical therapy for the patient with obesity. Circulation. 2012;125:1695–703.
86. Nathan DM, Cleary PA, Backlund JY, et al. Intensive diabetes treatment and cardiovascular disease in patients with type 1 diabetes. N Engl J Med. 2005; 353:2643–53.
87. Coll AP, Yeo GS, Farooqi IS, O'Rahilly S. SnapShot: the hormonal control of food intake. Cell. 2008; 135:572.e1–2.
88. Pantoja C, Huff JT, Yamamoto KR. Glucocorticoid signaling defines a novel commitment state during adipogenesis in vitro. Mol Biol Cell. 2008;19: 4032–41.
89. Deshmukh-Taskar P, Nicklas TA, Morales M, Yang SJ, Zakeri I, Berenson GS. Tracking of overweight status from childhood to young adulthood: the Bogalusa Heart Study. Eur J Clin Nutr. 2006;60: 48–57.
90. Smith DE, Lewis CE, Caveny JL, Perkins LL, Burke GL, Bild DE. Longitudinal changes in adiposity associated with pregnancy. The CARDIA Study. Coronary Artery Risk Development in Young Adults Study. JAMA. 1994;271:1747–51.
91. Sowers M, Zheng H, Tomey K, et al. Changes in body composition in women over six years at midlife: ovarian and chronological aging. J Clin Endocrinol Metab. 2007;92:895–901.
92. Winer DA, Luck H, Tsai S, Winer S. The intestinal immune system in obesity and insulin resistance. Cell Metab. 2016;23:413–26.
93. Gerber JS, Bryan M, Ross RK, et al. Antibiotic exposure during the first 6 months of life and weight gain during childhood. JAMA. 2016;315:1258–65.
94. Vrieze A, Van Nood E, Holleman F, et al. Transfer of intestinal microbiota from lean donors increases insulin sensitivity in individuals with metabolic syndrome. Gastroenterology. 2012;143:913–6. e7.
95. Patel CJ, Ioannidis JP. Studying the elusive environment in large scale. JAMA. 2014;311:2173–4.
96. Huang T, Hu FB. Gene–environment interactions and obesity: recent developments and future directions. BMC Med Genomics. 2015;8 Suppl 1:S2.
97. Marigorta UM, Gibson G. A simulation study of gene-by-environment interactions in GWAS implies ample hidden effects. Front Genet. 2014;5:225.
98. Demerath EW, Lutsey PL, Monda KL, et al. Interaction of FTO and physical activity level on adiposity in African-American and European-American adults: the ARIC study. Obesity (Silver Spring). 2011;19:1866–72.
99. Kilpelainen TO, Qi L, Brage S, et al. Physical activity attenuates the influence of FTO variants on obesity risk: a meta-analysis of 218,166 adults and 19,268 children. PLoS Med. 2011;8:e1001116.
100. Qi Q, Chu AY, Kang JH, et al. Sugar-sweetened beverages and genetic risk of obesity. N Engl J Med. 2012;367:1387–96.
101. Qi Q, Chu AY, Kang JH, et al. Fried food consumption, genetic risk, and body mass index: gene–diet interaction analysis in three US cohort studies. BMJ. 2014;348:g1610.
102. Garber JR, Cobin RH, Gharib H, et al. Clinical practice guidelines for hypothyroidism in adults: cosponsored by the American Association of Clinical

Endocrinologists and the American Thyroid Association. Endocr Pract. 2012;18:988–1028.
103. Nieman LK, Biller BM, Findling JW, et al. Treatment of Cushing's syndrome: an Endocrine Society Clinical Practice Guideline. J Clin Endocrinol Metab. 2015;100:2807–31.
104. Holmer H, Pozarek G, Wirfalt E, et al. Reduced energy expenditure and impaired feeding-related signals but not high energy intake reinforces hypothalamic obesity in adults with childhood onset craniopharyngioma. J Clin Endocrinol Metab. 2010;95:5395–402.
105. Muller HL, Emser A, Faldum A, et al. Longitudinal study on growth and body mass index before and after diagnosis of childhood craniopharyngioma. J Clin Endocrinol Metab. 2004;89:3298–305.

Insecure Attachment and Trauma in Obesity and Bariatric Surgery

4

R.G. Maunder, J.J. Hunter, and Tho Lan Le

The purpose of this chapter is to discuss an aspect of the psychosocial context of obesity that transcends diagnostic categories and is especially relevant to the management of severely obese patients. In particular, we will describe the relational context of obesity and the importance of insecure attachment and interpersonal trauma. In doing so we will try to make the case that patient-centered care (and perhaps surgical outcomes) can be improved by attending to the consequences of trauma and to ways in which the treatment of obesity is influenced by feelings of interpersonal security or insecurity.

R.G. Maunder (✉) • J.J. Hunter, M.D., F.R.C.P.C.
Division of Consultation-Liaison Psychiatry, Department of Psychiatry, Mount Sinai Hospital, University of Toronto, Room 1285-B, 600 University Ave., Toronto, ON, Canada M5G 1X5
e-mail: Robert.Maunder@sinaihealthsystem.ca; Jon.Hunter@sinaihealthsystem.ca

T.L. Le, Ph.D. Candidate
Institute of Medical Science, University of Toronto, Toronto, ON, Canada
e-mail: thaolan.le@gmail.com

4.1 Defining the Field

4.1.1 Trauma

In considering the impact of trauma on health outcomes, one needs to start by defining what the word means. All lives come with adversity, challenge, and stress, but trauma refers to something more. Furthermore, the prevalence and consequences of past trauma may vary with the how it is defined, so research methods matter. By far, most studies of the links between obesity and trauma have focused on developmental trauma, differentiating between two types of childhood exposure.

The first category of childhood trauma refers to physical and sexual abuse. There is a great deal of research studying one or both of these types of exposure. Definitions vary between studies, but are usually explicit about the type of behavior that is being surveyed. For example, the Canadian Community Health Survey [1], which uses items from the Childhood Experiences of Violence Questionnaire, classifies physical abuse into three categories of increasing severity: "(1) being slapped on the face, head or ears, or hit or spanked with something hard 3 or more times; (2) being pushed, grabbed or shoved, or having something thrown at the respondent to hurt them 3 or more times; and (3) being kicked, bit,

S. Sockalingam, R. Hawa (eds.), *Psychiatric Care in Severe Obesity*,
DOI 10.1007/978-3-319-42536-8_4

punched, choked, burned, or physically attacked." With similar clarity, sexual abuse is defined as "experiencing attempts or being forced into unwanted sexual activity by being threatened, held down or hurt in some way, and/or sexually touched, meaning unwanted touching or grabbing, kissing or fondling against the respondent's will." Different research instruments also define childhood differently, usually by specifying an age ("before you were sixteen") or simply asking respondents to report experiences "when you were a child."

Within these definitions, results from various populations produce fairly consistent results. Exposure to physical and/or sexual abuse during childhood is reported by about 25–30 % of adults, a shockingly high prevalence [1–3]. The type of exposure experienced is gendered; girls are more likely than boys to experience sexual abuse, boys more likely than girls to experience physical abuse. However, both boys and girls are exposed to each type of abuse and the overall prevalence is about the same in each gender. While child abuse is common in all demographic groups, there are some factors that increase risk, including low family income, maternal youth, maternal sociopathy, presence of a stepfather, children with disability, and other negative life events. The presence of multiple risk factors increases the risk quite substantially [4].

Distinguishing between levels of severity of traumatic exposure demonstrates that even less severe exposures cause harm. For example, in the 2012 Canadian Community Health Survey: Mental Health, the strength of correlation of physical abuse with adult problems rose with the severity of abuse for some adult problems, including diagnosis of depression or generalized anxiety, or the occurrence of suicide attempts [1]. For other problems, such as alcohol or drug dependence, the risk was similar for each category of abuse. In each of these cases, however, even the least severe type of exposure is associated with significantly increased risk compared to no exposure. The implication is that severity of exposure matters, but that there is no degree of exposure to abuse that is not potentially harmful.

The second category of childhood trauma is broader. Taking our cue from Vincent Felitti and colleagues [2], we refer to this category as "childhood adversity" in order to distinguish it from narrower studies of physical and sexual abuse. In addition to physical and sexual abuse, childhood adversity includes exposure to emotional or psychological abuse, various forms of neglect, family dysfunction as a result of members with mental illness, addictions or criminal behavior, exposure to violence, and parental separation. Studying these more diverse types of adverse experience, especially studying them all at the same time, is valuable because it allows a window into the potentially potent additive (or interactive) effects of multiple types of exposure [5].

The prevalence of childhood adversity depends, of course, on which types of adverse experience are included in a particular measure. One of the more prominent measures is the Adverse Childhood Experience (ACE) survey developed by the ACE Study [2]. This questionnaire probes ten types of childhood adversity and yields an ACE score (0–10), consisting of one point for each type of adversity that is reported. In the original report from the ACE Study, a population of over 8000 attendees of the Appraisal Clinic of a San Diego HMO, approximately half of the population was reported to be exposed to at least one of these broader categories of adversity. More precisely, the prevalence of exposure was: 0 ACEs 50 %, 1 ACE 25 %, 2 ACEs 13 %, 3 ACEs 7 %, 4 or more ACEs 6 % [2]. Similar prevalence has since been confirmed in other samples, including 48,526 adults from the Center for Disease Control's Behavioral Risk Factor Surveillance System survey of five US states [6].

4.1.2 Trauma and Obesity

The ACE Study found that adult obesity, as defined as a body mass index (BMI) ≥30, was more common among people who reported childhood verbal, physical, and sexual abuse [7]. The prevalence of severe obesity (BMI ≥35) by ACE score was: 0 ACE 5.4 %, 1 ACE 7.0 %, 2 ACE 9.5 %, 3 ACE 10.3 %, 4 or more ACE 12 % [2].

The "dose–response" gradient illustrated by these statistics is significant. This graded risk is important because a dose–response suggests that exposure to ACE makes incremental contributions to obesity with every step, not just in cases of extreme exposure. Since about half of adults are exposed to ACE, it is a risk factor for obesity that potentially has a wide impact. From a public health perspective, even relatively small increments of added risk to what is recognized as a growing epidemic of obesity may have very substantial overall costs, because the risk affects so many people.

Other studies have provided similar and complementary evidence. A consistent finding is that multiple exposures add increased risk. For example, in the National Longitudinal Study of Adolescent Health, severe obesity (defined as above the 95th percentile) was especially prevalent in adolescents who were exposed to both physical and sexual abuse [8], and the rate of growth of BMI from childhood to adolescence was most pronounced in adolescents who had experienced both physical abuse and neglect [9]. In addition, more severe exposure may have a stronger effect. In the 2007 Adult Psychiatric Morbidity Survey ($N=3486$), women who had experienced childhood sexual abuse involving intercourse were twice as likely to be obese as women with no childhood sexual abuse [10]. On average, those experiencing both sexual and physical abuse in childhood were over 11 kg heavier than those who experienced neither type of abuse [11].

Importantly, there are inconsistencies in the results of different studies. For one, the several studies cited here indicate that the relationship between childhood adversity is most relevant in people exposed to severe adversity or in people with severe obesity could stand in contrast to the graded "dose–response" relationship found in the ACE study. For another, studies differ in their findings about the age at which obesity becomes apparent in maltreated children [12, 13]. These inconsistencies may indicate heterogeneity in different populations. Furthermore, as we will discuss below, processes that differ between individuals may mediate the link between early adversity and obesity. As one example, binge eating disorder is more strongly related to early adversity than some other causes of obesity. Perhaps because of such heterogeneity between different populations, meta-analyses of studies of child sexual abuse (the most widely studied of the childhood adversities that may be related to obesity) have reached differing conclusions about the overall relationship between child abuse and obesity [14, 15].

4.1.3 Insecure Attachment

A lens on interpersonal dynamics that includes subtler influences than whether or not trauma occurs is also valuable. Attachment theory has provided a robust scientific basis from which to understand the role of close interpersonal relationships in health and healthcare [16]. Attachment theory describes how close bonds between infants and parents develop in a way that allows a parent's proximity and responsiveness to infant signals of distress to regulate the child's sense of safety and security [17]. Individual differences in attachment behavior emerge from these interactions that manifest as stable preferences for expression vs. suppression of separation protest, or a greater or lesser tendency towards seeking proximity. In particular, "non-validating" early environments [18] and low parental responsiveness to infant cues [19] often result in insecure patterns of attachment.

Attachment bonds are also found in adulthood, usually between committed romantic partners [20]. These patterns of attachment are relatively stable, representing preferred positions in the balance between expression vs. suppression of affect and dependency vs. distancing in intimate relationships. Often, adult attachment patterns are measured on two dimensions of insecure attachment: attachment anxiety and attachment avoidance. Attachment anxiety measures the degree to which a person seeks emotional closeness, fears rejection, and feels uncomfortable or unhappy when alone. People with high attachment anxiety may lack assertiveness and be willing to accommodate to others' wishes in order to achieve acceptance. They typically also seek reassurance and support energetically. Attachment avoidance measures the degree to which a person seeks autonomy, avoids vulnerability, suppresses expressions of distress, and mistrusts others. People with high attachment avoidance may minimize personal problems and avoid situations in which they may have to cede autonomy or depend on others.

These dimensions are not mutually exclusive. The uncomfortable co-occurrence of the opposing forces of attachment anxiety and attachment avoidance is often called fearful attachment [21]. At the other end of the spectrum, a person who has relatively little attachment anxiety and attachment avoidance has the flexibility to balance expression and suppression, intimacy and autonomy as suits the circumstances. This comfortable and well-balanced pattern of attachment is called secure attachment.

Patterns of attachment influence health and healthcare in a number of ways. There is consistent evidence that patterns of attachment affect the reporting of symptoms and rates of healthcare utilization. This occurs in opposing directions with attachment anxiety being linked to experiencing more symptoms and seeing healthcare providers more often, while attachment avoidance is associated with reporting fewer symptoms and receiving less healthcare [22]. Patterns of attachment also influence communication, which may be a reason that clinicians are more likely to find patients with higher attachment insecurity to be "difficult" [23, 24].

Importantly, patterns of attachment are related to physiological processes. In particular, there are various lines of evidence that indicate that insecure patterns of attachment are linked to difficulties with the regulation of stress in both the hypothalamic–pituitary–adrenal system and the autonomic nervous system [25–27].

4.1.4 Attachment and Obesity

Attachment insecurity is associated with both biological and psychological processes that could promote unhealthy eating and obesity, and thus several studies have examined the correlation. Fearful attachment, in particular, is associated with higher BMI and with higher waist–hip ratio [28]. This association is stronger when obesity is more severe. For example, in Thao Lan Le's study of 351 primary care patients at Mount Sinai Hospital in Toronto, the prevalence of fearful attachment (defined as being in the top third of both attachment anxiety and attachment avoidance) was 25 % in people with BMI >25, 37 % in people with BMI >30, and 58 % in people with BMI >35 (T. L. Le, personal communication).[1] These correlational studies support the possibility of a relationship between attachment insecurity and obesity, but of course correlations do not prove causality. It is important therefore that there is also data from prospective studies of early development to provide greater depth to the correlations.

In developmental studies, a child's BMI is predicted by both maternal BMI and the quality of the mother–infant attachment bond. In one longitudinal study that began during a mother's pregnancy and continued through the first 3 years of the baby's development, it was found that both mothers' emotional dysregulation and mother's prepregnancy BMI predicted the child's BMI at age 3 years [30]. Similarly, a study of 31 obese and 31 normal weight mothers with children aged 19–58 months found that obese mother–infant dyads had a lower quality of mother–child attachment than normal weight mother–infant dyads. In this study, mother–child attachment contributed to the prediction of the child's BMI above and beyond the predictive power of the child's BMI at birth and the BMI of the child's parents [31]. Furthermore, in a prospective

[1] Since fearful attachment among these primary care patients increased with ACE exposure, from 11 % in those with no exposure to ACE to 46 % in those exposed to four or more ACE categories ($p<0.001$), it is reasonable to wonder if insecure attachment could serve as a mediator between childhood adversity and subsequent obesity. Indeed, in this sample, we used PROCESS [29] to test the indirect effect of exposure to ACE on BMI, through insecure attachment and found a significant indirect effect through attachment avoidance (95 % confidence interval 0.13–0.75), and a nonsignificant effect through attachment anxiety (95 % confidence interval –0.25–0.21).

developmental study, low maternal sensitivity at 6 months of age (an important contributor to subsequent insecure attachment) predicted girls' (but not boys') BMI 2 years of age [32].

A qualitative study of attachment in the lives of obese adolescent girls gives some indication of the attachment processes that may be at work as children get older. Girls, who were 13–16 years of age, were interviewed using the Childhood Attachment Interview and reported family conflicts in which they adopted the role of caring for others and took a self-reliant stance which minimized acknowledgement of personal emotional needs or vulnerability [33]. These themes suggest the attachment pattern that Bowlby called compulsive caregiving [34]. Compulsive caregiving is a variant of dismissing attachment (high attachment avoidance plus low attachment anxiety [21]) in which emotional vulnerability is suppressed or masked by persistently assuming the role of the one who cares for others. All of these study participants described eating for comfort and using food to manage emotions such as boredom, loneliness, and depression.

4.2 Causal Mechanisms and the Roots of Obesity

How do we move from the evidence that obesity is associated with both childhood adversity and insecure attachment to evaluate if these early experiences contribute to the *causes* of obesity? One strategy is to examine potential mechanisms. The hypothesis that there is a causal link from interpersonal factors to obesity will be more convincing if there are plausible psychological and biological pathways by which this could occur.

It is a complex question. We eat because our bodies need fuel and provide biological signals of hunger and satiation in order to maintain the necessary intake of calories. Beyond that, of course, we eat for pleasure and comfort, to explore new tastes and bond with friends, to reward ourselves, and to pass the time. The causes of obesity, similarly, are many and interact in complex ways. We highlight here some contributors to obesity that may be linked to trauma and insecure attachment.

4.2.1 Patterns of Eating

The overlapping constructs of *disinhibited eating*, *emotional eating*, and *food addiction* all describe patterns of food consumption in which eating is a response to signals other than hunger and the pleasure of consumption. In each of these constructs, periodic over-eating is linked to obesity. Emotional eating refers to eating in response to negative emotions and is often considered a strategy to reduce those emotions, to feel better. Disinhibited eating is a broader construct. It includes emotional eating but also refers to difficulty resisting the urge to eat, either from within or from others. Food addiction is a more biological construct, based on neurological pathways for wanting (dopaminergic paths) and liking (opiate paths) that are shared between the rewarding properties of high fat and high sugar foods and various addictive substances. While the construct is biological, measures of food addiction draw on behaviors and attitudes that overlap disinhibited eating (e.g., "I find that when I start eating certain foods, I end up eating much more than I had planned" in the Yale Food Addiction Scale) [35]. For our purposes, distinctions between these constructs are less important than what they have in common. In a study of obese children and teenagers, the prevalence of "loss of control over eating" was found to be about 40 % in people who sought treatment for their weight and about 20 % in those that did not [36].

From the perspective of attachment insecurity, emotional eating is expected to function as an external regulator of affect [37]. External regulators of affect (including the use of various substances) are valued when internalized strategies for self-soothing are not well developed and interpersonal sources of solace and support are unavailable or ineffective. In addition to making it difficult to tolerate distress, insecure attachment often co-occurs with difficulty delaying gratification, a need to seek acceptance, and a lack of assertiveness [16], which may all contribute to disinhibited eating. This hypothesis has not received very much direct study as it applies to emotional eating, although the links between attachment insecurity and other external regulators of affect have been confirmed [38, 39].

Furthermore, in bariatric surgery patients, it has been found that emotion regulation serves as a mediator between insecure attachment and emotional eating [40], which is consistent with the attachment hypothesis. Insecure attachment is also linked to other aspects of unhealthy eating, for instance predicting high caloric food intake in both children and adults [41].

With respect to early life trauma, a study of 1650 adults from the National Survey of Midlife in the U.S. found that greater use of food in response to stress mediated between the early life experiences of combined, frequent psychological and physical violence from parents and adult obesity [42]. On the other hand, a population study of 4641 women in a large US health plan found that although binge eating was related to both early life sexual and physical abuse and to obesity, binge eating did not statistically mediate the relationship between abuse and obesity [43].

4.2.2 Body Image

Early adversity is associated with subsequent body dissatisfaction [44, 45]. Children and adults with insecure styles are also more concerned about body shape, more dissatisfied with their own bodies, and more interested in cosmetic surgery than those with secure attachment [46–48]. The need for approval that is inherent in attachment anxiety is, thus, one force that may increase vulnerability to social norms and influence body dissatisfaction. As a result, insecurity leads some people to feel that being loved and approved of depends on looking differently than they do. A person with high attachment anxiety can find herself in the conflicted position of being dissatisfied with how she looks, on one hand, and yet eating excessively in response to distressing feelings, on the other. This may create a vicious circle of negative emotions and negative self-image.

4.2.3 Psychopathology

Several mental illnesses are associated with obesity, including depression [49] and schizophrenia [50]. The causal forces behind these correlations may go in different directions. For example, in schizophrenia, obesity is likely to be a result of the drugs used to treat the disease [51]. On the other hand, since the risk of adult depression is higher in those who have been exposed to childhood adversity [1] and who have an insecure pattern of attachment [52, 53], depression may be a link between early life factors and adult overweight in some cases. This, however, is a mediating relationship in search of a mechanism. The relationship is only explanatory to the extent that the effects of depression can be further explicated through it impact on food consumption [54], caloric output [55], or metabolism [56]. It is also noteworthy that posttraumatic stress disorder is associated with "food addiction" in women, although it is not clear if the risk of obesity is related to posttraumatic stress disorder per se, or to some other consequence of trauma [57]. It is noteworthy that a prospective study of court-documented child physical abuse found that abuse was associated with adult depression, generalized anxiety disorder and anxiety posttraumatic stress disorder, and that among these consequences of trauma it was generalized anxiety disorder that served as a mediator with BMI—but as a suppressor; anxiety was associated with lower BMI [58].

Among mental illnesses, eating disorders are especially relevant to obesity. A history of childhood adversity and/or insecure attachment is common in eating disorders in general [59] and in binge eating [60] and binge eating disorder [61] in particular and is linked to affect dysregulation [62, 63]. The importance of attachment insecurity in this group is given further credence by the positive impact of group-based treatment for binge eating disorder on patterns of attachment [64].

4.2.4 Biological Mechanisms

Although the psychological consequences of early life adversity are clearly important to the subsequent risk of obesity, they do not entirely explain the link between early experience and obesity [65]. The biological mechanisms that may mediate between early adversity and/or insecure attachment and obesity, however, are far from well understood. While it would go beyond the scope of this chapter to explore potential biological mechanisms in depth, it is worth highlighting some intriguing results.

First, dysregulation in the hypothalamic–pituitary–adrenal (HPA) axis is implicated as a cause of obesity, although the hypothesized directions of dysregulation are complex and the evidence is inconclusive [66]. Indeed, both under-reactivity and over-reactivity of the HPA are associated with health risks. On one hand, over-reactivity of the HPA to stress, which results in chronically (or frequently) high levels of serum cortisol, is associated with central obesity and metabolic syndrome [66, 67]. On the other hand, low cortisol or under-reactive cortisol responses to stress are associated with early life adversity and may also promote obesity [66, 68, 69].

Second, there is evidence that early life adversity is subsequently associated with abnormal levels of leptin ("the satiety hormone") [70, 71]. Similarly, interpersonal stressors and loneliness may be related to levels of leptin and ghrelin ("the hunger hormone"), although this has only been found in nonobese women [72, 73]. These findings suggest one possible path by which interpersonal processes may result in physiological changes that promote weight gain.

Finally, there is very interesting evidence from a longitudinal, developmental study of differential susceptibility to obesogenic patterns of eating based on an interaction between a susceptibility gene (the hypoactive 7-repeat allele of the DRD4 gene) *plus* early life adversity [74]. Studies such as this may allow us to disentangle the individual differences in susceptibility that otherwise lead to inconsistent results when all subjects are assumed to be similar.

4.3 How a Relational View of Obesity Can Shape Assessment and Care in Bariatric Surgery

People who seek and then receive bariatric surgery are involved in a complex, long-term program of assessment, treatment, and follow-up that involves multiple professionals interacting on a team. At each step, insecure patterns of attachment and previous experiences of trauma may challenge effective engagement in the treatment program. This can occur in many ways, from the impact of trauma on trust or fear of invasive procedures to the impact of insecure attachment on treatment adherence, perceived difficulty in treatment relationships, and patient–provider communication [23, 75–78].

Psychiatrists are often routinely involved in the assessment and sometimes the ongoing management of bariatric surgery patients. Psychopathology is common among candidates seeking bariatric surgery, with up to 40 % experiencing a current psychiatric syndrome [79] and about one third having a lifetime history of substance use disorder. Adopting a relational approach to care, however, extends the psychological context of bariatric surgery substantially beyond the identification and treatment of psychiatric disorders.

Beyond assessing diagnoses, a relational lens on assessment helps to identify and respond to the impact of insecure attachment. Attachment anxiety may interfere with assessment because it leads a person to emphasize emotion over facts, to be unassertive or indecisive, and to require more reassurance than is the norm. The result of these forces is that a healthcare provider finds him- or herself in an exchange that is centered on providing interpersonal support or comfort that goes beyond (and may interfere with) the instrumental tasks of assessing, for example, surgical risks. On the other hand, attachment avoidance may complicate assessment because it leads a person to truncate his or her narrative and to provide self-descriptions in terms of clichés and social norms rather than clear expressions of his or her own experience and attitudes [80, 81]. So, attachment anxiety leads to conversations that are interpersonally intense and convey a great deal of extraneous information, whereas attachment avoidance leads to conversations that are interpersonally disengaged and convey too little information. In either case, assessment and care becomes complicated by the inherent communication biases created by attachment states. One study of bariatric surgery patients has confirmed that their assessment was influenced by their attachment style [82].

After bariatric surgery, maintenance of weight loss requires adherence to a diet regimen and benefits from ongoing contact with the bariatric surgery team. At this stage as well, a relational approach responds to barriers to success that go beyond psychiatric syndromes. Both a history of childhood adversity [83] and insecure attachment predict poor outcomes and, therefore, suggest an additional need for support and adaptions in care. In particular, attachment insecurity is a risk factor for poor adherence, which leads to poor weight loss results [84]. Beyond weight loss, insecure attachment is also associated with reduced quality of life after bariatric surgery [85].

4.3.1 A Relational Approach to Care in Bariatric Surgery

Sockalingam and Hawa have described their success in incorporating an attachment focus into an integrated multidisciplinary approach to bariatric surgery at the Toronto Western Hospital Bariatric Surgery Program (TWH-BSP) [86]. We summarize key components of their approach here, starting from comprehensive assessment [87] and continuing through postsurgical follow-up.

A key aspect of assessment at the TWH-BSP is the use of standardized measures to identify areas of vulnerability. Among other self-report instruments, they use a self-report measure of attachment insecurity that has been validated in a medical population, the ECR-M16 [88], to assess attachment anxiety and attachment avoidance. Treatment team members of all disciplines have received education that allows them to appreciate what these measures reveal and to use common language and common principles in responding to interpersonal vulnerability. This is reinforced at weekly team meetings when patients' attachment styles are discussed amongst all of the other relevant aspects of their care.

Measurement and a shared set of principles allow team members to tailor a menu of treatment and support options to patients' individual needs. Patients who are challenging to engage with are understood in terms of their particular relational patterns. For example, a patient may be high in attachment avoidance and have difficulty establishing a treatment alliance with most team members, but be able to form a stronger alliance with a particular member of the team. In such an instance, the "well-matched" staff member may serve as the patient's primary contact for longitudinal care to take advantage of the trust that the patient has established. Allowing the patient to effectively "choose" the treatment team in this way is an accommodation to an avoidant patient's need to maintain control and autonomy and promotes both a greater sense of security for the patient and better treatment. Patients with high attachment avoidance are also offered telephone or online CBT if they wish it. These modalities allow the patient to receive psychological treatment on their own schedule and without the experience of clinicians becoming "too close for comfort." Furthermore, dietitians provide these patients with e-mail access to facilitate the patient's control over communication during the postoperative phase.

Patients with high attachment anxiety also receive tailored care, often involving more frequent appointments. Regularly scheduled contact can help reduce frequent e-mails or calling which are manifestations of the anxiously attached patient's fear of managing alone. Attention to continuity of contact with core team members is also important, especially the contact with a familiar dietician for patients with high attachment anxiety who experience loss of control over eating and have trouble following the postsurgical diet regimen. The dieticians of the TWH-BSP are trained in cognitive-behavior therapy techniques and use these skills to help patients examine patterns of emotional eating. When this is not enough, a psychologist or psychiatrist is available.

When the expertise of another team member is required, patients with insecure attachment often benefit from a "warm handoff" in which the familiar team members walks them over to the new team member and provides an introduction. This helps to minimize the predictable feelings of insecurity that are triggered by relationship change.

Finally, the importance of relationship styles to bariatric care has been incorporated into a biweekly bariatric surgery support group at the TWH-BSP. Healthcare professionals facilitate not only to provide information, but also to foster interpersonal learning. Attachment theory is taught to patients as relevant for understanding how people relate to one another and is sometimes used to provide insights into how group members' attachment styles affect their efforts to lose weight.

4.4 Conclusion

For many people, developmental and relational processes play a substantial role in gaining weight. In living with obesity and in its treatment with bariatric surgery, the vulnerabilities that are set in motion by early life adversity and by the interpersonal conditions that produce insecure attachment can influence outcomes negatively. Fortunately, taking a relational perspective on the planning and follow-up of bariatric surgery patients also opens new possibilities for providing effective support, improving adherence to necessary lifestyle changes and, one hopes, to improving quality of life and health after surgery.

References

1. Afifi TO, MacMillan HL, Boyle M, Taillieu T, Cheung K, Sareen J. Child abuse and mental disorders in Canada. CMAJ. 2014;186(9):E324–32. doi:10.1503/cmaj.131792.
2. Felitti VJ, Anda RF, Nordenberg D, Williamson DF, Spitz AM, Edwards V, et al. Relationship of childhood abuse and household dysfunction to many of the leading causes of deaths in adults: the adverse childhood experiences (ACE) study. Am J Prev Med. 1998;14:245–58.
3. Briere J, Elliott DM. Prevalence and psychological sequelae of self-reported childhood physical and sexual abuse in a general population sample of men and women. Child Abuse Negl. 2003;27(10):1205–22.
4. Brown J, Cohen P, Johnson JG, Salzinger S. A longitudinal analysis of risk factors for child maltreatment: findings of a 17-year prospective study of officially recorded and self-reported child abuse and neglect. Child Abuse Negl. 1998;22(11):1065–78.
5. Finkelhor D, Ormrod RK, Turner HA. Poly-victimization: a neglected component in child victimization. Child Abuse Negl. 2007;31(1):7–26.
6. Campbell JA, Walker RJ, Egede LE. Associations between adverse childhood experiences, high-risk behaviors, and morbidity in adulthood. Am J Prev Med. 2016;50(3):344–52.
7. Williamson DF, Thompson TJ, Anda RF, Dietz WH, Felitti V. Body weight and obesity in adults and self-reported abuse in childhood. Int J Obes Relat Metab Disord. 2002;26(8):1075–82.
8. Richardson AS, Dietz WH, Gordon-Larsen P. The association between childhood sexual and physical abuse with incident adult severe obesity across 13 years of the National Longitudinal Study of Adolescent Health. Pediatr Obes. 2014;9(5):351–61.
9. Shin SH, Miller DP. A longitudinal examination of childhood maltreatment and adolescent obesity: results from the National Longitudinal Study of Adolescent Health (AddHealth) Study. Child Abuse Negl. 2012;36(2):84–94.
10. Mamun AA, Lawlor DA, O'Callaghan MJ, Bor W, Williams GM, Najman JM. Does childhood sexual abuse predict young adult's BMI? A birth cohort study. Obesity (Silver Spring). 2007;15(8):2103–10.
11. McCarthy-Jones S, McCarthy-Jones R. Body mass index and anxiety/depression as mediators of the effects of child sexual and physical abuse on physical health disorders in women. Child Abuse Negl. 2014;38(12):2007–20.
12. Whitaker RC, Phillips SM, Orzol SM, Burdette HL. The association between maltreatment and obesity among preschool children. Child Abuse Negl. 2007;31(11–12):1187–99.
13. Schneiderman JU, Negriff S, Peckins M, Mennen FE, Trickett PK. Body mass index trajectory throughout adolescence: a comparison of maltreated adolescents by maltreatment type to a community sample. Pediatr Obes. 2015;10(4):296–304.
14. Irish L, Kobayashi I, Delahanty DL. Long-term physical health consequences of childhood sexual abuse: a meta-analytic review. J Pediatr Psychol. 2010; 35(5):450–61.
15. Paras ML, Murad MH, Chen LP, Goranson EN, Sattler AL, Colbenson KM, et al. Sexual abuse and lifetime diagnosis of somatic disorders: a systematic review and meta-analysis. JAMA. 2009;302(5): 550–61.
16. Maunder R, Hunter J. Love, fear, and health: how our attachments to others shape health and health care. Toronto: University of Toronto Press; 2015.
17. Bowlby J. Attachment and loss: attachment, vol. 1. New York: Basic Books; 1969.
18. Leszcz M, Pain C, Hunter J, Maunder R, Ravitz P. Achieving psychotherapy effectiveness. New York: W.W. Norton; 2014.
19. Belsky J. Precursors of attachment security. In: Cassidy J, Shaver PR, editors. Handbook of attachment: theory, research and clinical applications. 2nd ed. New York: Guilford; 2008. p. 295–316.
20. Mikulincer M, Shaver PR. Attachment in adulthood: structure, dynamics, and change. New York: Guilford; 2007.

21. Bartholomew K, Horowitz LM. Attachment styles among young adults: a test of a four-category model. J Pers Soc Psychol. 1991;61:226–44.
22. Ciechanowski P, Walker EA, Katon WJ, Russo JE. Attachment theory: a model for health care utilization and somatization. Psychosom Med. 2002;64(4): 660–7.
23. Maunder RG, Panzer A, Viljoen M, Owen J, Human S, Hunter JJ. Physicians' difficulty with emergency department patients is related to patients' attachment style. Soc Sci Med. 2006;63(2):552–62.
24. Taylor RE, Mann AH, White NJ, Goldberg DP. Attachment style in patients with unexplained physical complaints. Psychol Med. 2000;30:931–41.
25. Luecken LJ. Childhood attachment and loss experiences affect adult cardiovascular and cortisol function. Psychosom Med. 1998;60:765–72.
26. Maunder RG, Lancee WJ, Nolan RP, Hunter JJ, Tannenbaum DW. The relationship of attachment insecurity to subjective stress and autonomic function during standardized acute stress in healthy adults. J Psychosom Res. 2006;60(3):283–90.
27. Kidd T. The psychobiology of attachment and the aetiology of disease. In: Hunter J, Maunder R, editors. Improving patient treatment with attachment theory: a guide for primary care practitioners and specialists. Switzerland: Springer; 2016. p. 145–54.
28. Hintsanen M, Jokela M, Pulkki-Raback L, Viikari JSA, Keltikangas-Jarvinen L. Associations of youth and adulthood body-mass index and waist-hip ratio with attachment styles and dimensions. Curr Psychol. 2010;29(3):257–71.
29. Hayes AF. PROCESS: a versatile computational tool for observed variable mediation, moderation, and conditional process modeling [White Paper]. 2012. http://afhayes.com/public/process2012.pdf
30. de Campora G, Larciprete G, Delogu AM, Meldolesi C, Giromini L. A longitudinal study on emotional dysregulation and obesity risk: from pregnancy to 3 years of age of the baby. Appetite. 2016;96:95–101.
31. Keitel-Korndorfer A, Sierau S, Klein AM, Bergmann S, Grube M, von Klitzing K. Insatiable insecurity: maternal obesity as a risk factor for mother-child attachment and child weight. Attach Hum Dev. 2015;17(4):399–413.
32. Wendland BE, Atkinson L, Steiner M, Fleming AS, Pencharz P, Moss E, et al. Low maternal sensitivity at 6 months of age predicts higher BMI in 48 month old girls but not boys. Appetite. 2014;82:97–102.
33. Holland S, Dallos R, Olver L. An exploration of young women's experiences of living with excess weight. Clin Child Psychol Psychiatry. 2012;17(4): 538–52.
34. Bowlby J. Making and breaking of affectional bonds: 1. aetiology and psychopathology in the light of attachment theory. Br J Psychiatry. 1977;130: 201–10.
35. Gearhardt AN, Corbin WR, Brownell KD. Preliminary validation of the Yale Food Addiction Scale. Appetite. 2009;52(2):430–6.
36. Goossens L, Braet C, Van Vlierberghe L, Mels S. Loss of control over eating in overweight youngsters: the role of anxiety, depression and emotional eating. Eur Eat Disord Rev. 2009;17(1):68–78.
37. Maunder RG, Hunter JJ. Attachment and psychosomatic medicine: developmental contributions to stress and disease. Psychosom Med. 2001;63(4):556–67.
38. Bahr SJ, Hoffmann JP, Yang X. Parental and peer influences on the risk of adolescent drug use. J Prim Prev. 2005;26(6):529–51.
39. DeFronzo J, Pawlak R. Effects of social bonds and childhood experience on alcohol abuse and smoking. J Soc Psychol. 1993;133:635–42.
40. Taube-Schiff M, Van Exan J, Tanaka R, Wnuk S, Hawa R, Sockalingam S. Attachment style and emotional eating in bariatric surgery candidates: the mediating role of difficulties in emotion regulation. Eat Behav. 2015;18:36–40.
41. Faber A, Dube L. Parental attachment insecurity predicts child and adult high-caloric food consumption. J Health Psychol. 2015;20(5):511–24.
42. Greenfield EA, Marks NF. Violence from parents in childhood and obesity in adulthood: using food in response to stress as a mediator of risk. Soc Sci Med. 2009;68(5):791–8.
43. Rohde P, Ichikawa L, Simon GE, Ludman EJ, Linde JA, Jeffery RW, et al. Associations of child sexual and physical abuse with obesity and depression in middle-aged women. Child Abuse Negl. 2008;32(9): 878–87.
44. Brooke L, Mussap AJ. Brief report: maltreatment in childhood and body concerns in adulthood. J Health Psychol. 2013;18(5):620–6.
45. Vartanian LR, Smyth JM, Zawadzki MJ, Heron KE, Coleman SR. Early adversity, personal resources, body dissatisfaction, and disordered eating. Int J Eat Disord. 2014;47(6):620–9.
46. Bosmans G, Goossens L, Braet C. Attachment and weight and shape concerns in inpatient overweight youngsters. Appetite. 2009;53(3):454–6.
47. Javo IM, Sorlie T. Psychosocial predictors of an interest in cosmetic surgery among young Norwegian women: a population-based study. Plast Reconstr Surg. 2009;124(6):2142–8.
48. Mayer B, Muris P, Meesters C, Zimmermann-van BR. Brief report: direct and indirect relations of risk factors with eating behavior problems in late adolescent females. J Adolesc. 2009;32(3):741–5.
49. de Wit L, Luppino F, van Straten A, Penninx B, Zitman F, Cuijpers P. Depression and obesity: a meta-analysis of community-based studies. Psychiatry Res. 2010;178(2):230–5.
50. Marder SR, Essock SM, Miller AL, Buchanan RW, Casey DE, Davis JM, et al. Physical health monitoring of patients with schizophrenia. Am J Psychiatry. 2004;161(8):1334–49.
51. Padmavati R, McCreadie RG, Tirupati S. Low prevalence of obesity and metabolic syndrome in never-treated chronic schizophrenia. Schizophr Res. 2010;121(1–3):199–202.

52. Bifulco A, Moran PM, Ball C, Bernazzani O. Adult attachment style. I: Its relationship to clinical depression. Soc Psychiatry Psychiatr Epidemiol. 2002;37: 50–9.
53. Bifulco A, Moran PM, Ball C, Lillie A. Adult attachment style. II: Its relationship to psychosocial depressive-vulnerability. Soc Psychiatry Psychiatr Epidemiol. 2002;37:60–7.
54. Michopoulos V, Powers A, Moore C, Villarreal S, Ressler KJ, Bradley B. The mediating role of emotion dysregulation and depression on the relationship between childhood trauma exposure and emotional eating. Appetite. 2015;91:129–36.
55. Vancampfort D, Stubbs B, Sienaert P, Wyckaert S, De Hert M, Rosenbaum S, et al. What are the factors that influence physical activity participation in individuals with depression? A review of physical activity correlates from 59 studies. Psychiatr Danub. 2015;27(3): 210–24.
56. Kiecolt-Glaser JK, Habash DL, Fagundes CP, Andridge R, Peng J, Malarkey WB, et al. Daily stressors, past depression, and metabolic responses to high-fat meals: a novel path to obesity. Biol Psychiatry. 2015;77(7):653–60.
57. Mason SM, Flint AJ, Roberts AL, Agnew-Blais J, Koenen KC, Rich-Edwards JW. Posttraumatic stress disorder symptoms and food addiction in women by timing and type of trauma exposure. JAMA Psychiatry. 2014;71(11):1271–8.
58. Francis MM, Nikulina V, Widom CS. A prospective examination of the mechanisms linking childhood physical abuse to body mass index in adulthood. Child Maltreat. 2015;20(3):203–13.
59. Tasca GA, Balfour L. Attachment and eating disorders: a review of current research. Int J Eat Disord. 2014;47(7):710–7.
60. Patton CJ. Fear of abandonment and binge eating. A subliminal psychodynamic activation investigation. J Nerv Ment Dis. 1992;180(8):484–90.
61. Caslini M, Bartoli F, Crocamo C, Dakanalis A, Clerici M, Carra G. Disentangling the association between child abuse and eating disorders: a systematic review and meta-analysis. Psychosom Med. 2016;78(1): 79–90.
62. Suejong H, Carole PM. College student binge eating: insecure attachment and emotion regulation. J Coll Stud Dev. 2014;55(1):16–29.
63. Shakory S, Van Exan J, Mills JS, Sockalingam S, Keating L, Taube-Schiff M. Binge eating in bariatric surgery candidates: the role of insecure attachment and emotion regulation. Appetite. 2015;91:69–75.
64. Maxwell H, Tasca GA, Ritchie K, Balfour L, Bissada H. Change in attachment insecurity is related to improved outcomes 1-year post group therapy in women with binge eating disorder. Psychotherapy (Chic). 2014;51(1):57–65.
65. D'Argenio A, Mazzi C, Pecchioli L, Di Lorenzo G, Siracusano A, Troisi A. Early trauma and adult obesity: is psychological dysfunction the mediating mechanism? Physiol Behav. 2009;98(5):543–6.
66. Incollingo Rodriguez AC, Epel ES, White ML, Standen EC, Seckl JR, Tomiyama AJ. Hypothalamic–pituitary–adrenal axis dysregulation and cortisol activity in obesity: a systematic review. Psychoneuroendocrinology. 2015;62:301–18.
67. Anagnostis P, Athyros VG, Tziomalos K, Karagiannis A, Mikhailidis DP. Clinical review: the pathogenetic role of cortisol in the metabolic syndrome: a hypothesis. J Clin Endocrinol Metab. 2009;94(8):2692–701.
68. Lovallo WR. Early life adversity reduces stress reactivity and enhances impulsive behavior: implications for health behaviors. Int J Psychophysiol. 2013; 90(1):8–16.
69. Ehlert U. Enduring psychobiological effects of childhood adversity. Psychoneuroendocrinology. 2013;38(9):1850–7.
70. Danese A, Dove R, Belsky DW, Henchy J, Williams B, Ambler A, et al. Leptin deficiency in maltreated children. Transl Psychiatry. 2014;4:e446.
71. Joung KE, Park KH, Zaichenko L, Sahin-Efe A, Thakkar B, Brinkoetter M, et al. Early life adversity is associated with elevated levels of circulating leptin, irisin, and decreased levels of adiponectin in midlife adults. J Clin Endocrinol Metab. 2014;99(6): E1055–60.
72. Jaremka LM, Belury MA, Andridge RR, Malarkey WB, Glaser R, Christian L, et al. Interpersonal stressors predict ghrelin and leptin levels in women. Psychoneuroendocrinology. 2014;48:178–88.
73. Jaremka LM, Fagundes CP, Peng J, Belury MA, Andridge RR, Malarkey WB, et al. Loneliness predicts postprandial ghrelin and hunger in women. Horm Behav. 2015;70:57–63.
74. Silveira PP, Gaudreau H, Atkinson L, Fleming AS, Sokolowski MB, Steiner M, et al. Genetic differential susceptibility to socioeconomic status and childhood obesogenic behavior: why targeted prevention may be the best societal investment. JAMA Pediatr. 2016;170(4):359–64.
75. Ciechanowski P, Russo J, Katon W, Von Korff M, Ludman E, Lin E, et al. Influence of patient attachment style on self-care and outcomes in diabetes. Psychosom Med. 2004;66(5):720–8.
76. Ciechanowski PS, Katon WJ, Russo JE, Walker EA. The patient-provider relationship: attachment theory and adherence to treatment in diabetes. Am J Psychiatry. 2001;158(1):29–35.
77. Clark L, Beesley H, Holcombe C, Salmon P. The influence of childhood abuse and adult attachment style on clinical relationships in breast cancer care. Gen Hosp Psychiatry. 2011;33(6):579–86.
78. Salmon P, Young B. Dependence and caring in clinical communication: the relevance of attachment and other theories. Patient Educ Couns. 2009;74(3): 331–8.
79. Kalarchian MA, Marcus MD, Levine MD, Courcoulas AP, Pilkonis PA, Ringham RM, et al. Psychiatric disorders among bariatric surgery candidates: relationship to obesity and functional health status. Am J Psychiatry. 2007;164(2):328–34. quiz 74.

80. Maunder RG, Hunter JJ. Assessing patterns of adult attachment in medical patients. Gen Hosp Psychiatry. 2009;31(2):123–30.
81. Maunder RG, Hunter JJ. A prototype-based model of adult attachment for clinicians. Psychodyn Psychiatry. 2012;40(4):549–73.
82. Aarts F, Hinnen C, Gerdes VE, Acherman Y, Brandjes DP. Psychologists' evaluation of bariatric surgery candidates influenced by patients' attachment representations and symptoms of depression and anxiety. J Clin Psychol Med Settings. 2014;21(1):116–23.
83. Grilo CM, White MA, Masheb RM, Rothschild BS, Burke-Martindale CH. Relation of childhood sexual abuse and other forms of maltreatment to 12-month postoperative outcomes in extremely obese gastric bypass patients. Obes Surg. 2006;16(4):454–60.
84. Aarts F, Geenen R, Gerdes VE, van de Laar A, Brandjes DP, Hinnen C. Attachment anxiety predicts poor adherence to dietary recommendations: an indirect effect on weight change 1 year after gastric bypass surgery. Obes Surg. 2015;25(4):666–72.
85. Sockalingam S, Wnuk S, Strimas R, Hawa R, Okrainec A. The association between attachment avoidance and quality of life in bariatric surgery candidates. Obes Facts. 2011;4(6):456–60.
86. Sockalingam S, Hawa R. Attachment style in bariatric surgery: a case study. In: Hunter J, Maunder R, editors. Improving patient treatment with attachment theory: a guide for primary care practitioners and specialists. Switzerland: Springer; 2016. p. 145–54.
87. Pitzul KB, Jackson T, Crawford S, Kwong JC, Sockalingam S, Hawa R, et al. Understanding disposition after referral for bariatric surgery: when and why patients referred do not undergo surgery. Obes Surg. 2014;24(1):134–40.
88. Lo C, Walsh A, Mikulincer M, Gagliese L, Zimmermann C, Rodin G. Measuring attachment security in patients with advanced cancer: psychometric properties of a modified and brief experiences in close relationships scale. Psychooncology. 2009; 18(5):490–9.

Medical Complications Resulting from Severe Obesity

5

Patti Kastanias, Karyn Mackenzie, Sandra Robinson, and Wei Wang

Obesity impacts every aspect of life and diminishes virtually all measures of health, from the ability to engage in meaningful work and relationships to cardiorespiratory function, memory, and fertility. Obesity increases the risk of several debilitating, and potentially fatal, diseases, including diabetes, cardiovascular disease, and some cancers (see Fig. 5.1 for medical conditions associated with obesity). It has been estimated one in ten premature deaths for Canadian adults aged 20–64 is directly caused by obesity [2, 3]. However, it can be difficult to accurately estimate this number because obesity is very closely related to many other potentially fatal diseases [3, 4]. It is anticipated that mortality rates associated with obesity will continue to increase in the coming years [5].

We are still learning how and why visceral obesity, excess intra-abdominal adipose tissue accumulation typically measured by waist circumference, leads to increased morbidity and mortality. Visceral obesity is associated with a chronic, low-grade inflammatory state and the pro-inflammatory theory has been proposed as a critical step contributing to the emergence of many of the pathologic features associated with obesity. This includes insulin resistance—a key component of metabolic syndrome (see Table 5.1 for diagnostic criteria). Other components of metabolic syndrome include elevated waist circumference, hypertension, hyperglycemia, and dyslipidemia. This cluster of symptoms is associated with increased prevalence of obesity and risk for diabetes and cardiovascular disease (CVD) [7, 8]. Adipose tissue is now recognized as an endocrine organ that secretes various immunomodulatory and inflammatory markers such as adipokines, cytokines, and hormones [9–12], which are involved in the pathogenesis of many medical complications resulting from severe obesity.

This chapter will give an overview of the vast array of health conditions caused by obesity in a review of systems framework. This overview will be followed by two case studies highlighting typical patient presentations in the primary care setting with workup suggestions. The goal of this chapter will be to provide health professionals with a summary of relevant medical conditions that should be considered in the management of obesity and comorbid mental illness.

P. Kastanias, M.Sc.(A.), N.P. (✉)
K. Mackenzie, M.N., N.P. • S. Robinson, M.N., N.P.
W. Wang, M.N., N.P.
Toronto Western Hospital Bariatric Surgery Program, University Health Network, 399 Bathurst Street, Toronto, ON, Canada M5T 2S8
e-mail: patti.kastanias@uhn.ca; sandra.robinson2@unh.ca

S. Sockalingam, R. Hawa (eds.), *Psychiatric Care in Severe Obesity*,
DOI 10.1007/978-3-319-42536-8_5

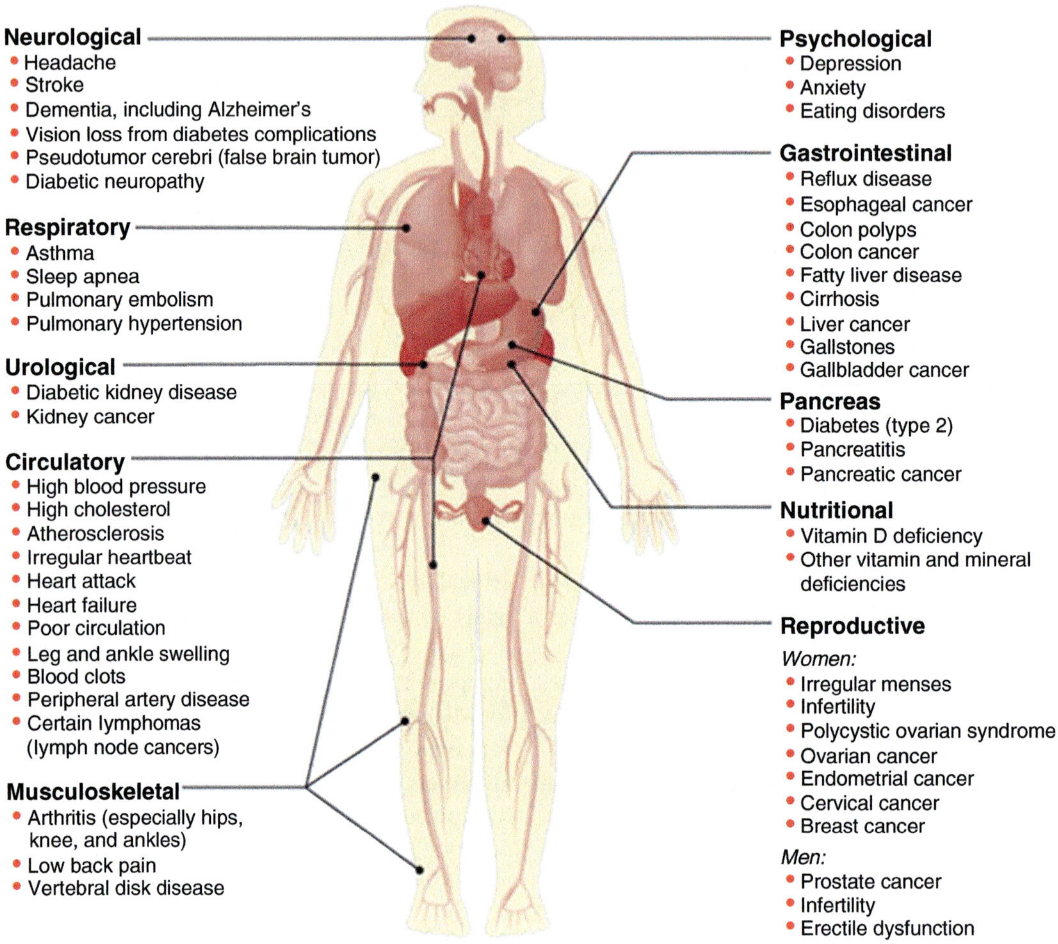

Fig. 5.1 Medical conditions associated with obesity [1]

Table 5.1 Diagnosis of metabolic syndrome

Criterion	Males	Females
Abdominal obesity		
• Canada, United States	≥40 in. (102 cm)	≥34 in. (88 cm)
• Europid, Middle Eastern, sub-Saharan African, Mediterranean	≥37 in. (94 cm)	≥31 in. (80 cm)
• Asian, Japanese, South and Central American	≥35 in. (90 cm)	≥31 in. (80 cm)
Low high-density lipoprotein (HDL)	<18.54 mg/dL (1.03 mmol/L)	<23.4 mg/dl (1.3 mmol/L)
Hypertriglyceridemia	≥30 mg/dL (1.7 mmol/L)	
High blood pressure (BP)	≥130/85 mmHg	
High fasting glucose (FPG)	≥100.8 mg/dL (5.6 mmol/L)	

A diagnosis of metabolic syndrome is made when three or more criteria are met
Adapted from CDA (2013) [6]

5.1 Endocrine

5.1.1 Type 2 Diabetes Mellitus

Type 2 diabetes mellitus (DM) is a disease commonly associated with obesity [13]. The incidence of developing type 2 DM increases with the degree of excess weight [13] with a prevalence rate as high as 49 % in patients who are obese [14]. It is a metabolic disorder primarily characterized by abnormal carbohydrate metabolism and the clinical presence of hyperglycemia. The disease may range from a relative defect in insulin secretion, insulin resistance at the cellular level, or varying degrees of both [6]. It is associated with many long-term macrovascular and microvascular complications affecting the eyes, kidneys, and nerves, as well as an increased risk for cardiovascular disease.

5.1.1.1 The Pathology of Type 2 Diabetes in Overweight/Obese People

Although research is still ongoing, there are currently three hypothesized mechanisms for the development of type 2 DM in adults: (1) increased circulation of free fatty acids (FFAs); (2) altered levels of adipocytokines; and (3) altered body fat distribution.

Persons with excess adipose tissue have an increase in circulating FFAs [15]. This chronic increase in FFAs has been linked with the onset of insulin resistance and beta cell dysfunction, leading to a defect in insulin secretion [15]. Elevated FFAs and intracellular lipids inhibit insulin signaling, leading to a reduction in insulin-stimulated muscle glucose transport [15]. In the liver, elevated FFAs may contribute to hyperglycemia by antagonizing the effects of insulin on endogenous glucose production [16].

Adipose tissue has been recognized as an endocrine organ, and produces a large number of cytokines, which include leptin, adiponectin, tumor necrosis factor-α (TNF-α), interleukin-6 (IL-6), and resistin. These cytokines serve as important factors in the pathogenesis of type 2 DM from obesity [17–20]. Leptin is predominantly involved in regulating metabolism peripherally as well as serving as a signal for satiety [21]. Research has suggested that obese individuals are insensitive to endogenous leptin production, which is thought to lead to altered metabolism and decreased satiety after meals [22, 23]. Adiponectin levels have been shown to be positively correlated with insulin sensitivity [24, 25]. However, plasma adiponectin levels are decreased in both obesity and type 2 DM, which leads to decreased insulin sensitivity [26, 27]. This is believed to be an important factor in the pathogenesis of insulin resistance. Pro-inflammatory cytokines, such as TNF-α and IL-6, are elevated in obesity and diabetes, which is also believed to contribute to insulin resistance [18, 28–30]. Resistin is also closely related to hepatic insulin resistance [31].

Increasing evidence has demonstrated that the pattern of body fat distribution plays an important role in the development of insulin resistance, glucose intolerance, and type 2 DM. Central obesity in which there is an increase in intra-abdominal fat, particularly subcutaneous and omental fat, leads to more insulin resistance and metabolic alterations than does primarily lower-body fat [32, 33]. Organ-specific deposition of fat is also related to insulin resistance. For instance, increased intramyocellular triglyceride content closely correlates with muscle insulin resistance [34] and intrahepatic fat accumulation is associated with hepatic insulin resistance [35].

5.1.1.2 Screening and Diagnosis of Type 2 diabetes

The development of type 2 DM is characterized by the progressive deterioration of glucose tolerance over a period of several years. Regular screening for type 2 DM in people with risk factors leads to earlier diagnosis, a reduction in associated complications, and overall cost savings [2]. According to the Canadian Diabetes Risk Questionnaire (CANRISK) developed by the Canadian Diabetes Association (CDA), overweight/obese (BMI >35) and increased waist circumference (men >102 cm/40 in., women >88 cm/35 in.) are the two major risk factors for the development of the disease.

The screening and diagnosis tools recommended by the CDA are fasting plasma glucose

Table 5.2 Diagnosis of type II diabetes mellitus

Test	Prediabetes	Diabetes
FPG mg/dL (mmol/L)	109–124 (6.1–6.9)	≥126 (7.0)
2 h PG after a 75 g OGTT mg/dL (mmol/L)	140–199 (7.8–11.0)	≥200 (11.1)
A1C (%)	6.0–6.4 %	≥6.5 %
Random PG mg/dL (mmol/L)		≥200 mg/dL (11.1)

Adapted from CDA (2013) [6]
In the absence of symptomatic hyperglycemia, a repeat confirmatory laboratory test (FPG, A1C, 2hPG in a 75 g OGTT) must be done on another day to confirm the diagnosis of diabetes

(FPG) and/or glycated hemoglobin (A1c). Two-hour plasma glucose (PG) after a 75 g oral glucose tolerate test (OGTT) or random PG can also aid in diagnosis. Diagnosis criteria can be found in Table 5.2.

5.1.1.3 Management of Type 2 Diabetes for Obese/Overweight Patients

A higher body mass index (BMI) in people with diabetes is associated with increased overall mortality; therefore, weight management is very crucial and is seen as the first step in disease management [6]. When choosing antihyperglycemic medications, the drug's effects on body weight should be considered. Many are associated with weight gain, while some are weight neutral or associated with weight loss [6]. Studies have shown that a weight loss of 5 kg or more can reduce the risk of developing type 2 DM by approximately 50 % [36], and more drastic weight loss may even cause remission of the disease, for instance, after bariatric surgery.

5.1.2 Thyroid Function

The relationship between obesity and thyroid disease is intertwined. Thyroid hormones regulate energy metabolism, which can affect body weight and composition. Both subclinical and overt hypothyroidism are frequently associated with weight gain [37]. Furthermore, evidence suggests that BMI has been positively associated with TSH level and negatively associated with serum free T4 (FT4) among euthyroid obese and overweight individuals [38, 39]. These alterations seem rather a consequence than a cause of obesity since weight loss leads to a normalization of elevated TSH [40, 41]. It has been hypothesized the correlation between TSH and BMI could be mediated by leptin through the following paths: (1) regulates energy homeostasis by informing the central nervous system about adipose tissue reserves [39]; (2) modulates the neuroendocrine and behavior responses to overfeeding; (3) has effects on hypothalamic–pituitary–thyroid axis [42]; and (4) affects thyroid deiodinase activities with activation of T4 to T3 conversion [43].

5.2 Cardiac

Obesity has many known undesirable effects on the cardiovascular system. Many risk factors for cardiovascular disease are also associated with obesity, such as poor diet, lack of physical activity, diabetes, hypertension, elevated waist circumference [44], and hyperlipidemia [45]. However, obesity alone, in the absence of such comorbidities, is an independent risk factor for cardiac disease [10]. Even a modest increase in body weight can lead to significant increase in cardiovascular morbidity and mortality [7]. The pro-inflammatory theory has been used to explain how obesity independently causes cardiovascular disease, i.e., cytokines secreted by adipocytes promote inflammation and atherosclerosis [12].

5.2.1 Hypertension and Hyperlipidemia

Obesity is a well-known cause of hypertension [8, 45, 46]. It is estimated that obesity accounts for 65–75 % of essential hypertension [46]. 50–60 % of obese persons have mild to moderate hypertension, while 5–10 % have severe hypertension [47]. Although the exact etiology is unknown, there are four suggestions to explain this causality: (1) a change in hemodynamics—

obese persons require a greater total blood volume in order to perfuse extra adipose tissue [8, 46]. This increase in blood volume leads to a greater cardiac output and stroke volume [8]. When combined with increased peripheral vascular resistance, this may lead to greater intravascular pressures [8], (2) physical compression of the kidneys—intra-abdominal pressure caused by excess abdominal fat physically compresses the kidneys, renal veins, and ureters which can further increase blood pressure [46]. This pressure leads to impaired renal-pressure natriuresis and increased sodium reabsorption [47]; (3) changes in the renin–angiotensin–aldosterone system (RAAS); and (4) increased sympathetic nervous system activity [46]—obesity is associated with increased plasma renin activity, angiotensinogen, angiotensin-converting enzyme activity, angiotensin II, and aldosterone [46]. This leads to vasoconstriction, sodium and fluid retention, and an increase in the sympathetic nervous system [46].

Obesity is also a well-known cause of dyslipidemia [48]. Typically obese individuals display increased triglycerides and free fatty acids, decreased high-density lipoprotein (HDL) cholesterol, with normal or slightly increased low-density lipoprotein (LDL) cholesterol [48]. Persons with a BMI over 40 are almost twice as likely to develop hyperlipidemia [49]. The decision to prescribe cholesterol lowering medication may be informed by the patient's Framingham Risk Score (FRS), which equates to their 10 year estimated risk of developing cardiovascular disease [50]. This score takes into account age, gender, total cholesterol, HDL cholesterol, smoking, diabetes, and blood pressure [50].

5.2.2 Coronary Artery Disease

Obesity and many of its comorbidities such as hypertension and dyslipidemia [51] accelerate the accumulation of intraluminal fatty plaques and therefore progression of atherosclerosis [52]. Plaques may cause stenosis, leading to angina or ischemia, or may also cause a thrombus or complete blockage leading to myocardial infarction or stroke [52]. Moreover, obese persons have increased levels of fibrinogen, factor VII, factor VIII, and plasminogen activator inhibitors, and decreased levels of antithrombin III and fibrinolytic activity [47]. This alteration in coagulation, when combined with increased abdominal pressures, venous stasis, valve incompetence, and decreased mobility, increases the risk for venous thromboembolism [8, 10] as well as dermatologic conditions in the lower extremities such as ulcers and cellulitis [10].

5.2.3 Cardiomyopathy

It is estimated that the risk for congestive heart failure increases by 5 % for men and 7 % for women for every 1 unit increase in BMI [8]. As mentioned above, obese persons have a greater total blood volume and cardiac output [45, 47]. Since the heart rate remains unchanged, this increase in cardiac output is mainly a result of an increase in stroke volume [43, 47]. The left ventricle becomes dilated and hypertrophic because it ejects more blood with each contraction [10, 45]. This leads to irreversible damage [10], impaired function, and an increased risk for cardiac failure [8, 10, 45]. To further complicate this problem, adipocytes may gradually infiltrate the cardiac myocytes and cause dysfunction and pressure-induced atrophy of cardiac muscle [8].

5.2.4 Sudden Cardiac Death

The risk for sudden cardiac death is 40 times higher in the obese population [8]. This increase in risk is most commonly as a result of coronary atherosclerosis [53] or arrhythmias related to cardiomyopathies [8, 51]. Autopsy studies indicate that up to 2/3 of sudden deaths are the result of cardiac dysfunction, 60 % of which are caused by coronary artery disease (CAD) or ischemic heart disease [53]. About 70 % of sudden cardiac deaths also show cardiomegaly, sometimes in the absence of CAD, which indicates left ventricular hypertrophy may cause sudden cardiac death related to arrhythmias [53].

5.3 Respiratory

Physiological and structural changes to the respiratory and ventilatory systems have been directly linked to the adverse effects of obesity. Lung volumes, gas exchange, and sleep are all negatively impacted by obesity [54–56]. As a result, the obese patient is at increased risk of pulmonary complications such as sleep disorders, asthma, pneumonia, pulmonary hypertension (PH), chronic obstructive lung disease (COPD), and pulmonary embolism [57].

The most consistently reported impact of obesity on the respiratory system is a decrease in lung volume, particularly the functional residual capacity (FRC) [54–56]. This is presumed to be due to an increase in adipose tissue around the chest wall, rib cage, abdomen, and visceral organs, which exert pressure on the lungs and diaphragm thereby decreasing the ability of the lungs to fully expand during inspiration. There is, however, conflicting evidence about whether the reduced compliance is as a result of decreased chest wall compliance, decreased lung compliance, or a combination of both [55, 58, 59].

To compensate for a decrease in lung volume, the work of breathing increases, with a resultant increase in the respiratory rate, carbon dioxide production, and oxygen and energy consumption [55, 59]. Although the bases of the lungs have an adequate blood supply, ventilation typically occurs in the upper areas of the lungs leaving the bases under-ventilated which leads to poor gas exchange and hypoxemia [54, 55].

5.3.1 Asthma

Asthma is a chronic airway disease characterized by airway inflammation, hypersensitivity, and reversible air flow obstruction [60]. There is growing evidence that links obesity and asthma [61]. Asthma symptoms in the obese individual can be more severe and difficult to treat as there is decreased responsiveness to traditional treatments [62]. According to Mokdad et al. [49], the risk of developing asthma for those with a BMI of 40 or greater is almost threefold. Although the exact mechanism is unknown, the following causes of asthma have been hypothesized: systemic inflammation due to increased adipose tissue; structural changes to the lungs due to decreased lung volumes; an increased genetic predisposition to the development of atopic allergies; the impact of pro-inflammatory markers such as leptin and adiponectin; and the effects of excessive macronutrients intake [61–63].

5.3.2 Pulmonary Hypertension

There is little data on the prevalence of pulmonary hypertension (PH) in obesity; however, one study showed that 38 % of patients with primary PH were obese [64]. PH is a potentially fatal condition. It results from an increase in pulmonary artery pressure which impedes blood flow to the lungs. Proposed mechanisms for the development of PH in obesity include obstructive sleep apnea (OSA), obesity hypoventilation syndrome (OHS), cardiomyopathy, pulmonary thromboembolic disease, endothelial dysfunction, hyperuricemia, and the use of appetite suppressants [65]. Patients with PH present with shortness of breath on exertion, chest pain, dizziness, and swelling of the legs [65].

5.3.3 Obstructive Sleep Apnea (Refer Chap. 12)

OSA is a sleep disorder that is characterized by episodes of breathing cessation interspersed with disordered breathing and snoring [57, 66]. Estimates are that 50 to 60 % of obese individuals have some degree of OSA [67]. A high BMI, hypertension, and male gender are several of the risk factors associated with the development of OSA (see Table 5.3 for screening criteria). Research has demonstrated that obese patients with OSA have excess fat around the soft and hard palate and tongue leading to a narrowing of the upper airway and increased airway resistance [69]. In addition to fragmented sleep, untreated OSA predisposes individuals to cardiac arrhythmias, CHF, hypertension, DM, and motor vehicle collisions [57, 70].

Table 5.3 STOP-Bang screening tool for OSA

Snoring	Do you snore loudly (louder than talking or loud enough to be heard through closed doors)?
Tired	Do you often feel tired, fatigued, or sleepy during daytime?
Observed	Has anyone observed you stop breathing during your sleep?
Blood Pressure	Do you have or are you being treated for high blood pressure?
BMI	BMI more than 35 kg/m^2?
Age	Age over 50 years old?
Neck circumference	Neck circumference greater than 40 cm?
Gender	Gender male?

High risk of OSA: answering yes to three or more items
Adapted from Chung (2008) [68]

5.3.4 Obesity Hypoventilation Syndrome (Refer Chap. 12)

OHS is characterized by a trio of features: obesity, low daytime blood oxygen levels (hypoxemia), and high serum concentration of carbon dioxide (hypercapnia) in the absence of an underlying cardiorespiratory cause [71]. The exact prevalence of OHS is unknown; however, one study estimated that OHS was present in approximately 31 % of hospitalized obese patients and the mortality rate was estimated to be 2.5 times higher at 18 months post discharge [72].

It is difficult to distinguish OHS from OSA because the clinical presentations of daytime somnolence, irritability, and mood disturbance are similar. As a result, many patients go undiagnosed until they have an episode of severe respiratory failure requiring ventilatory support in an intensive care unit setting [71]. The chronic effects of hypoxia and hypercapnia are polycythemia, PH, cardiac disturbances, and CHF, which contribute to increased mortality in this population [57].

5.4 Gastrointestinal

There is an increased risk of gastrointestinal (GI) disorders in people who are obese. Both the upper and lower GI system, including the esophagus, pancreas, liver, and colon, are affected by disorders such as gastroesophageal reflux disease (GERD), non-alcoholic fatty liver disease (NAFLD), gallbladder disease, and certain types of cancer [73]. Additionally, GI symptoms such as irritable bowel syndrome (IBS) and dyspepsia are more prevalent [74].

GERD is a spectrum of disorders that includes gastroesophageal reflux and reflux esophagitis which can lead to precancerous changes such as Barrett's esophagus or even progress to esophageal adenocarcinoma [73, 75, 76]. Severe obesity has been identified as a contributing factor to the development of GERD [73, 76]. The symptoms of heartburn and regurgitation are due to the reflux of gastric contents into the esophagus and have been attributed to mechanisms such as a high fat diet, increased intra-abdominal pressure, decreased clearance of the esophagus, a relaxed lower esophageal sphincter and alterations in the gastroesophageal junction, such as hiatus hernia [77].

Obese individuals, particularly women, are at increased risk for gallbladder disease. This is thought to be due to the increased secretion of cholesterol, excess bile production, increased gallbladder size, and impaired contractility [78].

Research has determined that there is a strong correlation between obesity and liver disease. In their 2009 study, Nguyen and El-Serag [79] found that there was a higher prevalence of NAFLD, cirrhosis, and liver cancer in obese individuals. They also found that the prevalence of NAFLD was in the range of 58–74 % in the obese individual, compared with 3–24 % in the general population.

The pro-inflammatory state related to obesity may trigger the progression of liver damage from NAFLD to non-alcoholic steatohepatitis (NASH), to steatofibrosis, to cirrhosis, possibly resulting in hepatocellular carcinoma [80].

Although research is still emerging, the secretion of several gut hormones has been found to play a key role in the regulation of food intake in keeping with the energy requirements of the body [81] (see Table 5.4 for the roles of gut hormones in obesity).

Table 5.4 Gut hormones and obesity

Gut Hormone	Role
Peptide tyrosine-tyrosine (PYY)	– Released from the L cells of the GI tract
	– Believed to play a role in satiety
	– An alteration in the release of PYY may be a factor in the development of obesity
Pancreatic polypeptide (PP)	– Released from Type F cells within the pancreatic islets
	– Stimulated by the intake of food
	– Slows the transport of food through the gut by delaying gastric emptying
	– The reduced secretion of PP after meals has been linked with obesity
Glucagon-like peptide-1 (GLP-1)	– Released from L cells of GI tract
	– Inhibits gastric acid secretion, delays gastric emptying, and stimulates the release of insulin by the pancreas
	– Released in response to food intake in quantities influenced by caloric intake
Oxyntomodulin (OXM)	– Released from L cells of GI tract
	– Functions as a satiety hormone
	– Released in response to food intake in quantities influenced by caloric intake
	– Slows the transport of food through the gut by delaying gastric emptying
Ghrelin	– Released by the gut, intestine, pancreas, pituitary, and colon
	– Hunger hormone which stimulates food intake and enhances gastric motility
	– Controls appetite, gastric motility, and body weight
	– Circulating levels of ghrelin in obese individuals remain high
Cholecystokinin (CCK)	– Released from the small intestine in response to food intake
	– Stimulates secretions from the pancreas and gallbladder, delays gastric emptying, and increases intestinal motility
Insulin	– Secreted by the islet cells of the pancreas
	– Promotes the storage of energy
	– Increased circulation in response to food intake and obesity
Leptin	– Released by adipocytes and circulates to the hypothalamus through a negative feedback loop
	– Controls appetite, gastric motility, and body weight

Adapted from Jayasena and Bloom (2008) [82] and Foxx-Orenstein (2010) [73]

5.5 Musculoskeletal Disorders

It has been known for some time that obesity increases the risk of musculoskeletal (MSK) disorders of both of bone and soft tissue. Compared with adults of normal weight, those with a BMI of 40 are more than four times more likely to develop arthritis [49]. Given both the rise in our ageing population and the expanding obesity epidemic, it is not surprising that the incidence of various types of arthritis is increasing. The mechanisms have not been completely elucidated but are thought to be multifactorial. Current research has focused on the mechanical stressors and pro-inflammatory nature of obesity as key factors [82–84]. A high BMI imposes structural and functional limitations on the musculoskeletal system resulting in increased joint loading pressures and altered biomechanics. This in turn increases the risk of soft tissue and bone injury. In addition, the systemic inflammation of obesity results in further deterioration of an already stressed musculoskeletal system. Obesity also appears to be a major contributing factor to the onset and progression of various autoimmune diseases such as rheumatoid arthritis (RA), psoriatic arthritis (PsA), and systemic lupus erythematous (SLE) [85].

Osteoarthritis (OA) is the most common type of arthritis. It is characterized by the breakdown of joint cartilage. There is a clear link between obesity and increased incidence and severity of OA. This link has been mainly studied in OA of the knee [86] but also occurs in OA of the hands, hip, and low back. A meta-analysis by Blagojevic et al. [87] demonstrated that there is an almost threefold increase in the risk of developing OA within an obese population.

RA is an autoimmune disease in which the body's immune system targets joint tissue. This creates systemic inflammation, which leads to joint erosion and pain. Adipokines released by visceral fat are thought to have a negative effect on this process by promoting inflammation. The reports of the impact of obesity on the risk of RA have been conflicting; however, the majority of studies indicate a positive association in women [88].

PsA is a type of arthritis that effects up to 30 % of people with psoriasis, an autoimmune condition that causes scaly, inflamed skin. Psoriasis usually precedes PsA. Recent evidence suggests that increased BMI in early adulthood increases the risk of PsA development in psoriatic patients [89].

SLE is a chronic, autoimmune disorder characterized by multisystem involvement which can range from relatively mild to serious life threatening complications. Several studies have found that rates of obesity are higher in SLE than in the general population. Obesity in SLE is also associated with more severe renal and cognitive involvement, increased cardiovascular risk, and reduced quality of life [85].

Gout is the most common inflammatory arthritis in men and is caused by elevated uric acid levels in blood. When uric acid crystallizes and deposits in tendons, joints, and surrounding tissues, it causes severe pain. A recent systematic review looking at the relationship between gout and obesity found a linear dose–response relationship; for every 5 unit increase in BMI, there was a 55 % increased risk of gout [90]. Interestingly, this association was independent of other risk factors such as hypertension, blood cholesterol, alcohol, diuretics, renal dysfunction, or intake of meat or seafood.

Carpal tunnel syndrome (CTS) is the most common upper extremity neuropathy. CTS is characterized by compression of the median nerve of the wrist, causing pain; numbness; and tingling of the fingers, wrist, upper and lower arms. It is a major cause of work disability [91, 92] and has been associated with obesity, diabetes, and thyroid disease [93]. Moreover, Bland [94] found that BMI is an independent risk factor in patients younger than 63 but this is a less important factor in those who were older.

5.6 Pain and Cognition

Pain is an unpleasant sensory and emotional experience associated with actual or potential tissue damage, or described in terms of such damage [95]. It is a highly subjective, multifactorial, and multidimensional experience. The prevalence of chronic pain is similar to the prevalence of obesity [96]—approximately 30 % worldwide [97], and both significantly impair function and quality of life.

Pain incidence and severity are positively correlated with increased BMI, especially in central obesity where individuals are twice as likely to have chronic pain [98–100]. The combination of obesity and pain may worsen functional status and quality of life more than each condition in isolation [96].

Unfortunately there is evidence that obesity is also associated with reduced benefits from behavioral and surgical pain treatments [101, 102]. Meta-analysis and systematic review evidence for specific pain states associated with obesity include fibromyalgia, lumbar radicular pain, sciatica [103], gout [90], general headaches and migraines, and idiopathic intracranial hypertension [104]. Interestingly, obesity appears to be only weakly linked to low back pain (LBP)—a widely prevalent cause of morbidity and occupational disability [105, 106].

The nature of the relationship between obesity and pain is complex and not fully understood. It has been theorized that inflammation may be a common pathway since obesity is a pro-inflammatory state and inflammatory mechanisms contribute to the development of pain [100, 107]. The increased mechanical stresses brought on by obesity may also be a key factor. In addition, pain causes an increase in cortisol levels through stimulation of the hypothalamic–pituitary–adrenal axis. High cortisol levels counteract insulin's action and may contribute to insulin resistance—a key pathway to metabolic syndrome. At least one study postulates that there may be a direct causal relationship between chronic pain and metabolic syndrome due to the high cortisol and catecholamine levels from inflammation and psychological stress [108]. In the elderly, however, Ray et al. [100] demonstrated that it was neither insulin resistance, inflammation, OA, nor neuropathy which showed the strongest independent association with pain, but rather central obesity.

Finally, both obesity and chronic pain are associated with mood disorders. Pain is worse among obese individuals with depression and anxiety [109–113]. Metabolic syndrome may be a unifying mechanism since it is associated with chronic pain [114], mood disorders [115], inflammation [116], and insulin resistance [117].

McVinnie [98] has proposed a useful conceptual framework that describes the complex, multifactorial, and cyclical relationship between pain and obesity (Fig. 5.2).

Interestingly, obesity may also negatively impact cognitive function, especially executive function. A recent systematic review [118] concluded that, across all ages, higher adiposity was consistently associated with gray matter atrophy in the frontal region, particularly in the prefrontal cortex. In middle and old age, higher adiposity was associated with gray matter atrophy in the parietal and temporal regions. In a related finding, adiposity has been linked to worse cognitive performance and higher risk for Alzheimer's disease [119] and vascular dementia [120].

5.7 Renal

Epidemiological evidence shows that obesity increases the risk for acute and chronic kidney disease (CKD) in the general population by 40 %, with a stronger association in women [121]. The link between obesity and CKD may be through comorbid conditions such as diabetes, hypertension, and dyslipidemia. However, in obese persons, CKD can occur in the absence of these risk factors [122–125]. There is a linear association between BMI and the progression of CKD to end stage renal disease [126].

Our current understanding of the mechanisms of obesity-induced renal damage is limited. Some proposed hypotheses are: (1) insulin resistance, which induces systemic and intraglomerular hypertension, leading to microalbuminuria and proteinuria [122, 127]; (2) increased serum leptin levels which stimulate cellular proliferation, leading to glomerulosclerosis [122, 127]; and (3) the pro-inflammatory state [122, 127].

5.8 Reproductive System

Obesity, specifically abdominal obesity, can lead to reproductive system disorders in both men and women, such as infertility and abnormal hormone levels. Obese men are more susceptible to a condition known as hyperestrogenic hypogonadotropic hypogonadism, characterized by reduced testosterone and adrenal androgens, and increased estrogen levels [128–130]. The decrease in free testosterone level in obese men is in proportional to their degree of obesity [131]. These hormonal changes lead to decreased sperm count and erectile dysfunction, which results in a marked impairment in reproductive function, sexual life, and fertility [132, 133].

The cause of hypogonadism is multifactorial. The primary attributable factor is an increase in circulating estrogens [130, 131]. Excess fatty tissue leads to an increase in available aromatase enzyme, and thus a higher conversion of androgens to estrogens [134]. The decrease in total testosterone is thought to be related to: (1) a reduction in the level of sex hormone binding globulin (SHBG); (2) an increase in estrogen levels without a compensatory increase in follicle stimulating hormone (FSH) [128]; and (3) insulin resistance [135].

The relationship between the female reproductive system and body weight is more complicated due to its cyclic nature. Increased reproductive risks associated with excess body weight include early onset of menstruation, menstrual irregularities, polycystic ovary syndrome (PCOS), subfertility, miscarriage, and adverse pregnancy outcomes [136].

The onset of menarche may occur at a younger age in obese girls. According to Frisch [137], menstruation begins when the body weight or fat

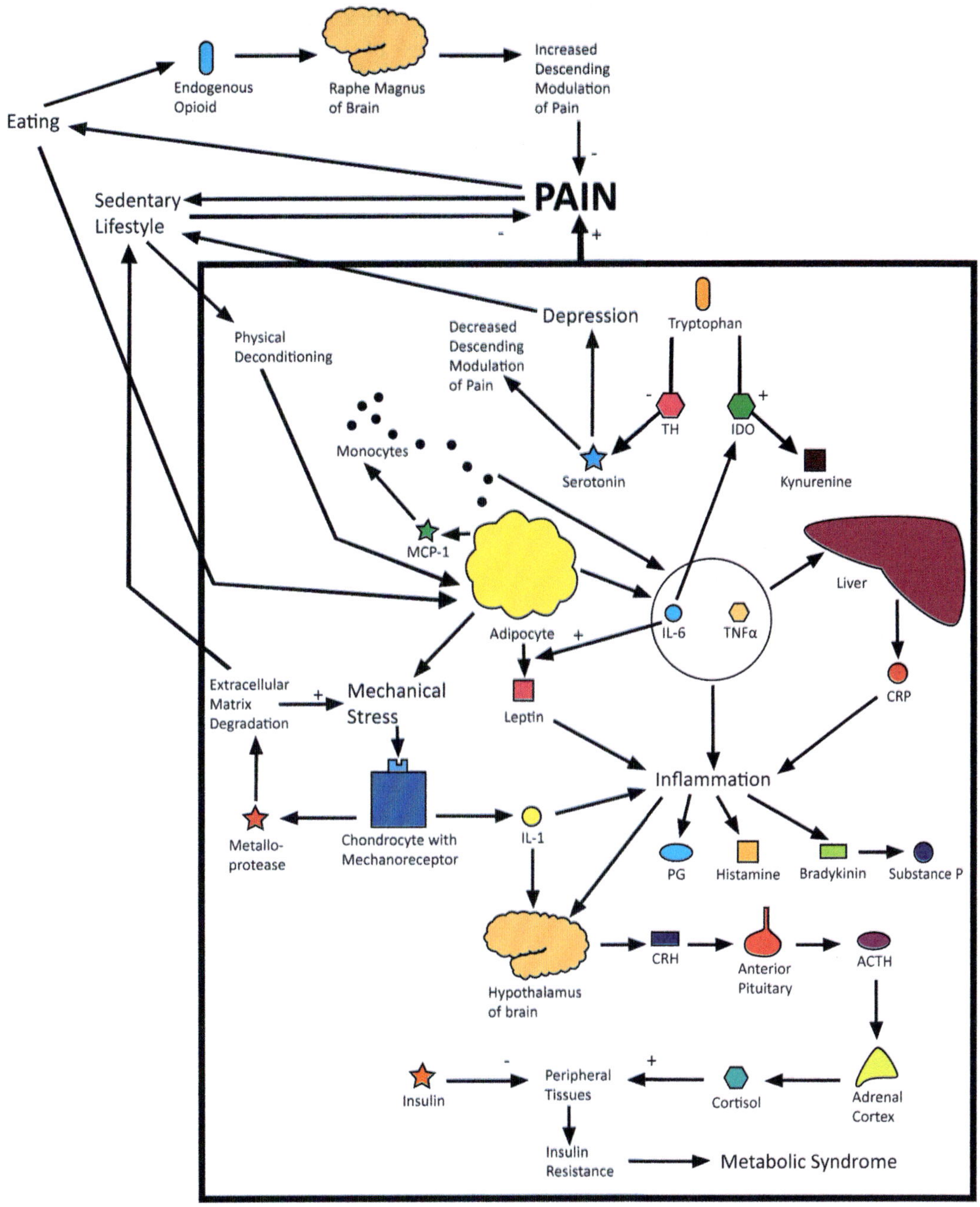

Fig. 5.2 Model of obesity and pain. Courtesy of McVinnie DS. Obesity and pain

percentage reaches a certain range (48 kg or 22 % of fat). Since obese girls enter this critical weight range at a younger age, menses usually occurs about a year earlier [137].

Obesity-related menstrual irregularities are often due to anovulation [136]. This may be related to abnormal adipokines in obese woman, which have effect on hypothalamic–pituitary signaling [138]. Metabolic abnormalities induced by excess weight, like insulin resistance, may promote the development of PCOS, a clinical condition characterized by overweight, hirsutism, oligomenorrhea, multiple cysts in the ovaries, and infertility [139]. The prevalence of overweight and obesity in women with PCOS may be as high as 80 % [139].

Reproductive disturbances are more common in obese women regardless of the diagnosis of PCOS. Anovulation contributes to subfertility in this population; however, even in obese women with regular cycles, time to pregnancy is increased [140]. An increased risk of miscarriage among obese women is also reported [141].

Evidence shows a link between alterations in adipokines and abnormal reproductive function [138]. For example, elevated FFA levels are associated with impaired oocyte maturation and decreased chances of pregnancy [142]. Leptin may affect reproductive function at the level of the hypothalamus [138]. Low adiponectin levels in obesity negatively impact implantation and embryonic development [143]. Additionally, obesity poses an increased antenatal risk for preeclampsia, gestational diabetes, fetal growth and congenital abnormalities, stillbiirth, and the need for cesarean section [144].

5.9 Cancer

It has been estimated that 14 % of all cancer deaths in men and 20 % of all cancer deaths in women are caused by overweight and obesity [145]. Obese individuals have a 1.5–3.5-fold increased risk of developing cancer (see Table 5.5 for types of cancers related to obesity).

The etiology for increased cancer risk in obesity is unclear and may vary depending on cancer type and site. For example, increased postmenopausal breast cancer may be related to increased circulating estradiol levels, while increased esophageal cancer may be due to acid reflux caused by obesity [147]. Some other hypothesized mechanisms are: (1) excessive intake of potentially carcinogenic foods [148]; (2) decreased energy output (i.e., loss of the protective effects of physical activity) [149]; (3) chronic hyperinsulinemia and production of insulin-like growth factors (IGFs) promote cell proliferation [150]; (4) increased bioavailability of steroid hormones promotes hormone-dependent cancers such as endometrial, breast, uterine, ovarian, and prostate [151, 152]; and (5) adipose tissue-derived hormones and cytokines (adipokines) may encourage tumorigenesis [153].

5.10 Anemia

There is a strong link between iron deficiency, a condition in which there is inadequate levels of iron necessary to maintain normal bodily functions, and a high BMI [154]. The health impact of iron deficiency includes fatigue, decreased brain function, a weakened immune system, decreased physical endurance, and impaired

Table 5.5 Risk of cancer in obesity

	Male	Female
Strong evidence to increased cancer risk related to overweight/obesity	Colorectal cancer	Colorectal cancer
	Esophageal adenocarcinoma	Endometrial Cancer
	Kidney cancer	Oesophageal adenocarcinoma
	Pancreatic cancer	Kidney cancer
	Thyroid cancer	Pancreatic cancer
		Postmenopausal breast cancer
Weaker evidence of increased cancer risk related to overweight/obesity	Leukemia	Leukemia
	Malignant melanoma	Thyroid cancer
	Multiple myeloma	
	Non-Hodgkin's Lymphoma	

Adapted from Basen-Engquist and Chang (2011) [146]

insulin sensitivity [155]. A meta-analysis found high hemoglobin and ferritin levels but low serum iron and transferrin saturation in obese individuals [156]. A combination of factors is felt to contribute to iron deficiency in obesity: chronic inflammation, decreased dietary iron intake and absorption, and increased adipose tissue [154]. Additionally, the hormone hepcidin which regulates iron homeostasis in a negative feedback loop has been found to be elevated in individuals with obesity [154, 156]. Treatment of iron deficiency in this population presents a challenge as oral supplementation is often ineffective, due to decreased absorption in the gut and as a result parenteral administration is often necessary [154].

Anemia of chronic disease (ACD) differs from iron deficiency in that ACD is thought to be the body's defensive response to invading bacteria [157]. Although there are adequate iron stores, the mobilization of iron from dietary intake and from the stores is impaired [157]. Ausk & Ioannou [158] hypothesized that the association between anemia of chronic disease is due to the existence of obesity-related chronic inflammation which can lead to high serum ferritin levels, low serum iron, and low transferrin saturation in response to infection or inflammation.

5.11 Integumentary

Due to the seriousness of other obesity-related health problems, the effects on the integumentary system are often minimized. The higher incidence of diabetes [159, 160], peripheral edema, venous stasis [10, 161], malnutrition [162], and inflammation [163] contributes to poor wound healing, ulcers, cellulitis, and general infections in this population [10, 160]. This is not only true of the lower extremities, but also in between skin folds, which can be a source for lesions, rashes, and bacterial or fungal infections due to excess moisture and friction [162, 164]. Other common integumentary conditions in obesity include: lymphedema [159, 160], acrochordons (skin tags) [161, 164], keratosis pilaris [161], hyperandrogenism [160], plantar hyperkeratosis [160, 161], xerosis (dry skin) [160], and atopic dermatitis (eczema) [160].

Case Vignettes

The case of Mr. W

Mr. W is a 42-year-old male with a BMI of 52 who presents to his family doctor with worsening GERD symptoms and chest discomfort. He states that he feels a pressure and a burning sensation mid-sternum, especially after a meal but sometimes occurs randomly. This occurs approximately 2 days per week. He takes over the counter antacids when he experiences the burning sensation but it doesn't really seem to help. He is concerned for his heart health as his father died of a myocardial infarction at age 48.

You look into his file and see that he has not had a formal history and physical for 2 years. He has a history of hypertension, erectile dysfunction, impaired fasting glucose, chronic back and knee pain. You notice you have treated him for right lower calf cellulitis twice in the past year. His paternal aunt and grandfather were diagnosed with colon cancer in their mid-40s and he has a family history of diabetes. He does not smoke and drinks alcohol rarely.

His prescribed medications include amlodipine 5 mg once daily, hydrochlorothiazide 25 mg OD, Celebrex 200 mg BID, and over the counter antacid. He tells you he doesn't like taking his blood pressure medications, especially the one that makes him urinate frequently.

The physical exam is difficult due to his body habitus. His blood pressure on exam is 153/94; however, he remarks that he has missed his blood pressure medication for 2 days in a row. His heart rate is 92, oxygen saturation 95 %, and respiratory rate is 18. His waist circumference is 156 cm. He has gained approximately 25 lbs in the past 2

(continued)

(continued)

years since you last weighed him. His cardiovascular, respiratory, and abdominal exam is relatively normal. You ask him to take off his shoes and socks so that you may assess his peripheral vascular system and you see that this is very challenging for him due to his large abdominal girth. You notice that the skin of his lower legs is dry and scaly, with large callouses to bilateral feet and overgrown toes nails. His lower legs are slightly red, with dark scarring of the skin where he has had cellulitis. When you press on his tibial bone you note 2+ pitting edema to lower legs and feet, however the right side looks much more edematous than the left. When you ask him about the skin of his lower legs, he also offers to show you the itchy "rashes" that he has under his skin folds. The area under his pannus is red, inflamed, and has an odor. He mentions that his erectile dysfunction is worse.

As an initial workup you decide to order some blood work, fasting glucose level, glycated hemoglobin (A1c), CBC, lipids, creatinine, liver enzymes, testosterone level, and Vitamin D level (see Table 5.6 for routine testing in the obese population). To rule out cardiac problems you decide to order an ECG, and you consider ordering bilateral leg dopplers to rule out DVT of the lower leg.

You see him again 2 days later to take a look at the blood work, ECG, and Doppler. His fasting glucose was 10.2 mmol/L, A1c is 11.1 %, his CBC was normal, and cholesterol was abnormal with high LDL and triglyceride levels. His creatinine was normal, and his liver enzymes were slightly elevated. His ECG was abnormal with a prolonged QT interval and low QRS voltage.

With a formal diagnosis of diabetes, you discuss with him the importance of lifestyle modification in management of his blood sugar. When considering medication choices for this obese individual, you may consider medications that are weight-neutral or weight losing agents. You decide to start with Metformin 500 mg BID, increasing the dose up to 1000 mg BID, and sitagliptin 100 mg once daily. A referral is made for diabetes education and opthalmology. You order a urine ACR to screen for renal disease. You will see him again to recheck his fasting and A1c levels in 2–3 months time. You introduce glucose monitoring and confirm with him that he will be taught more in depth about this at the diabetes education center.

Based on his abnormal lipid levels he should be started on cholesterol medication and levels reevaluated in 2–3 months. Based on his high liver enzymes he should have an abdominal ultrasound to assess for fatty liver disease. You discuss with him that his urinary frequency might be a symptom of his high blood glucose. You decrease the dose of hydrochlorothiazide to 12.5 mg once daily and add ramipril 10 mg to add benefit of kidney protection in type 2 DM patients. Based on abnormal ECG and his risk factors for CAD you decide to order persantine stress test (since he is not physically able to run for the treadmill test) and refer him to cardiology. You consider starting him on ASA 81 mg/day. You also consider referral to a chiropodist to help him with foot care. You prescribe him a proton pump inhibitor to see if it helps with his GERD symptoms. You also recommend that he start taking Vitamin D 2000 IU per day. You ask him if he would like to talk about his weight. In collaboration with the patient, both you and Mr. W decide you will refer him for a medical weight loss program.

The case of Ms. H

Ms. H is a 39-year-old female who is a new client at your family health team (FHT).

(continued)

Table 5.6 Routine testing for obese population

Laboratory investigations	Frequency	Normal values	Rationale
Fasting glucose (NPO × 8 h)	Every 3 years or more frequently for those at very high risk according to CANRISK [14]	≤108 mg/dL (6.0 mmol/L)—normal	Obesity is risk factor for type 2 diabetes mellitus
OR		110–125 mg/dL (6.1–6.9 mmol/L)—impaired fasting glucose	
Glycated hemoglobin (HbA1c)		≥126 mg/dL (7.0 mmol/L)—diabetes	
		≤5.9—normal	
		6.0–6.4 %—prediabetes	
		≥6.5—diabetes [14]	
Lipid profile	May screen at any age in the presence of obesity [50]	LDL is primary target and depends on risk according to FRS	Obesity is risk factor for hyperlipidemia
	Framingham risk score (FRS)	High risk: FRS ≥20 % target is ≤77 mg/dL (2.0 mmol/L) or 50 % decrease. Start therapy regardless of LDL level	
	<5 % repeat every 3–5 years	Intermediate risk: FRS 10–19 % target is LDL ≤77 mg/dL (2.0 mmol/L). Start therapy if LDL ≥135 mg/dL (3.5 mmol/L)	
	≥5 % repeat every year [50]	Low risk: FRS <10 % target is 50 % decrease in LDL. Start therapy if LDL >193 mg/dL (5 mmol/L) or family history of hypercholesterolemia	
		Other targets:	
		Total cholesterol <201 mg/dL (5.2 mmol/L)	
		Triglycerides <66 mg/dL (1.7 mmol/L)	
		HDL ≥50 mg/dL (1.3 mmol/L) [50]	
Serum 25-hydroxy vitamin D	Levels should not be measured in the general population [165, 166]	Optimal levels are >0.075 μmol/L (75 nmol/L)	Obesity is risk factor for Vitamin D deficiency [166]. They may need larger doses to reach optimal levels [165, 166]. Low Vitamin D levels are a risk factor for bone loss and osteoporosis [165, 166]
	May screen for deficiency in obese population if deficiency is suspected, and every 3–4 months thereafter to recheck levels [165, 166]		Obese persons may require 800–2000 IU daily to achieve optimal doses [165, 166]

(continued)

Table 5.6 (continued)

Laboratory investigations	Frequency	Normal values	Rationale
Liver enzymes: ALT, AST, ALP	Annually in all ages [167]	Alanine aminotransferase (ALT): 7–40 U/L	Obesity is risk factor for progressive liver disease [167]
		Aspartate aminotransferase (AST): 5–34 U/L	ALT: both sensitive and specific for liver disease of a hepatocellular injury type [167]
		Alkaline phosphatase (ALP): 40–150 U/L	AST: less sensitive [167]
			ALT:AST ratio can suggest cause or extent of disease [167]
			ALP: elevated in all forms of liver disease [167]
Complete blood count (CBC) for serum hemoglobin (Hb) and serum ferritin as needed	Routine screening in general population not recommended [168]	Anemia, microcytosis, and hypochromia are suggestive of iron deficiency [168]	Obesity has been linked with anemia [154]
	All women should be screened for anemia between ages 15 and 25, and every 5–10 years thereafter if no risk factors [169]	Serum Ferritin (μg/L):	CBC: can suggest cause and severity of anemia, should be correlated with ferritin [168]
		<15—iron deficiency	
		15–50—probable iron deficiency	Ferritin: diagnostic test of choice, however higher levels do not exclude iron deficiency [168]
		50–100—possible iron deficiency	
		100—iron deficiency unlikely	

Thyroid stimulating hormone (TSH)	Expert panels have disagreed about TSH screening in the general population who are asymptomatic; however, weight gain may warrant screening [170]	TSH: 0.2–4.0 mU/L	Hypothyroidism can contribute to weight gain in obese population
Random urine albumin-to-creatinine ratio (ACR)	Insufficient evidence to warrant screening in asymptomatic adults, however obesity is risk factor for CKD [171]	Urine ACR (mg/mmol):	Obesity is risk factor for CKD [171]
		<2—normal	
		2–20—microalbuminuria	ACR: predicts 24 h urinary albumin excretion [14]. Need at least two of three urine samples over time to be diagnostic [14]. Can be inaccurate as urinary albumin concentration can vary due to urine concentration; however, the 24-h urine collection is cumbersome [14]
		>20—overt nephropathy	
	Type 2 DM: screen at time of diagnosis and annually [14]	eGFR (mL/min/1.73 m^2):	
	Hypertension: recommendation is to screen routinely	≥90 mL/min/1.73 m^2—normal, stage 1	
		60–89—mild CKD, stage 2	
		30–59—moderate CKD, stage 3	
		15–29—severe CKD, stage 4	
Or Serum creatinine converted into estimated glomerular filtration rate (eGFR)		<15 or dialysis—end stage renal disease, stage 5	eGFR: uses the 4-variable MDRD (modification of diet in renal disease) equation, requires knowledge of patient's age, sex, serum creatinine, and race, and is automatically computed [14]. Is generally a better estimate than serum creatinine [14]

Adapted from Lau et al. (2007) [2]

(continued)

She has been seeing a social worker at the FHT for supportive counselling related to a relationship breakdown. During team rounds, the social worker reports that Ms. H has a history of depression but this has been well controlled with an antidepressant and Ms. H's current low mood is probably situational. However, the social worker raises concerns about Ms. H's increasing weight. She has gained 20 lbs in the last 2 months and reports of increasing fatigue and daytime sleepiness. The social worker (SW) was concerned that Ms. H almost fell asleep at the wheel while driving her kids home from school last week. The social worker (SW) has advised Ms. H not to drive until she is referred to the medical team for a complete history and physical.

Upon reviewing her file, it is noted that she has a history of menorrhagia, dysmenorrhea, irregular periods, and difficulty getting pregnant. She was diagnosed with fibromyalgia 3 years ago and She was also recently diagnosed with hypertension. Her history is negative for asthma or COPD. She has a positive family history of obesity and first- and second-degree relatives diagnosed with uterine cancer.

Ms. H reports that she has been feeling increasingly sleepy for the last 6 weeks. She notes that she has not been sleeping well, but attributes this to the stress she is experiencing as a result of her 6-year relationship breakdown. She indicates that her fibromyalgia pain has been getting worse with severity, up to 8/10, which interferes with her ability to care for her two children at times. She also reports that she gets very short of breath after climbing 1/2 a flight of stairs. She notes that she is currently menstruating, but that this is her first menstruation in 6 months and that it is very heavy, with clots and is now into its tenth day.

Her current medications are Cipralex 40 mg OD, Lyrica 25 mg qhs, Naproxen 250 mg prn, and Lisinopril 20 mg OD.

On physical examination, Ms. H appears her stated age. She is noted to have hirsutism, most notably on her upper lip and chin. Her vital signs are as follows: BP 132/80, HR87, RR 24, O2 sat on room air 93 %. She is notably obese with much of her weight concentrated centrally. Her BMI is calculated at 39 kg/m^2 with a waist circumference of 151 cm. She states that she has gained most of her weight in the last 2 years after she stopped smoking.

Her respiratory exam reveals clear air entry bilaterally, slightly decreased to the bases. Her abdominal exam revealed that she had tenderness in the suprapubic region, a non-palpable liver, and no rebound tenderness. Her JVP is normal and she has mild, non-pitting ankle and lower leg edema. There are no lesions or discoloration of her lower legs. Pedal pulses are palpable but tibial pulses are not palpable mainly due to ankle edema.

A STOP-BANG screening for sleep apnea is completed and Ms. H scores 6/8 which indicates probable sleep apnea. She is referred for a diagnostic sleep study. Ms. H is asked if she would like to discuss her weight as this may be contributing to her low energy. She is happy to discuss it but doesn't know what to do because she states that she has tried "everything" and always regains the weight "and more." On hearing that there are some medical and surgical weight loss options that are covered by provincial healthcare, Ms. H agrees to be referred to a medical weight loss program.

Ms. H's sleep study reveals severe apnea (AHI of 32) with desaturations down to 81 % especially while supine. She is prescribed CPAP at 10 cm H_2O. She is having difficulty tolerating the CPAP mask and is

(continued)

(continued)

working with the retail outlet that she rented the CPAP machine from to find a type of mask that she is able to wear at least 4 h per night. At her 3 month follow-up, she reveals that she is using a nasal pillow mask for most of the night and is feeling a little more rested. She no longer falls asleep while driving. However, her energy level is still not very good.

You order CBC, ferritin, TSH, bHCG, and CR. The results come back as: Hemoglobin 112 (range 120–160 g/L), MCV 78.4 (range 80–95 fL), ferritin 9 (range 11–307 μg/L), TSH 6.76 (range 0.2–4.0 mU/L), bHCG negative, CR clearance 85 (range 50–98 mL/min). You have also completed a pap smear that was negative for abnormal cells. To r/o mild heart failure (which is low on the differential), you have also ordered a 2D Echo which was within normal limits. Although the TSH is high, you will just monitor this since it is not high enough to warrant supplementation at this time. You had also considered referring Ms. H to a rheumatologist to rule out autoimmune disease such as lupus based on her history of obesity and recent fatigue symptoms. However based on the findings of severe OSA and iron deficiency anemia, you choose to defer this for now.

Ms. H's iron deficiency anemia is presumably due to anemia of chronic disease exacerbated by her recent menorrhagia. You decide to start an iron supplement such as ferrous fumarate (Palafer) 300 mg once daily and order a pelvic ultrasound. This reveals multiple ovarian cysts and a fairly large uterine mass, most likely a fibroid. You decide to refer Ms. H to a gynecologist to r/o polycystic ovarian syndrome (PCOS) and endometrial fibroids. Gynecological CA is also on the differential.

The gynecologist rules out CA with a biopsy of her uterine mass but diagnoses Ms. H with PCOS and endometriosis. She starts Ms. H on Metformin 500 mg BID and schedules her for a uterine artery ablation procedure.

To better manage her pain, you increase her Lyrica dosing to 25 mg BID. This helps somewhat so you consider referring her to a chronic pain clinic for further titration of the Lyrica as well as other pharmacological and non-pharmacological therapies such as Tai Chi, acupuncture, and CBT.

References

1. HelpGuide.Org. Help yourself to greater health and happiness. How excess weight affects your health: Understanding the increased risks to your health. [image on the internet]. No date. [cited 2016 April 26]. http://www.helpguide.org/harvard/how-excess-weight-affects-your-health.htm
2. Lau DC, Douketis JD, Morrison KM, Hramiak IM, Sharma AM, Ur E, Members of the Obesity Canada Clinical Practice Guidelines Expert Panel. 2006 Canadian clinical practice guidelines on the management and prevention of obesity in adults and children [summary]. Can Med Assoc J. 2007;176(8):S1–3.
3. Corscadden L, Taylor A, Sebold A, Maddocks E, Pearson C, Harvey J. Obesity in Canada: a joint report from the Public Health Agency of Canada and the Canadian Institute for Health Information. Public Health Agency of Canada; 2011.
4. Flegal KM, Williamson DF, Pamuk ER, Rosenberg HM. Estimating deaths attributable to obesity in the United States. Am J Public Health. 2004;94(9):1486–9.
5. Katzmarzyk PT, Ardern CI. Overweight and obesity mortality trends in Canada, 1985–2000. Can J Public Health. 2004;1:16–20.
6. Wherrett D, Huot C, Mitchell B, Pacaud D. Canadian Diabetes Association 2013 Clinical Practice Guidelines for the Prevention and Management of Diabetes in Canada: type I diabetes in children and adolescents. Can J Diabetes. 2013;37:S1–216.
7. Zhang Y, Sowers JR, Ren J. Pathophysiological insights into cardiovascular health in metabolic syndrome. Exp Diabetes Res. 2012;2012:320534.
8. Poirier P, Giles TD, Bray GA, Hong Y, Stern JS, Pi-Sunyer FX, et al. Obesity and cardiovascular disease: pathophysiology, evaluation, and effect of weight loss. Arterioscler Thromb Vasc Biol. 2006;26(5):968–76.

9. Kershaw EE, Flier JS. Adipose tissue as an endocrine organ. J Clin Endocrinol Metab. 2004;89(6):2548–56.
10. Peavy WC. Cardiovascular effects of obesity: implications for critical care. Crit Care Nurs Clin North Am. 2009;21(3):293–300.
11. Wisse BE. The inflammatory syndrome: the role of adipose tissue cytokines in metabolic disorders linked to obesity. J Am Soc Nephrol. 2004;15(11):2792–800.
12. Northcott JM, Yeganeh A, Taylor CG, Zahradka P, Wingle JT. Adipokines and the cardiovascular system: mechanisms mediating health and disease. Can J Physiol Pharmacol. 2012;90(8):1029–59.
13. Field AE, Coakley EH, Must A, Spadano JL, Laird N, Dietz WH, Rimm E, Colditz GA. Impact of overweight on the risk of developing common chronic diseases during a 10-year period. Arch Intern Med. 2001;161(13):1581–6.
14. Nguyen NT, Nguyen X-MT, Lane J, Wang P. Relationship between obesity and diabetes in a US adult population: findings from the National Health and Nutrition Examination Survey, 1999–2006. Obes Surg. 2011;21(3):351–5.
15. Boden G, Shulman GI. Free fatty acids in obesity and type 2 diabetes: defining their role in the development of insulin resistance and β-cell dysfunction. Eur J Clin Invest. 2002;32(s3):14–23.
16. Fanelli C, Calderone S, Epifano L, De Vincenzo A, Modarelli F, Pampanelli S, Perriello G, De Feo P, Brunetti P, Gerich JE. Demonstration of a critical role for free fatty acids in mediating counterregulatory stimulation of gluconeogenesis and suppression of glucose utilization in humans. J Clin Invest. 1993;92(4):1617.
17. Zhang Y, Proenca R, Maffei M, Barone M, Leopold L, Friedman JM. Positional cloning of the mouse obese gene and its human homologue. Nature. 1994;372(6505):425–32.
18. Hotamisligil GS, Arner P, Caro JF, Atkinson RL, Spiegelman BM. Increased adipose tissue expression of tumor necrosis factor-α in human obesity and insulin resistance. J Clin Invest. 1995;95(5):2409–15.
19. Steppan CM, Bailey ST, Bhat S, Brown EJ, Banerjee RR, Wright CM, et al. The hormone resistin links obesity to diabetes. Nature. 2001;409(6818):307–12.
20. Mora S, Pessin JE. An adipocentric view of signaling and intracellular trafficking. Diabetes Metab Res Rev. 2002;18(5):345–56.
21. Lönnqvist F, Nordfors L, Schalling M. Leptin and its potential role in human obesity. J Intern Med. 1999;245(6):643–52.
22. Van Heek M, Compton DS, France CF, Tedesco RP, Fawzi AB, Graziano MP, et al. Diet-induced obese mice develop peripheral, but not central, resistance to leptin. J Clin Invest. 1997;99(3):385–90.
23. Considine RV, Sinha MK, Heiman ML, Kriauciunas A, Stephens TW, Nyce MR, et al. Serum immunoreactive-leptin concentrations in normal-weight and obese humans. N Engl J Med. 1996;334(5):292–5.
24. Hotta K, Funahshi T, Bodkin NL, Ortmeyer HK, Arita Y, Hansen BC, et al. Circulating concentrations of the adipocyte protein adiponectin are decreased in parallel with reduced insulin sensitivity during the progression to type 2 diabetes in rhesus monkeys. Diabetes. 2001;50(5):1126–33.
25. Weyer C, Funahashi T, Tanaka S, Hotta K, Matsuzawa Y, Pratley RE, et al. Hypoadiponectinemia in obesity and type 2 diabetes: close association with insulin resistance and hyperinsulinemia. J Clin Endocrinol Metab. 2001;86(5):1930–5.
26. Arita Y, Kihara S, Ouchi N, Takahashi M, Maeda K, Miyagawa J, et al. Paradoxical decrease of an adipose-specific protein, adiponectin, in obesity. Biochem Biophys Res Commun. 1999;257(1):79–83.
27. Hotta K, Funahashi T, Arita Y, Takahashi M, Matsuda M, Okamoto Y, et al. Plasma concentration of a novel adipose-specific protein, adiponectin, in type 2 diabetic patients. Arterioscler Thromb Vasc Biol. 2000;20(6):1595–9.
28. Miyazaki Y, Pipek R, Mandarino LJ, DeFronzo RA. Tumor necrosis factor α and insulin resistance in obese type 2 diabetic patients. Int J Obes Relat Metab Disord. 2003;27(1):88–94.
29. Pradhan AD, Manso JE, Rifai N, Buring JE, Ridker PM. C-reactive protein, interleukin 6 and the risk of developing type 2 diabetes. JAMA. 2001;286(3):327–34.
30. Pickup JC, Chusney GD, Thomas SM, Burt D. Plasma interleukin 6, tumor necrosis factor and blood cytokine production in type 2 diabetes. Life Sci. 2000;67(3):291–300.
31. Vidal-Puig A, O'Rahilly S. Resistin: a new link between obesity and insulin resistance? Clin Endocrinol (Oxf). 2001;55(5):437–8.
32. Albu JB, Kovera AJ, Johnson JA. Fat distribution and health in obesity. Ann N Y Acad Sci. 2000;904:491–501.
33. Despres JP, Lemieux S, Lamarche B, Prud'homme D, Moorjani S, Brun LD, et al. The insulin resistance-dyslipidemic syndrome: contribution of visceral obesity and therapeutic implications. Int J Obes Relat Metab Disord. 1995;19 Suppl 1:S76–86.
34. Bajaj M, Surramornkul S, Pratipanawatr T, Hardies LJ, Pratipanawatr W, Glass L, et al. Pioglitazone reduces hepatic fat content and augments splanchnic glucose uptake in patients with type 2 diabetes mellitus. Diabetes. 2003;52(6):1364–70.
35. Oral EA, Simha V, Ruiz E, Andewelt A, Premkumar A, Snell P, et al. Leptin-replacement therapy for lipodystrophy. N Engl J Med. 2002;346(8):57–8.
36. Colditz GA, Willett WC, Rotnitzky A, Manson JE. Weight gain as a risk factor for clinical diabetes mellitus in women. Ann Intern Med. 1995;122(7): 481–6.
37. Hoogwerf BJ, Nuttall FQ. Long-term weight regulation in treated hyperthyroid and hypothyroid subjects. Am J Med. 1984;76:963–70.
38. Knudsen N, Laurberg P, Rasmussen LB, Bülow I, Perrild H, Ovesen L, Jørgensen T. Small differences in thyroid function may be important for body mass index and the occurrence of obesity in the population. J Clin Endocrinol Metab. 2005;82:1118–25.

39. Reinehr T. Obesity and thyroid function. Mol Cell Endocrinol. 2010;316(2):165–71.
40. Reinehr T, De Sousa G, Andler W. Hyperthy rotropinemia in obese children is reversible after weight loss and in not related to lipids. J Clin Endocrinol Metab. 2006;91:3088–91.
41. De Pergola G, Ciampolillo A, Paolotti S, Trerotoli P, Giorgino R. Free triiodothyronine and thyroid stimulating hormone are directly associated with waist circumference, independently of insulin resistance, metabolic parameters and blood pressure in overweight and obese woman. Clin Endocrinol (Oxf). 2007;67:265–9.
42. Oge A, Bayraktar F, Saygili F, Guney E, Demir S. TSH influences serum leptin levels independent of thyroid hormones in hypothyroid and hyperthyroid patients. Endocr J. 2005;52:213–7.
43. Zimmermann-Belsing T, Brabant G, Holst JJ, Feldt-Rasmussen U. Circulating leptin and thyroid dysfunction. Eur J Endocrinol. 2003;149:257–71.
44. Zhao J, Liu GL, Wei Y, Jiang LH, Bao PL, Yang QY, et al. Association of plasma glucose, insulin, and cardiovascular risk factors in overweight and obese children. Saudi Med J. 2014;35(2):132–7.
45. Kuchta KF. Pathophysiologic changes of obesity. Anesthesiol Clin North America. 2005;23(3):421–9.
46. Hall JE, do Carmo JM, da Silva AA, Wang Z, Hall M. Obesity-induced hypertension: interaction of neurohumoral and renal mechanisms. Circ Res. 2015;116(6):991–1006.
47. Garrett K, Lauer K, Christopher BA. The effects of obesity on the cardiopulmonary system: implications for critical care nursing. Prog Cardiovasc Nurs. 2004;19(4):155–61.
48. Klop B, Elte JW, Cabezas MC. Dyslipidemia in obesity: mechanisms and potential targets. Nutrients. 2013;5(4):1218–40.
49. Mokdad AH, Ford ES, Bowman BA, Dietz WH, Vinicor F, Bales VS, Marks JS. Prevalence of obesity, diabetes, and obesity-related health risk factors, 2001. JAMA. 2003;289(1):76–9.
50. Anderson TJ, Grégoire J, Hegele RA, Couture P, Mancini GB, McPherson R, Francis GA, Poirier P, Lau DC, Grover S, Genest Jr J, Carpentier AC, Dufour R, Gupta M, Ward R, Leiter LA, Lonn E, Ng DS, Pearson GJ, Yates GM, Stone JA, Ur E. 2012 Update of the Canadian Cardiovascular Society Guidelines for the diagnosis and treatment of dyslipidemia for the prevention of cardiovascular disease in the adult. Can J Cardiol. 2013;29(2):151–67.
51. Reisin E, Jack AV. Obesity and hypertension: mechanisms, cardio-renal consequences, and therapeutic approaches. Med Clin North Am. 2009;93(3):733–51.
52. Insull W. The pathology of atherosclerosis: plaque development and plaque responses to medical treatment. Am J Med. 2009;122(1):S3–14.
53. Tavora F, Zhang Y, Zhang M, Li L, Ripple M, Fowler D, et al. Cardiomegaly is a common arrhythmogenic substrate in adult sudden cardiac deaths, and is associated with obesity. Pathology. 2012;44(3):187–91.
54. Salome C, King G, Berend N. Physiology of obesity and effects on lung function. J Appl Physiol. 2009;108(1):206–11.
55. Bahammam A, Al-Jawder S. Managing acute respiratory decompensation in the morbidly obese. Respirology. 2012;17(5):759–71.
56. Yaegashi M. Outcome of morbid obesity in the intensive care unit. J Intensive Care Med. 2005;20(3):147–54.
57. Murugan A, Murugan G. Obesity and respiratory diseases. Chron Respir Dis. 2008;5:233–42.
58. Koening S. Pulmonary complications of obesity. Am J Med Sci. 2001;321(4):249–79.
59. Littleton S. Impact of obesity on respiratory function. Respirology. 2011;17(1):43–9.
60. Masoli M, Fabian D, Holt S, Beasley R. The global burden of asthma: executive summary of the GINA Dissemination Committee report. Allergy. 2004;59(5):469–78.
61. Beuther DA, Weiss ST, Sutherland ER. Obesity and asthma. Am J Respir Crit Care Med. 2006;174(2):112–9.
62. Dixon A, Holguin F, Sood A, Salome C, Pratley R, Beuther D, et al. An official American Thoracic Society Workshop report: obesity and asthma. Proc Am Thorac Soc. 2010;7(5):325–35.
63. Sin D, Sutherland E. Obesity and the lung: 4 {middle dot} Obesity and asthma. Thorax. 2008;63(11):1018–23.
64. Taraseviciute A, Voelkel NF. Severe pulmonary hypertension in postmenopausal obese women. Eur J Med Res. 2006;11(5):198.
65. Friedman SE, Andrus BW. Obesity and pulmonary hypertension: a review of pathophysiologic mechanisms. J Obes. 2012;2012:1–9.
66. Chung F. Obstructive sleep apnea and anesthesia—what an anesthesiologist should know? 2014. www.stopbang.ca/pdf/refresher.pdf
67. Resta O, Foschino-Barbaro MP, Legari G, Talamo S, Bonfitto P, Palumbo A, et al. Sleep-related breathing disorders, loud snoring and excessive daytime sleepiness in obese subjects. Int J Obes Relat Metab Disord. 2001;25(5):669–75.
68. Basen-Engquist K, Chang M. Obesity and cancer risk: recent review and evidence. Curr Oncol Rep. 2011;13(1):71–6.
69. Horner RL, Mohiaddin RH, Lowell DG, Shea SA, Burman ED, Longmore DB, et al. Sites and sizes of fat deposits around the pharynx in obese patients with obstructive sleep apnoea and weight matched controls. Eur Respir J. 1989;2(7):613–22.
70. Vasu TS, Grewal R, Doghramji K. Obstructive sleep apnea syndrome and perioperative complications: a systematic review of the literature. J Clin Sleep Med. 2012;8(2):199–207.
71. Berger K, Goldring R, Rapoport D. Obesity hypoventilation syndrome. Semin Respir Crit Care Med. 2009;30:253–61.
72. Nowbar S, Burkart KM, Gonzales R, Fedorowicz A, Gozansky WS, Gaudio JC, et al. Obesity-

associated hypoventilation in hospitalized patients: prevalence, effects, and outcome. Am J Med. 2004; 116(1):1–7.
73. Foxx-Orenstein A. Gastrointestinal symptoms and diseases related to obesity: an overview. Gastroenterol Clin North Am. 2010;39(1):23–37.
74. Ho W, Spiegel B. The relationship between obesity and functional gastrointestinal disorders: causation, association, or neither? Gastroenterol Hepatol. 2008;4(8):572–8.
75. Jones R, Galmiche JP. Review: what do we mean by GERD?—definition and diagnosis. Aliment Pharmacol Ther. 2005;22(s1):2–10.
76. Fujimoto A, Hoteya S, Iizuka T, Ogawa O, Mitani T, Kuroki Y, et al. Obesity and gastrointestinal diseases. Gastroenterol Res Pract. 2013;2013(2013):1–6.
77. Suter M, Dorta G, Giusti V, Calmes J. Gastro-esophageal reflux and esophageal motility disorders in morbidly obese patients. Obes Surg. 2004;14(7):959–66.
78. Dittrick GW, Thompson JS, Campos D, Bremers D, Sudan D. Gallbladder pathology in morbid obesity. Obes Surg. 2005;15(2):238–42.
79. Nguyen D, El-Serag H. The big burden of obesity. Gastrointest Endosc. 2009;70(4):752–7.
80. Tran A, Gual P. Non-alcoholic steatohepatitis in morbidly obese patients. Clin Res Hepatol Gastroenterol. 2013;37(1):17–29.
81. Jayasena CN, Bloom SR. Role of gut hormones in obesity. Endocrinol Metab Clin North Am. 2008;37(3):769–87.
82. Thijssen E, van Caam A, van der Kraan PM. Obesity and osteoarthritis, more than just wear and tear: pivotal roles for inflamed adipose tissue and dyslipidaemia in obesity-induced osteoarthritis. Rheumatology. 2015;54(4):588–600.
83. Kerekes G, Nurmohamed MT, González-Gay MA, Seres I, Paragh G, Kardos Z, Baráth Z, Tamási L, Soltész P, Szekanecz Z. Rheumatoid arthritis and metabolic syndrome. Nat Rev Rheumatol. 2014;10(11):691–6.
84. Berenbaum F, Eymard F, Houard X. Osteoarthritis, inflammation and obesity. Curr Opin Rheumatol. 2013;25(1):114–8.
85. Versini M, Jeandel PY, Rosenthal E, Shoenfeld Y. Obesity in autoimmune diseases: not a passive bystander. Autoimmun Rev. 2014;13(9):981–1000.
86. Felson DT, Anderson JJ, Naimark A, Walker AM, Meenan RF. Obesity and knee osteoarthritis: the Framingham Study. Ann Intern Med. 1988;109(1):18–24.
87. Blagojevic M, Jinks C, Jeffery A, Jordan KP. Risk factors for onset of osteoarthritis of the knee in older adults: a systematic review and meta-analysis. Osteoarthr Cartil. 2010;18(1):24–33.
88. Finckh A, Turesson C. The impact of obesity on the development and progression of rheumatoid arthritis. Ann Rheum Dis. 2014;73(11):1911–3.
89. Russolillo A, Iervolino S, Peluso R, Lupoli R, Di Minno A, Pappone N, Di Minno MN. Obesity and psoriatic arthritis: from pathogenesis to clinical outcome and management. Rheumatology. 2013;52(1):62–7.
90. Aune D, Norat T, Vatten LJ. Body mass index and the risk of gout: a systematic review and dose–response meta-analysis of prospective studies. Eur J Nutr. 2014;53(8):1591–601.
91. Katz JN, Lew RA, Bessette L, Punnett L, Fossel AH, Mooney N, Keller RB. Prevalence and predictors of long-term work disability due to carpal tunnel syndrome. Am J Ind Med. 1998;33(6):543–50.
92. Ohnari K, Uozumi T, Tsuji S. Occupation and carpal tunnel syndrome. Brain Nerve (Shinkei kenkyu no shinpo). 2007;59(11):1247–52.
93. Karpitskaya Y, Novak CB, Mackinnon SE. Prevalence of smoking, obesity, diabetes mellitus, and thyroid disease in patients with carpal tunnel syndrome. Ann Plast Surg. 2002;48(3):269–73.
94. Bland JD. The relationship of obesity, age, and carpal tunnel syndrome: more complex than was thought? Muscle Nerve. 2005;32(4):527–32.
95. Merksey H, Bogduk N, editors. Pain terms: a current list with definitions and notes on usage. Seattle: ISAP Press; 1994. p. 209–14.
96. Narouze S, Souzdalnitski D. Obesity and chronic pain: systematic review of prevalence and implications for pain practice. Reg Anesth Pain Med. 2015;40(2):91–111.
97. Elzahaf RA, Tashani OA, Unsworth BA, Johnson MI. The prevalence of chronic pain with an analysis of countries with a Human Development Index less than 0.9: a systematic review without meta-analysis. Curr Med Res Opin. 2012;28(7):1221–9.
98. McVinnie DS. Obesity and pain. Br J Pain. 2013;7(4):163–70.
99. Stone AA, Broderick JE. Obesity and pain are associated in the United States. Obesity. 2012;20(7):1491–5.
100. Ray L, Lipton RB, Zimmerman ME, Katz MJ, Derby CA. Mechanisms of association between obesity and chronic pain in the elderly. Pain. 2011;152(1):53–9.
101. Sellinger JJ, Clark EA, Shulman M, Rosenberger PH, Heapy AA, Kerns RD. The moderating effect of obesity on cognitive–behavioral pain treatment outcomes. Pain Med. 2010;11(9):1381–90.
102. Rihn JA, Kurd M, Hilibrand AS, Lurie J, Zhao W, Albert T, Weinstein J. The influence of obesity on the outcome of treatment of lumbar disc herniation. J Bone Joint Surg Am. 2013;95(1):1–8.
103. Shiri R, Lallukka T, Karppinen J, Viikari-Juntura E. Obesity as a risk factor for sciatica: a meta-analysis. Am J Epidemiol. 2014;179(8):929–37.
104. Chai NC, Scher AI, Moghekar A, Bond DS, Peterlin BL. Obesity and headache: part I–a systematic review of the epidemiology of obesity and headache. Headache. 2014;54(2):219–34.
105. Leboeuf-Yde C. Body weight and low back pain: a systematic literature review of 56 journal articles reporting on 65 epidemiologic studies. Spine. 2000;25(2):226.

106. Shiri R, Karppinen J, Leino-Arjas P, Solovieva S, Viikari-Juntura E. The association between obesity and low back pain: a meta-analysis. Am J Epidemiol. 2010;171(2):135–54.
107. Watkins LR, Maier SF, Goehler LE. Immune activation: the role of pro-inflammatory cytokines in inflammation, illness responses and pathological pain states. Pain. 1995;63(3):289–302.
108. Rezania K, Soliven B, Rezai KA, Roos RP. Impaired glucose tolerance and metabolic syndrome in idiopathic polyneuropathy: the role of pain and depression. Med Hypotheses. 2011;76(4):538–42.
109. De Wit LM, Van Straten A, Van Herten M, Penninx BW, Cuijpers P. Depression and body mass index, a u-shaped association. BMC Public Health. 2009;9(1):14.
110. Luppino FS, de Wit LM, Bouvy PF, Stijnen T, Cuijpers P, Penninx BW, Zitman FG. Overweight, obesity, and depression: a systematic review and meta-analysis of longitudinal studies. Arch Gen Psychiatry. 2010;67(3):220–9.
111. Ohayon MM, Schatzberg AF. Chronic pain and major depressive disorder in the general population. J Psychiatr Res. 2010;44(7):454–61.
112. Tietjen GE, Peterlin BL, Brandes JL, Hafeez F, Hutchinson S, Martin VT, Dafer RM, Aurora SK, Stein MR, Herial NA, Utley C. Depression and anxiety: effect on the migraine–obesity relationship. Headache. 2007;47(6):866–75.
113. Vogelzangs N, Kritchevsky SB, Beekman AT, Brenes GA, Newman AB, Satterfield S, Yaffe K, Harris TB, Penninx BW. Obesity and onset of significant depressive symptoms: results from a prospective community-based cohort study of older men and women. J Clin Psychiatry. 2009;71(4):1–478.
114. Loevinger BL, Muller D, Alonso C, Coe CL. Metabolic syndrome in women with chronic pain. Metabolism. 2007;56(1):87–93.
115. Räikkönen K, Matthews KA, Kuller LH. Depressive symptoms and stressful life events predict metabolic syndrome among middle-aged women a comparison of World Health Organization, Adult Treatment Panel III, and International Diabetes Foundation definitions. Diabetes Care. 2007;30(4):872–7.
116. Lee IT, Lee WJ, Huang CN, Sheu WH. The association of low-grade inflammation, urinary albumin, and insulin resistance with metabolic syndrome in nondiabetic Taiwanese. Metabolism. 2007;56(12):1708–13.
117. Lann D, LeRoith D. Insulin resistance as the underlying cause for the metabolic syndrome. Med Clin North Am. 2007;91(6):1063–77.
118. Willette AA, Kapogiannis D. Does the brain shrink as the waist expands? Ageing Res Rev. 2015;20:86–97.
119. Elias MF, Goodell AL, Waldstein SR. Obesity, cognitive functioning and dementia: back to the future. J Alzheimers Dis. 2012;30(s2):S113–25.
120. Bischof GN, Park DC. Obesity and aging: consequences for cognition, brain structure, and brain function. Psychosom Med. 2015;77(6):697–709.
121. Wang Y, Chen X, Song Y, Caballero B, Cheskin LJ. Association between obesity and kidney disease: a systematic review and meta-analysis. Kidney Int. 2008;73(1):19–33.
122. De Jong PE, Verhave JC, Pinto-Sietsma SJ, Hillege HL. Obesity and target organ damage: the kidney. Int J Obes Relat Metab Disord. 2002;2:26.
123. Fox CS, Larson MG, Leip EP, Culleton B, Wilson PW, Levy D. Predictors of new-onset kidney disease in a community-based population. JAMA. 2004;291(7):844–50.
124. Kramer H, Luke A, Bidani A, Cao G, Cooper R, McGee D. Obesity and prevalent and incident CKD: the hypertension detection and follow-up program. Am J Kidney Dis. 2005;46(4):587–94.
125. Gelber RP, Kurth T, Kausz AT, Manson JE, Buring JE, Levey AS, Gaziano JM. Association between body mass index and CKD in apparently healthy men. Am J Kidney Dis. 2005;46(5):871–80.
126. Hsu CY, McCulloch CE, Iribarren C, Darbinian J, Go AS. Body mass index and risk for end-stage renal disease. Ann Intern Med. 2006;144(1):21–8.
127. Ting SM, Nair H, Ching I, Taheri S, Dasgupta I. Overweight, obesity and chronic kidney disease. Nephron Clin Pract. 2009;112(3):c121–7.
128. Kley HK, Edelman P, Krushemper HL. Relationships of plasma sex hormones to different parameters of obesity in male subjects. Metabolism. 1980;29:1041–5.
129. Schneider G, Kirschner MA, Berkowitz R, Ertel NH. Increased estrogen production in obese men. J Clin Endocrinol Metab. 1979;48:633–8.
130. Zumoff B, Strain GW, Miller LK, et al. Plasma free and non-sex-hormone-binding-globulin-bound testosterone are decreased in obese men in proportion to their degree of obesity. J Clin Endocrinol Metab. 1990;71:929–31.
131. Magnusdottir EV, Thorsteinsson T, Thorsteinsdottir S, Heimisdottir M, Olafsdottir K. Persistent organochlorines, sedentary occupation, obesity and human male subfertility. Hum Reprod. 2005;20:208–15.
132. Feldman HA, Johannes CB, Derby CA, Kleinman KP, Mohr BA, Araujo AB, McKinlay JB. Erectile dysfunction and coronary risk factors, prospective results from the Massachusetts male aging study. Prev Med. 2000;30:328–38.
133. de Boer H, Verschoor L, Ruinemans-Koerts J, Jansen M. Letrozole normalizes serum testosterone in severely obese men with hypogonadotropic hypogonadism. Diabetes Obes Metab. 2005;7:211–5.
134. Haffner SM, Katz MS, Dunn JF. The relationship of insulin sensitivity and metabolic clearance of insulin to adiposity and sex-hormone binding globulin. Endocr Rev. 1990;16:361–76.
135. Jungheim ES, Travieso JL, Carson KR, Moley KH. Obesity and reproductive function. Obstet Gynecol Clin North Am. 2012;39(4):479–93.
136. Frisch RE. Pubertal adipose tissue: is it necessary for normal sexual maturation? Evidence from the rat and human female. Fed Proc. 1980;39:2390–400.

137. Gosman GG, Katcher HI, Legro RS. Obesity and the role of gut and adipose hormones in female reproduction. Hum Reprod Update. 2006;12(5):585–601.
138. Sam S, Dunaif A. Polycystic ovary syndrome: syndrome XX? Trends Endocrinol Metab. 2003; 14:365–70.
139. Wise LA, Rothman KJ, Mikkelsen EM, Sorensen HT, Riis A, Hatch EE. An internet-based prospective study of body size and time to pregnancy. Hum Reprod. 2010;25(1):253–64.
140. Boots C, Stephenson MD. Does obesity increase the risk of miscarriage in spontaneous conception: a systemic review. Semin Reprod Med. 2011;29:507–13.
141. Jungheim ES, Macones GA, Odem RR, et al. Associations between free fatty acids, cumulus oocyte complex morphology and ovarian function during in vitro fertilization. Fertil Steril. 2011;95(6):1970–4.
142. Kim ST, Marquard K, Stephens S, Louden E, Allsworth J, Moley KH. Adiponectin and adiponectin receptors in the mouse preimplantation embryo and uterus. Hum Reprod. 2011;26(1):82–95.
143. Catalano PM, Ehrenberg HM. The short- and long-term implications of maternal obesity on the mother and her offspring. BJOG. 2006;113(10): 1126–33.
144. Calle EE, Rodrigues C, Walker-Thurmond K, Thun MJ. Overweight, obesity and mortality from cancer in a prospectively studied cohort of US adults. N Engl J Med. 2003;348:1625–38.
145. Pischon T, Nöthlings U, Boeing H. Obesity and cancer. Proc Nutr Soc. 2008;67(02):128–45.
146. Hanley DA, Cranney A, Jones G, Whiting SJ, Leslie WD, Cole DE, Atkinson SA, Josse RG, Feldman S, Kline GA, Rosen C. Vitamin D in adult health and disease: a review and guideline statement from Osteoporosis Canada. Can Med Assoc J. 2010;182(12):E610–8.
147. Pan SY, DesMeules M. Energy intake, physical activity, energy balance, and cancer: epidemiologic evidence. Methods Mol Biol. 2009;472:191–215.
148. Thompson HJ. Obesity as a cancer risk factor: potential mechanisms. In: Nutrition and cancer prevention. Boca Raton, FL: Taylor & Francis; 2006. pp 565–57.
149. Calle EE, Kaaks R. Overweight, obesity and cancer: epidemiological evidence and proposed mechanisms. Nat Rev Cancer. 2004;4:579–91.
150. Roberts DL, Dive C, Renehan AG. Biological mechanisms linking obesity and cancer risk: new perspectives. Annu Rev Med. 2010;61:301–16.
151. Nock NL, Berger NA. Obesity and cancer: overview of mechanisms. In: Berger NA, editor. Cancer and energy balance, epidemiology and overview. New York: Springer; 2010. p. 129–79.
152. van Kruijsdijk RC, van der Wall E, Visseren FL. Obesity and cancer: the role of dysfunctional adipose tissue. Cancer Epidemiol Biomarkers Prev. 2009;18:2569–78.
153. Aigner E, Feldman A, Datz C. Obesity as an emerging risk factor for iron deficiency. Nutrients. 2014;6(9):3587–600.
154. Beard J. Iron biology in immune function, muscle metabolism and neuronal functioning. J Nutr. 2016;131(2):568s–80.
155. Cheng HL, Bryant C, Cook R, O'Connor H, Rooney K, Steinbeck K. The relationship between obesity and hypoferraemia in adults: a systematic review. Obes Rev. 2012;13(2):150–61.
156. Tussing-Humphreys L, Pustacioglu C, Nemeth E, Braunschweig C. Rethinking iron regulation and assessment in iron deficiency, anemia of chronic disease, and obesity: introducing hepcidin. J Acad Nutr Diet. 2012;112(3):391–400.
157. Ausk K, Ioannou G. Is obesity associated with anemia of chronic disease? A population-based study. Epidemiology. 2008;16(10):2356–61.
158. Wilkins C, Swain G, Cooke C. Facing up to the obesity crisis: outcomes of a bariatric lymphoedema clinic. J Lymphoedema. 2014;9(2):27–9.
159. Shipman AR, Millington GW. Obesity and the skin. Br J Dermatol. 2011;165(4):743–50.
160. Plascencia Gomez A, Vega Memije ME, Torres Tamayo M, Rodriguez Carreon AA. Skin disorders in overweight and obese patients and their relationship with insulin. Actas Dermosifiliogr. 2014;105(2):178–85.
161. Rush A, Muir M. Maintaining skin integrity in bariatric patients. Br J Community Nurs. 2012;17(4):154. 156–9.
162. Nino M, Franzese A, Perrino NR, Balato N. The effect of obesity on skin disease and epidermal permeability barrier status in children. Pediatr Dermatol. 2012;29(5):567–70.
163. Boza JC, Trindade EN, Peruzzo J, Sachett L, Rech L, Cestari TF. Skin manifestations of obesity: a comparative study. J Eur Acad Dermatol Venereol. 2012;26(10):1220–3.
164. Chung F, Yegneswaran B, Liao P, Chung SA, Vairavanathan S, Islam S, et al. STOP questionnaire: a tool to screen patients for obstructive sleep apnea. Anesthesiology. 2008;108(5):812–21.
165. Toward Optimized Practice (TOP) Working Group for Vitamin D. Guideline for vitamin D testing and supplementation in adults. Edmonton, AB: Toward Optimized Practice; 2012.
166. Minuk GY. Canadian Association of Gastroenterology Practice Guidelines: evaluation of abnormal liver enzyme tests. Can J Gastroenterol Hepatol. 1998;12(6):417–21.
167. Guidelines and Protocols Advisory Committee, Doctors of British Columbia and the Ministry of Health in British Columbia, 2010.
168. Earl R, Woteki CE, editors. Iron deficiency anemia: recommended guidelines for the prevention, detection, and management among US children and women of childbearing age. Washington, DC: National Academies Press; 1994.

169. Toward Optimized Practice Clinical Practice Guideline Working Group. Clinical Practice Guideline: investigation and management of primary thyroid dysfunction. Edmonton, AB: Toward Optimized Practice Program; 2008.
170. U.S. Preventive Services Task Force (USPSTF). Screening for chronic kidney disease: U.S. Preventive Services Task Force recommendation statement. Ann Intern Med. 2012;157(8):567–70.
171. Daskalopoulou SS, Rabi DM, Zarnke KB, Dasgupta K, Nerenberg K, Cloutier L, Gelfer M, Lamarre-Cliche M, Milot A, Bolli P, McKay DW. The 2015 Canadian Hypertension Education Program recommendations for blood pressure measurement, diagnosis, assessment of risk, prevention, and treatment of hypertension. Can J Cardiol. 2015;31(5):549–68.

6 Overview of Medical and Surgical Treatment of Severe Obesity

Kristel Lobo Prabhu and Timothy Jackson

This chapter will explore medical treatments and potential surgical options for treating severe obesity. Medications commonly used for weight loss will be summarized including potential limitations. A brief description of bariatric surgery procedures will be illustrated followed by a summary of the risk-adjusted outcomes as well as rates of improvement of obesity-related comorbidities.

K.L. Prabhu, M.D., F.R.C.S.C.
University of Toronto, Toronto, ON, Canada

Minimally Invasive and Bariatric Surgery, Division of General Surgery, Department of Surgery and Institute of Health Policy, Management and Evaluation, Faculty of Medicine, University Health Network, Toronto Western Hospital, University of Toronto, 399 Bathurst St, 8MP-322, Toronto, ON, Canada M5T 2S8
e-mail: kristelprabhu@gmail.com

T. Jackson, B.Sc., M.D., M.P.H., F.R.C.S., F.A.C.S. (✉)
Minimally Invasive and Bariatric Surgery, Division of General Surgery, Department of Surgery and Institute of Health Policy, Management and Evaluation Faculty of Medicine, University Health Network, Toronto Western Hospital, University of Toronto, 399 Bathurst St, 8MP-322, Toronto, ON, Canada M5T 2S8
e-mail: timothy.jackson@uhn.ca

6.1 Evidence for Medical Treatments of Obesity

The management of an obese adult should begin with the determination of the patient's BMI and waist circumference. If the BMI is found to be greater than 25 or the waist circumference is above the cut-off point for the patient's ethnicity, investigations must be undertaken to assess for the presence of comorbidities [1]. Major obesity-related medical problems include type 2 diabetes mellitus, hypertension, dyslipidemia, cardiovascular disease, and sleep apnea [2].

The first step in the management of the obese patient is lifestyle modification with interventions aimed at diet, exercise, and behavioural modification. Pharmacotherapy may be used as an adjunct to lifestyle modification in patients with a BMI ≥27 with one of more obesity-related comorbidities or in patients with a BMI ≥30 with or without associated risk factors [1].

Drugs currently approved by the United States Food and Drug Administration (FDA) for the treatment of obesity include orlistat, lorcaserin, and noradrengeric agents including phentermine, diethylpropion, phendimetrazine, and benzphetamine [3].

6.1.1 Orlistat

Orlistat inhibits the actions of gastric and pancreatic lipases, thus decreasing the absorption of

S. Sockalingam, R. Hawa (eds.), *Psychiatric Care in Severe Obesity*,
DOI 10.1007/978-3-319-42536-8_6

dietary fat [4]. A systematic review by Yanovski et al., analyzing Orlistat 120 mg trails, found that 35–73 % of participants in the treatment group achieved a ≥5 % weight loss at 1 year [3]. Weight loss was found to be maintained up to 24–36 months with continued use of Orlistat [5]. The XENDOS trial which followed 3305 patients treated for up to 4 years found that Orlistat decreased body weight by 2.7 % more than placebo [6]. They also found a 37 % reduction in the conversion from impaired glucose tolerance to diabetes mellitus [6]. In a systematic review and metanalysis of randomized control trials (RCT) conducted by Zhou et al., Orlistat was found improve cardiovascular risk factors by decreasing total cholesterol, low density lipoprotein, fasting glucose, and systolic and diastolic blood pressure [7]. The major side effects resulting from the use of orlistat are gastrointestinal and include flatus with discharge, oily spotting, fecal urgency, fatty/oily stool, oily evacuation, fecal incontinence, and increased defacation [8]. Rare cases of severe liver injury have been reported with the use of Orlistat [9].

6.1.2 Lorcaserin

Lorcaserin is a selective agonist of the serotonin 2C receptor resulting in appetite suppression [10]. In a large, multi-centre, placebo-controlled trial, Smith et al. showed that 47.5 % of patients in the lorcaserin group compared to 20.3 % of patients in the placebo group achieved ≥5 % of their body weight at 1 year [11]. Furthermore, this weight loss was maintained in a greater proportion of patients who continued lorcaserin use (67.9 %) compared to placebo (50.3 %) at the end of 2 years [11]. A second large RCT of 4008 participants similarly found that significantly more patients treated with lorcaserin 10 mg BID (47.2 %) versus placebo (25.0 %) had lost at least 5 % of their baseline body weight [12]. Lorcaserin use was associated with a significant decrease in blood pressure, total cholesterol, low density lipoprotein, and triglycerides; as well as improved glycated hemoglobin concentrations in diabetic patients [3, 13]. The most commonly reported side effects of the drug were headache, nausea, and dizziness [12].

6.1.3 Noradrenergic Agents

Phentermine, diethylpropion, benzphetamine, and phendimetrazine are sympathomimetic drugs that induce weight loss by reducing appetite through the activation of adrenergic and dopaminergic receptors [14]. They are all approved for short-term (12 weeks) treatment of obesity [3]. There is limited high-quality data on the efficacy of this class of drugs for the treatment of obesity. Phentermine is the commonly prescribed drug obesity medication in the United States [15]. The longest double-blind trial on the use of phentermine evaluated its continuous and intermittent use compared to placebo over a 36-week period [16]. Greater weight loss was seen in those who received phentermine continuously (12.2 kg) or intermittently (13.0 kg) compared to placebo (4.8 kg) [16].

Phentermine and diethylpropion are classified as schedule IV drugs by the United States Drug Enforcement Agency (DEA). Benzphetamine and phendimetrazine are classified as schedule III drugs [9]. This regulatory classification indicates potential for abuse, though this potential is low. Common adverse effects of this drug class include insomnia, elevated heart rate, dry mouth, dizziness, and headache [3].

6.2 Types of Weight Loss Surgery

The National Institutes of Health consensus statement on gastrointestinal surgery for severe obesity (1991) recommends the consideration of bariatric surgery in patients with BMI ≥40 or BMI ≥35 with severe comorbid disease [17].

Several high-quality studies have demonstrated the superiority of bariatric surgery compared to conventional medical treatment options for obesity. A systematic review of randomized control trials by Gloy et al. demonstrated that bariatric surgery resulted in greater weight loss and higher remission rates of Type 2 diabetes and metabolic syndrome compared to non-surgical treatments [18]. A randomized control trial by Schauer et al. assessed 3-year outcomes of intensive medical therapy alone or in combination with Roux-en-Y gastric bypass or sleeve gastrectomy [19]. Five percent of patients in the medical therapy group achieved glycemic control compared to 38 % of patients who underwent a Roux-en-Y gastric bypass and 24 % of those who received a sleeve gastrectomy [19]. Additionally, patients in the surgical group had a greater reduction in body weight and improvement in quality of life compared to the medical group [19]. Most recently, Mingrone et al. published the results of a randomized control trial comparing the 5-year outcomes of bariatric surgery to conventional medical treatment in obese patients with Type 2 diabetes [20]. In this study, 50 % of patients in the surgical group maintained remission of their diabetes at 5 years compared to none of the patients in the medical treatment group [20]. The surgical group also experienced greater weight loss, along with significant reductions in plasma lipids, cardiovascular risk, and overall medication use [20].

The two primary mechanisms by which bariatric surgery results in weight loss are restriction and malabsorption. Currently performed procedures may rely on a single mechanism or a combination of the two. Restrictive procedures reduce the number of calories the patient can ingest by limiting the size of the gastric reservoir. Malabsorptive procedures result in weight loss by bypassing a portion of the intestine where calories are absorbed. Laparoscopic adjustable gastric banding (LAGB) and sleeve gastrectomy (LSG) are purely restrictive procedures currently in use. Roux-en-Y gastric bypass combines features of restriction and malabsorption.

6.3 Contemporary Procedure Descriptions

6.3.1 Laparoscopic Sleeve Gastrectomy

In this technique, most of the greater curve of the stomach is removed laparoscopically, thus decreasing the volume of the gastric reservoir (Fig. 6.1) [21]. The gastric antrum is divided 5–6 cm from the pylorus and a stapled sleeve is then created around a 32–50F bougie [22]. The sleeve gastrectomy originated as the initial part of the duodenal switch operation. It was offered as the first stage procedure to super obese patients (BMI ≥60) and was noted to result in weight loss sufficient enough to make the second stage of the duodenal switch unnecessary [22]. The major but rare complication of this procedure is leakage along the staple line that may require revision [23]. LSG has morbidity and effectiveness positioned between LAGB and laparoscopic Roux-en-Y gastric bypass (LRYGB) [24].

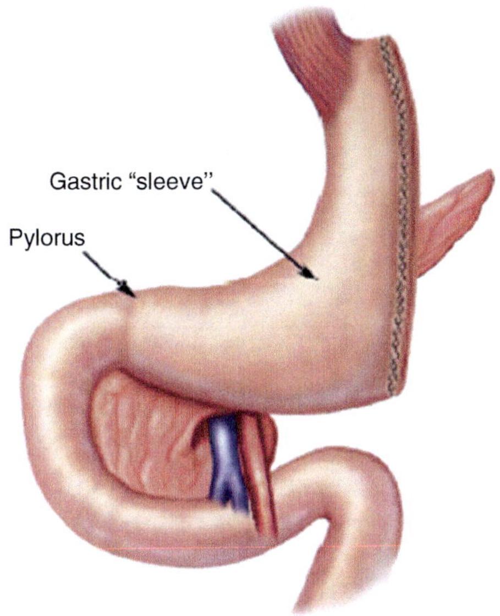

Fig. 6.1 Sleeve gastrectomy. From Jones DB, Maithel SK, Schneider BE. Atlas of minimally invasive surgery. Woodbury CT: Cine-Med; 2006. Copyright Cine-Med Inc.; with permission

6.3.2 Laparoscopic Adjustable Gastric Banding

An adjustable silicone band is placed laparoscopically around the cardia of the stomach, 1–2 cm below the gastroesophageal junction and locked into place (Fig. 6.2) [21]. The band is connected to a port located in the subcutaneous tissue. Injection and withdrawal of saline via the port controls the tightness of the band and thus the degree of restriction offered by it [25, 26]. LAGB placement accounted for 46 % of all bariatric procedures performed in American College of Surgery accredited centres in 2011 [24]. Early complications of the procedure are rare and include slippage, obstruction, gastric or esophageal perforation, and port site

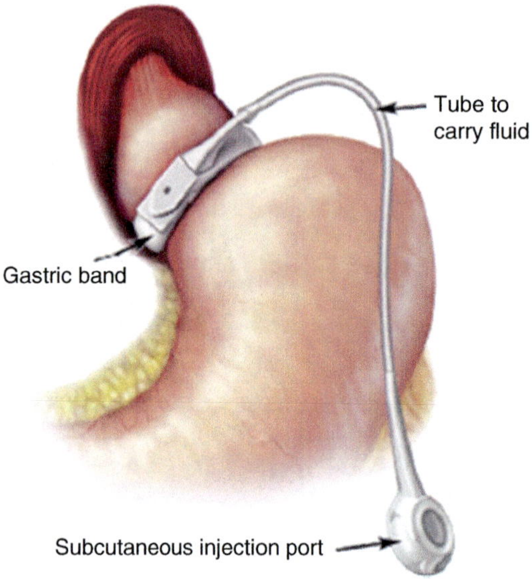

Fig. 6.2 Laparoscopic adjustable gastric band. From Jones DB, Maithel SK, Schneider BE. Atlas of minimally invasive surgery. Woodbury CT: Cine-Med; 2006. Copyright Cine-Med Inc.; with permission

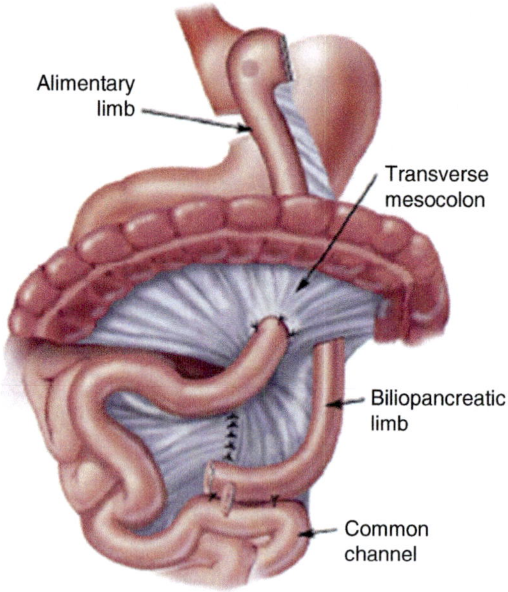

Fig. 6.3 Laparoscopic Roux-en-Y gastric bypass. From Jones DB, Maithel SK, Schneider BE. Atlas of minimally invasive surgery. Woodbury CT: Cine-Med; 2006. Copyright Cine-Med Inc.; with permission

infection [27]. The long-term safety and efficacy of LAGB is less clear with reported rates of surgical failure of up to 40 % at 5 years [28].

6.3.3 Laparoscopic Roux-en-Y Gastric Bypass

The restrictive portion of this procedure involves the creation of a 20–30 mL gastric pouch from the proximal lesser curve of the stomach through the sequential firing of a linear stapler [29]. A biliopancreatic limb, an alimentary limb, and a common channel result from the creation of the Roux-en-Y anastomosis (Fig. 6.3) [21]. The biliopancreatic limb extends from the ligament of Treitz to the jejunojejunostomy and is generally 30–60 cm in length. The alimentary limb extends from the gastrojejunostomy to the jejunojejunostomy. It is typically 75–150 cm long and carries the ingested food without biliary and pancreatic secretions. The common channel refers to the remainder of the small intestine extending from the jejunojejunostomy to the ileocecal valve [26]. LRYGB results in greater reduction in BMI than the LSG or the LAGB. The specific surgical complications associated with this procedure include anastomotic leak, bleeding, internal hernia, marginal ulcer, and staple line failure [30]. LRYGB is associated with a 30-day mortality of 0.14 % and a 30-day morbidity of 5.91 % [24].

6.3.4 Biliopancreatic Diversion

This procedure consists of a distal gastrectomy combined with a long Roux-en-Y reconstruction [31]. In a variation of the procedure called biliopancreatic diversion (BPD) with duodenal switch, the pylorus is preserved and an ileoduodenostomy is created distal to the pylorus. In this procedure, the length of the common channel varies between 50 and 125 cm from the ileocecal valve and determines the degree of malabsorption [26]. There are no clear indications for when to perform BPD. It can be considered in super obese patients, given its superior weight loss results compared to LRYGB [32].

6.4 Outdated Procedures

6.4.1 Jejunoileal Bypass

In this procedure, the jejunum is divided proximally; variable lengths of small intestine are then excluded before this segment of jejunum is anastomosed distally to the ileum. The jejunoileal bypass has been abandoned due to reports that greater than 20 % of patients who underwent this procedure developed life-threatening complications [33]. These complications include progressive liver disease, intractable diarrhea and electrolyte abnormalities, kidney stones and renal failure resulting from hyperoxaluria, and migrating arthralgias [33].

6.4.2 Vertical Band Gastroplasty

A vertical staple line is used to partition the upper portion of the stomach, which results in the formation of a tight outlet. This outlet is then wrapped with a band or mesh to prevent dilation over time [26]. This procedure has been abandoned due to failure to maintain weight loss over time [34]. Furthermore, up to 56 % of patients undergoing this procedure ultimately require revisional surgery due to complications such as leakage and fistula formation, scarring and stricture formation, and gastroesophageal fistula formation [26, 35].

6.5 Evidence for Treating Severe Obesity

The prospective, controlled Swedish Obesity Subjects study followed over 4000 obese patients, with half undergoing a bariatric procedure and a matched control group undergoing conventional treatment [36]. The study reported on mortality over a 10.9 year period, with a 99.9 % follow-up rate. The hazard ratio (adjusted for sex, age, and risk factors) for the surgery group was 0.71 compared to the control group [36]. Thus, the study demonstrated that bariatric surgery is associated with decreased overall mortality [36].

In 2011, the American College of Surgeons—Bariatric Surgery Centre Network (ACS-BSCN) published its first report on the safety and efficacy of LAGB, LSG, and LRYGB [24]. At 1 year, patients undergoing LAGB, LSG, and LRYGB had a BMI reduction of 7.05, 11.87, and 15.34, respectively [24]. Additionally, the clinical efficacy of these procedures for the treatment of five weight-related comorbidities was assessed; these included diabetes, hypertension, hyperlipidemia, obstructive sleep apnea (OSA), and gastroesophageal reflux disease (GERD). In diabetic patients, 44 % had resolution or improvement of their disease following LAGB, 55 % following LSG, and 83 % following LRYGB [24]. Forty-four percent of hypertensive patients had disease resolution or improvement after LAGB, 68 % after LSG, and 79 % after LRYGB [24]. Similar results were seen for the remaining three comorbidities studied with the efficacy of LSG lying intermediate between that of the LAGB and the LRYGB (Table 6.1) [24]. In obese patients with uncontrolled Type 2 diabetes mellitus, Schauer et al. reported that 3 years of intensive medical therapy combined with bariatric surgery resulted in better glycemic control than medical therapy alone [19]. In a study by Pournaras et al., 72 % of diabetic patients undergoing gastric bypass were deemed to be in remission from their disease and

Table 6.1 Rates of improvement or resolution of obesity-related comorbidities by bariatric surgery type [8]

1 year outcome	Laparoscopic RYGB	Lap sleeve gastrectomy	Lap band
Reduction in BMI (kg/m^2)	−15.34	−11.87	-7.05
Diabetes	83 %	55 %	44 %
Hyperlipidemia	66 %	35 %	33 %
Hypertension	79 %	68 %	44 %
Obstructive sleep apnea	66 %	62 %	38 %
GERD	70 %	50 %	64 %

Table 6.2 Risk-adjusted outcomes for bariatric cases performed at ACS-BSCN accredited centres [8]

	Laparoscopic RYGB (%)	Lap sleeve gastrectomy (%)	Lap band (%)
30-day mortality	0.14	0.11	0.05
1-year mortality	0.34	0.21	0.08
30-day morbidity	5.91	5.61	0.92
Readmission	6.47	5.40	1.71
Reoperation	5.02	2.97	0.76

improvements in insulin resistance have been found to precede weight loss [37]. Bariatric surgery is also found to be associated with improved glycemic control in non-morbidly obese patients with BMIs between 30 and 35 [38].

A large, prospective, multicentre, observational study of 30-day outcomes by the Longitudinal Assessment of Bariatric Surgery (LABS) consortium demonstrated a low 30-day rate of death among patients undergoing Roux-en-Y gastric bypass or LAGB of 0.3 % [39]. The rate of 30-day morbidity was also found to be low with 4.3 % of patients having at least one major adverse outcome [39]. The advent of laparoscopic bariatric procedures has greatly improved the safety profile of these interventions. 30-day rate of death was 2.1 % for open Roux-en-Y gastric bypass compared to 0.2 % for LRYGB [39]. Of the three most commonly performed laparoscopic bariatric procedures, the morbidity associated with LSG (5.61 %) is intermediate between that of LAGB (0.92 %) and LRYGB (5.91 %) [8]. Similarly, the mortality risk associated with LSG (0.11 %) is intermediate between than of LAGB (0.05 %) and LRYGB (0.14 %) [24] (Table 6.2).

Case Vignettes

Mr. Z has struggled with his weight for years. He has tried different diet programs and different medications, including Orlistat and Phentermine, with initial reduction in his weight followed by regain of his weight and more. He is frustrated with his weight, physical limitations, and uncontrolled hypertension. At his last medical appointment, he noted further weight gain and his most recent BMI is 55 kg/m^2.

Mr. Z is concerned about the idea of weight loss surgery and is particularly anxious about the risks of surgery. He meets with the bariatric surgery program's surgeon and has an opportunity to discuss the risks and available procedures. After completing a series of pre-surgery assessments through the bariatric surgery program, Mr. Z decides with his surgeon that the LSG is the most suitable procedure considering his concerns about complications, long-term effects of malabsorption, and the treatment effect on his poorly controlled hypertension.

Three months later, Mr. Z underwent laparoscopic sleeve surgery with no complications. His hypertension resolved within the first 6 months of the procedure. His mobility has improved and he feels more energetic. He started incorporating daily walks and attending a regular support group for eating healthy.

6.6 Summary and Take Home Messages

In this chapter, we have reviewed common medical treatments for obesity and have provided an overview of bariatric surgery procedures, specifically contrasting contemporary and older procedures. The following are key points outlined in this chapter:

- Pharmacotherapy can help in the treatment of obesity; however, it has better outcomes when combined with diet, lifestyle changes, and exercise.
- There are a number of bariatric procedures for the treatment of obesity and each procedure has its unique mechanism of action—be it restrictive, malabsorptive, or combined.

- Each bariatric procedure has different rates of improvement of obesity-related comorbidities with the evidence favouring LRYGB.
- Risk-adjusted outcomes for mortality, morbidity, and readmission favour LAGB; however, this lower risk should be balanced against its reduced obesity-related comorbidity treatment effect.

References

1. Lau DCW, Douketis JD, Morrison KM, Hramiak IM, Sharma AM, Ur E. 2006 Canadian clinical practice guidelines on the management and prevention of obesity in adults and children. Can Med Assoc J. 2007;176(8 Suppl):s1–13.
2. Khaodhiar L, McCowen KC, Blackburn GL. Obesity and its comorbid conditions. Clin Cornerstone. 1999;2(3):17–28.
3. Yanovski SZ, Yanovski JA. Long-term drug treatment for obesity. JAMA. 2013;311(1):1–13.
4. Heck AM, Yanovski JA, Calis KA. Orlistat, a new lipase inhibitor for the management of obesity. Pharmacotherapy. 2000;20(3):270–9.
5. LeBlanc E, O'Connor E, Whitlock E, Patnode C, Kapka T. Effectiveness of primary care-relevant treatments for obesity in adults: a systematic evidence review for the U.S. Preventive Services Task Force. Ann Intern Med. 2011;155:434–47.
6. Jarl S, Mark N. XENical in the prevention of diabetes in obese subjects (XENDOS) study. Diabetes Care. 2004;27(1):155–61.
7. Zhou Y-H, Ma X-Q, Wu C, et al. Effect of anti-obesity drug on cardiovascular risk factors: a systematic review and meta-analysis of randomized controlled trials. PLoS One. 2012;7(6):e39062.
8. Hollander PA, Elbein SC, Hirsch IB, Kelley D, McGill J, Taylor T, Weiss SR, Crockett SE, Kaplan RA, Comstock J, Lucas CP, Lodewick PA, Canovatchel W, Chung J, Hauptman J. Role of orlistat in the treatment of obese patients with type 2 diabetes. A 1-year randomized double-blind study. Diabetes Care. 1998;21(8):1288–94.
9. Bray GA, Ryan DH. Medical therapy for the patient with obesity. Circulation. 2012;125(13):1695–703.
10. Gustafson A, King C, Rey JA. Lorcaserin (Belviq): a selective Serotonin 5-HT2C agonist in the treatment of obesity. P T. 2013;38(9):525–34.
11. Smith SR, Weissman NJ, Anderson CM, et al. Multicenter, placebo-controlled trial of lorcaserin for weight management. N Engl J Med. 2010;363(3):245–56.
12. Fidler MC, Sanchez M, Raether B, et al. A one-year randomized trial of lorcaserin for weight loss in obese and overweight adults: the BLOSSOM trial. J Clin Endocrinol Metab. 2011;96(10):3067–77.
13. O'Neil PM, Smith SR, Weissman NJ, et al. Randomized placebo-controlled clinical trial of lorcaserin for weight loss in type 2 diabetes mellitus: the BLOOM-DM Study. Obesity. 2012;20(7):1426–36.
14. Ioannides-Demos LL, Piccenna L, McNeil JJ. Pharmacotherapies for obesity: past, current, and future therapies. J Obes. 2011;2011:179674.
15. Hampp C, Kang EM, Borders-Hemphill V. Use of prescription antiobesity drugs in the United States. Pharmacotherapy. 2013;33(12):1299–307.
16. Munro JF, MacCuish AC, Wilson EM, Duncan LJ. Comparison of continuous and intermittent anorectic therapy in obesity. Br Med J. 1968;1(5588):352–4.
17. National Institutes of Health. Gastrointestinal surgery for severe obesity. NIH Consens Statement Online. 1991;9(9):1–20.
18. Gloy VL, Briel M, Bhatt DL, et al. Bariatric surgery versus non-surgical treatment for obesity: a systematic review and meta-analysis of randomised controlled trials. Br Med J. 2013;347(oct22_1):f5934.
19. Schauer P. Bariatric surgery versus intensive medical therapy for diabetes. N Engl J Med. 2014;371(7):680–2.
20. Mingrone G, Panunzi S, De Gaetano A, et al. Bariatric-metabolic surgery versus conventional medical treatment in obese patients with type 2 diabetes: 5 year follow-up of an open-label, single-centre, randomised controlled trial. Lancet. 2015;386(9997):964–73.
21. Jackson TD, Hutter MM. Morbidity and effectiveness of laparoscopic sleeve gastrectomy, adjustable gastric band, and gastric bypass for morbid obesity. Adv Surg. 2012;46(1):255–68.
22. Deitel M, Gagner M, Erickson AL, Crosby RD. Third International Summit: current status of sleeve gastrectomy. Surg Obes Relat Dis. 2011;7(6):749–59.
23. Felberbauer FX, Langer F, Shakeri-Manesch S, et al. Laparoscopic sleeve gastrectomy as an isolated bariatric procedure: Intermediate-term results from a large series in three Austrian centers. Obes Surg. 2008;18(7):814–8.
24. Hutter M, Schirmer B, Jones D. First Report from the American College of Surgeons—Bariatric Surgery Center Network: laparoscopic sleeve gastrectomy has morbidity and effectiveness positioned between the band and the bypass. Ann Surg. 2011;254(3):410–22.
25. Belachew M, Legrand M, Vincent V, et al. Laparoscopic placement of adjustable silicone gastric band in the treatment of morbid obesity: how to do it. Obes Surg. 1995;5(1):66–70.
26. Elder KA, Wolfe BM. Bariatric surgery: a review of procedures and outcomes. Gastroenterology. 2007;132(6):2253–71.
27. Finks JF, Kole KL, Yenumula PR, et al. Predicting risk for serious complications with bariatric surgery: results from the Michigan Bariatric Surgery Collaborative. Ann Surg. 2011;254(4):633–40.
28. Boza C, Gamboa C, Perez G, et al. Laparoscopic adjustable gastric banding (LAGB): surgical results and 5-year follow-up. Surg Endosc. 2011;25(1):292–7.

29. Brunicardi CF, Andersen DK, Billiar TR, Dunn DL, Hunter JG, Pollock RE. Schwartz's manual of surgery. 8th ed. New York: McGraw-Hill; 2006.
30. Zuegel NP, Lang RA, Hüttl TP, et al. Complications and outcome after laparoscopic bariatric surgery: LAGB versus LRYGB. Langenbecks Arch Surg. 2012;397(8):1235–41.
31. Scopinaro N, Gianetta E, Adami GF, et al. Biliopancreatic diversion for obesity at eighteen years. Surgery. 1996;119(3):261–8.
32. SAGES Guidelines Committee Society of American Gastrointestinal Endoscopic Surgeons. Guidelines for Clinical Application of Laparoscopic Bariatric Surgery SAGES Guidelines Committee. SAGES. 2008:1–31.
33. Chousleb E, Patel S, Szomstein S, Rosenthal R. Reasons and operative outcomes after reversal of gastric bypass and jejunoileal bypass. Obes Surg. 2012;22(10):1611–6.
34. Balsiger BM, Poggio JL, Mai J, Kelly KA, Sarr MG. Ten and more years after vertical banded gastroplasty as primary operation for morbid obesity. J Gastrointest Surg. 2000;4(6):598–605.
35. Van Gemert WG, Van Wersch MM, Greve JWM, Soeters PB. Revisional surgery after failed vertical banded gastroplasty: restoration of vertical banded gastroplasty or conversion to gastric bypass. Obes Surg. 1998;8(1):21–8.
36. Rerks-Ngarm S, Pitisuttithum P, Nitayaphan S, Kaewkungwal J, Chiu J, Paris R, Premsri N, Namwat C, de Souza M, Adams E, Benenson M, Gurunathan S, Tartaglia J, McNeil JG, Francis DP, Stablein D, Birx DL, Chunsuttiwat S, Khamboonruang C, Thongcharoen P, Robb ML, Michael NL, Kunasol P, Kim JH; MOPH-TAVEG Investigators. Vaccination with ALVAC and AIDSVAX to prevent HIV-1 infection in Thailand. N Engl J Med. 2009; 361(23):2209–2220.
37. Pournaras DJ, Osborne A, Hawkins SC, et al. Remission of type 2 diabetes after gastric bypass and banding: mechanisms and 2 year outcomes. Ann Surg. 2010;252(6):966–71.
38. Maggard-Gibbons M, Maglione M, Livhits M, Ewing B, Maher AR, Hu J, Li Z, Shekelle PG. Bariatric surgery for weight loss and glycemic control in nonmorbidly obese adults with diabetes a systematic review. JAMA. 2013;309(21):2250–61.
39. Bhargava SK, Sachdev HS, Fall CH, Osmond C, Lakshmy R, Barker DJ, Biswas SK, Ramji S, Prabhakaran D, Reddy KS. Relation of serial changes in childhood body-mass index to impaired glucose tolerance in young adulthood. N Engl J Med. 2004;350(9):865–75.

Integrated Models for Severe Obesity Management: Role for Psychosocial Teams

7

Wynne Lundblad, Alexis M. Fertig, and Sanjeev Sockalingam

7.1 Introduction

Severe obesity has significant comorbidity with a range of psychiatric disorders. Untreated psychiatric disorders have a significant negative impact on health outcomes, including the management of obesity. There is increasing recognition that integrated behavioral health care improves both health and psychological outcomes while remaining cost-effective. This chapter provides a brief overview of the history of integrated behavioral health care and discusses possible applications to the treatment of severe obesity. We also review the limited literature examining integrated and collaborative care for patients with obesity.

Case Vignettes

Mrs. R is a 38-year-old separated woman who presents to a family medicine clinic to establish care as her previous provider recently retired. Her medical history is notable for hypertension and migraine headaches. Her medications are lisinopril 40 mg daily, fluoxetine 20 mg daily, and a multivitamin. She has no complaints on review of systems. Her height is 64 in/162.56 cm and her weight is 271 lb/123 kg, BMI 46.5. Her PHQ-9 is 10, indicating moderate depression, with which she was diagnosed two months ago. Her blood pressure is 148/92 and all other vital signs are within normal limits. Her exam is notable only for obesity. She had been overweight as a teenager and has not been able to sustain weight loss for any period as an adult. After the birth of her son 5 years ago, she "just kept gaining" and estimates that her weight has been relatively steady over the past year despite attempts to lose weight by reducing sugar intake and not snacking after dinner. She states that she wants to lose weight, but struggles to "be good" and will overeat in social situations and when she has a deadline at work and has to work late. Since separating from her husband 3 months ago, she estimates that she has gained 15 lbs/6.8 kg.

(continued)

W. Lundblad, M.D. (✉) • A. Fertig, M.D., M.P.H.
Department of Psychiatry, Western Psychiatric Institute and Clinic, University of Pittsburgh Medical Center, 3811 O'Hara Street, E8013, Pittsburgh, PA 15203, USA
e-mail: lundbladwr@upmc.edu; fertigam@upmc.edu

S. Sockalingam
Toronto Western Hospital Bariatric Surgery Program, Centre for Mental Health, University Health Network, 200 Elizabeth Street, Toronto, ON, Canada M5G 2C4

Department of Psychiatry, University of Toronto, Toronto, ON, Canada
e-mail: sanjeev.sockalingam@uhn.ca

S. Sockalingam, R. Hawa (eds.), *Psychiatric Care in Severe Obesity*,
DOI 10.1007/978-3-319-42536-8_7

(continued)
She has considered bariatric surgery, but worries about possible medical complications as well as lifetime behavioral changes. She does not wish to pursue pharmacological treatments, saying that she "knows what to do, I just have to do it." She has never sought group or individual therapy and denies a history of anxiety, mania, substance use, or other psychiatric illness.

Severe obesity is a complicated medical condition with implications for physical and psychological health. As with many other complicated chronic conditions, it is virtually impossible for a primary care provider to satisfactorily address all potential comorbidities within a single 15-min office visit. Further, primary care physicians often lack confidence and training to address behavioral and psychological issues that frequently occur in the severely obese.

While obesity is not itself a psychiatric disorder, patients with severe obesity are more likely than controls to have more than one mental health diagnosis as compared to non-obese controls (17.1 vs. 62.5 %) [1]. As discussed later in this book, the risk for suicidal ideation and suicide attempts is higher in obese patients than in those who are normal weight or overweight [2].

The directionality of the obesity-mental health relationship is unknown, but some work suggests that the stigma of being obese may contribute to some psychiatric burden [3]. While reduction in weight has been associated with improvement in mental health [4], multiple studies suggest the presence of untreated or undertreated psychiatric illness may hinder weight loss efforts. Further, many psychiatric medications are associated with weight gain, perhaps contributing to obesity in patients with mental illness [5].

Given both the high rates of psychiatric illness in the severely obese as well as the potential contribution of psychiatric illness to obesity, psychosocial providers (e.g. therapists, psychiatric nurses, psychologists, and psychiatrists) play an important role in the treatment of obesity and comorbid psychiatric disorders. Models exist for incorporating psychosocial treatment into the management of chronic illness, although little has been written specifically about psychosocial care for obesity in the medical setting. There is sufficient evidence for the chronic care model (CCM) in the management of diabetes and major depressive disorder, conditions that share psychological, behavioral, and physical characteristics with severe obesity. Several models for integrating psychosocial care into the management of the severely obese patient will be examined.

7.2 Opportunities with Integrated Care

The Institute of Medicine specifically added mental and emotional health to its definition of primary care in 1996; and the World Health Organization emphasizes behavioral health as part of a population-based primary care strategy. The American Psychiatric Association, American Society of Addiction Medicine, American Psychological Association, and American Academy of Family Physicians all support integration of behavioral health care in the medical setting. A movement toward the patient-centered medical home (PCMH) has emerged as one way to integrate behavioral and medical health services. In the United States, the Affordable Care Act incentivizes the development of Medicaid health homes, with behavioral health care as part of the primary care delivery system.

Medical providers (particularly PCPs) provide most of the mental health care in the United States [6]. One third of patients with a mental health diagnosis receive care exclusively from their primary care physician [6]; 56 % of patients would initially go to their primary care provider for mental health treatment compared to 26 % who would go to a mental health provider [7]. Among the reasons for preferentially seeing a PCP for mental health concerns are the stigma associated with receiving mental health treatment, limited mental health, and limited access to mental health providers.

Integrating medical and behavioral health care addresses these issues and enhances the ability to meet more of a patient's needs.

The high rates of mental health treatment in the primary care setting match current prescribing practices. In 1993–4, PCPs prescribed 55 % of anxiolytics, 40 % of antidepressants, 54 % of stimulants, and 30 % of antipsychotics in the United States [8]. A 2009 survey of a national prescribing database found an increase in these numbers: primary care providers prescribed 65 % of anxiolytics, 62 % of antidepressants, 52 % of stimulants, 37 % of antipsychotics, and 22 % of antimanic agents [9]. In this survey, psychiatrists prescribed only 23 % of psychotropic medications in the United States.

Yet many with psychiatric illness receive no care at all: 60 % of patients with a mental condition do not receive any behavioral health services [10]. Reasons for this include poor behavioral health insurance coverage, lack of mental health providers, and patients' belief that their symptoms do not require treatment [2, 11, 12].

7.3 Barriers to Integrated Care

Historically, behavioral and physical health care have operated in silos, with primary care providers reporting low levels of knowledge and comfort with respect to treating mental health conditions [13]. In addition, training and care delivery in each area are remarkably different and most providers require specific training to enable them to work in an integrated setting. There will need to be more emphasis on providing this training and experience to providers before they enter the work force [14].

Regulatory requirements, which vary by location and discipline, present another potential hurdle in the integration of mental health in the medical setting. Credentialing, restrictions on sharing protected health information, and reimbursement are all complex processes in behavioral health settings. These factors must be taken into account in the development of integrated programs. Cohen provides an in-depth discussion of key areas for consideration of the successful integration of primary care and behavioral health [15].

SAMHSA estimates that the Affordable Care Act will provide behavioral health coverage to 60 million US citizens, increasing the demand for therapists, psychologists, and psychiatrists [16]. Unfortunately, this comes at a time when there is a pronounced workforce shortage of 1800 psychiatrists and 6000 core mental health professionals, including social workers, therapists, psychologists, and psychiatric nurses [17]. As with other fields of medicine, this shortage is most pronounced in rural areas; of the 55 % of counties with no practicing mental health providers, all are rural. An examination of the distribution of primary care providers, psychiatrists, and psychologists shows that many rural areas do not have mental health providers rendering integrated care an unattainable option [18]. The reasons for this are numerous: low compensation, limited behavioral health insurance coverage in rural areas, high turnover, uneven concentration of providers in urban and suburban areas, and negative stigma associated with mental illness and the mental health profession [19].

The stigma associated with behavioral health treatment is a compelling barrier that persists for a significant minority of patients, particularly older patients, those from ethnic and racial minorities, and those in rural settings [6, 20]. Integration of behavioral health into the primary care setting is likely to increase access for patients who do not wish to be seen at a behavioral health-only clinic. Further, decision support services allow the PCP to treat the patient in consultation with a mental health provider (frequently a psychiatrist); this allows for high quality, empirically supported expert care while preserving patient comfort with their PCP.

7.4 Models of Integrated Care

There is variability in the degree of collaboration and integration between behavioral and physical health programs, ranging from primary care and behavioral health discussing shared patients as needed to providing services simultaneously [13]. Blount described three different levels of collaboration and integration to help clarify different options and to enhance understanding of research [21]. The first category Blount addresses is coordinated services, which entail communication when necessary about shared patients even though care delivery is in separate settings. The success of this category is dependent on the commitment of providers to this practice and is quite variable. Colocation is the next category described and consists of shared space for medical and mental health providers. This enhanced proximity results in improved communication, education, and quality of patient care, but does not necessarily involve structured communication and coordination between teams. Finally, Blount discusses true integrated care which involves a team approach resulting in one, joint treatment plan [21].

Wagner initially described the chronic care model (CCM) in 1996, recognizing that most primary care delivery systems were designed for acute issues rather than management of chronic conditions. In reviewing programs that successfully manage chronic illnesses, he found four key factors [22]:

1. Patients and providers collaborate on treatment priorities,
2. A clear plan is developed to target priorities and reach goals,
3. Education and behavioral support are provided, and
4. There is regular follow-up.

Bernstein describes the use of patient-centered medical homes (PCMH) to treat patients with obesity and associated complications. The team would potentially consist of a primary care provider, behavioral health provider, dietician, professionals to help with levels of physical activity, and case managers [23].

7.5 Evidence in Support of Collaborative Care Models Outside of Obesity

While the available evidence does not specifically address collaborative care for patients with severe obesity, much has been published on integrated care for depression, anxiety, at-risk alcohol use, and ADHD. A 2012 Cochrane Review found significantly greater improvement in anxiety and depression outcomes for adults treated under a collaborative model of care than those treated by traditional means [24]. A randomized trial of adolescents with depressive disorders was similarly encouraging, demonstrating greater improvement with integrated care than care as usual at 12 months [25]. Several specific models have been extensively researched and warrant further discussion:

7.5.1 IMPACT: Depression Care Management

The Improving Mood-Promoting Access to Collaborative Treatment (IMPACT) model for depression has been found effective in numerous high-quality studies [26, 27]. These studies have spanned a range of health care settings and have been consistent with a variety of chronic medical illnesses, including cancer and diabetic populations [28]. This model incorporates depression screening with a depression care manager (typically a mid-level provider) who provides evidence-based treatment and monitoring. A psychiatrist consults on patients who do not respond to care as expected [26, 27].

7.5.2 SBIRT: At-Risk Substance Use

The Screening, Brief Interventions, Referral to Treatment (SBIRT) model is effective with substance use disorders in primary care settings [29]. In this model, an evidence-based screening (i.e. AUDIT) is used to determine the risk of the patient's alcohol use. Patients with moderate to high-risk drinking receive a brief intervention (based on the principles of Motivational Interviewing), while patients who meet criteria for a substance use disorder are referred to specialty treatment. Few studies have looked at MI/SBIRT in obesity and weight management; those that have been published suggest a dose response, with greatest weight loss in patients who received intensive behavioral interventions [29].

7.5.3 PRISM-E: Enhanced Referral vs. Integrated Care

The Primary Care Research in Substance Abuse and Mental Health Care for the Elderly (PRISM-E) study compares outcomes in patients seen at the primary care office by an integrated behavioral health team (including licensed therapists, psychiatric nurses, and psychiatrists) against those referred to specialty mental health care services. While 6-month outcomes were the same for those in both groups, patients with major depressive disorder assigned to integrated care had superior symptom reduction [30].

7.6 Evidence for Collaborative Care in Obesity Management

Severe obesity is a condition that responds to multidisciplinary chronic care management, which includes integrated behavioral health services. Challenges with peri-operative patient adherence and medical follow-up underscore the need for an integrated care approach to bariatric surgery after care [31, 32]. Studies have demonstrated that psychosocial factors, such as a history of a substance use disorder or living a longer distance from surgical centers, may decrease patient completion of pre-bariatric surgery assessments [33]. Moreover, post-operative follow-up with bariatric surgery care may be decreased in individuals with more avoidant relationship styles [32]. Therefore, collaborative care approaches to severe obesity management are paramount to addressing challenges with patient engagement and psychiatric comorbidity, which may complicate patient follow-up care.

While large scale studies of integrated care in obesity management are still evolving, there are clear recommendations from obesity management consensus guidelines, reinforcing the importance of a multidisciplinary approach to obesity clinical care [34]. Using a chronic care model, Baillargeon et al. describe a protocol for using preceptorships and virtual communities to improve primary care management of obesity and weight loss [35]. Preliminary data on this model has shown improvements in primary care physicians' and nurses' self-efficacy in managing obesity within their community settings.

In the Netherlands, the Partnership Overweight Netherlands (PON) is a collaborative network with multiple healthcare systems and professions and was created to facilitate the development and implementation of an integrated health standard for the management and prevention of obesity [36]. The model utilizes a stepped care approach to obesity care, matching the level of treatment intervention to the level of weight-related health risk based on evidence from national clinical guidelines. Moreover, these types of integrated models of care in severe obesity management provide opportunities for establishing standardized and common pathways of care crossing multiple disciplines and healthcare sectors [37].

Future collaborative care models in severe obesity management should explore the role of integrating professional development programs to build capacity in primary care. For example, Project Extension for Community Healthcare Outcomes (Project ECHO) is a model of healthcare education and delivery providing primary and specialty care to chronic disease patient populations in rural areas [38]. The Project ECHO models have been expanded to obesity management and could serve as an additional collaborative care resource for patients across the severe obesity management spectrum, including after bariatric surgery [39]. As these models emerge, evaluation of program results including cost-effectiveness will be critical to discerning program scalability and the feasibility of broad-scale implementation.

7.7 Technology and Integrated Care

Telephone care management and telepsychiatry have allowed patients in rural or other resource-poor settings to access high-quality care without travel to a larger medical center. Fortney et al. developed a collaborative care model within small VA community clinics, in which patients with PHQ-9 scores of 12 or greater were enrolled in an intervention with both telepsychiatry and depression care management. This combination increased odds that patients would be both adherent and responsive to treatment at 6 and 12 months

[40]. Several models have been developed for obesity treatment, with one study of telepsychiatry for pediatric patients with obesity demonstrating both feasibility and comparable outcomes with respect to BMI reduction and the child behavior checklist [41]. Telephone care management, in which a provider (usually a nurse) speaks with a patient on a regular basis (usually every 2 weeks in the acute phase and every 4 weeks thereafter), has been found to reduce symptoms of depression and increase patient-reported quality of life, while remaining acceptable to providers and patients [42, 43]. Moreover, telephone-based cognitive behavioral therapy provides additional interventions that could be used in an integrated stepped care pathway for post-bariatric surgery care [44, 45].

7.8 Cost

Cost emerges as a concern with any new intervention in health care. It has long been established that patients with depression and other mental health diagnoses have higher rates of utilization and higher health care costs than age-matched peers [26]. Diabetes treatment costs are 50% higher in patients with mental health diagnoses; and one study estimated the cost of medical care for patients with depression to be up to 100% greater than patients without depression [46]. Several cost-effectiveness studies have been conducted on integrated care models [47, 48]. These cost benefits have been found in patients with complex chronic medical issues as well as in patients with severe and persistent mental illness.

Back to the Case Vignette

As part of the multidisciplinary evaluation, Mrs. R underwent dietary, behavioral, and psychological evaluation. Given her persistent depressive symptoms after 8 weeks of treatment with fluoxetine, the decision was made to increase the medication to 40 mg daily. She also agreed to a short course of CBT for depression and binge eating, which was discovered by the dietitian and psychologist in the office. She reported a long history of loss-of-control eating with an average of two subjective binge episodes per week since age 18, when she started university. In the months leading up to her marital separation, she found that the frequency and size of her binge episodes increased and have not abated.

Mrs. R's case was reviewed at the weekly care conference, where the psychiatrist recommended increasing her fluoxetine to 40 mg and beginning CBT to address binge eating and residual depressive symptoms. She participated in weekly telephone coaching with a psychiatric nurse, and kept food logs, which were electronically shared with the interdisciplinary team. In the subsequent 3 months, her binge frequency decreased by 50% and binge size decreased 25% overall. She lost 6 lb (2.7 kg) and reports less distress around food and mealtimes. Her PHQ-9 at 3 months was 4, indicating that her depression was in remission.

7.9 Take Home Points

Severe obesity is a condition that responds to multidisciplinary chronic care management, which includes integrated behavioral health services. Further research is needed to determine which models are the most feasible, successful, and cost-effective. In addition, further clarification of which components of programs are critical to integrated care treatment in obese patient populations is needed. Nonetheless, the following key points should be considered as part of an integrated approach to obesity management:

- Several models for integrated care exist in various mental health and physical health settings and can serve as models for integrated care in obesity management.

- Given the complexity of obesity, an integrated care approach can facilitate appropriate post-operative screening and treatment of patient concerns.
- Integration of technology-enhanced interventions, such as telepsychiatry and telephone-based psychosocial treatments, can support stepped-care models targeting reduced psychiatric burden and supporting long-term weight loss.
- Further research evaluating the effectiveness and cost of these collaborative care models in obesity care are needed to determine long-term benefit.

References

1. Black DW, Goldstein RB, Mason EE. Prevalence of mental disorder in 88 morbidly obese bariatric clinic patients. Am J Psychiatry. 1992;149(2):227–34.
2. Carpenter KM, Hasin DS, Allison DB, Faith MS. Relationships between obesity and DSM-IV major depressive disorder, suicide ideation, and suicide attempts: results from a general population study. Am J Public Health. 2000;90(2):251–7.
3. Friedman KE, Reichmann SK, Costanzo PR, Musante GJ. Body image partially mediates the relationship between obesity and psychological distress. Obes Res. 2002;10(1):33–41.
4. Dixon JB, Dixon ME, O'Brien PE. Depression in association with severe obesity: changes with weight loss. Arch Intern Med. 2003;163(17):2058–65.
5. Schwartz TL, Nihalani N, Jindal S, Virk S, Jones N. Psychiatric medication-induced obesity: a review. Obes Rev. 2004;5(2):115–21.
6. Russell L. Mental health care services in primary care: tackling the issues in the context of health care reform. Washington, DC: Center for American Progress; 2010.
7. Mickus M, Colenda CC, Hogan AJ. Knowledge of mental health benefits and preferences for type of mental health providers among the general public. Psychiatr Serv. 2000;51(2):199–202.
8. Pincus HA, Tanielian TL, Marcus SC, Olfson M, Zarin DA, Thompson J, et al. Prescribing trends in psychotropic medications: primary care, psychiatry, and other medical specialties. JAMA. 1998;279(7):526–31.
9. Mark TL, Levit KR, Buck JA. Datapoints: psychotropic drug prescriptions by medical specialty. Psychiatr Serv. 2009;60(9):1167.
10. Garfield RL. Mental health financing in the United States: a primer. Washington, DC: Kaiser Family Foundation; 2011.
11. Substance Abuse and Mental Health Services Administration. Results from the 2012 National Survey on drug use and health: mental health findings. Substance Abuse and Mental Health Services Administration: Rockville, MD; 2013.
12. Blount FA, Miller BF. Addressing the workforce crisis in integrated primary care. J Clin Psychol Med Settings. 2009;16(1):113–9.
13. Crowley RA, Kirschner N, Health, Public Policy Committee of the American College of Physicians. The integration of care for mental health, substance abuse, and other behavioral health conditions into primary care: executive summary of an American College of Physicians position paper. Ann Intern Med. 2015;163(4):298–9.
14. Fisher L, Dickinson WP. Psychology and primary care: new collaborations for providing effective care for adults with chronic health conditions. Am Psychol. 2014;69(4):355–63.
15. Cohen DJ, Davis MM, Hall JD, Gilchrist EC, Miller BF. A guidebook of professional practices for behavioral health and primary care integration: observations from exemplary sites. Rockville, MD: Agency for Healthcare Research and Quality; 2015.
16. Substance Abuse and Mental Health Services Administration. Health financing. 2014. Accessed at http://www.samhsa.gov/health-financing on 9 September 2016
17. Heisler EJ, Bagalman E. The mental health workforce: a primer. Washington, DC: Congressional Research Service; 2015.
18. Miller BF, Petterson S, Burke BT, Phillips Jr RL, Green LA. Proximity of providers: colocating behavioral health and primary care and the prospects for an integrated workforce. Am Psychol. 2014;69(4):443–51.
19. Hyde PS. Report to Congress on the Nation's substance abuse and mental health workforce issues. Rockville, MD: Substance Abuse and Mental Health Services Administration; 2013.
20. Chapa T. Mental health services in primary care settings for racial and ethnic minority populations. U.S. Department of Health and Human Services Office of Minority Health: Rockville, MD; 2004.
21. Blount A. Integrated primary care meets health reform. Fam Syst Health. 2010;28(2):77.
22. Wagner EH, Austin BT, Von Korff M. Organizing care for patients with chronic illness. Milbank Q. 1996; 74(4):511–44.
23. Bernstein KM, Manning DA, Julian RM. Multidisciplinary teams and obesity: role of the modern patient-centered medical home. Prim Care. 2016;43(1):53–9.
24. Archer J, Bower P, Gilbody S, Lovell K, Richards D, Gask L, et al. Collaborative care for depression and anxiety problems. Cochrane Database Syst Rev. 2012;10:CD006525.
25. Richardson LP, Ludman E, McCauley E, Lindenbaum J, Larison C, Zhou C, et al. Collaborative care for adolescents with depression in primary care: a randomized clinical trial. JAMA. 2014;312(8):809–16.
26. Unutzer J, Harbin H, Schoenbaum M, Druss B. The collaborative care model: an approach for integrating physical and mental health care in medicaid health homes. Health Home Information Resource Center

Brief. Washington, DC: Centers for Medicare & Medcaid Services; 2013.

27. Unutzer J, Katon W, Williams Jr JW, Callahan CM, Harpole L, Hunkeler EM, et al. Improving primary care for depression in late life: the design of a multicenter randomized trial. Med Care. 2001;39(8):785–99.
28. Unutzer J, Park M. Strategies to improve the management of depression in primary care. Prim Care. 2012;39(2):415–31.
29. Leblanc ES, O'Connor E, Whitlock EP, Patnode CD, Kapka T. Effectiveness of primary care-relevant treatments for obesity in adults: a systematic evidence review for the U.S. Preventive Services Task Force. Ann Intern Med. 2011;155(7):434–47.
30. Krahn DD, Bartels SJ, Coakley E, Oslin DW, Chen H, McIntyre J, et al. PRISM-E: comparison of integrated care and enhanced specialty referral models in depression outcomes. Psychiatr Serv. 2006;57(7):946–53.
31. Larjani S, Spivak I, Hao Guo M, Aliarzadeh B, Wang W, Robinson S, et al. Preoperative predictors of adherence to multidisciplinary follow-up care postbariatric surgery. Surg Obes Relat Dis. 2016;12(2):350–6.
32. Sockalingam S, Cassin S, Hawa R, Khan A, Wnuk S, Jackson T, et al. Predictors of post-bariatric surgery appointment attendance: the role of relationship style. Obes Surg. 2013;23(12):2026–32.
33. Diamant A, Milner J, Cleghorn M, Sockalingam S, Okrainec A, Jackson TD, et al. Analysis of patient attrition in a publicly funded bariatric surgery program. J Am Coll Surg. 2014;219(5):1047–55.
34. Lau DC, Douketis JD, Morrison KM, Hramiak IM, Sharma AM, Ur E, et al. 2006 Canadian clinical practice guidelines on the management and prevention of obesity in adults and children [summary]. CMAJ. 2007;176(8):S1–13.
35. Baillargeon JP, St-Cyr-Tribble D, Xhignesse M, Grant A, Brown C, Langlois MF. Impact of an integrated obesity management system on patient's care—research protocol. BMC Obes. 2014;1:19.
36. Seidell JC, Halberstadt J, Noordam H, Niemer S. An integrated health care standard for the management and prevention of obesity in the Netherlands. Fam Pract. 2012;29 Suppl 1:i153–6.
37. Pronk NP, Boucher J. Systems approach to childhood and adolescent obesity prevention and treatment in a managed care organization. Int J Obes Relat Metab Disord. 1999;23 Suppl 2:S38–42.
38. Arora S, Kalishman S, Thornton K, Dion D, Murata G, Deming P, et al. Expanding access to hepatitis C virus treatment—Extension for Community Healthcare Outcomes (ECHO) project: disruptive innovation in specialty care. Hepatology. 2010;52(3):1124–33.
39. Arora S, Kalishman S, Dion D, Som D, Thornton K, Bankhurst A, et al. Partnering urban academic medical centers and rural primary care clinicians to provide complex chronic disease care. Health Aff (Millwood). 2011;30(6):1176–84.
40. Fortney JC, Pyne JM, Edlund MJ, Williams DK, Robinson DE, Mittal D, et al. A randomized trial of telemedicine-based collaborative care for depression. J Gen Intern Med. 2007;22(8):1086–93.
41. Davis AM, Sampilo M, Gallagher KS, Dean K, Saroja MB, Yu Q, et al. Treating rural paediatric obesity through telemedicine vs. telephone: outcomes from a cluster randomized controlled trial. J Telemed Telecare. 2016;22(2):86–95.
42. Rollman BL, Belnap BH, Mazumdar S, Houck PR, Zhu F, Gardner W, et al. A randomized trial to improve the quality of treatment for panic and generalized anxiety disorders in primary care. Arch Gen Psychiatry. 2005;62(12):1332–41.
43. Simon GE, Von Korff M, Saunders K, Miglioretti DL, Crane PK, van Belle G, et al. Association between obesity and psychiatric disorders in the US adult population. Arch Gen Psychiatry. 2006;63(7):824–30.
44. Cassin SE, Sockalingam S, Du C, Wnuk S, Hawa R, Parikh SV. A pilot randomized controlled trial of telephone-based cognitive behavioral therapy for preoperative bariatric surgery patients. Behav Res Ther. 2016;80:17–22.
45. Cassin SE, Sockalingam S, Wnuk S, Strimas R, Royal S, Hawa R, et al. Cognitive behavioral therapy for bariatric surgery patients: preliminary evidence for feasibility, acceptability, and effectiveness. Cogn Behav Pract. 2013;20(4):529–43.
46. Nardone M, Snyder S, Paradise J. Integrating physical and behavioral health care: promising medicaid models. Washington, DC: Kaiser Commission on Medicaid and the Uninsured; 2014.
47. Katon W, Russo J, Lin EH, Schmittdiel J, Ciechanowski P, Ludman E, et al. Cost-effectiveness of a multicondition collaborative care intervention: a randomized controlled trial. Arch Gen Psychiatry. 2012;69(5):506–14.
48. Katon W, Unutzer J, Fan MY, Williams Jr JW, Schoenbaum M, Lin EH, et al. Cost-effectiveness and net benefit of enhanced treatment of depression for older adults with diabetes and depression. Diabetes Care. 2006;29(2):265–70.

Part III

Assessment of Psychosocial Domains in Severe Obesity Care

Weight-Based Stigma and Body Image in Severe Obesity

8

Stephanie E. Cassin and Aliza Friedman

Case Vignettes

Ms. Smith is a 30-year-old woman referred by her primary care physician for a psychosocial assessment of body image concerns, emotional eating, and depression. She also reports currently experiencing a number of medical complications associated with obesity (current body mass index [BMI] = 40 kg/m^2), including type 2 diabetes and sleep apnea. Ms. Smith describes a long-standing history of mental health issues beginning at age 7 when she first began being bullied by her peers for being overweight. She also reports being criticized by her parents as being "fat" and "lazy" throughout her childhood and adolescence. Ms. Smith states that these comments precipitated a vicious cycle of chronic dieting and emotional overeating, which has continued throughout her adult life. Ms. Smith also describes her weight as an impediment in romantic relationships, stating that former romantic partners have ended relationships with her because "they are embarrassed to have an obese girlfriend". Similarly, she reports a recent experience of discrimination in the workplace, in which her boss threatened to fire Ms. Smith if she did not lose weight to "look better in her uniform". When asked to describe how she currently feels about her body image and weight, Ms. Smith endorses internalizing anti-fat attitudes, stating, "I feel depressed and disgusted with myself every time I look in the mirror. I am incompetent and unlovable because I cannot seem to lose weight and keep it off".

S.E. Cassin, Ph.D., C.Psych. (✉)
Department of Psychology, Ryerson University, 350 Victoria St, Toronto, ON, Canada M5B 2K3

Department of Psychiatry, University of Toronto, Toronto, ON, Canada

Centre for Mental Health, University Health Network, Toronto, ON, Canada
e-mail: stephanie.cassin@psych.ryerson.ca

A. Friedman, M.A.
Department of Psychology, Ryerson University, 350 Victoria St, Toronto, ON, Canada M5B 2K3
e-mail: aliza.friedman@psych.ryerson.ca

8.1 Introduction

In this chapter, we first review the negative effects associated with weight-based stigma and discrimination in individuals with severe obesity, challenges with the assessment of these constructs, and some promising psychosocial interventions for stigma reduction. We then provide

S. Sockalingam, R. Hawa (eds.), *Psychiatric Care in Severe Obesity*,
DOI 10.1007/978-3-319-42536-8_8

an overview of body image in individuals with severe obesity, including body image concerns, the impact of weight loss and psychosocial interventions on body image, and issues regarding the assessment of body image in individuals with severe obesity. Finally, we return to the case example and discuss some tools that can be used to assess weight-related stigma/discrimination and body image in individuals with severe obesity.

8.2 Weight-Based Stigma in Individuals with Severe Obesity

Weight-based stigma, defined as negative attitudes towards individuals on the basis of their weight and shape, is often considered to be the last socially acceptable form of bias [1, 2]. Commonly endorsed stereotypes about individuals with obesity include beliefs that they are lazy, overemotional, sexually inexperienced, and lacking self-control [2]. These biases are pervasive, and have been reported in numerous populations, including children [3], high school teachers [4], and college students [5]. Even healthcare professionals are not immune to weight-based stigma; in fact, anti-fat biases have been endorsed by dietetics students [6], registered nurses [7], psychologists [8], primary care physicians [9], and healthcare professionals specializing in obesity [10].

Although some researchers have proposed that stigma could be harnessed as an effective strategy for targeting public health concerns such as obesity [11, 12], there is little evidence to suggest that being a target of weight-based stigma improves weight loss outcomes. Experiencing weight-based stigma instead produces a paradoxical effect [13], such that targeted individuals have been found to demonstrate poorer weight loss outcomes in a behavioural weight loss treatment program [14], as well as avoidance of exercise [15]. Experimental studies highlight the same phenomenon: exposure to weight-based stigmatizing news articles actually increases caloric consumption among women who self-identify as overweight or obese [13]. In addition to poorer weight loss outcomes, experiencing weight-based stigma is also associated with numerous adverse psychological and physical health outcomes, including increased rates of psychological distress [16], disordered eating [16], and suicide ideation [17].

8.2.1 Stigma, Perceived Discrimination, and Internalized Weight Bias

8.2.1.1 Stigma

According to sociologist Erving Goffman [18], stigma is defined as an “attribute that is deeply discrediting” for the individual (p. 3). Goffman states that there are three different types of stigma: “abominations of the body” (i.e. stigmas associated with physical disfigurement), “blemishes of individual character” (i.e. characterological stigmas such as sexual orientation or mental illness), and “tribal stigmas” (i.e. stigmas such as race that are passed on from one generation to the next; p. 4). Given that obesity is associated with physical unattractiveness [19, 20] and a host of negative personality characteristics [2], obesity can be conceptualized as both a physical and characterological stigma [21]. Additionally, unlike many other forms of stigma, individuals who are overweight or obese are typically considered to be personally responsible for their condition [22], which in turn makes them more vulnerable to the experience of discrimination [21]. These findings are consistent with attribution theory, which proposes that both stigmatized individuals and their observers undergo a process whereby they seek to determine the cause of a stigma (i.e. the reason why an individual is obese). Weiner and colleagues [22] describe that often the stigma itself (i.e. obesity) is associated with an attribution (e.g. laziness, poor self-control), which then prevents individuals from looking for other plausible causes of an individual’s condition (e.g. genetics, differences in metabolism).

Although the majority of research studies thus far have focused on individuals’ (both obese and non-obese) attitudes towards those with obesity

[3–10], more recent studies have begun to focus on the experiences of individuals who are overweight or obese. With respect to stigma specifically, researchers have begun exploring individuals' concerns over experiencing weight stigma [13, 23], suggesting that even suspecting or anticipating weight stigma may lead to deleterious outcomes [23].

8.2.1.2 Perceived Discrimination

Weight-based stigma often leads to discriminatory treatment against individuals with obesity, which can be defined as "the inappropriate and potentially unfair treatment of individuals due to group membership" ([24], p. 8). Individuals with obesity report experiencing discriminatory treatment in a number of situations, including healthcare, employment, and educational settings, as well as within interpersonal relationships [25]. Andreyeva, Puhl, and Brownell [26] measured the prevalence of perceived discrimination in the United States related to individuals' weight or height, and found that the prevalence of perceived weight/height discrimination has increased by 66% in recent years, from 7.3% in 1996 to 12.2% in 2006. Although average BMI remained relatively stable across weight categories over the 10-year period (aside from the category of BMI ≥ 45 kg/m^2), the prevalence of weight/height discrimination nevertheless increased for each BMI category for people with a BMI of 27–29 kg/m^2 (overweight) and 31–40 kg/m^2 (obese).

Prevalence ratings of perceived discrimination increase substantially when considering individuals who are severely obese. Puhl, Andreyeva, and Brownell [27] found that 40% of individuals with a BMI ≥ 35 kg/m^2 reported experiencing either some major form of lifetime weight/height discrimination (e.g. being denied a bank loan) or daily interpersonal discrimination (e.g. being called names or insulted), with discrimination in employment-based settings occurring most frequently. When comparing the prevalence of weight/height discrimination to other types of discrimination, weight/height discrimination was the third most prevalent form of perceived discrimination for women (following gender and age) and the fourth most prevalent form of discrimination among men and women combined (following gender, age, and race) [27]. Taken together, these findings demonstrate that perceived weight discrimination is highly prevalent within society today, and is growing at a rate that exceeds the rising prevalence of obesity.

8.2.1.3 Internalized Weight Bias

In addition to examining concerns regarding weight-based stigma and perceived discrimination in individuals with obesity, researchers have also begun to assess whether they internalize negative attitudes regarding weight. Unlike other minority groups (e.g. Asians, gay/bisexual men and women), individuals who are overweight or obese do not demonstrate a favourable in-group bias [1, 28, 29], and instead actually internalize anti-fat stereotypes [1, 30, 31].

There are a number of differences between individuals with obesity and other stigmatized groups (e.g. race, sexual orientation) that may account for the lack of favourable in-group bias. First, Major, Eliezer, and Rieck [32] highlight that individuals often become obese later in life, which allows them a substantial amount of time to internalize the negative stereotypes against those with obesity prior to becoming obese and joining that group themselves. Second, individuals who are obese might perceive that they can disassociate from the stigmatized group at any time by losing weight, which may prevent them from connecting to the group and learning to dispel negative obesity stereotypes [28]. Finally, although most diets do not lead to long-term positive health or weight loss benefits [33], obesity is often perceived to be within an individual's personal control [22]. Given that stigmas associated with greater perceived controllability have been found to engender less pity, greater levels of anger, and less willingness to assist [34], individuals who are obese must cope with this additional contributor to stigma not present in many other stigmatized groups (e.g. race, gender, age).

8.2.2 Weight-Based Stigma and Negative Outcomes

Research conducted to date demonstrates that weight stigma concerns, perceived weight-based discrimination, and weight bias internalization are each associated with a host of negative outcomes among individuals who are overweight or obese. Controlling for BMI, adverse outcomes include increased rates of depression and anxiety [35], poorer weight loss treatment outcomes in a behavioural weight loss treatment program [14], as well as greater impairment in mental and physical quality of life [36]. Accordingly, Puhl and Heuer [37] highlight that weight stigma is a serious public health concern that must be properly addressed in order to target the obesity epidemic.

Much of the research examining the relations between weight-based stigma and binge eating has focused specifically on weight bias internalization. Weight bias internalization has been associated with objective binge eating episodes in adolescents seeking bariatric surgery [38], and with increased binge eating in adult men and women with obesity [39], including those seeking weight loss treatment [40]. Similarly, Durso and Latner [30] demonstrated that weight bias internalization was associated with greater binge frequency over a 6-month period in a group of adults who were overweight or obese.

The effects of experiencing weight-based stigma and perceiving weight-based discrimination have also been examined in relation to binge eating and emotional eating. For example, in a sample of adults seeking bariatric surgery, Friedman and colleagues [35] found that the frequency of stigmatizing situations experienced within the past month predicted greater emotional eating and a current diagnosis of Binge Eating Disorder (BED). Furthermore, increased frequency of stigmatizing situations has also been associated with higher rates of binge eating and poorer weight loss treatment outcomes in adults enrolled in a behavioural weight loss treatment programme [14]. Finally, Ashmore and colleagues [16] found that lifetime occurrence of weight stigmatization was associated with increased rates of binge eating in adults with obesity. Regarding perceived discrimination, Farrow and Tarrant [41] found that perceived weight-based discrimination among college students with varied BMIs was associated with greater emotional eating. Similarly, in a sample of adults with varied BMIs, Durso and colleagues [42] found that perceived interpersonal discrimination (e.g. everyday encounters in interpersonal settings) and institutional discrimination (e.g. perceived job loss due to one's weight) predicted greater emotional eating and higher binge eating frequency at 3 months, with stronger relations for interpersonal discrimination.

Taken together, these findings demonstrate that there is a positive association between experiencing weight-based stigma, perceiving weight-based discrimination, and internalizing anti-fat attitudes with negative psychological outcomes across a variety of populations (e.g. adults with obesity, weight loss treatment-seeking adults, bariatric surgery-seeking adolescents).

8.2.3 Assessment of Weight-Based Stigma and Discrimination in Individuals with Severe Obesity

There are a number of challenges that impact assessment of weight-based stigma and discrimination. First, although constructs such as weight stigma concerns, perceived discrimination, and internalized weight bias are related, these terms are often erroneously used interchangeably. For example, until the development of the Weight Bias Internalization Scale (WBIS) [30], which measures the extent to which individuals who are overweight or obese endorse negative attributions about obesity as being true for themselves specifically, measures of anti-fat attitudes were understood as representing weight bias internalization. Durso and Latner [30] posit that holding negative attributions towards individuals who are overweight or obese does not necessarily indicate that individuals hold these beliefs for themselves, necessitating the separation of holding anti-fat attitudes towards individuals who are overweight or obese, and weight bias internalization (i.e. holding these negative attributions about oneself).

Second, measures assessing weight stigma experiences (i.e. experiencing others making negative weight-related assumptions) are often confounded with perceived discrimination (i.e. the behavioural manifestation of stigma). For example, the Stigmatizing Situations Inventory (SSI; [43]) is a self-report scale that measures frequency of stigmatizing experiences. Three of the items on the scale assess the experience of having others make negative weight-related assumptions (e.g. "having people assume you have emotional problems because you are overweight"), whereas the remaining items refer to experiencing a variety of stigmatizing situations such as interpersonal interactions (e.g. "nasty comments from children"), physical barriers (e.g. "not being able to fit into seats at restaurants, theatres, and other public places"), and job discrimination (e.g. "losing a job because of your size"). Perceived discrimination is typically assessed in a similar manner, using self-report inventories that measure experiences of discrimination in employment, healthcare, and educational settings (e.g. "not given a job promotion"), as well as in interpersonal interactions (e.g. "receive poorer service than other people at restaurants or stores") [26]. Thus, the experience of stigmatizing situations and perceived discrimination are *both* primarily measuring perceptions of interpersonal and institutional discrimination, suggesting that the experience of weight-based stigma (as it is currently measured) and perceived discrimination may in fact represent the same phenomenon.

Third, constructs including weight stigma concerns, perceived discrimination, and internalized weight bias are not typically assessed simultaneously within one research study, which hinders the interpretation of findings within and across research studies. For example, in a sample of women who were overweight or obese, Pearl, Puhl, and Dovidio [44] found that weight bias internalization was negatively correlated with motivation to exercise and self-efficacy to engage in exercise, whereas weight stigma experiences were positively correlated with current exercise frequency. These findings suggest that varied weight stigma constructs may be associated with differential health-related outcomes.

Finally, a major limitation with the current assessment of weight-based stigma and discrimination is the lack of widely used measures with good psychometric properties. Researchers often develop their own individual measures to assess the desired constructs within their studies, which further hinders cross-study comparisons.

8.2.4 Treatment of Internalized Weight-Based Stigma

Studies evaluating the effectiveness of weight-based stigma reduction interventions have been described as the most needed studies to advance society's understanding of weight-based stigma [25]. To date, only one study has examined the impact of a therapeutic intervention on internalized stigma and perceived discrimination reduction in individuals with obesity. Lillis and colleagues [45] found that a 6-hour mindfulness and acceptance-based workshop that focused on teaching participants to mindfully accept (rather than avoid) their stigmatizing experiences was effective in improving obesity-related stigma and psychological distress 3 months following the workshop in treatment-seeking adults with obesity. These preliminary results suggest that acceptance and mindfulness-based therapeutic interventions may help to reduce internalized stigma and perceived discrimination in individuals with severe obesity. Furthermore, interventions that incorporate compassion-focused techniques, psychoeducation, and cognitive restructuring have all demonstrated promising results in other stigmatized populations (e.g. HIV-positive gay and bisexual men; individuals with mental illness; [46, 47]), and could potentially be modified for individuals with severe obesity.

8.3 Body Image in Individuals with Severe Obesity

Body image refers to an individual's beliefs, perceptions, cognitions, emotions, and behaviours pertaining to his/her physical appearance [48, 49]. The factors contributing to body image are complex and multidimensional [50]. Historical influences on body image include factors such as cultural socialization, interpersonal experiences, physical characteristics and changes, and personality factors [50]. Cultural socialization includes messages that are disseminated regarding the cultural ideal of attractiveness—for example, thinness is valued whereas obesity is stigmatized; therefore, people are expected to engage in body modification through diet, exercise, and medical procedures to achieve the societal expectation. Interpersonal experiences contributing to body image include weight-based teasing, rejection, or criticism by family, peers, and others, as well as weight-based discrimination. The extent of discrepancy that exists between a person's actual physical characteristics and the cultural ideal impacts not only how the person is evaluated and treated by others, but also how the person evaluates him- or herself. In addition, the evaluation depends on changes in physical characteristics, such as whether a person has recently been gaining or losing weight [51]. Moreover, those with predisposing personality characteristics, such as low self-esteem and perfectionism, are at heightened risk of developing negative body image. These historical influences are not mutually exclusive, but rather, interact in complex ways to influence body image. Moreover, the historical influences are helpful in understanding the ways in which weight-based stigma and discrimination contribute to body image.

8.3.1 Body Image Concerns in Individuals with Obesity

There is a strong link between obesity and poor body image [51]; however, substantial heterogeneity exists among individuals with obesity. Some of the factors that have been shown to increase the risk of body image concerns include female gender, presence of binge eating disorder, current weight gain trajectory, and the subjective experience of weight cycling (more so than objective weight fluctuations) [51].

Much of the research examining body image in individuals with obesity has focused on women, likely because they are over-represented among treatment-seeking samples. However, studies including both men and women suggest that body image concerns are greater among women [51]. The majority of women with obesity report negative body image concerning their weight, and approximately half identify their abdomen and waist region as the greatest area of concern [52]. Although body image concerns are prevalent among women in the community, the concerns reported by women with obesity exceed those reported by non-obese women [51–53]. For example, women seeking weight loss surgery report less appearance satisfaction, greater body image dysphoria, and greater impairment in body image quality of life relative to normative samples [54].

8.3.2 The Impact of Negative Body Image

Individuals with obesity do not necessarily have higher rates of psychological distress than non-obese individuals; however, negative body image has been proposed as a potential mediator of the relationship between obesity and psychological distress [55]. That is, individuals with obesity and poor body image will be at increased risk of psychological symptoms relative to those without significant body image concerns. Body image has indeed been shown to partially mediate the relationship between obesity and psychological symptoms (depression and low self-esteem) in treatment-seeking men and women [35].

It is a dangerous misconception that the psychological distress associated with weight-based stigma and discrimination should motivate individuals with obesity to lose weight. Some psychological distress is likely required for most people (including healthy weight individuals) to persist in making all types of behavioural changes. However, high levels of distress (e.g. negative body image, depression, low self-esteem) can be very counterproductive to weight loss efforts because it can cause people to feel self-conscious while engaging in physical activity and doubt their likelihood of successful weight loss through diet and exercise, which in turn makes it difficult to persist with healthy behavioural changes [51, 53]. In fact, body dissatisfaction and psychological distress can actually be a trigger for eating and weight-related problems [56].

8.3.3 The Impact of Weight Loss on Body Image

The desire to improve appearance and body image is often reported as being among the most important motives for weight loss [57]. A recent systematic review and meta-analysis reported that body image improves in individuals with obesity enrolled in weight loss programmes [58]. A recent study found that women with severe obesity participating in a 6-month behavioural intervention focused on nutrition and physical activity improved their weight, and that weight loss was a mediator of improved body satisfaction [59]. Importantly, improvements in body image are typically observed with modest weight loss, and prior to achieving a healthy weight. For example, significant improvements in body image have been reported in individuals who lose 5–10 % of their body weight through a behavioural weight loss program; however, improvements in body image observed during weight loss treatment begin to deteriorate if weight regain occurs [60]. Even for previously overweight individuals who are able to maintain a healthy weight, their body image typically remains lower relative to individuals who have never been overweight. This phenomenon of residual body image concerns following weight loss has been termed "phantom fat" [61].

Significant improvements in body image have also been reported following surgical weight loss treatment, including improvements in appearance evaluation and reductions in body dissatisfaction, weight/shape concerns, and feelings of fatness [62–65]. Moreover, the improvements in body image following surgery are associated with a number of positive outcomes, including improvements in physical and mental quality of life [64, 66], as well as sexual functioning and psychological functioning [67].

The impact of bariatric surgery on body image is not uniformly positive. Although body image does improve following surgery, it remains more negative than body image reported in the general population [62, 64]. This finding could be due in part to the "phantom fat" phenomenon described above. However, another major contributing factor is the excess skin that develops in most patients due to the dramatic weight loss that occurs within a very short period of time [68]. As a result, many patients feel conflicted about their body image—on the one hand, they feel satisfied with the overall reduction in their body weight and size, and on the other hand, they feel dissatisfied with the appearance of the redundant and hanging skin which leaves them feeling "abnormal" or "deformed" and susceptible to stereotypes and discrimination from others [69, 70]. Patients often report engaging in a number of avoidance behaviours as a result of the excess skin, such as wearing certain clothes, showing their bodies to others, and participating in social activities. Despite the excess skin, most patients report that the overall benefits of bariatric surgery outweigh the costs. However, a small minority of patients find the excess skin so distressing that they regret their decision to have surgery [68], and other patients report intentionally regaining some weight because they prefer the appearance of a larger body over excess skin [69].

In addition to the development of excess skin, the "mind–body lag" is another issue that occurs in many patients as a result of losing a substantial amount of weight in a short time period [69]. This phenomenon refers to the time lag that often occurs between the physical changes to the body, and the cognitive and behavioural changes associated with weight loss. That is, despite losing a substantial amount of weight, patients continue to perceive themselves as obese—a finding that has been attributed to a failure to update the "body schema" following weight loss [71]. As a result, patients continue to behave in ways consistent with their body distortions. For example, some patients report bringing seat belt extenders, searching for seats without arm rests, turning sideways through turnstiles, and shopping in plus size stores long after weight loss has occurred.

8.3.4 The Impact of Psychosocial Interventions on Body Image

Psychosocial interventions have demonstrated that it is possible to improve body image independent of weight loss. Cognitive behavioural interventions focused on body image and weight acceptance typically include cognitive strategies such as cognitive restructuring (e.g. identifying, challenging, and altering negative thoughts concerning body image), and behavioural strategies such as exposure to situations that are typically avoided as a result of poor body image. Given the multidimensional nature of body image concerns, clinicians are advised to target multiple facets of body image, including cognitive, behavioural, and affective components [54].

Cognitive behavioural interventions have been shown to improve body image-related distress and psychological distress (e.g. self-esteem, depression) [72–74]. One study that compared a behavioural weight control intervention to a combined behavioural weight control plus cognitive behavioural body image intervention reported that the combined treatment did not confer additional benefit [75]. Given that weight loss alone appears to have a powerful impact on body image, some have recommended that cognitive behavioural body image interventions be offered during the weight maintenance phase for optimal benefit [76, 77]. A cognitive behavioural intervention enhanced with virtual reality has been found to improve body image and weight loss outcomes in individuals with severe obesity and BED [78], and virtual reality-based treatments appear promising for individuals with obesity who experience significant body distortion [79].

8.3.5 Assessment of Body Image Concerns in Individuals with Severe Obesity

Body image is a multidimensional construct, making the assessment of body image quite complex. It consists of both a perceptual component (i.e. accuracy of body size estimation) and attitudinal component. The attitudinal component comprises global satisfaction, as well as affective, cognitive, and behavioural components [80]. Global satisfaction refers to overall body satisfaction/dissatisfaction (e.g. body weight or shape, or particular body sites), and is typically assessed using questionnaires or figural ratings (i.e. the discrepancy between their perceived "actual" body and "ideal" body figures). The affective component includes feelings such as anxiety, discomfort, or shame related to appearance. The cognitive component includes beliefs, thoughts, and appraisals related to appearance, such as the importance that people place on their appearance and the influence it has on their overall self-worth (i.e. appearance investment). The behavioural component includes the behavioural manifestations of body image, such as body checking (e.g. frequent weighing and mirror checking) and avoidance of body image triggers (e.g. avoidance of scales or mirrors). The affective, cognitive, and behavioural components of body image are typically assessed using questionnaires.

The complexity in assessing body image is further complicated by the fact that many existing measures have significant limitations when used to assess body image in individuals with severe obesity. Most of the commonly used measures [80] were designed for women with eating disorders or non-obese individuals, which has a number of implications for the assessment of body image in individuals (and particularly men) with obesity. First, many questions may have different meanings for individuals with severe obesity. An individual with a body mass index of 55 kg/m^2 may endorse the item, "My stomach is too big", for reasons other than body image concerns, including being aware of the medical issues associated with abdominal adiposity. It is possible for a person to prefer a thinner body or desire to lose weight for health reasons while still generally feeling positive towards his or her current body [51]. Unfortunately, the questionnaires do not distinguish between these various factors. As a result, two individuals with a body mass index of 55 and 19 kg/m^2 may receive the same high score on a measure of body dissatisfaction; however, this score would be more pathological for an individual with a low to healthy body weight. Unfortunately, given that most commonly used measures were developed for women with eating disorders and non-obese individuals, normative data are not available for individuals with severe obesity, which makes it difficult to interpret their scores on these measures. This limitation is further amplified in men with obesity.

Second, the measures simply may not be suitable for individuals with severe obesity. For example, scales commonly used to assess body image estimation and body dissatisfaction include figures or silhouettes ranging from underweight to overweight. Respondents are asked to indicate their current body size and ideal body size. However, the respondent may have a different distribution of weight (e.g. relatively smaller upper body and larger lower body) than the well-proportioned figures presented in the rating scale. In addition, the respondent's size might actually exceed the largest figure on the rating scale (even after significant weight loss) because the scales do not include adequate coverage of obese bodies. Not only would such a measure be unhelpful in the assessment of body image, but it could also be perceived as a stigmatizing experience that could trigger additional weight-related concerns in respondents.

Third, the existing measures used to assess body image do not take into consideration excess skin resulting from radical weight loss. As noted earlier, many bariatric surgery patients feel ambivalent about their post-surgical bodies. They are generally satisfied with their reduced weight and size and feelings of "fatness", but feel that the excess skin is a "deformity", which in some cases leaves them feeling more body-conscious and causes them to avoid more body image triggers than they did at a higher weight. As a result, many measures may overestimate positive body image following radical weight loss because the measures tend to focus on the aspects that these individuals are most satisfied with and neglect other aspects (i.e. excess skin) that contribute to great distress. Commonly used body image measures are typically not suitable for many individuals with appearance-altering medical conditions [81], and the excess skin that results from radical weight loss could be considered an appearance-altering medical condition. Altering the instructions, items, and response format of existing validated body image measures can change the psychometric properties [81]; thus, it will be important for future research to create body image measures suitable for individuals with severe obesity, including those who experience radical weight loss, and to collect normative data for these populations.

Case Vignettes: Assessment of Weight-Based Stigma and Body Image

In working with Ms. Smith, it would be helpful to assess her experiences with weight-based stigma and discrimination, as well as her body image. Given the current lack of commonly used measures to assess concerns regarding weight-based stigma and perceived discrimination, many studies have developed weight stigma-specific modified versions of well-established scales utilized in other populations. For example, the Stigma-Consciousness Questionnaire [82] and the Everyday Discrimination Scale [83] have been modified to assess for weight stigma concerns and perceived discrimination, respectively [13, 23, 84]. The Stigmatizing Situations Inventory [43] could also be used to assess the frequency with which Ms. Smith has experienced stigmatizing experiences; however, it is important to note this measure's limitation of conflating weight-based stigma and perceived discrimination. Furthermore, the Weight Bias

(continued)

(continued)

Internalization Scale [30] or the Weight Self-Stigma Questionnaire [85] could be used to assess Ms. Smith's acceptance of anti-fat attitudes as being true for herself. In order to evaluate Ms. Smith's attitudes towards individuals who are overweight or obese, the clinician could administer the Anti-Fat Attitudes Questionnaire [28], the Universal Measure of Bias-FAT version (UMB-FAT) [1], or the Fat Phobia Scale-short form [86].

Keeping in mind the caveats noted above regarding the assessment of body image in severe obesity, it is important to select measures suitable for Ms. Smith. To assess global body image, the clinician could use the Body Shape Questionnaire [87], Body Satisfaction Scale [88], or Multidimensional Body Self-Relations Questionnaire—Appearance Evaluation Body Areas Satisfaction Scale [89]. The Situational Inventory of Body Image Dysphoria [90] could be used to assess the affective component of body image. The Multidimensional Body Self-Relations Questionnaire—Appearance Orientation Scale [89] or Appearance Schemas Inventory-Revised [91] could be used to assess the cognitive component of body image. The Body Checking Questionnaire [92] and Body Image Avoidance Questionnaire [93] could be used to assess the behavioural component of body image. In addition, the Body Image Quality of Life Inventory [94] would be helpful in determining the impact of body image on quality of life. Although none of these measures were developed specifically for use with individuals with obesity, they have been used in populations with obesity. In addition to administering these measures of body image, it would be beneficial to inquire about distress and avoidance behaviours associated with excess skin from previous weight loss attempts if that issue is relevant to Ms. Smith.

8.4 Summary and Take-Home Messages

- Individuals with severe obesity have greater body image and weight stigma concerns relative to non-obese individuals
- Weight-based stigma and discrimination have been associated with disordered eating, suicide ideation, and psychological distress
- The assessment of weight-based stigma and discrimination is limited by conflation among constructs and a lack of widely used measures with good psychometric properties
- Acceptance- and mindfulness-based therapeutic interventions appear to offer promising results for weight-based stigma reduction
- Weight loss and cognitive behavioural body image interventions have both been shown to improve body image
- The assessment of body image is complex due to the multidimensional nature of body image and the unique issues in assessing body image in populations with severe obesity

8.5 Appendix: Helpful Tips for Healthcare Professionals

- Consider the physical space of a medical office environment. Purchasing larger blood pressure cuffs and gowns as well as seats that accommodate individuals who are overweight or obese will help ensure that a space is more inclusive.

- Be aware of any biases that you may have towards individuals who are overweight or obese, and work towards overcoming them.
- Recognize that stigmatizing comments and discriminatory treatment do not promote weight loss and instead contribute to increased levels of disordered eating and psychological distress.

References

1. Latner JD, O'Brien KS, Durso LE, Brinkman LA, MacDonald T. Weighing obesity stigma: the relative strength of different forms of bias. Int J Obes. 2008;32(7):1145–52.
2. Puhl R, Brownell KD. Bias, discrimination, and obesity. Obes Res. 2001;9(12):788–805.
3. Davison KK, Birch LL. Predictors of fat stereotypes among 9-year-old girls and their parents. Obes Res. 2004;12(1):86–94.
4. Neumark-Sztainer D, Story M, Harris T. Beliefs and attitudes about obesity among teachers and school health care providers working with adolescents. J Nutr Educ. 1999;31(1):3–9.
5. Regan PC. Sexual outcasts: the perceived impact of body weight and gender on sexuality. J Appl Soc Psychol. 1996;26(20):1803–15.
6. Berryman DE, Dubale GM, Manchester DS, Mittelstaedt R. Dietetics students possess negative attitudes towards obesity similar to nondietetics students. J Am Diet Assoc. 2006;106(10):1678–82.
7. Poon MY, Tarrant M. Obesity: attitudes of undergraduate student nurses and registered nurses. J Clin Nurs. 2009;18(16):2355–65.
8. Davis-Coelho K, Waltz J, Davis-Coelho B. Awareness and prevention and bias against fat clients in psychotherapy. Prof Psychol Res Pr. 2000;31(6):682–4.
9. Hebl MR, Xu J. Weighing the care: physicians' reactions to the size of a patient. Int J Obes. 2001;25:1246–52.
10. Schwartz MB, Chambliss HO, Brownell KD, Blair SN, Billington C. Weight bias among health professionals specializing in obesity. Obes Res. 2003;11(9):1033–9.
11. Bayer R. Stigma and the ethics of public health: not can we but should we. Soc Sci Med. 2008;67(3):463–72.
12. Stuber J, Meyer I, Link B. Stigma, prejudice, discrimination and health. Soc Sci Med. 2008;67(3):351–7.
13. Major B, Hunger JM, Bunyan DP, Miller CT. The ironic effects of weight stigma. J Exp Soc Psychol. 2014;51:74–80.
14. Wott CB, Carels RA. Overt weight stigma, psychological distress and weight loss treatment outcomes. J Health Psychol. 2009;15(4):608–14.
15. Vartanian LR, Novak SA. Internalized societal attitudes moderate the impact of weight stigma on avoidance of exercise. Obesity (Silver Spring). 2011;19(4):757–62.
16. Ashmore JA, Friedman KE, Reichmann SK, Musante GJ. Weight-based stigmatization, psychological distress, and binge-eating behavior among obese treatment-seeking adults. Eat Behav. 2008;9(2):203–9.
17. Chen EY, Fettich KC, McCloskey MS. Correlates of suicidal ideation and/or behavior in bariatric-surgery-seeking individuals with severe obesity. Crisis. 2012;33(3):137–43.
18. Goffman E. Stigma: notes on the management of spoiled identity. New York: Simon & Schuster; 1963.
19. Harris MB, Harris RJ, Bochner S. Fat, four-eyed and female: stereotypes of obesity, glasses, and gender. J Appl Soc Psychol. 1982;12(6):503–16.
20. Wigton RS, McGaghie WC. The effect of obesity on medical students' approach to patients with abdominal pain. J Gen Intern Med. 2001;16(4):262–5.
21. DeJong W. The stigma of obesity: the consequences of naive assumptions concerning the causes of physical deviance. J Health Soc Behav. 1980;21(1):75–87.
22. Weiner B, Perry RP, Magnusson J. An attributional analysis of reactions to stigmas. J Pers Soc Psychol. 1988;55(2):738–48.
23. Hunger JM, Major B, Blodorn A, Miller C. Weighed down by sigma: how weight-based social identity threat contributes to weight gain and poor health. Soc Personal Psychol Compass. 2015;9(6):255–68.
24. Dovidio JF, Hewstone M, Glick P, Esses VM. Prejudice, stereotyping, and discrimination: theoretical and empirical overview. In: Dovidio JF, Hewstone M, Glick P, Esses VM, editors. The SAGE handbook of prejudice, stereotyping, and discrimination. London: Sage; 2010. p. 3–28.
25. Puhl RM, Heuer CA. The stigma of obesity: a review and update. Obesity (Silver Spring). 2009;17(5):941–64.
26. Andreyeva T, Puhl RM, Brownell KD. Changes in perceived weight discrimination among Americans, 1995–1996 through 2004–2006. Obesity (Silver Spring). 2008;16(5):1129–34.
27. Puhl RM, Andreyeva T, Brownell KD. Perceptions of weight discrimination: prevalence and comparison to race and gender discrimination in America. Int J Obes. 2008;32(6):992–1000.
28. Crandall CS. Prejudice against fat people: ideology and self-interest. J Pers Soc Psychol. 1994;66(5):882–94.
29. Rudman LA, Feinberg J, Fairchild K. Minority members' implicit attitudes: automatic ingroup bias as a function of group status. Soc Cogn. 2002;20(4):294–320.
30. Durso LE, Latner JD. Understanding self-directed stigma: development of the weight bias internalization scale. Obesity (Silver Spring). 2008;16 Suppl 2:S80–6.

31. Wang SS, Brownell KD, Wadden TA. The influence of the stigma of obesity on overweight individuals. Int J Obes. 2004;28(10):1333–7.
32. Major B, Eliezer D, Rieck H. The psychological weight of weight stigma. Soc Psychol Personal Sci. 2012;3(6):651–8.
33. Mann T, Tomiyama AJ, Westling E, Lew AM, Samuels B, Chatman J. Medicare's search for effective obesity treatments: diets are not the answer. Am Psychol. 2007;62(3):220–33.
34. Menec VH, Perry RP. Reactions to stigmas among Canadian students: testing an attribution-affect-help judgment model. J Soc Psychol. 1998;138(4):443–53.
35. Friedman KE, Reichmann SK, Costanzo PR, Zelli A, Ashmore JA, Musante GJ. Weight stigmatization and ideological beliefs: relation to psychological functioning in obese adults. Obes Res. 2005;13(5):907–16.
36. Latner JD, Durso LE, Mond JM. Health and health-related quality of life among treatment-seeking overweight and obese adults: associations with internalized weight bias. J Eat Disord. 2013;1:3.
37. Puhl RM, Heuer CA. Obesity stigma: important considerations for public health. Am J Public Health. 2010;100(6):1019–28.
38. Roberto CA, Sysko R, Bush J, Pearl R, Puhl RM, Schvey NA, Dovidio JF. Clinical correlates of the weight bias internalization scale in a sample of obese adolescents seeking bariatric surgery. Obesity (Silver Spring). 2012;20(3):533–9.
39. Puhl RM, Moss-Racusin CA, Schwartz MB. Internalization of weight bias: implications for binge eating and emotional well-being. Obesity (Silver Spring). 2007;15(1):19–23.
40. Carels RA, Wott CB, Young KM, Gumble A, Koball A, Oehlhof MW. Implicit, explicit, and internalized weight bias and psychosocial maladjustment among treatment-seeking adults. Eat Behav. 2010;11(3): 180–5.
41. Farrow CV, Tarrant M. Weight-based discrimination, body dissatisfaction and emotional eating: the role of perceived social consensus. Psychol Health. 2009;24(9):1021–34.
42. Durso LE, Latner JD, Hayashi K. Perceived discrimination is associated with binge eating in a community sample of non-overweight, overweight, and obese adults. Obes Facts. 2012;5(6):869–80.
43. Myers A, Rosen JC. Obesity stigmatization and coping: relation to mental health symptoms, body image, and self-esteem. Int J Obes. 1999;23(3):221–30.
44. Pearl RL, Puhl RM, Dovidio JF. Differential effects of weight bias experiences and internalization on exercise among women with overweight and obesity. J Health Psychol. 2015;20(12):1626–32.
45. Lillis J, Hayes SC, Bunting K, Masuda A. Teaching acceptance and mindfulness to improve the lives of the obese: a preliminary test of a theoretical model. Ann Behav Med. 2009;37(1):58–69.
46. Mittal D, Sullivan G, Chekuri L, Allee E, Corrigan PW. Empirical studies of self-stigma reduction strategies: a critical review of the literature. Psychiatr Serv. 2012;63(10):974–81.
47. Skinta MD, Lezama M, Wells G, Dilley JW. Acceptance and compassion-based group therapy to reduce HIV stigma. Cogn Behav Pract. 2015; 22(4):481–90.
48. Cash TF. The body image workbook: an eight-step program for learning to like your looks. 2nd ed. Oakland: New Harbinger; 2008.
49. Grogan S. Body image: understanding body dissatisfaction in men, women, and children. London: Routledge; 1999.
50. Cash TF. Cognitive behavioral perspectives on body image. In: Cash TF, Smolak L, editors. Body image: a handbook of science, practice, and prevention. 2nd ed. New York: The Guilford Press; 2011. p. 39–47.
51. Schwartz MB, Brownell KD. Obesity and body image. Body Image. 2004;1(1):43–56.
52. Sarwer DB, Wadden TA, Foster GD. Assessment of body image dissatisfaction in obese women: specificity, severity, and clinical significance. J Consult Clin Psychol. 1998;66(4):651–4.
53. Sarwer DB, Thomspon JK, Cash TF. Body image and obesity in adulthood. Psychiatr Clin North Am. 2005;28(1):69–87.
54. Ghai A, Milosevic I, Laliberte M, Taylor VH, McCabe RE. Body image concerns in obese women seeking bariatric surgery. Ethn Inequalities Health Soc Care. 2014;7(2):96–107.
55. Friedman MA, Brownell KD. Psychological correlates of obesity: moving to the next research generation. Psychol Bull. 1995;117(1):3–20.
56. Bucchianeri MM, Neumark-Sztainer D. Body dissatisfaction: an overlooked public health concern. J Public Ment Health. 2014;13(2):64–9.
57. Levy AS, Heaton AW. Weight control practices of US adults trying to lose weight. Ann Intern Med. 1993;119(7 Pt 2):661–6.
58. Chao H-L. Body image change in obese and overweight persons enrolled in weight loss intervention programs: a systematic review and meta-analysis. PLoS One. 2015;10(5):e0124036.
59. Annesi JJ, Porter KJ. Reciprocal effects of exercise and nutrition treatment-induced weight loss with improved body image and physical self-concept. Behav Med. 2015;41(1):18–24.
60. Foster GD, Wadden TA, Vogt RA. Body image in obese women before, during, and after weight loss treatment. Health Psychol. 1997;16(3):226–9.
61. Cash TF, Counts B, Huffine CE. Current and vestigial effects of overweight among women: fear of fat, attitudinal body image, and eating behaviors. J Psychopathol Behav Assess. 1990;12(2):157–67.
62. Adami GF, Meneghelli A, Bressani A, Scopinaro N. Body image in obese patients before and after stable weight reduction following bariatric surgery. J Psychosom Res. 1999;46(3):275–81.
63. Camps MA, Zervos E, Goode S, Rosemurgy AS. Impact of bariatric surgery on body image perception and sexuality in morbidly obese patients and their partners. Obes Surg. 1996;6(4):356–60.
64. Dixon JB, Dixon ME, O'Brien PE. Body image: appearance orientation and evaluation in the severely

obese. Changes with weight loss. Obes Surg. 2002;12(1):65–71.
65. Hrabosky JI, Masheb RM, White MA, Rothschild BS, Burke-Martindale CH, Grilo CM. A prospective study of body dissatisfaction and concerns in extremely obese gastric bypass patients: 6- and 12-month postoperative outcomes. Obes Surg. 2006;16(12):1615–21.
66. Sarwer DB, Wadden TA, Moore RH, Eisenberg MH, Raper SE, Williams NN. Changes in quality of life and body image after gastric bypass surgery. Surg Obes Relat Dis. 2010;6(6):608–14.
67. Pujols Y, Seal BN, Meston CM. The association between sexual satisfaction and body image in women. J Sex Med. 2010;7(2 Pt 2):905–16.
68. Kitzinger HB, Abayev S, Pittermann A, Karle B, Bohdjalian A, Langer FB, et al. After massive weight loss: patients' expectations of body contouring surgery. Obes Surg. 2012;22(4):544–8.
69. Lyons K, Meisner BA, Sockalingam S, Cassin SE. Body image after bariatric surgery: a qualitative study. Bariatr Surg Pract Patient Care. 2014;9(1): 41–9.
70. Magdaleno R Jr, Chaim EA, Pareja JC, Turato ER. The psychology of bariatric patient: what replaces obesity? A qualitative research with Brazilian women. Obes Surg. 2011;21(3):336–9.
71. Guardia D, Metral M, Pigeyre M, Bauwens I, Cottencin O, Luyat M. Body distortions after massive weight loss: lack of updating of the body schema hypothesis. Eat Weight Disord. 2013;18(3):333–6.
72. Bacon L, Keim NL, Van Loan MD, Derricote M, Gale B, Kazaks A, et al. Evaluating a 'non-diet' wellness intervention for improvement of metabolic fitness, psychological well-being and eating and activity behaviors. Int J Obes Relat Metab Disord. 2002;26(6):854–65.
73. Rosen JC, Orosan P, Reiter J. Cognitive behavioural therapy for negative body image in obese women. Behav Ther. 1995;26(1):25–42.
74. Roughan P, Seddon E, Vernon-Roberts J. Long-term effects of a psychologically based group programme for women preoccupied with body weight and eating behaviour. Int J Obes. 1990;14(2):135–47.
75. Ramirez EM, Rosen JC. A comparison of weight control and weight control plus body image therapy for obese men and women. J Consult Clin Psychol. 2001;69(3):440–6.
76. Cooper Z, Fairburn CG. Cognitive behavioural treatment of obesity. In: Wadden TA, Stunkard AJ, editors. Handbook of obesity treatment. New York: The Guilford Press; 2002. p. 465–79.
77. Sarwer DB, Thompson JK. Obesity and body image disturbance. In: Wadden TA, Stunkard J, editors. Handbook of obesity treatment. New York: The Guilford Press; 2002. p. 447–64.
78. Cesa GL, Manzoni GM, Bacchetta M, Castelnuovo G, Conti S, Gaggioli A, et al. Virtual reality for enhancing the cognitive behavioral treatment of obesity with binge eating disorder: randomized controlled study with one-year follow-up. J Med Internet Res. 2013;15(6):e113.
79. Ferrer-Garcia M, Gutierrez-Maldonado J, Giuseppe R. Virtual reality based treatments in eating disorders and obesity: a review. J Contemp Psychother. 2013;43(4):207–21.
80. Menzel JE, Krawczyk R, Thompson JK. Attitudinal assessment of body image for adolescents and adults. In: Cash TF, Smolak L, editors. Body image: a handbook of science, practice, and prevention. 2nd ed. New York: The Guilford Press; 2011. p. 154–69.
81. Cash TF. Crucial considerations in the assessment of body image. In: Cash TF, Smolak L, editors. Body image: a handbook of science, practice, and prevention. 2nd ed. New York: The Guilford Press; 2011. p. 129–37.
82. Pinel EC. Stigma consciousness: the psychological legacy of social stereotypes. J Pers Soc Psychol. 1999;76(1):114–28.
83. Williams DR, Yan Y, Jackson JS, Anderson NB. Racial differences in physical and mental health: socio-economic status, stress, and discrimination. J Health Psychol. 1997;2(3):335–51.
84. Sutin AR, Terracciano A. Perceived weight discrimination and obesity. PLoS One. 2013;8(7):e70048.
85. Lillis J, Luoma JB, Levin ME, Hayes SC. Measuring weight self-stigma: the weight self-stigma questionnaire. Obesity (Silver Spring). 2010;18(5):971–6.
86. Bacon JG, Scheltema KE, Robinson BE. Fat Phobia Scale revisited: the short form. Int J Obes. 2001;25(2):252–7.
87. Cooper PJ, Taylor MJ, Cooper Z, Fairburn CG. The development and validation of the Body Shape Questionnaire. Int J Eat Disord. 1987;6(4):485–94.
88. Slade PD, Dewey ME, Newton T, Brodie D, Kiemle G. Development and preliminary validation of the Body Satisfaction Scale. Psychol Health. 1990;4(3):213–20.
89. Brown TA, Cash TF, Mikulka PJ. Attitudinal body-image assessment: factor analysis of the Body-Self Relations Questionnaire. J Pers Assess. 1990;55(1–2):135–44.
90. Cash TF. The situational inventory of body-image dysphoria: psychometric evidence and development of a short form. Int J Eat Disord. 2002;32(3):362–6.
91. Cash TF, Melnyk SE, Hrabosky JL. The assessment of body image investment: an extensive revision of the Appearance Schemas Inventory. Int J Eat Disord. 2004;35(3):305–16.
92. Reas DL, Whisenhunt BL, Netemeyer R, Williamson DA. Development of the body checking questionnaire: a self-report measure of body checking behaviors. Int J Eat Disord. 2002;31(3):324–33.
93. Rosen JC, Srebnik D, Saltzberg E, Wendt S. Development of a body image avoidance questionnaire. J Consult Clin Psychol. 1991;3(1):32–7.
94. Cash TF, Fleming EC. The impact of body image experiences: development of the body image quality of life inventory. Int J Eat Disord. 2002;31(4):455–60.

9 Mood Disorders and Severe Obesity: A Case Study

Giovanni Amodeo, Mehala Subramaniapillai, Rodrigo B. Mansur, and Roger S. McIntyre

Case Vignettes

Lisa is a 28-year-old Caucasian female. She is single, unemployed and lives with her parents. She has been receiving long-term disability due to her severe depression. She is diagnosed with major depressive disorder (MDD) and she visits a mood disorder clinic for a comprehensive second opinion, as requested by her current psychiatrist. There is a history of mental health problems in her family. Lisa's mother also suffered from MDD and her uncle died by suicide at the age of 33. Furthermore, her sister is diagnosed with generalized anxiety disorder. Lisa was first diagnosed with MDD in her early twenties, during the latter years of her undergraduate studies. She noted long periods of low energy, lack of pleasure in the activities she used to enjoy and inability to go to class and fulfill her course requirements. As a result of these symptoms, she discontinued enrollment at university.

Lisa currently weighs 120 kg, with a BMI of 32 kg/m^2. She has been struggling with increased body weight throughout her life, which has been an enduring source of guilt and shame. Notwithstanding, Lisa finds food comforting when she is faced with the various challenges and notes it to temporarily reduce her anxiety. Lisa sleeps 10 hours per night and often finds that she needs to nap during the day. She reports having an insatiable appetite, often eating two dinners—one in the early evening and again before bed, in order to satisfy her hunger.

(continued)

G. Amodeo, M.D.
Department of Psychiatry, Department of Molecular Medicine and Development, University of Siena School of Medicine, Viale Bracci, 1, Via XXIV Maggio, 23, Siena 53100, Italy
e-mail: giovanniamodeo86@gmail.com

M. Subramaniapillai, H.B.Sc., M.Sc. (✉)
R.B. Mansur, M.D.
Mood Disorders Psychopharmacology Unit, University Health Network, 399 Bathurst Street, MP 9-325, Toronto, ON, Canada M5T 2S8
e-mail: m.subram@mail.utoronto.ca; Rodrigo.Mansur@uhn.ca

R.S. McIntyre, M.D., F.R.C.P.C.
Mood Disorders Psychopharmacology Unit, University Health Network, 399 Bathurst Street, MP 9-325, Toronto, ON, Canada M5T 2S8

Department of Psychiatry and Pharmacology, University of Toronto, Toronto, ON, Canada

Executive Director, Brain and Cognition, Discovery Foundation (BCDF), University of Toronto, Toronto, ON, Canada
e-mail: roger.mcintyre@uhn.ca

S. Sockalingam, R. Hawa (eds.), *Psychiatric Care in Severe Obesity*,
DOI 10.1007/978-3-319-42536-8_9

(continued)

During her visit to the clinic, Lisa also reports having difficulty concentrating on her day-to-day tasks, such as difficulty focusing on what she is reading and holding conversations with others. She is a heavy smoker, consuming a more than half-a-pack per day for the past 5 years. Lisa also noted that she has sought treatment for her inflammatory bowel disorder.

At the present visit, she denies drug or alcohol misuse. She denies suicidal or homicidal ideation, although she reports that she has had suicidal ideation in the past. She is currently taking 150 mg of venlafaxine XR once daily.

9.1 Introduction

Mood disorders, including major depressive disorder (MDD) and bipolar disorder (BD), have a high prevalence and morbidity. MDD has a 4.33 % overall global point prevalence [1], whereas BD has an estimated lifetime prevalence of 1.5 % [2]. Collectively, mood disorders are common and serious mental illnesses associated with substantial costs to individuals and society. "Burden of illness" studies provide replicated evidence that mood disorders are leading categories of the indicators of high disability-adjusted life years (DALYs) and years lived with disability (YLDs).

In addition to mood disorders, overweight and obesity are also a public health priority. Epidemiological studies have estimated that about 50 % of individuals in the Organization for Economic Co-operation and Development (OECD) countries are currently overweight and 18 % are affected by mild-to-severe obesity [3]. In addition, obesity is linked to numerous metabolic and physical health complications, such as type 2 diabetes, dyslipidemia, increased risk of cardiovascular events, diseases of the musculoskeletal system, and different forms of cancer [4].

As mentioned previously in this book, mood disorders and obesity frequently co-exist [148]. Individuals with MDD have an increased probability of obesity, notably abdominal obesity that is up to 50 % greater than the matched general population [5]. In addition to the extensive overlap of MDD and obesity, the prevalence of obesity is also increased in individuals with BD [6,144]. Conversely, obese patients also have a higher risk of incident depressive and manic symptoms/episodes [7–9]. Individually, both mood disorders and obesity have a high rate of morbidity and the co-occurrence often incurs a more severe and complicated illness presentation [10]. Consequently, comorbid obesity in persons with a mood disorder is not only a proxy of elevated risk of mortality and increased public health costs, but also a primary therapeutic target [11].

Although traditionally mood disorders and obesity have been considered as two separate entities, epidemiological, longitudinal, and clinical studies have shown that the co-occurrence of both conditions do bi-directionally influence each other and alter illness trajectory, presentation, and outcome. Although there may not yet be definitive evidence to support this view, some authors have proposed a "metabolic-mood syndrome," highlighting the relationship between these two diseases with features of bi-directionality and convergence [12, 13].

This chapter intends to provide an overview of both mood disorders and obesity, followed by studies examining the presence of obesity in mood disorders and mood disorders in obesity. The subsequent section will examine the emerging paradigm of the "metabolic-mood syndrome" and the various factors that characterize this relationship between mood and metabolism, including genetic, and environment risk factors. An examination of antidepressants and their impact on obesity will also be provided, specifically examining the serotonin norepinephrine re-uptake inhibitors (SNRIs) and selective serotonin re-uptake inhibitors (SSRIs). This chapter will conclude by revisiting the case study presented at the beginning of this chapter.

9.2 Mood Disorders

Mood disorders represent a category of illness characterized by pathological changes in mood, both positive (manic and hypomanic) and negative (depressive episodes). These changes in mood are also often accompanied by cognitive deficits, changes in neuro-vegetative function and physical health. A longstanding interest in psychiatry has been to sub-classify different subtypes of mood disorders with an overarching aim of providing prognostication and informing treatment selection. Achieving the foregoing goal, however, is belied by the clinical and pathoetiological heterogeneity of these disorders. Although the DSM-5 [14] has separate chapters for depressive disorders and bipolar disorders, recognition of overlap in both disorders is well established. Each mood disorder may be characterized by varying rates of severity, and specific features of onset (e.g., seasonal, postpartum), course (e.g., remitting, recurrent), and etiology (exogenous, endogenous) [15].

The etiology of mood disorders is polygenic and multifactorial. According to preclinical and clinical studies, data-driven hypothesis indicates that mood disorders are the result of multiple interacting risk factors (genetic, environmental, biological) [16–18, 147]. Given this heterogeneity, it is not surprising that patient response to existing multimodality therapies is variable and unpredictable [19–21].

9.3 Obesity

Overweight and obesity are defined as abnormal or excessive fat accumulation that represents a risk to health. The National Heart, Lung, and Blood Institute (NHLBI) guidelines define overweight as a body mass index (BMI) between 25.0 and 29.9 kg/m^2, obesity as a BMI of ≥30 kg/m^2, and extreme obesity as a BMI of ≥40 kg/m^2. Most people develop obesity from a combination of excessive food intake and a sedentary lifestyle. However, risk factors, such as genetic and environmental factors, are involved in the regulation of body weight, appetite, adiposity, as well as levels of physical activity. As such, there are wide individual differences around the mechanism of weight gain [22–24, 143]. Furthermore, there is also ample evidence to demonstrate that hormonal pathways and insulin resistance are involved in the development of obesity [25, 26] (see Chapter 3).

Overweight and obesity are major risk factors for a number of chronic diseases, including type 2 diabetes, hypertension, dyslipidemia, cardiovascular diseases, and severe cancers. However, there seem to be specific subgroups of obese patients that are lacking these comorbidities, termed "Metabolically Healthy Obese" (MHO), with a risk of cardiovascular disease similar to healthy subjects [27]. Conversely, individuals with healthy body weight can display obesity-associated illnesses, which have been called "Normal-Weight Obese" (NWO) [28, 29]. Another interesting phenomenon is the "Obese Paradox," where several clinical trials have shown that in patients with type 2 diabetes, kidney failure or heart failure, increased body weight appeared to be a protective factor, decreasing the patients' rate of mortality when compared with normal-weight subjects [30, 31]. There are divergent opinions about the validity of this paradox [32], but emerging data suggest that body weight is a correlate of metabolic abnormalities with tremendous variation between individuals in their metabolic signature.

9.4 Clinical Studies of Obesity in Mood Disorders

Community studies have been conducted with an aim of exploring the correlation between mood disorders and obesity. Kendler et al. [33] performed a community retrospective study using the data from 1,029 pairs of female twins, assessing depressive symptoms and BMI values. They concluded that a high percentage (28.9 %) of individuals with atypical depressive symptoms also had a higher BMI (>28.6 kg/m^2) than individuals with typical or severe depressive symptoms [33]. A prospective community study performed in adolescents investigated the relationship between mood disorders in youth and obesity in early adulthood. Patients were evaluated first in 1983 (adolescence) and again in 1992 (young adulthood). The authors described a correlation between those with a high BMI in adolescence and incident depression in adulthood ($p<0.01$). Furthermore, there was also a significant correlation between women with obesity in adulthood with an increased prevalence of depression symptoms in youth [34]. In another study, Roberts et al. [35] evaluated 1,886 patients (≥50 years of age) in 1994 (MDD = 7.3 %), with a repeat evaluation in 1999. They reported a 65 % higher rate of obesity when compared to those without depression. Moreover, the presence of depression at index evaluation also predicted obesity at the follow-up visit 5 years later (OR = 1.92; 95 % CI = 1.31–2.80) [35]. Another community study was performed in 591 young adults (292 males, 299 females) between the ages of 18 and 19 years, comparing those with mood disorders to their healthy peers, and then following them until the age of 40 years. At the first assessment, 19 % of the sample was defined as overweight. The results show a significant association between atypical depression and overweight in both men and women (OR = 2.8, 95 % CI = 1.6, 4.8; $p<0.01$). Specifically, women with a history of childhood depressive symptoms had higher mean BMI (21.9 %; 95 % CI = 0.5, 2.0; $p<0.01$) and higher average weight gain between the ages of 20 and 40 years than women without childhood depressive symptoms. It was further noted that hypomanic symptoms were associated with weight gain only in men [36].

A cross-sectional study with a sample of 49 patients with mood disorders (29 BD) treated with long-term lithium had a higher rate of severe obesity (12 %) than the general population (5.7 %) [37]. In addition, there are large differences in the reported correlation of obesity and mood disorders as a function of gender. For instance, McElroy et al. [38] assessed a sample of 644 individuals with BD (type I and II) across the United States and Europe and found that 57 % of patients were overweight or obese (31 % overweight, 21 % obese, and5 % severely obese). When compared with the healthy population, this sample showed that BD females have a high rate of obesity or severe obesity (BMI >40 kg/m^2). Males with BD instead showed a high rate of overweight and obesity but not an elevated rate of severe obesity [38]. With a large sample (n = 175), Fagiolini et al. [39] demonstrated that, compared with non-obese BD patients, obese BD patients had fewer years of schooling, earlier depressive and manic episodes, higher depressive symptoms at baseline, and required a longer course of treatment during the acute phase to achieve remission. Furthermore, obese patients experienced a relapse (n = 25, 54 %) at a higher rate than non-obese patients and the time-to-relapse was shorter than among patients who were not obese at baseline. Specifically, recurrences of depressive symptoms were significantly greater for obese patients (n = 15, 33 %) than for non-obese patients (n = 11, 14 %) [39]. In an analysis of data from a Canadian community survey (n = 36,984), McIntyre et al. [40] reported that individuals with a lifetime history of a mood disorder were more likely to be obese (19 %) than those without a mood disorder (15 %, $p<0.05$). The age-adjusted rate of overweight or obesity (BMI ≥25 kg/m^2) in persons with BD I was significantly higher than that of the general population (55 % vs. 48 %, $p<0.01$) [40].

In an analysis of data from 9,125 respondents in the National Comorbidity Survey-Replication (NCS-R), obesity was significantly associated with a lifetime diagnosis of BD (OR = 1.47; 95 % CI: 1.12–1.93) and this association was greater for BD present in the last 12 months (OR = 1.61; 95 % CI: 1.07–2.43) [41]. Furthermore, evaluating data from 43,093 respondents in the National Epidemiological Survey on Alcohol and Related Conditions (NESARC) revealed that adults with lifetime BD had a significantly greater age-, race-, and sex-adjusted prevalence of obesity compared to control subjects (OR = 1.65, 95 % CI:1.45–1.89; $p<0.01$) [42]. Conversely, in the same dataset, obesity was associated with any mood disorder, including a manic episode (OR = 1.55; 95 % CI: 1.29–1.86 for obesity and OR = 2.70; 95 % CI: 2.00–3.66 for severe obesity) [43].

9.5 Clinical Studies of Mood Disorders in Obesity

There are also numerous studies assessing mood disorders in patients with severe obesity. However, most of these studies have reported mood disorders based on informal clinical interview, self-report scales, and/or psychological tests. Only a few studies have used clinician-administered structured diagnostic interviews, such as the Mini International Neuropsychiatric Interview (M.I.N.I.), to diagnose mood disorders in study participants. Several studies have assessed symptoms of depression, anxiety, distress, or stress among obese patients and individuals seeking treatment for obesity (e.g., ileal bypass, gastric bypass operations, bariatric surgery, and other forms of anti-obesity treatments). A review of 11 studies, with a combined sample of 837 obese patients, found that mood disorders were assessed with DSM criteria (any edition) among ten studies. The review demonstrated that a large percentage (32 %, n = 294) of obese patients met DSM criteria for lifetime mood disorders (MDD, BD I, BD II, dysthymia). Specifically, among studies that used structured clinical interviews to assess syndromal mood disorders, 41 % of patients had a mood disorder in their lifetime, compared with 24 % of patients in studies that did not use structured clinical interviews [44].

Similarly, Black et al. [45] reported a significantly high proportion of MDD (19 % vs. 5 %) and other mood disorders (31 % vs. 9 %) among a sample of 88 obese patients undergoing bariatric surgery, compared to individuals of normal weight. Furthermore, a clinical study performed on a sample of 47 adolescents and young adult patients receiving inpatient treatment for severe obesity (mean BMI = 42.2 kg/m^2) found that 19 obese adolescents (43 %) met DSM-IV criteria for mood disorders (14 MDD, 5 BD) compared with 8 (17 %) out of the 47 mild obese patients (mean BMI = 29.8 kg/m^2) and 247 (15 %) of 1,608 healthy control subjects [46].

9.6 The Metabolic-Mood Syndrome

Taken together, the overlap of mood disorders and obesity provides the basis for proposing a patho-etiological framework that has both discrete and shared pathophysiological substrates that subserve both phenotypes. Herein, we describe the features of this bidirectional and convergent relationship.

9.6.1 Phenomenology

The presentation and the clinical features of mood disorders are frequently different and more complicated when a patient is obese. Overweight or obese patients tend to present atypical depressive symptoms with greater frequency (e.g., reactive mood, increased appetite, hypersomnia, leaden paralysis) when compared to depressed patients of normal weight. Conversely, depression with melancholic features, depression that is not meeting criteria for any existing DSM5-defined specifier, has a prevalence of association with obesity similar to the general population [5, 47–50]. Although it could be postulated that obesity is a mere consequence of the food intake and lack of physical activity associated with atypical depression, results described above indicate that obesity in itself subsequently increases the risk of developing depressive symptoms as well the risk of suicide and cognitive impairment [51–53].

Furthermore, when obesity co-occurs with depression, it usually has a more chronic course [54]. Similarly, the co-occurrence of obesity with BD is linked to a predominance of depressive symptoms and need for hospitalization, with longer depressive phases when compared to BD patients with normal body weight [42]. Obesity also adversely affects the response to pharmacological treatment of mood disorders. Clinical trials have shown that obese patients with BD have a reduced probability of response to antidepressants and to lithium/valproate, respectively [55–60]. In addition, comorbid mood disorders have a negative impact on both the pharmacological and surgical interventions of obesity [61].

9.6.2 Genetic Factors

Genetic factors are involved in both mood disorders and obesity. Major depressive disorder and BD are illnesses with elevated rates of heritability (30–50 % and 50–70 %, respectively) [62, 63]. The genetics of both mood disorders and obesity are considered polygenic, with alterations being described in a large number of genes [64–66].

Surprisingly, there are specific genes that are involved in both diseases and, in some instances, there is evidence of interactions. For example, the FTO (fat mass and obesity-associated) gene is related to the development of obesity, and a recent study has shown that this correlation is mitigated by the presence of depressive symptoms [67].

9.6.3 Environmental Risk Factors

Obesity and mood disorders have several environmental risk factors (i.e., social determinants of health) in common and the bi-directionality between the two clinical entities is evident. Generally, psychosocial stress is considered to be one of the biggest risk factors for developing a mood disorder and consequential emotional eating behaviors, leading to overweight and obesity [68–70]. Sedentary lifestyle and unhealthy diet can also lead to the development of obesity, but recent results have proffered a possible causative role of mood disorders [71, 72]. However, the most replicated epidemiological factor that precedes a mood disorder is childhood trauma (sexual, emotional, or physical) [73]. Emerging data have underscored the involvement of this risk factor in obesity [74].

9.6.4 Metabolic Systems

Endocrinological and inflammatory mechanisms have been recognized as factors that contribute to the development of both obesity and mood disorders. The hypothalamic–pituitary–adrenal (HPA) axis is involved in the mobilization of energy reserves to restore energy homeostasis through its hormonal action on various regions of the body, including adipose tissue. Obese individuals often have a dysfunctional HPA axis, which can lead to increased food intake and lack of hunger satisfaction. Individuals with mood disorders also have alterations in the HPA axis. In fact, BD patients have an increased secretion of cortisol during euthymic, depressive, and manic periods, and show a reduced response and reactivity to stress. The relationship between mood disorders and inflammatory disorders has been a significant focus of research during the last decade. Several meta-analyses have shown high levels of pro-inflammatory cytokines (e.g. TNF-α, IL-6) in the blood of patients with MDD and BD [75–77]. Excess adipose tissue can lead to inflammatory dysregulation, with the body being in a chronic and persistent low-grade inflammatory state, with select studies noting persistently high levels of C-reactive protein (CRP) in obese patients [78]. Interestingly, Milaneschi et al. [79] found a relationship between leptin, an adipose-derived hormone involved in the regulation of food intake and energy expenditure, and depressive symptoms. In particular, they found that elevated levels of leptin secretion by central adiposity could facilitate the development of depressive mood over a 9-year follow-up period [79].

9.6.5 Brain Substrates

Mood disorders are clinical conditions associated with alterations in brain structures and functions. It has been shown that MDD and BD are subserved by abnormalities in the structure and function of neural circuits that govern reward/emotion regulation and cognitive functions. For example, neuroimaging studies have reported alterations in functional connectivity at different levels of brain networks, such as frontal-occipital, frontal-amygdala, and subcortical regions [80–82]. Recently, it has been suggested that obesity could have pathological brain biomarkers involved in the regulation of motivation and reward (e.g. in fronto-occipital and fronto-amygdala networks) both at resting-state and in response to food and non-food rewarding stimuli, indicating that abnormalities extend beyond appetite regulation [83, 84]. Furthermore, data from neuroimaging studies have shown that a reduction in white matter, often present in MDD, is significantly linked to a higher BMI value [85]. More prominent alterations of temporal, parietal, and occipital structures were also found in patients with depression and higher BMIs [86].

Several studies implicate the monoamine systems (e.g. dopamine and serotonin) in the regulation of reward mechanisms and control of food intake [87–89]. Mood disorders are characterized by dopamine dysfunction—induction of abnormal mood changes by manipulating dopamine and its receptors is well documented in animal and pharmacological studies [90]. In addition, medications targeting the dopamine receptors (e.g. antipsychotics or antidepressants) are effective in dealing with heterogeneous symptoms that characterize mood disorders [91]. Neuroimaging studies have shown an involvement of dopaminergic circuits in patients with MDD and BD [92–94]. Obese subjects, both in preclinical and clinical studies, have a reduced availability of dopamine receptors in direct proportion to their BMI value. In particular, dopamine receptors are highly sensitive to stimuli, such as high-calorie food, but they have poor sensitivity to reward and feelings of hunger satisfaction.

An alteration in energy metabolism is also a common factor to mood disorders and obesity. The mitochondria system is the cellular network responsible for energy metabolism. Neuroimaging studies have shown that mitochondrial function is impaired in mood disorders, leading to altered concentrations of creatine, lactate, and *n*-acetylaspartate in the brain [95–99]. Studies in obese patients have demonstrated similar alterations in brain concentrations of these components [100–102]. An important factor involved in regulating energy metabolism is the neurotrophin Brain-Derived Neurotropic Factor (BDNF). The dysregulation of BDNF plays a significant role in the etiopathogenesis of mood disorders. Multiple studies have illustrated that many antidepressants stimulate an increased production in BDNF that is involved in processes of neuroplasticity, such as dendritic arborization, axonal growth, neuronal differentiation mechanisms, and neurodegeneration functions [103, 104]. Patients with MDD and BD, in all phases, have reduced serum concentrations of BDNF compared to healthy individuals [105, 106]. BDNF is also involved in regulating energy metabolism by modulating neuronal transport of glucose, mitochondrial function, and by regulating the intercellular energy homeostasis [107, 108]. Preclinical studies have shown that a reduction in BDNF in the periphery produces hyperphagia and body weight gain. In contrast, BDNF appears to be inhibited in patients with severe anorexia or those with significant food restriction and enhanced by energy availability [109, 110].

Finally, it is also important to consider the role of the endocannabinoid system (ECS), as it also seems to be involved in energy metabolism. Rimonabant, a medication with antagonistic action on the endocannabinoid type 1 receptor (CB1), has recently been discontinued as an anti-obesity agent due to the emergence of depressive and anxiety symptoms and suicidal ideation [111, 112]. Several animal studies demonstrated antidepressant-like and anxiolytic-like effects of endocannabinoids [113–115]. Furthermore, clinical studies indicate an endocannabinoid dysregulation in obesity, with altered concentrations of endocannabinoids in serum, saliva, and adipose tissue of obese patients [116–119].

9.7 Antidepressant Medications and Severe Obesity: An Overview

The FDA-approved drugs for the treatment of mood disorders are anticonvulsants, antipsychotics, and antidepressants. Many of these drugs are linked to weight gain, leading to severe obesity and contributing to the development of metabolic diseases by altering metabolic parameters (i.e. lipids, insulin-resistance, glucose). Antipsychotic agents can be classified based on their risk for weight gain and subsequent development of metabolic diseases. Different antipsychotics confer high (clozapine and olanzapine), medium (risperidone and quetiapine) or low (amisulpride, asenapine, aripiprazole, lurasidone, and ziprasidone) risk [120]. The treatment with lithium and valproate is also linked with weight gain/obesity and thus, may also influence metabolic parameters. Lamotrigine appears to have a low risk of inducing weight gain/obesity. In an 18-month, multicenter, placebo-controlled study where patients were treated with lamotrigine for the last 8 weeks of an open-label phase, obese patients with BD I (n = 155) had significant weight loss with lamotrigine when compared with the placebo group [121]. Weight gain associated with anticonvulsants and antipsychotics are discussed in detail in a subsequent chapter (Chap. 22).

The following section provides an overview of two classes of antidepressants used to treat MDD and BD: serotonin norepinephrine re-uptake inhibitors and selective serotonin re-uptake inhibitors as they relate to obesity. Generally, second-generation, atypical antidepressant medications have a neutral or a beneficial role in body weight, inducing weight loss. Herein, we provide evidence from clinical trials that have evaluated the most commonly used antidepressant medications, examining their potency to induce weight changes. Interestingly, most of these clinical trials have samples composed of overweight and obese patients who were affected by Binge Eating Disorder (BED). At the moment, there are no studies that have evaluated antidepressants among participants who have a co-occurrence of both mood disorders and obesity. However, this type of evaluation is necessary in the future to have a comprehensive view of the relationship between body weight management and antidepressant drugs.

9.7.1 Serotonin Norepinephrine Re-Uptake Inhibitors

9.7.1.1 Venlafaxine

A 4-month retrospective clinical study involving 35 obese patients with BED found that venlafaxine (from 75 to 300 mg/day) is able to induce changes in body weight. The patients had significant reduction in their BMI values (M=2.00 kg/m^2; range: −2.75–1.25 kg/m^2) and body weight (M= −10.90 kg; range −15.18 to −6.62 kg) [122]. On the contrary, a recent clinical trial, investigating the relationship of long-term antidepressant use with weight gain/obesity, found that a high percentage of patients in treatment with venlafaxine (67 %) experienced a 7 % increase in body weight from baseline [123]. It is likely that the difference in body weight outcomes is correlated with other factors, such as age of onset, environmental risk factors, and gender.

9.7.1.2 Duloxetine

A 12-week open-label study involving 45 patients with a diagnosis of BED and obesity treated with flexible doses of duloxetine (30–90 mg/day) showed a statistically significant reduction in weight [124]. Recently, a 12-week randomized-controlled trial (RCT) by Guerdjikova et al. [125] assessed the efficacy of a flexible dose of duloxetine vs. placebo in 40 patients with a diagnosis of BED according to the DSM–IV–TR criteria and a concurrent comorbid depressive disorder. In their initial longitudinal analysis, duloxetine was found to be superior to the placebo in reducing weight (p = 0.04). However, the endpoint analysis results did not confirm these findings.

9.7.2 Selective Serotonin Re-Uptake Inhibitors

9.7.2.1 Fluvoxamine

Gardiner et al. [126] conducted a 9-week open-label study involving five patients with BED treated with fluvoxamine at 100–200 mg/day and reported significant weight loss and BMI reductions. Hudson et al. [127] found similar results in a study with 85 obese BED patients, who were randomized to receive either placebo or fluvoxamine at 300 mg/day (starting dose 50 mg/day). Results show a statistically significant reduction in BMI (M = −0.167 kg/m^2; SD = 0.08). The estimated mean weight loss after 9 weeks of fluvoxamine treatment was 2.7 lbs, compared with 0.3 lbs for placebo (p<0.04). Notwithstanding, both studies have methodological limitations, such as small sample sizes and short treatment durations. However, a longer-term (12-week) double-blind, placebo-controlled trial (n = 20) performed by Pearlstein et al. [128] found no statistical differences in weight change between fluvoxamine at 150 mg/day and a placebo.

9.7.2.2 Sertraline

McElroy et al. [129] conducted a 6-week clinical trial, with 34 patients affected by obesity and BED using sertraline at 50 mg/day. A statistically significant reduction in BMI (M = 0.596 kg/m^2; SD = 0.189) was observed at the end of the trial. Similar results were found in a 12-week RCT (n = 20) 5 years later [130]. Patients who received sertraline at 100 mg/day showed a 9 % reduction in body weight after 2 weeks of treatment [130]. In another 24-week study with a sample of 32 obese patients with BED, sertraline was administered in doses ranging from 100 to 200 mg/day [131]. At the 12-week follow-up, a reduction of more than 5 % in body weight was recorded in 64 % of the sample. These intermediate results were confirmed at the conclusion of the study, after 24 weeks.

9.7.2.3 Fluoxetine

In 1996, Greeno and Wing [132] conducted a study on 79 patients with a BMI between 30 and 45 kg/m^2, who were assigned to treatment with a placebo or fluoxetine at 60 mg/day. After 6 days of treatment, the subjects receiving fluoxetine showed a significant reduction in their caloric intake from baseline compared to those treated with placebo. Similar results were found by Arnold et al. [133] after a 6-week RCT of 60 patients with BED and obesity comparing fluoxetine at 20–80 mg/day to a placebo. A significant reduction in BMI and weight was reported at the endpoint analysis, but not a reduction in the number of binge eating episodes.

9.7.2.4 Citalopram and Escitalopram

McElroy et al. [134] assessed the efficacy of citalopram for treatment of BED using a placebo-controlled design. Patients with BED (n = 38) received either placebo or citalopram (from 20 to 60 mg/day) for 6 weeks. The endpoint analysis showed a statistically significant reduction in BMI (M = −0.81 kg/m^2; SD = 0.25) and weight loss (M = −2.49 kg; SD = 0.66). Guerdjikova et al. [135] evaluated the efficacy of escitalopram at 30 mg/day vs. placebo in 44 obese patients with BED over a 12-week study. The main results were a significant reduction in BMI and binge eating episodes per week.

9.7.2.5 Bupropion

Several studies [136, 137] report that bupropion is effective in the treatment of hyperplasic depressed patients and overweight/obese subjects. Calandra et al. [138] conducted a retrospective cohort study to compare the effectiveness of sertraline and bupropion over a period of 24 weeks in obese depressed patients with BED. The study assessed 15 patients treated with bupropion at 150 mg/day and 15 with sertraline at 200 mg/day. After 24 weeks of treatment, greater weight loss was recorded in the bupropion group (p<0.01) compared with the sertraline group. It is also notable that, in the bupropion group, the patients with a higher BMI showed greater weight loss. Combinations of bupropion and naltrexone are currently being used for the treatment of obesity and are well described in detail in a subsequent chapter regarding anti-obesity agents and relative effects on psychiatric symptoms [139, 140].

This overview of select clinical trials highlights the wide variability of antidepressant agents on influencing weight gain. It is strongly recommended that psychiatrists choose antidepressants with a low metabolic risk profile in patients with known metabolic risk factors (e.g., clinical history, eating behavior, BMI, genetic, environmental, and biologic), as these factors could be predictive of increases in body weight for select agents.

Back to the Case Vignettes

Lisa's diagnosis of MDD is confirmed at the Mood Disorders Clinic. She is advised to continue taking 150 mg of venlafaxine XR once daily. Lisa can also try adding another antidepressant, such bupropion, to help with her ongoing depressive symptoms. However, the effectiveness of a combined antidepressant treatment strategy, or other medication combinations (e.g., psychostimulants), to mitigate weight gain is not well established. Lisa is strongly encouraged to engage in physical activity and participate in a behavioral weight-loss intervention, as these programs for individuals with a serious mental illness have been shown to be effective [141]. We also advised Lisa to seek behavioral and weight loss counseling to manage her weight.

9.8 Conclusion

During the past two decades, the connection between mood disorders and obesity has been widely highlighted and this focus has been greatly investigated by researchers. Both conditions share considerable overlap in their phenomenology, patho-etiology, social determinants, and illness course (i.e. chronicity).

Clinical studies reviewed herein indicate that patients with mood disorder have a higher risk of developing weight gain/obesity, and obese patients have an increased risk of developing mood disorders, with an overrepresentation of MDD characterized by atypical features, anxiety symptoms, and chronic course. The involvement of common risk factors (genetic, environmental, developmental); brain substrates surrounding reward, emotion regulation and cognitive functions; and common metabolic mechanisms suggest the existence of unique pathophysiological processes underlying both illnesses (e.g., immune-inflammatory, stress-correlated). For instance, anhedonia, a central symptom of depression, has been linked to obesity through mechanisms of reward and emotional control. Furthermore, recent evidence suggests that anhedonia is strongly associated with eating behavior, increasing food intake in uncontrolled, emotional, and binge eating [142].

The recognition of a syndrome that unifies the two diseases into a single entity, the "metabolic-mood syndrome," would serve to create a subtype of patients on whom to perform further investigations in order to improve outcomes, ameliorate course, and personalize treatments. In order to propose and confirm this new concept, clinical studies, based on the several psychopathological domains and considering multidimensional metabolic dysfunctions, are necessary.

9.9 Take Home Messages

- There is a strong, bi-directional relationship between mood disorders and obesity.
- When treating mood disorders, health care providers are strongly encouraged to assess and address metabolic-related risk factors, particularly obesity.
- Where possible, psychiatrists should choose to treat mood disorders with a low risk for weight gain and help the patient manage their weight.
- Conversely, when considering avenues to address a patient's weight, the possible presence of mood disorders should be evaluated and addressed.
- Health care providers should strongly encourage their patients to engage in regular physical activity.

References

1. Vos T, Flaxman AD, Naghavi M, et al. Years lived with disability (YLDs) for 1160 sequelae of 289 diseases and injuries 1990–2010: a systematic analysis for the Global Burden of Disease Study 2010. Lancet. 2012;380(9859):2163–96.
2. Perala J, Suvisaari J, Saarni SI, et al. Lifetime prevalence of psychotic and bipolar I disorders in a general population. Arch Gen Psychiatry. 2007;64(1):19–28.
3. OECD. Health at a glance 2013: OECD indicators. Paris: OECD Publishing; 2013. doi:10.1787/health_glance-2013-en
4. Flegal KM, Kit BK, Orpana H, Graubard BI. Association of all-cause mortality with overweight and obesity using standard body mass index categories: a systematic review and meta-analysis. JAMA. 2013;309(1):71–82.
5. Toups MS, Myers AK, Wisniewski SR, et al. Relationship between obesity and depression: characteristics and treatment outcomes with antidepressant medication. Psychosom Med. 2013;75(9):863–72.
6. McIntyre RS, Danilewitz M, Liauw SS, et al. Bipolar disorder and metabolic syndrome: an international perspective. J Affect Disord. 2010;126(3):366–87.
7. Luppino FS, de Wit LM, Bouvy PF, et al. Overweight, obesity, and depression: a systematic review and meta-analysis of longitudinal studies. Arch Gen Psychiatry. 2010;67(3):220–9.
8. Mather AA, Cox BJ, Enns MW, Sareen J. Associations of obesity with psychiatric disorders and suicidal behaviors in a nationally representative sample. J Psychosom Res. 2009;66(4):277–85.
9. Vannucchi G, Toni C, Maremmani I, Perugi G. Does obesity predict bipolarity in major depressive patients? J Affect Disord. 2014;155:118–22.
10. Kemp DE, Sylvia LG, Calabrese JR, et al. General medical burden in bipolar disorder: findings from the

LiTMUS comparative effectiveness trial. Acta Psychiatr Scand. 2014;129(1):24–34.
11. Finkelstein EA, Trogdon JG, Cohen JW, Dietz W. Annual medical spending attributable to obesity: payer-and service-specific estimates. Health Aff (Millwood). 2009;28(5):w822–31.
12. Mansur RB, Brietzke E, McIntyre RS. Is there a "metabolic-mood syndrome"? A review of the relationship between obesity and mood disorders. Neurosci Biobehav Rev. 2014;52:89–104.
13. McIntyre RS, Soczynska JK, Konarski JZ, et al. Should depressive syndromes be reclassified as "metabolic syndrome type II"? Ann Clin Psychiatry. 2007;19(4):257–64.
14. American Psychiatric Association. DSM 5—Diagnostic and statistical manual of mental disorders. 5th ed. Washington, DC: APA; 2013
15. Harald B, Gordon P. Meta-review of depressive subtyping models. J Affect Disord. 2012;139(2):126–40.
16. Moylan S, Maes M, Wray NR, Berk M. The neuroprogressive nature of major depressive disorder: pathways to disease evolution and resistance, and therapeutic implications. Mol Psychiatry. 2013;18(5):595–606.
17. Pfaffenseller B, Fries GR, Wollenhaupt-Aguiar B, et al. Neurotrophins, inflammation and oxidative stress as illness activity biomarkers in bipolar disorder. Expert Rev Neurother. 2013;13(7):827–42.
18. Strakowski SM, Adler CM, Almeida J, et al. The functional neuroanatomy of bipolar disorder: a consensus model. Bipolar Disord. 2012;14(4):313–25.
19. Bowden CL, Perlis RH, Thase ME, et al. Aims and results of the NIMH systematic treatment enhancement program for bipolar disorder (STEP-BD). CNS Neurosci Ther. 2012;18(3):243–9.
20. Nierenberg AA, Husain MM, Trivedi MH, et al. Residual symptoms after remission of major depressive disorder with citalopram and risk of relapse: a STAR*D report. Psychol Med. 2010;40(1):41–50.
21. Perlis RH, Ostacher MJ, Patel JK, et al. Predictors of recurrence in bipolar disorder: primary outcomes from the systematic treatment enhancement program for bipolar disorder (STEP-BD). Am J Psychiatry. 2006;163(2):217–24.
22. Despres JP. Health consequences of visceral obesity. Ann Med. 2001;33(8):534–41.
23. Field AE, Camargo Jr CA, Ogino S. The merits of subtyping obesity: one size does not fit all. JAMA. 2013;310(20):2147–8.
24. Naukkarinen J, Rissanen A, Kaprio J, Pietilainen KH. Causes and consequences of obesity: the contribution of recent twin studies. Int J Obes (Lond). 2012;36(8):1017–24.
25. Hussain SS, Bloom SR. The regulation of food intake by the gut–brain axis: implications for obesity. Int J Obes (Lond). 2013;37(5):625–33.
26. Kahn SE, Hull RL, Utzschneider KM. Mechanisms linking obesity to insulin resistance and type 2 diabetes. Nature. 2006;444(7121):840–6.
27. Morkedal B, Vatten LJ, Romundstad PR, Laugsand LE, Janszky I. Risk of myocardial infarction and heart failure among metabolically healthy but obese individuals: HUNT (Nord-Trondelag Health Study), Norway. J Am Coll Cardiol. 2014;63(11):1071–8.
28. Marques-Vidal P, Pecoud A, Hayoz D, et al. Prevalence of normal weight obesity in Switzerland: effect of various definitions. Eur J Nutr. 2008;47(5):251–7.
29. Oliveros E, Somers VK, Sochor O, Goel K, Lopez-Jimenez F. The concept of normal weight obesity. Prog Cardiovasc Dis. 2014;56(4):426–33.
30. Jialin W, Yi Z, Weijie Y. Relationship between body mass index and mortality in hemodialysis patients: a meta-analysis. Nephron Clin Pract. 2012;121(3–4):c102–11.
31. Oreopoulos A, Padwal R, Kalantar-Zadeh K, Fonarow GC, Norris CM, McAlister FA. Body mass index and mortality in heart failure: a meta-analysis. Am Heart J. 2008;156(1):13–22.
32. Tobias DK, Pan A, Jackson CL, et al. Body-mass index and mortality among adults with incident type 2 diabetes. N Engl J Med. 2014;370(3):233–44.
33. Kendler KS, Eaves LJ, Walters EE, Neale MC, Heath AC, Kessler RC. The identification and validation of distinct depressive syndromes in a population-based sample of female twins. Arch Gen Psychiatry. 1996;53:391–9.
34. Pine DS, Cohen P, Brook J, et al. Psychiatry symptoms in adolescence as predictors of obesity in early adulthood: a longitudinal study. Am J Public Health. 1997;97:1303–10.
35. Roberts RE, Deleger S, Strawbridge WJ, et al. Prospective association between obesity and depression: evidence from Alameda County Study. Int J Obes Relat Metab Disord. 2003;27:514–21.
36. Hasler G, Merikangas K, Eich D, et al. Psychopathology as a risk factor for being overweight. In: New Research Abstracts of the 156th Annual Meeting of the American Psychiatry Association, San Francisco, CA, 17–22 May 2003. NR106:39–40.
37. Muller-Oelinghausen B, Passoth P-M, Poser W, et al. Imapaired glucose tolerance in long-term lithium-treated patients. Int Pharmacopsychiatry. 1979;14:350–62.
38. McElroy SL, Frye MA, Suppes T, et al. Correlates of overweight and obesity in 644 patients with bipolar disorder. J Clin Psychiatry. 2002;63:207–13.
39. Fagiolini A, Kupfer DJ, Houck PR, et al. Obesity as a correlate of outcome in patients with bipolar I disorder. Am J Psychiatry. 2003;60:112–7.
40. McIntyre RS, Konarski JZ, Wilkins K, et al. Obesity in bipolar disorder and major depressive disorder: results from a national community health survey on mental health and well-being. Can J Psychiatry. 2006;51(5):274–80.
41. Simon GE, Von Korff M, Saunders K, et al. Association between obesity and psychiatric disorders in the US adult population. Arch Gen Psychiatry. 2006;63:824–30.

42. Goldstein BI, Liu SM, Zivkovic N, et al. The burden of obesity among adults with bipolar disorder in the United States. Bipolar Disord. 2011;13:387–95.
43. Petry NM, Barry D, Pietrzak RH, et al. Overweight and obesity are associated with psychiatric disorders: results from the National Epidemiologic Survey on Alcohol and Related Conditions. Psychosom Med. 2008;70:288–97.
44. McElroy SL, Kotwal R, Malhotra S, Nelson EB, Keck PE, Nemeroff CB. Are mood disorders and obesity related? A review for the mental health professional. J Clin Psychiatry. 2004;65(5):634–51.
45. Black DW, Goldstein RB, Mason EE. Prevalence of mental disorders in 88 morbidly obese bariatric clinic patients. Am J Psychiatry. 1992;149:227–34.
46. Britz B, Siegfried W, Ziegler A, et al. Rates of psychiatry disorders in a clinical study group of adolescents with extreme obesity and in obese adolescents ascertained via a population based study. Int J Obes. 2000;24:1707–14.
47. Cizza G, Ronsaville DS, Kleitz H, et al. Clinical subtypes of depression are associated with specific metabolic parameters and circadian endocrine profiles in women: the power study. PLoS One. 2012;7(1):e28912.
48. Glaus J, Vandeleur C, Gholam-Rezaee M, et al. Atypical depression and alcohol misuse are related to the cardiovascular risk in the general population. Acta Psychiatr Scand. 2013;128(4):282–93.
49. Lamers F, de Jonge P, Nolen WA, et al. Identifying depressive subtypes in a large cohort study: results from the Netherlands Study of Depression and Anxiety (NESDA). J Clin Psychiatry. 2010;71(12):1582–9.
50. Levitan RD, Davis C, Kaplan AS, Arenovich T, Phillips DI, Ravindran AV. Obesity comorbidity in unipolar major depressive disorder: refining the core phenotype. J Clin Psychiatry. 2012;73(8):1119–24.
51. Byers AL, Vittinghoff E, Lui LY, et al. Twenty-year depressive trajectories among older women. Arch Gen Psychiatry. 2012;69(10):1073–9.
52. Marijnissen RM, Bus BA, Holewijn S, et al. Depressive symptom clusters are differentially associated with general and visceral obesity. J Am Geriatr Soc. 2011;59(1):67–72.
53. Simon GE, Ludman EJ, Linde JA, et al. Association between obesity and depression in middle-aged women. Gen Hosp Psychiatry. 2008;30(1):32–9.
54. Vogelzangs N, Kritchevsky SB, Beekman AT, et al. Obesity and onset of significant depressive symptoms: results from a prospective community-based cohort study of older men and women. J Clin Psychiatry. 2010;71(4):391–9.
55. Kemp DE, Gao K, Chan PK, Ganocy SJ, Findling RL, Calabrese JR. Medical comorbidity in bipolar disorder: relationship between illnesses of the endocrine/metabolic system and treatment outcome. Bipolar Disord. 2010;12(4):404–13.
56. Khan A, Schwartz KA, Kolts RL, Brown WA. BMI, sex, and antidepressant response. J Affect Disord. 2007;99(1–3):101–6.
57. Kloiber S, Ising M, Reppermund S, et al. Overweight and obesity affect treatment response in major depression. Biol Psychiatry. 2007;62(4):321–6.
58. Oskooilar N, Wilcox CS, Tong ML, Grosz DE. Body mass index and response to antidepressants in depressed research subjects. J Clin Psychiatry. 2009;70(11):1609–10.
59. Papakostas GI, Petersen T, Iosifescu DV, et al. Obesity among outpatients with major depressive disorder. Int J Neuropsychopharmacol. 2005;8(1):59–63.
60. Uher R, Mors O, Hauser J, et al. Body weight as a predictor of antidepressant efficacy in the GENDEP project. J Affect Disord. 2009;118(1–3):147–54.
61. Busch AM, Whited MC, Appelhans BM, et al. Reliable change in depression during behavioral weight loss treatment among women with major depression. Obesity (Silver Spring). 2013;21(3): E211–8.
62. Kendler KS, Gatz M, Gardner CO, Pedersen NL. A Swedish national twin study of lifetime major depression. Am J Psychiatry. 2006;163(1):109–14.
63. Sullivan PF, Neale MC, Kendler KS. Genetic epidemiology of major depression: review and meta-analysis. Am J Psychiatry. 2000;157(10):1552–62.
64. Afari N, Noonan C, Goldberg J, et al. Depression and obesity: do shared genes explain the relationship? Depress Anxiety. 2010;27(9):799–806.
65. Jokela M, Elovainio M, Keltikangas-Jarvinen L, et al. Body mass index and depressive symptoms: instrumental-variables regression with genetic risk score. Genes Brain Behav. 2012;11(8):942–8.
66. Samaan Z, Anand SS, Zhang X, et al. The protective effect of the obesity-associated rs9939609 A variant in fat mass- and obesity-associated gene on depression. Mol Psychiatry. 2013;18(12):1281–6.
67. Rivera M, Cohen-Woods S, Kapur K, et al. Depressive disorder moderates the effect of the FTO gene on body mass index. Mol Psychiatry. 2012;17(6):604–11.
68. Altman S, Haeri S, Cohen LJ, et al. Predictors of relapse in bipolar disorder: a review. J Psychiatr Pract. 2006;12(5):269–82.
69. Horesh N, Iancu I. A comparison of life events in patients with unipolar disorder or bipolar disorder and controls. Compr Psychiatry. 2010;51(2):157–64.
70. Kyrou I, Chrousos GP, Tsigos C. Stress, visceral obesity, and metabolic complications. Ann N Y Acad Sci. 2006;1083:77–110.
71. Lai JS, Hiles S, Bisquera A, Hure AJ, McEvoy M, Attia J. A systematic review and meta-analysis of dietary patterns and depression in community-dwelling adults. Am J Clin Nutr. 2014;99(1):181–97.
72. Lopresti AL, Hood SD, Drummond PD. A review of lifestyle factors that contribute to important pathways associated with major depression: diet, sleep and exercise. J Affect Disord. 2013;148(1):12–27.
73. Nanni V, Uher R, Danese A. Childhood maltreatment predicts unfavorable course of illness and treatment outcome in depression: a meta-analysis. Am J Psychiatry. 2012;169(2):141–51.

74. Lee C, Tsenkova V, Carr D. Childhood trauma and metabolic syndrome in men and women. Soc Sci Med. 2014;105:122–30.
75. Dowlati Y, Herrmann N, Swardfager W, et al. A meta-analysis of cytokines in major depression. Biol Psychiatry. 2010;67(5):446–57.
76. Howren MB, Lamkin DM, Suls J. Associations of depression with C-reactive protein IL-1, and IL-6: a meta-analysis. Psychosom Med. 2009;71(2):171–86.
77. Munkholm K, Vinberg M, Vedel Kessing L. Cytokines in bipolar disorder: a systematic review and meta-analysis. J Affect Disord. 2013;144(1–2):16–27.
78. Choi J, Joseph L, Pilote L. Obesity and C-reactive protein in various populations: a systematic review and meta-analysis. Obes Rev. 2013;14(3):232–44.
79. Milaneschi Y, Sutin AR, Terracciano A, et al. The association between leptin and depressive symptoms is modulated by abdominal adiposity. Psychoneuroendocrinology. 2014;42:1–10.
80. Liao Y, Huang X, Wu Q, et al. Is depression a disconnection syndrome? Meta-analysis of diffusion tensor imaging studies in patients with MDD. J Psychiatry Neurosci. 2013;38(1):49–56.
81. Lin F, Weng S, Xie B, Wu G, Lei H. Abnormal frontal cortex white matter connections in bipolar disorder: a DTI tractography study. J Affect Disord. 2011;131(1–3):299–306.
82. Vederine FE, Wessa M, Leboyer M, Houenou J. A meta-analysis of whole-brain diffusion tensor imaging studies in bipolar disorder. Prog Neuropsychopharmacol Biol Psychiatry. 2011;35(8):1820–6.
83. Garcia-Garcia I, Jurado MA, Garolera M, et al. Functional connectivity in obesity during reward processing. Neuroimage. 2012;66C:232–9.
84. Kullmann S, Heni M, Veit R, et al. The obese brain: association of body mass index and insulin sensitivity with resting state network functional connectivity. Hum Brain Mapp. 2012;33(5):1052–61.
85. Cole JH, Boyle CP, Simmons A, et al. Body mass index, but not FTO geno-type or major depressive disorder, influences brain structure. Neuroscience. 2013;252:109–17.
86. Kuswanto CN, Sum MY, Yang GL, Nowinski WL, McIntyre RS, Sim K. Increased body mass index makes an impact on brain white-matter integrity in adults with remitted first-episode mania. Psychol Med. 2014;44(3):533–41.
87. Cota D, Tschop MH, Horvath TL, Levine AS. Cannabinoids, opioids and eating behavior: the molecular face of hedonism? Brain Res Rev. 2006;51(1):85–107.
88. Russo SJ, Nestler EJ. The brain reward circuitry in mood disorders. Nat Rev Neurosci. 2013;14(9): 609–25.
89. Volkow ND, Wang GJ, Baler RD. Reward, dopamine and the control of food intake: implications for obesity. Trends Cogn Sci. 2011;15(1):37–46.
90. D'Aquila PS, Collu M, Gessa GL, Serra G. The role of dopamine in the mechanism of action of antidepressant drugs. Eur J Pharmacol. 2000;405(1–3):365–73.
91. Jann MW. Diagnosis and treatment of bipolar disorders in adults: a review of the evidence on pharmacologic treatments. Am Health Drug Benefits. 2014;7(9):489–99.
92. Anand A, Barkay G, Dzemidzic M, et al. Striatal dopamine transporter availability in unmedicated bipolar disorder. Bipolar Disord. 2011;13(4):406–13.
93. Camardese G, Di Giuda D, Di Nicola M, et al. Imaging studies on dopamine transporter and depression: a review of literature and suggestions for future research. J Psychiatr Res. 2014;51:7–18.
94. Chang TT, Yeh TL, Chiu NT, et al. Higher striatal dopamine transporters in euthymic patients with bipolar disorder: a SPECT study with [Tc] TRODAT-1. Bipolar Disord. 2010;12(1):102–6.
95. Brady Jr RO, Cooper A, Jensen JE, et al. A longitudinal pilot proton MRS investigation of the manic and euthymic states of bipolar disorder. Transl Psychiatry. 2012;2:e160.
96. Chu WJ, Delbello MP, Jarvis KB, et al. Magnetic resonance spectroscopy imaging of lactate in patients with bipolar disorder. Psychiatry Res. 2013;213(3):230–4.
97. Iosifescu DV, Renshaw PE. 31P-magnetic resonance spectroscopy and thyroid hormones in major depressive disorder: toward a bioenergetic mechanism in depression? Harv Rev Psychiatry. 2003;11(2):51–63.
98. Kraguljac NV, Reid M, White D, et al. Neurometabolites in schizophrenia and bipolar disorder—a systematic review and meta-analysis. Psychiatry Res. 2012;203(2–3):111–25.
99. Stork C, Renshaw PF. Mitochondrial dysfunction in bipolar disorder: evidence from magnetic resonance spectroscopy research. Mol Psychiatry. 2005;10(10):900–19.
100. Gazdzinski S, Kornak J, Weiner MW, Meyerhoff DJ. Body mass index and magnetic resonance markers of brain integrity in adults. Ann Neurol. 2008;63(5):652–7.
101. Gazdzinski S, Millin R, Kaiser LG, et al. BMI and neuronal integrity in healthy, cognitively normal elderly: a proton magnetic resonance spectroscopy study. Obesity (Silver Spring). 2010;18(4):743–8.
102. Schmoller A, Hass T, Strugovshchikova O, et al. Evidence for a relationship between body mass and energy metabolism in the human brain. J Cereb Blood Flow Metab. 2010;30(7):1403–10.
103. Cowansage KK, LeDoux JE, Monfils MH. Brain-derived neurotrophic factor: a dynamic gatekeeper of neural plasticity. Curr Mol Pharmacol. 2010;3(1):12–29.
104. Zagrebelsky M, Korte M. Form follows function: BDNF and its involvement in sculpting the function and structure of synapses. Neuropharmacology. 2014;76(Pt C):628–38.
105. Bocchio-Chiavetto L, Bagnardi V, Zanardini R, et al. Serum and plasma BDNF levels in major depression: a replication study and meta-analyses. World J Biol Psychiatry. 2010;11(6):763–73.

106. Fernandes BS, Gama CS, Cereser KM, et al. Brain-derived neurotrophic factor as a state-marker of mood episodes in bipolar disorders: a systematic review and meta-regression analysis. J Psychiatr Res. 2011;45(8):995–1004.
107. Burkhalter J, Fiumelli H, Allaman I, Chatton JY, Martin JL. Brain-derived neurotrophic factor stimulates energy metabolism in developing cortical neurons. J Neurosci. 2003;23(23):8212–20.
108. Markham A, Cameron I, Bains R, et al. Brain-derived neurotrophic factor-mediated effects on mitochondrial respiratory coupling and neuroprotection share the same molecular signalling pathways. Eur J Neurosci. 2012;35(3):366–74.
109. Unger TJ, Calderon GA, Bradley LC, Sena-Esteves M, Rios M. Selective deletion of BDNF in the ventromedial and dorsomedial hypothalamus of adult mice results in hyperphagic behavior and obesity. J Neurosci. 2007;27(52):14265–74.
110. Xu B, Goulding EH, Zang K, et al. Brain-derived neurotrophic factor regulates energy balance downstream of melanocortin-4 receptor. Nat Neurosci. 2003;6(7):736–42.
111. Christopoulou FD, Kiortsis DN. An overview of the metabolic effects of rimonabant in randomized controlled trials: potential for other cannabinoid 1 receptor blockers in obesity. J Clin Pharm Ther. 2011;36(1):10–8.
112. Di Marzo V, Despres JP. CB1 antagonists for obesity—what lessons have we learned from rimonabant? Nat Rev Endocrinol. 2009;5(11):633–8.
113. Gobbi G, Bambico FR, Mangieri R, et al. Antidepressant-like activity and modulation of brain monoaminergic transmission by blockade of anandamide hydrolysis. Proc Natl Acad Sci U S A. 2005;102(51):18620–5.
114. Mitchell PB, Morris MJ. Depression and anxiety with rimonabant. Lancet. 2007;370(9600):1671–2.
115. Moreira FA, Kaiser N, Monory K, Lutz B. Reduced anxiety-like behaviour induced by genetic and pharmacological inhibition of the endocannabinoid-degrading enzyme fatty acid amide hydrolase (FAAH) is mediated by CB1 receptors. Neuropharmacology. 2008;54(1):141–50.
116. Bennetzen MF, Wellner N, Ahmed SS, et al. Investigations of the human endocannabinoid system in two subcutaneous adipose tissue depots in lean subjects and in obese subjects before and after weight loss. Int J Obes (Lond). 2011;35(11):1377–84.
117. Bluher M, Engeli S, Kloting N, et al. Dysregulation of the peripheral and adipose tissue endocannabinoid system in human abdominal obesity. Diabetes. 2006;55(11):3053–60.
118. Di Marzo V, Cote M, Matias I, et al. Changes in plasma endocannabinoid levels in viscerally obese men following a 1 year lifestyle modification programme and waist circumference reduction: associations with changes in metabolic risk factors. Diabetologia. 2009;52(2):213–7.
119. Matias I, Gatta-Cherifi B, Tabarin A, et al. Endocannabinoids measurement in human saliva as potential biomarker of obesity. PLoS One. 2012; 7(7):e42399.
120. McElroy SL, Keck PE. Metabolic syndrome in bipolar disorder. J Clin Psychiatry. 2014; 75(January):46–61.
121. Bowden CL, Calabrese JR, Ketter TA, et al. Impact of lamotrigine and lithium on weight in obese and nonobese patients with bipolar I disorder. Am J Psychiatry. 2006;163(7):1199–201.
122. Malhotra S, King KH, Welge JA, et al. Venlafaxine treatment of binge-eating disorder associated with obesity: a series of 35 patients. J Clin Psychiatry. 2002;63:802–6.
123. Uguz F, Sahingoz M, Gungor B, Akosv F, Askin R. Weight gain and associated factors in patients using newer antidepressant drugs. Gen Hosp Psychiatry. 2015;37(1):46–8.
124. Leombruni P, Lavagnino L, Gastaldi F, et al. Duloxetine in obese binge eater outpatients: preliminary results from a 12-week open trial. Hum Psychopharmacol. 2009;24:483–8.
125. Guerdjikova AI, McElroy SL, Winstanley EL, et al. Duloxetine in the treatment of binge eating disorder with depressive disorder: a placebo controlled trial. Int J Eat Disord. 2012;45(2):281–9.
126. Gardiner HM, Freeman CP, Jesinger DK, et al. Fluvoxamine: an open pilot study in moderate obese female patients suffering from atypical eating disorders and episodes of bingeing. Int J Obes Relat Metab Disord. 1993;17(5):301–5.
127. Hudson JI, McElroy SL, Raymond NC, et al. Fluvoxamine in the treatment of binge-eating disorder: a multicenter placebo-controlled, double-blind trial. Am J Psychiatry. 1998;155:1756–62.
128. Pearlstein T, Spurell E, Hohlstein LA, et al. A double-blind, placebo-controlled trial of fluvoxamine in binge eating disorder: a high placebo response. Arch Womens Ment Health. 2003;6: 147–51.
129. McElroy SL, Casuto LS, Nelson EB, et al. Placebo-controlled trial of sertraline in the treatment of binge eating disorder. Am J Psychiatry. 2000;157:1004–46.
130. Milano W, Petrella C, Capasso A. Treatment of binge eating disorder with sertraline: a randomized controlled trial. Biomed Res. 2005;16:89–91.
131. Leombruni P, Pierò A, Brustolin A, et al. A 12 to 24 weeks pilot study of sertraline treatment in obese women binge eaters. Hum Psychopharmacol. 2006;21:181–8.
132. Greeno CG, Wing RR. A double blind, placebo-controlled trial of fluoxetine on dietary intake in overweight women with and without binge-eating disorder. Am J Clin Nutr. 1996;64:267–73.
133. Arnold LM, McElroy SL, Hudson JI, et al. A placebo-controlled, randomized trial of fluoxetine in the treatment of binge-eating disorder. J Clin Psychiatry. 2002;63:1028–33.

134. McElroy SL, Hudson JI, Malhotra S, et al. Citalopram in the treatment of binge-eating disorder: a placebo-controlled trial. J Clin Psychiatry. 2003;64:807–13.
135. Guerdjikova AL, McElroy SL, Kotwal R, et al. High-dose escitalopram in the treatment of binge-eating disorder with obesity: a placebo-controlled monotherapy trial. Hum Psychopharmacol. 2008;23:1–11.
136. Gadde KM, Parker CB, Maner LG, et al. Bupropion for weight loss: an investigation of efficacy and tolerability in overweight and obese women. Obes Res. 2001;9:544–51.
137. Jain AK, Kaplan RA, Gadde KM, et al. Bupropion SR vs placebo for weight loss in obese patients with depressive symptoms. Obes Res. 2002;10:1049–56.
138. Calandra C, Russo RG, Luca M. Bupropion versus Sertraline in the treatment of depressive patients with binge eating disorder: retrospective cohort study. Psychiatr Q. 2012;83:177–85.
139. Greenway FL, Fujioka K, Plodkowski RA, et al. Effect of naltrexone plus bupropion on weight loss in overweight and obese adults (COR-I): a multi-centre, randomised, double-blind, placebo-controlled, phase 3 trial. Lancet. 2010;376:595–606.
140. Halpern B, Oliveira ESL, Faria AM, et al. Combinations of drugs in the treatment of obesity. Pharmaceuticals. 2010;3:2398–415.
141. Daumit GL, Dickerson FB, Wang NY, Dalcin A, Jerome GJ, Anderson CA, Young DR, Frick KD, Yu A, Gennusa JV, Oefinger M, Crum RM, Charleston J, Casagrande SS, Guallar E, Goldberg RW, Campbell LM, Appel LJ. A behavioral weight-loss intervention in persons with serious mental illness. N Engl J Med. 2013;368(17):1594–602.
142. Keranen AM, Rasinaho E, Hakko H, Savolainen M, Lindeman S. Eating behavior in obese and overweight persons with and without anhedonia. Appetite. 2010;55(3):726–9.
143. Bell CG, Walley AJ, Froguel P. The genetics of human obesity. Nat Rev Genet. 2005;6(3):221–34.
144. Calkin C, van de Velde C, Ruzickova M, et al. Can body mass index help predict outcome in patients with bipolar disorder? Bipolar Disord. 2009;11(6):650–6.
145. Gardner A, Boles RG. Beyond the serotonin hypothesis: mitochondria, inflammation and neurodegeneration in major depression and affective spectrum disorders. Prog Neuropsychopharmacol Biol Psychiatry. 2011;35(3):730–43.
146. Jackson MB, Ahima RS. Neuroendocrine and metabolic effects of adipocyte-derived hormones. Clin Sci (Lond). 2006;110(2):143–52.
147. Kendler KS, Aggen SH, Neale MC. Evidence for multiple genetic factors underlying DSM-IV criteria for major depression. JAMA Psychiatry. 2013;70(6):599–607.
148. McElroy SL. Obesity in patients with severe mental illness: overview and management. J Clin Psychiatry. 2009;70 suppl 3:12–21.
149. McIntyre RS, Muzina DJ, Kemp DE, et al. Bipolar disorder and suicide: research synthesis and clinical translation. Curr Psychiatry Rep. 2008;10(1):66–72.
150. Raison CL, Rutherford RE, Woolwine BJ, et al. A randomized controlled trial of the tumor necrosis factor antagonist infliximab for treatment-resistant depression: the role of baseline inflammatory biomarkers. JAMA Psychiatry. 2013;70(1):31–41.
151. van de Giessen E, Celik F, Schweitzer DH, van den Brink W, Booij J. Dopamine D2/3 receptor availability and amphetamine-induced dopamine release in obesity. J Psychopharmacol. 2014;28(9):866–73.
152. Volkow ND, Wang GJ, Fowler JS, Telang F. Overlapping neuronal circuits in addiction and obesity: evidence of systems pathology. Philos Trans R Soc Lond B Biol Sci. 2008;363(1507):3191–200.

Eating Disorders in Severe Obesity

10

Susan Wnuk, Jessica Van Exan, and Raed Hawa

10.1 Introduction

In this chapter, we review and recommend strategies for assessing eating disorders in patients with obesity who present for treatment in settings that are not specialized to treat eating disorders. Our purpose is to equip clinicians working with obese individuals or in general community practices with the tools to understand eating disorder symptoms and make appropriate recommendations to patients with obesity. A case example of a common clinical presentation will be used to illustrate the assessment and triage process. We will begin by reviewing prevalence data and providing an overview of the research literature on eating disorders typically found in individuals with obesity, namely binge eating disorder (BED) and night eating syndrome (NES). We will then summarize recent diagnostic changes in the DSM-5 criteria for eating disorders. We discuss interview and self-report instruments and recommend how best to incorporate these into clinical practice so as to reliably and accurately assess for eating disorders. Although other chapters in this volume describe specific psychological treatments for obesity, we outline a plan for triaging patients with obesity who also suffer from eating disorders to more intensive treatment. Finally, we review medications for eating disorders found in patients with obesity.

S. Wnuk, B.A., M.A., Ph.D. (✉)
J. Van Exan, Ph.D., C.Psych.
Toronto Western Hospital Bariatric Surgery Program, University Health Network, Toronto, ON, Canada
e-mail: susan.wnuk@gmail.com; jessica.vanexan@uhn.ca; jessica.vanexan@rogers.com

R. Hawa
Toronto Western Hospital Bariatric Surgery Program, University Health Network, 399 Bathurst Street, Toronto, ON, Canada M5T 2S8

Department of Psychiatry, University of Toronto, Toronto, ON, Canada
e-mail: Raed.Hawa@uhn.ca

Case Vignettes

Mark is a 48-year-old male with a body mass index of 43 kg/m^2 (with a weight of 310 lbs and height of 5′11″). He was diagnosed with type 2 diabetes 3 years ago and is followed by an endocrinologist. His blood sugar is poorly controlled and his hemoglobin A1c is abnormally elevated. In addition, he was diagnosed with obstructive sleep apnea 7 years ago and uses a continuous positive airway pressure (CPAP) machine at night. Mark reports difficulty adhering to diet and exercise recommendations though he takes his medications as prescribed. Mark told his endocrinologist

(continued)

S. Sockalingam, R. Hawa (eds.), *Psychiatric Care in Severe Obesity*,
DOI 10.1007/978-3-319-42536-8_10

(continued)
that he is frustrated by his increasing weight, especially since his diabetes diagnosis, and wants help with weight loss. Over the past 15 years he has repeatedly lost up to 50 lbs through various commercial weight loss programs and by exercising at a gym with a personal trainer. He has maintained this weight loss for up to 1 year, only to regain the weight plus an additional 10–15 lbs each time. Mark reported that his tendency with these weight loss programs is to be "all in," following the diet programs exactly or exercising for 2 h a day at least four times a week. He explained that as soon as he ate a food not endorsed by a diet plan or missed working out for more than a week, he would return to his old eating habits and give up on his weight loss goals.

Mark has been married for 22 years and has two children in their teens. He describes his marriage and family life as "solid" but noted that work stress often leads him to eat for comfort. He works full time as a warehouse manager but gained a significant amount of weight 8 years ago after a layoff. He was unemployed for a year and experienced significant financial hardship. Mark reported that during this time he also experienced an episode of depression and took venlafaxine for 6 months. After he found his current job his depression remitted and he discontinued his antidepressant. He played team sports throughout high school in his early twenties but with mounting family and work responsibilities in his late twenties he became significantly less physically active. He describes himself as a "lifelong big eater" who ate larger portions than others beginning in late childhood but the high levels of physical activity in his early life helped prevent significant weight gain. Mark also binges in the evenings 2–3 times a week after having a stressful day at work. He usually purchases takeout food that he eats while watching television, after his wife and children have gone to bed. Although he feels embarrassed about this eating because it "proves my eating is out of control" and he is aware of the negative consequences to his diabetes, this eating is his main source of enjoyment and distraction from his responsibilities. He received education from his endocrinologist about the importance of exercise for blood sugar control, but finds it difficult to find time in his schedule for exercise. Although Mark is proud of his adherence to his medication regimen and blood sugar monitoring, he feels he needs more support with his eating habits.

10.2 Epidemiology of Eating Disorders in Obesity

Binge eating disorder (BED) and night eating syndrome (NES) are the most common eating disorders reported in severely obese populations [1, 2]. The general lifetime prevalence of BED across countries worldwide is estimated at 1.4 %, ranging from 0.8 to 1.9 % [3]. The prevalence of NES in the general community is estimated to be approximately 1.5 %, ranging from 1 to 5.7 % [4–6]. Prevalence rates for BED and NES are substantially higher in obese samples and vary widely depending on the population and method of assessment [7]. Specifically, prevalence rates for BED range from 1 to 30 % [7] and for NES obese patients seeking weight loss range from 6 to 16 % [5, 8]. For bariatric surgery candidates, the range for BED is greater with a prevalence from 2 to 49 % [7] and 2 to 31 % for NES [5, 7–9].

In terms of demographic characteristics, both BED and NES have been found to emerge between the late teens to early twenties [6, 10, 11], which is later than the age of onset for anorexia or bulimia nervosa [3]. An earlier onset of binge eating has been found to predict worse outcomes in terms of treatment of BED [10].

Compared to other eating disorder diagnoses, the gender differences for BED and NES are less pronounced [10, 12]. Lifetime prevalence rates of BED are slightly higher in women than men with ratios between 2:1 and 6:1 [13, 14]. Generally the rates are comparable among men and women with NES [6, 15]. One distinct difference between obese men and women with eating disorders is that women are more likely to report shape and weight concerns [10, 16, 17], which is associated with greater impairment and poorer quality of life [10]. Few cultural differences have been found for BED [12] and NES [18]. In recent studies examining cultural differences in treatment-seeking adults with BED [12, 19], African-American adults were found to have higher BMIs than Hispanic and Caucasian adults. Regarding eating disorder symptoms however, research has been inconsistent in terms of whether there are differences in binge eating frequency and eating pathology across ethnic groups [12, 19] and further research is warranted.

The underlying etiology of BED and NES remains unclear and is likely multifaceted in terms of both predisposing and environmental factors contributing to the onset of eating pathology [20]. The course of these disorders tends to be stable and there is little crossover with other eating disorders [10].

10.3 Eating Disorders and Body Mass Index

The results are inconclusive as to whether disordered eating leads to obesity or obesity leads to disordered eating [1], but both BED and NES are thought to contribute to problems associated with obesity. Specifically, the loss of control and overeating associated with binge eating and the delayed eating pattern associated with night eating are thought to contribute to weight gain and at the least make weight loss and the prevention of further weight gain more difficult [21]. Both BED and NES have been found to be more prevalent in obese compared to nonobese samples when examining rates cross-sectionally [10, 22–25]. In addition, among obese patients, bariatric surgery candidates report higher BMIs, more objective and subjective binge eating, and higher rates of night eating compared to nonsurgical overweight controls [8, 26].

For NES, some studies have found a positive association between NES and body weight (e.g., [8, 27–29]); however, a number of studies have found no correlation (e.g., [15, 18, 30]). The inconsistency in NES criteria used across studies greatly impacts the interpretation and generalizability of findings [23]. Also, most of the research on NES has included samples with small BMI ranges where there would be inadequate power to detect differences [8]. Colles, Dixon, and O'Brien's [8] is the only study to date that has examined NES across a broad spectrum of BMI and they found significant differences in prevalence of NES based on BMI category such that higher rates of NES were associated with higher BMIs. Overall, this suggests that both BED and NES are associated with obesity, but the nature and direction of this relationship remains unclear [23].

When examining differences between normal-weight and obese adults with BED, one study found that while there were no differences in age of onset of binge eating or frequency of binge episodes, normal-weight individuals were significantly younger [31]. Dingemans and Furth [32] similarly found that nonobese individuals with BED were younger and were less likely to have received treatment. Marshall et al. [33] found that compared to obese patients with NES, normal-weight individuals were again considerably younger. Normal-weight individuals with BED have also been found to be more likely to engage in weight-control behaviors [31] and to have higher dietary restraint [34], which may partly explain differences in weight status. These findings suggest that the risk of obesity for BED and NES may increase with age due to the longer duration of these eating patterns [31].

10.4 Psychiatric and Medical Comorbidity

Prevalence rates for BED and NES have been found to be higher in obese patients with serious mental illness compared to the general population [9, 35] and BED and NES are associated with higher psychiatric comorbidity compared with individuals without eating disorders. Depression and anxiety are the most common associated disorders [9, 15, 27, 36, 37] followed by substance use disorders [27]. Specifically, Grilo et al. [38] found that 67 % of treatment-seeking BED patients had at least one lifetime DSM-IV axis I psychiatric disorder. Similarly, De Zwaan et al. [39] found that over half of NES patients reported a lifetime history of major depressive disorder and 66 % reported problems related to insomnia. Higher rates of personality disorders have also been reported in individuals with BED and NES [10, 40, 41]. The findings are similar in bariatric surgery candidates. Mitchell et al. [42] reported that 68.7 % of bariatric candidates had a lifetime history and 33.7 % met criteria for a current axis 1 disorder. Bariatric surgery candidates with BED report greater depressive symptoms than non-BED bariatric surgery patients [43]. Also, loss of control with respect to binge eating has been found to be associated with higher rates of night eating, general eating pathology, and depressive symptoms in pre-bariatric surgery patients [43].

Psychiatric comorbidity in BED and NES patients has been found to be associated with greater severity of eating pathology and poorer functioning in general [38, 44, 45]. Specifically, eating disorders are associated with low self-esteem [46] as well as a reduced quality of life [24, 36, 47]. Overevaluation of weight and shape has been found to be related to greater eating disorder pathology and poorer psychological functioning in obese patients with BED [38]. In bariatric candidates with BED, lower self-esteem is reported compared to those without BED [43] as well as greater eating pathology and higher levels of body dissatisfaction [48, 49]. These findings suggest that when considering the degree of severity in terms of BED and NES, it is important to consider the degree of comorbid psychiatric conditions as well as factors such as self-esteem, quality of life, and the degree of overevaluation of weight and shape [10].

Medical comorbidity is also common in obese individuals. BED has been associated with an increased risk for various medical problems including hypertension, Type 2 diabetes, cardiovascular disease, and physical mobility limitations [50]. In bariatric surgery patients, the presence of at least one axis 1 disorder was related to greater severity of obesity and worse functional health status [51]. In general, there is a high degree of psychiatric and medical comorbidity in individuals with BED and NES that needs to be assessed as it may impact treatment considerations and outcome.

10.5 Measurement and Assessment

10.5.1 Classification of Eating Disorders in DSM-5

The purpose of this section is to briefly review the DSM-5 criteria for BED and NES, the eating disorders most commonly found in obesity. We will also briefly discuss BN and Avoidant Restrictive Food Intake Disorder (ARFID). While BN and ARFID are not as prevalent, it is important to be familiar with these disorders as well as they may present in patients with obesity.

10.5.2 Binge Eating Disorder

The disorder of most interest to clinicians working with patients with obesity is BED. It features repeated eating binges during which an individual consumes an excessively large amount of food and experiences a subjective loss of control over their eating, but does not engage in methods to compensate for the excess calories. Binges need to occur weekly and symptoms need to persist only for 3 months to reach diagnostic threshold. Severity specifiers, from mild to severe, are based on frequency of binge episodes.

Although overvaluation of weight and shape is not a diagnostic criterion for BED as it is for BN and anorexia nervosa (AN), in research this feature has been found in 60 % of BED patients, a level significantly higher than in non-BED obese patients, though lower than in AN and BN [38]. This is a feature that should be assessed as it is a marker of greater psychosocial impairment

Table 10.1 Differentiating objective binge eating from other eating pathology/normal eating patterns

	Control	Loss of control
Large amount of food eaten	Overeating	Objective binge eating
Average amount of food eaten	Normal eating	Subjective binge eating

Source: Fairburn and Cooper [52]

and poorer quality of life [38]. BED should also be differentiated from other eating patterns often found in individuals with obesity like snacking or grazing throughout the day regardless of hunger, eating in response to emotional states, eating in response to strong cravings for certain types of foods like sweets, morning undereating [52, 53], and subjective binge eating ([54], see Table 10.1). Subjective binge eating, defined as eating an amount of food that is not excessively large while feeling out of control, has been associated with increased psychopathology and distress [54]. These eating patterns may coexist with BED, but in the absence of objective eating binges with loss of control, do not in themselves constitute BED. If present in concert with sufficient additional eating disorder symptoms however, a diagnosis of OSFED or USFED may be warranted.

10.5.3 Bulimia Nervosa

Although seen less frequently in obese individuals than BED and NES, BN does occur in obese individuals [55] and thus should be assessed. In addition to regular binge eating episodes as defined in BED, a diagnosis of BN requires the use of problematic methods to prevent weight gain such as inducing vomiting, misuse of laxatives, prolonged fasting, and excessive exercise. The frequency of binge episodes and compensatory behaviors occur at least weekly and symptoms persist for at least 3 months.

10.5.4 Night Eating Syndrome

Whereas the core feature of BED is episodes of overeating accompanied by a lack of control without the use of inappropriate compensatory behaviors, the core feature of NES is the delayed circadian shift of eating [8, 56]. First described by Stunkard et al. in 1955 [57], awareness of NES amongst clinicians and researchers has only recently emerged. It is now listed in the DSM-5 as an Other Specified Feeding or Eating Disorder but diagnostic criteria have not yet been fully quantified. Allison et al. [28] propose that for NES, as established by the International NES Working group, the core criterion is an abnormally increased food intake in the evening and/or at night, manifested by (1) consumption of at least 25 % of intake after the evening meal and before bedtime and/or (2) nocturnal awakenings with eating at least twice per week. In addition to distress or impairment in functioning, NES involves awareness of the eating episodes as this feature differentiates NES from sleep-related eating disorder (SRED), a parasomnia in which individuals do not recall their night-time eating [28]. Allison et al. [28] propose additional criteria for NES that involves the endorsement of at least three of five additional symptoms: (1) lack of eating in the morning; (2) strong desire to eat between dinner and sleep or upon awakening from sleep; (3) insomnia; (4) belief that one must eat in order to get to sleep; and (5) low mood in the evening. These criteria must be met for a minimum duration of 3 months. These additional criteria are not required by the DSM-5 given that further research on night eating is needed; however, the criteria outlined by Allison et al. [28] are useful for differentiating NES from other disorders such as BED and SRED.

10.5.5 Differentiating Between BED and NES

BED and NES are thought to be distinct disorders; however, they share the common feature of evening hyperphagia ([28], see Fig. 10.1). The rates of co-occurring BED and NES range from 7 to 25 % and approximately 9 % for BN and NES [28, 58].

NES can be distinguished from BED in that individuals with NES demonstrate a phase delay in the circadian pattern of eating leading them to consume more of their total energy intake later in the day and at night compared to individuals

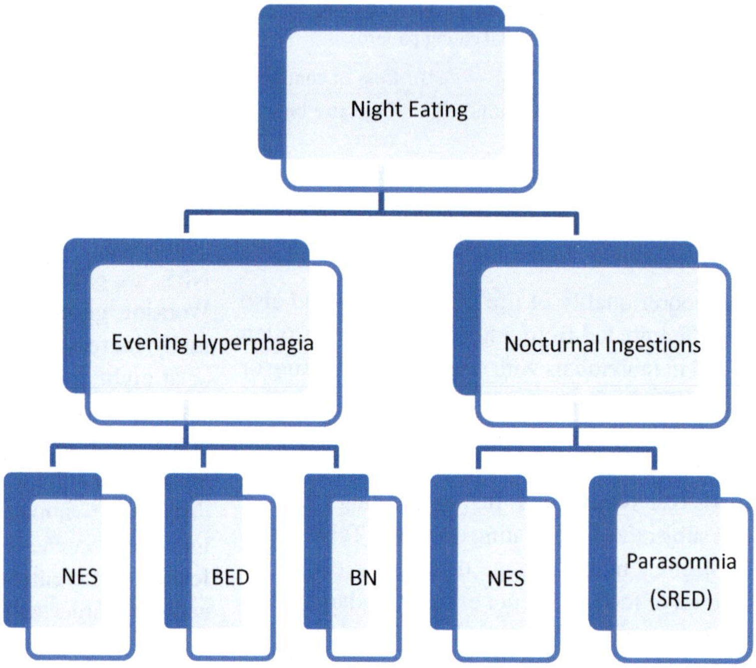

Fig. 10.1 Differentiating NES from other eating and sleep disorders

without NES [36, 46, 59]. Gluck et al. [46] found that after fasting for 8 h, night eaters reported less hunger before a daytime test meal. In terms of waking to eat, Birketvedt et al. [59] found that night eaters woke on average 3.6 times per night compared to only 0.3 times in controls and 52 % of awakenings in night eaters were accompanied by food intake. NES participants have been found to have lower disinhibition scores than individuals with BED, but higher than controls [60], and those with both BED and NES scored the highest. One difference that has been highlighted in the literature is that sleep disturbance is less common in individuals with BED compared to those with NES [4, 36].

Individuals with NES have also been found to exhibit less general psychological distress than individuals with BED [8]. Allison et al. [37] in their study comparing individuals with BED and NES found the BED group exhibited greater eating pathology and experienced many more objective binge eating episodes with loss of control. Some of the NES participants reported a loss of control during their night eating episodes, but this was rarely objectively large in terms of quantity of food. The eating patterns of the groups differed significantly as well, with the NES group eating far fewer meals during the first half of the day. The BED and NES groups ate a similar number of evening snacks after the main evening meal, indicating that both groups have some trouble regulating their eating in the evening hours before bedtime. The BED group had higher scores on the Eating Disorders Exam-Questionnaire ([61], please see Table 10.3 for a description of this measure) weight concern and shape concerns subscales than the NES group even after controlling for BMI differences. Allison et al. [37] note that since both the NES and BED groups were characterized by disordered eating, clinicians should attend to the assessment and regulation of meal patterns. For nocturnal ingestions, NES can also be distinguished from sleep-related eating disorder in that individuals with NES are awake when eating and can recall these episodes compared to individuals with SRED who are asleep when these eating episodes occur [5].

10.5.6 Avoidant Restrictive Food Intake Disorder

ARFID is characterized by an apparent lack of interest in eating or food, avoidance of food based on the food's sensory characteristics, and avoidance of particular foods due to concerns about the negative consequences of eating, like abdominal discomfort. Unlike other eating disorders, the motivation to avoid eating is not to achieve or maintain a certain body weight or shape. ARFID can co-occur with a number of other mental disorders, in particular, with autism spectrum disorder and other neurodevelopmental disorders, as well as anxiety disorders [62]. Little research on ARFID in adults has been published and the prevalence of ARFID in obese individuals has not been documented. However, sufficient numbers of post-bariatric surgery patients across different countries and settings have been documented with problematic food aversions to have generated several publications and research studies (e.g., [63–67]. Although these studies do not diagnose these individuals with ARFID, the presentation may be similar to that of ARFID. Foods that are typically avoided after bariatric surgery tend to be tougher or denser in texture, particularly meats, rice, and pasta. These aversions usually develop after the foods in question lead to an episode of abdominal discomfort. However, these food avoidances tend to disappear over time and do not usually indicate a diagnosis of ARFID.

10.5.7 Assessment Methods

As with other psychiatric disorders, the eating disorders involve symptoms that are behavioral (e.g., bingeing, restriction), cognitive (e.g., prioritization of dietary restraint, negative body image), and affective (e.g., eating to regulate emotional distress) in nature and a complete, valid, and reliable assessment must consider all of these. Table 10.2 lists the symptoms and features that are typically found in eating disorders that should be assessed in all patients.

Table 10.2 Characteristic features and symptoms by DSM-5 disorder, to be assessed in all patients

Feature	BED	BN	NES	ARFID
Objective binge eating	✓	✓		
Loss of control over eating	✓	✓	✓	
Extreme compensatory methods		✓		
Overvaluation of weight and shape	✓	✓		
Excessive evening eating	✓	✓	✓	
Nocturnal eating upon awakening			✓	
Irregular/chaotic eating pattern	✓	✓	✓	✓
Dietary restriction	✓	✓	✓	✓

Regardless of whether the assessment is conducted for treatment or research purposes, a clinical interview should be the foundation of any valid eating disorders assessment. Based on the available research evidence and our clinical experience, clinician interviews are critical for understanding past and present eating behaviors and for obtaining accurate diagnoses in both bariatric surgery [68–71] and non-bariatric surgery populations [61]. The choice of particular interview and questionnaire instruments can then be based on factors such as time available to conduct the assessment and the type of information that is useful in a particular setting. Please see Table 10.3 for a description of the recommended eating disorder-specific interview and self-report assessment instruments.

The Eating Disorders Exam-Interview [72] is the most used and widely recognized interview used to diagnose eating disorders. The eating disorders modules of the Structured Clinical Interview [73] and the MINI Neuropsychiatric Interview are also available [74]. However, as of yet these measures do not include questions to assess NES or ARFID. The Night Eating Syndrome History and Inventory (NESHI) is a more recent addition to the field and can be used to guide the assessment of NES [75]. Currently there are no validated instruments for assessing ARFID. Therefore, a thorough understanding of

Table 10.3 Recommended instruments

Measure	Description
Clinical interview	
Eating disorder examination—interview [54]	Takes ~45–75 min and is freely available; diagnoses eating disorders according to the DSM-IV and provides scores on eating disorder pathology via four subscales: dietary restraint, eating concern, weight concern, shape concern, plus a global score are computed
Night eating syndrome history and inventory (NESHI) [78]	A semi-structured interview used to diagnose NES. It assesses a typical 24-h food intake, including a recall of all meals and snacks, and sleeping patterns. A total score of 25 can be used as the threshold for diagnosing NES
Self-report	
Binge eating scale [124]	16 items; computes a total score reflecting severity of binge behaviors to screen for binge eating disorder; measures the behavioral, emotional, and cognitive symptoms associated with binge eating. Participants with scores ≥17 can be classified "binge eaters." [131]. Cut scores of binge eating severity [132]: no binge eating (score ≤17), mild to moderate binge eating (score of 18–26), severe binge eating (score ≥27)
The Dutch eating behaviors questionnaire [125]	33 items, developed to measure aspects of eating found through research to be common in obese individuals: restrained eating, emotional eating, external eating, with emotional and external eating characteristic of individuals with obesity; not diagnostic
Eating disorders exam—questionnaire [75]	28 items; adapted from the EDE-I to assess symptoms of eating disorders according to the DSM-IV; four subscales: restraint, eating concern, shape concern, weight concern, and a global score
Eating disorders inventory-3 [126]	91 items organized into 12 primary scales: Drive for Thinness, Bulimia, Body Dissatisfaction, Low Self-Esteem, Personal Alienation, Interpersonal Insecurity, Interpersonal Alienation, Interoceptive Deficits, Emotional Dysregulation, Perfectionism, Asceticism, and Maturity Fears. Yields six composite scores: one that is eating disorder specific (i.e., Eating Disorder Risk) and five that are general integrative psychological constructs (i.e., Ineffectiveness, Interpersonal Problems, Affective Problems, Overcontrol, General Psychological Maladjustment)
Questionnaire for eating disorder diagnoses [127]	50 items that operationalize the DSM (fourth edition) eating disorder diagnoses into (a) those with and without an eating disorder diagnosis, (b) eating-disordered, symptomatic, and asymptomatic individuals, and (c) those with anorexia and bulimia diagnoses
Questionnaire of eating and weight patterns (revised) [128]	28 items; assesses symptoms and history of BED and BN as per the DSM-IV
Night eating questionnaire [129]	17 items; assesses presence and severity of symptoms of night eating
Night eating diagnostic questionnaire [47]	21 items to diagnose NES as per Allison et al. [30]
Three-factor eating questionnaire/eating inventory [130]	51 items; measures three aspects of eating behavior found in research to be common in individuals with obesity, through three scales: Cognitive restraint, disinhibition, hunger. High scores on disinhibition and hunger are characteristic of BED. Not diagnostic

when and how the food aversion developed, the persistence of the avoidance and associated distress and/or impairment are needed to inform diagnosis.

Self-report instruments are useful to screen for particular disorders like binge eating disorder or night eating syndrome and features like shape- and weight-related concerns. However, binge eating, which is necessary for diagnosing BED and BN, is difficult to assess accurately through self-report instruments. The bulk of the research conducted on the concordance between self-report and interview measures have compared the Eating Disorders Exam-Interview (EDE-I) to the Eating Disorders Exam-Questionnaire (EDE-Q) [76–79]. In summary, this research shows that self-report measures yield higher levels of binge eating compared to clinical interviews [61, 76–80]. As Fairburn and Beglin [61] note and our experience supports, this is because patients generally lack the knowledge required for accurately defining a binge. The term “binge eating” has entered the cultural lexicon, but individuals who do not have an understanding of the clinically defined features of a binge, such as the amount of food required for an objective binge, cannot accurately report on these symptoms. Clinical interviews thus allow for the probing that is needed to determine whether a patient who reports “binge eating” truly is binge eating according to the DSM-5.

In addition to binge eating, self-report measures as compared to clinical interviews tend to yield higher scores on weight- and shape-related concerns [81]. Fairburn and Beglin [61] posit that similarly to binge eating, laypersons lack the knowledge needed to assess clinically defined weight- and shape-related distress. The ability to differentiate normative dissatisfaction about shape and weight from the more extreme concerns typical in eating disorders requires clinical experience. However, they found little discrepancy between the EDE-Q and EDE-I in assessing the frequency of self-induced vomiting and laxative misuse, likely because these are behaviors that are simply either present or absent. The overall pattern of findings in this study suggested that self-report questionnaires can be used to assess clearly defined behavioral symptoms like self-induced vomiting, laxative misuse, and dietary restraint, but interviews should be used to assess binge eating and body dissatisfaction.

10.6 Considerations for Triaging to Treatment

Once an obese patient has been diagnosed with an eating disorder, planning for treatment involves several considerations (see Table 10.4 for steps for triage following a diagnosis of an eating disorder).

10.6.1 Dieting

Weight loss diets are often a first choice option for obese individuals who want to lose weight; however, for individuals who are obese and have an eating disorder, there are some important cautions. Individuals who diet typically only lose 5–10 % of their total body weight [82–84]. Also, the long-term maintenance of weight loss is typically minimal with only approximately 7 lbs with diet alone or 8 lbs with diet and exercise [85–87]. There are numerous different types of diets available and there is no consensus on which diets work best; however, diet and exercise combined has been found to increase the likelihood of maintaining weight loss at 1 year [88]. Very low calorie diets demonstrate the greatest efficacy in terms of amount of initial weight loss (approximately 20 %), but these diets are difficult to sustain [83]. Long-term studies suggest that many dieters regain more weight than they lost initially

Table 10.4 Steps for triage following diagnosis of an eating disorder

1.	Complete diagnostic assessment
2.	Communicate diagnosis to patient
3.	Provide psychoeducation
4.	Assess motivation to change
5.	Consider medications
6.	Involve other health care providers
7.	Monitor medical status
8.	Refer to evidence-based psychotherapy

and lifestyle changes alone have not been found to produce significant long-term weight reductions [82]. When examining individuals who are successful at maintaining weight loss, findings from the National Weight Control Registry have found that factors associated with weight loss maintenance include having a weight loss goal, more weight loss initially, increased physical activity, a regular eating pattern, self-monitoring, and flexible control over eating [89, 90].

Depression and other psychiatric disorders can be obstacles to weight loss and weight loss maintenance [89]. There has also been concern raised that dietary restriction may in fact increase binge eating frequency or night eating in individuals who have an eating disorder. Research has not found a consistent association between severe dietary restriction and binge eating or night eating [39, 91]. Binge episodes generally decline during the weight loss attempts [83, 92]. Even with very low calorie diets, binge eaters can lose a similar amount of weight to those without binge eating [83]. It is important to note that binge eating may return when the severe energy restriction or the diet is terminated, but it has not necessarily been found to increase binge eating [83]. While dieting has not been a proven risk factor for BED, weight cycling is associated with binge eating and thus psychological treatments are likely best as first-line interventions to address the eating disorder pathology [10]. Also, in terms of addressing problems associated with obesity in individuals with eating disorders, a focus on normalizing food intake and physical activity with only moderate calorie restrictions is suggested [10, 83].

10.6.2 Psychological Approaches

Cognitive Behavior Therapy (CBT; [72]), Interpersonal Therapy (IPT; [93]), Dialectical Behavior Therapy (DBT; [94]), Motivational Interviewing (MI; [95]), and mindfulness approaches [96] have all been used in treatment studies of BED. CBT is the most studied modality and both CBT and IPT are currently considered empirically validated treatments for BED [21]. Psychological interventions have generally been found to be superior to behavioral interventions in terms of reducing eating pathology and improving psychological functioning, but weight loss has been minimal with these approaches [22]. Grilo et al. [97] found that when substantial improvements in reducing binge eating symptoms occurred within the first 4 weeks of treatment, this rapid response predicted remission at post-treatment in obese patients with BED. Regarding night eating, Berner and Allison [58] reviewed treatments available and found two case studies that suggested that behavioral interventions improved night eating and another study found that progressive muscle relaxation helped to reduce evening appetite [98]. CBT for NES has recently been developed and integrates elements of CBT for insomnia. The preliminary results of a pilot study suggest that a decrease in nocturnal ingestions and NES symptoms were found using this ten-session protocol [28]. While psychological interventions have not been found to reduce weight per se, they are effective first-line interventions for treatment of eating disorder symptoms and may in fact prevent further weight gain by reducing eating disorder pathology [99].

10.7 Psychopharmacology

10.7.1 Stimulants, Antidepressants, and Antiepileptic Medications Have Been Tried Successfully in Treatment of BED

Lisdexamfetamine dimesylate (Vyvanse) is now the first FDA-approved medication to treat moderate to severe binge eating disorder (defined as having at least 3 binge days a week for 2 weeks). The recommended starting dose for Vyvanse is 30 mg to be titrated upwards in 20 mg increments up to 70 mg.

In two studies [100] involving more than 700 people, Vyvanse (50 and 70 mg studied over 12 weeks) decreased the average number of binge days more than a placebo. Vyvanse cut the average number of binge days per week from nearly 5 to less than 1 at the end of the 12-week study.

In another clinical trial [101], half of those taking the 70-mg dose of Vyvanse stopped binge eating during the 4-week period studied, compared to 21 % of those taking placebo. The most common side effects reported were dry mouth, sleeplessness, increased heart rate, a jittery feeling, and anxiety. Caution should be exercised regarding the use of stimulants as they can cause or exacerbate psychosis, mania, or seizures as well as sudden death in people who have existing heart problems. Abuse potential is another consideration.

The efficacy of antidepressant agents in the treatment of BED has been examined. In a meta-analysis of seven RCTs [102], treatment with antidepressants (six with selective serotonin reuptake inhibitors and one with a tricyclic antidepressant) was associated with significantly higher binge eating remission rates (40.5 %) compared with the placebo group (22.2 %). There were no significant differences between the antidepressant and placebo groups in change in mean frequency of binge eating episodes, BMI, or treatment discontinuation. Bupropion [103], however, when compared to placebo did not show any improvement in binge eating frequency but rather weight loss whereas duloxetine demonstrated greater improvement in binge eating, body weight and global measures of improvement when compared to placebo [104].

Two large placebo-controlled RCTs of topiramate in BED found that topiramate treatment was superior to placebo in reducing binge eating frequency, obsessive-compulsive features of binge eating, global severity of illness, body weight, and BMI [105, 106].

Zonisamide was superior to placebo in reducing binge eating frequency, body weight, BMI, measures of global severity, disinhibition of eating, and obsessive-compulsive characteristics of binge eating in a 12-week randomized controlled trial [107].

10.7.2 Antidepressants, Melatonergic Medications, Topiramate, and Light Therapy Might Help in the Treatment of NES

Collectively, limited double-blind controlled studies and case reports suggest that SSRI medications, (particularly sertraline and escitalopram), melatonergic medications, topiramate, and light therapy may be effective for the treatment of NES.

Two double blinded placebo-controlled studies are available studying the impact of antidepressants on NES. Sertraline (mean dose of 126.5 mg over 8 weeks) has improved NES symptoms and quality of life indicators with significant weight loss (2.9+/−3.8 kg) compared to placebo [108]. However, escitalopram (10–20 mg over 12 weeks) did fare better than placebo in terms of NES symptom improvement or weight loss [109].

In open-label studies, there was evidence of improvement in NES symptoms when patients were tried on sertraline [110] and escitalopram [111].

Agomelatine (50 mg/day) was shown in one case report [112] used over 3 months and in a case series of five patients [113] given over 10 weeks to improve NES and depressive symptoms with decrease in average weight change.

Topiramate (75 mg to 125 mg/day) in few case reports [114–116] has shown over 3–9 months trial positive results improving patients' NES, sleep walking, and nocturnal eating. Two weeks treatment with 10,000 lux of light therapy over 30 min daily has been documented in two case reports to improve NES and depressive symptoms [117, 118].

10.7.3 Bariatric Surgery and Eating Disorders

In terms of weight loss interventions, bariatric surgery is the most effective in that individuals typically lose between 20–40 % of their excess weight [22]. While weight loss surgery rates are increasing, approximately 20–30 % of individuals have difficulty maintaining weight loss post-surgery and will regain weight [119], with postoperative weight regain typically occurring between 18 and 24 months post-surgery [120]. Factors that contribute to weight regain include poor adherence to diet recommendations, a return to unhealthy eating patterns, lack of physical activity, substance abuse, and potential resolution of dumping syndrome [119]. When examining pre-op predictors of weight loss post-surgery, there is little evidence that pre-op disordered eating or other psychiatric disorders predicts post-op weight outcomes [7, 22, 119] and currently, the most robust predictor of postoperative weight loss is postoperative eating behavior and adherence to diet and physical activity recommendations [121]. The longest longitudinal study to date with a 10-year follow-up found that individuals with higher hunger and disinhibition scores 10 years post-surgery were more likely to have gained weight or have lost less than 10 % of baseline weight [122].

Eating disorders have been found to emerge post-bariatric surgery; however, disordered eating presents differently than classic eating disorder behaviors, which makes it more difficult to classify using DSM-5 criteria. For example, after bariatric surgery it is difficult to eat large amounts of food at one time and thus grazing with a loss of control is more typical of binge eating after surgery. De Zwaan [22] found that 25 % of post-bariatric surgery patients report subjective binge eating 2 years after surgery with more than half reporting weekly episodes, but only 3.4 % met full criteria for BED. Similarly, vomiting is common after surgery due to gastric discomfort, particularly during the first several months after surgery, but some individuals may vomit for compensatory reasons. De Zwaan [22] found that while 62.7 % reported vomiting due to gastric discomfort, 12 % reported vomiting for shape- and weight-related concerns. Lastly, many post-bariatric surgery individuals overly restrict their food intake but do not necessarily achieve the very low weights typical of anorexia patients. Therefore, detecting the presence of an eating disorder can be difficult in post-bariatric surgery patients as changes in eating after surgery may appear to mimic eating disorder symptoms.

Disordered eating (e.g., grazing, emotional eating, night eating, binge eating, loss of control) has been found to predict poorer weight loss and higher levels of distress in post-bariatric patients [121]. White et al. [123] found that higher post-surgery depressive symptoms not only predicted poorer weight loss, but also greater eating disorder pathology and lower quality of life. Most of the research to date on postsurgical eating disorders has been based on case studies. A report on five case studies of patients with symptoms of anorexia and bulimia post-surgery noted that post-op anxiety about weight regain and body image concerns were prominent [66]. A review of 12 cases of anorexia and bulimia post-surgery [124] found that 50 % had complications after surgery and eating disorder symptoms included intense restriction, a marked fear of weight regain, and body image disturbance related to loose skin. In this case study series, all patients reported a history of dieting and 66 % had a history of an eating disorder. Of note, women who develop eating disorders after bariatric surgery tend to be considerably older than typical eating disorder populations. Conceicao et al. [124] suggest that the eating changes required by bariatric surgery and the accelerated weight loss may result in some individuals being vulnerable to developing eating disorders post-surgery. Body image dissatisfaction, difficulty recognizing weight loss, and concern about loose skin have been reported in case studies describing eating disorders post-surgery [66]. The authors also highlight that the risk of severe restrictive behaviors tends to increase when weight loss slows. Further research is needed to better understand the risk factors for developing eating disorders post-surgery as there are likely moderating and mediating factors.

It is important to first consider psychological treatments for patients considering bariatric surgery and who also have an eating disorder. While the current literature does not demonstrate a direct association between eating disorder pathology pre-surgery and problems with weight loss or eating disorders post-surgery, the limited research does suggest that when eating disorder symptoms emerge post-surgery, they can be more complicated and contribute to further problems with weight loss. Such individuals would likely benefit from developing skills to reduce eating disorder symptoms pre-surgery. Surgical assessment centers that assess eating disorder pathology when considering individuals for surgery may recommend that eating disorder treatment is pursued prior to surgery. For individuals that are accepted and decide to have surgery, it is important to closely monitor these patients both in terms of depression and eating disorder symptoms post-surgery, especially within the first 2 years as this is typically the time period when problems may occur. If eating disorder symptoms emerge post-surgery, it is important to accurately assess and diagnose eating disorders in this population. Specifically, understanding the motivation for engaging in eating behaviors is instrumental in differentiating between typical post-bariatric surgery eating practices versus eating disorder symptoms. Furthermore, the level of preoccupation and related distress are often indicators of severity. Individuals who engage in significant dietary restriction may not present as significantly underweight; thus, assessing physical health is essential as these patients may be at increased risk of nutritional deficiencies given the malabsorption that accompanies some bariatric surgeries.

Case Vignettes Revisited

Mark completed an assessment with a psychologist who specializes in eating disorders. In addition to screening for other psychiatric disorders, the psychologist used the EDE-I to diagnose eating disorders, and Mark completed the Binge Eating Scale and Night Eating Questionnaire. Based on these measures, the psychologist diagnosed him with Binge Eating Disorder, but not Night Eating Disorder. During the clinical interview, the psychologist ascertained that while Mark did consume a significant amount of food 1–2 h before bedtime, which may be indicative of NES, he also ate medium to large portions of food for breakfast, lunch, and dinner in an attempt to adhere to recommendations to eat regularly as a way to manage his diabetes. In the interview as well as on the Binge Eating Scale, he endorsed feeling out of control of his eating, frequent cravings, and being preoccupied with eating.

Based on the assessment, the psychologist referred Mark to a course of individual CBT to address BED. Treatment involved identifying the factors contributing to Mark's weight gain and maintenance, daily food tracking and establishing a regularly eating pattern, thought monitoring, and problem-solving. He was also referred to a registered dietitian familiar with diabetes management for nutritional counseling. Mark was engaged and motivated to implement the CBT strategies. Initially his binges decreased in size, then in frequency to once per week from two to three times each week. He and a friend from work who wanted to improve his fitness committed to going to a gym together once a week after work for 1–2 h. In contrast to previous weight loss attempts that consumed most of Mark's free time but were unsustainable long-term, the CBT program helped him find more reasonable and sustainable solutions to his eating habits. After 3 months of identifying and learning to problem-solve the triggers for his binge eating, Mark's blood sugar control improved, his mood and energy improved, and he reported sleeping better at night. Although he still uses his CPAP, the pressure requirement was reduced due to weight loss.

10.8 Summary

- Binge eating disorder (BED) and night eating syndrome (NES) are commonly reported in severely obese populations and eating disorders contribute to problems associated with obesity. There is a high degree of psychiatric comorbidity (depression, anxiety, substance abuse) with eating disorders in obese individuals. Psychiatric comorbidity contributes to greater severity of eating disorder pathology and poorer functioning in general.

- A comprehensive assessment is required to determine the presence and nature of eating disorder pathology. While there are various valid self-report measures that are useful for screening, these cannot replace the value of a thorough clinical interview. Body image disturbance should be assessed as well and can be a marker of severity despite that it is not a criterion for BED or NES. Also, assessing self-esteem, quality of life, and psychiatric comorbidity is important when considering factors that may influence the degree of severity of eating pathology.
- Psychological treatments should be a priority for addressing eating disorders, and various treatments including CBT and IPT have been found to be successful in reducing eating disorder symptoms. If weight loss is a secondary treatment goal, the various weight loss approaches available need to be carefully considered given the individual's presentation in order to reduce the chance of weight cycling, which is associated with binge eating. When considering bariatric surgery, it is important to be aware of the risks of eating pathology post-surgery and the challenges associated with assessment and treatment.

References

1. Tanofsky-Kraff M, Yanovski SZ. Eating disorder or disordered eating? Non-normative eating patterns in obese individuals. Obes Res. 2004;12(9):1361–6.
2. Urquhart CS, Mihalynuk TV. Disordered eating in women: implications for the obesity pandemic. Can J Diet Pract Res. 2011;72(50):e115–25.
3. Kessler RC, Berglund PA, Tat Chiu W, et al. The prevalence and correlates of binge eating disorder in the world health organization world mental health surveys. Biol Psychiatry. 2013;73:904–14.
4. Colles SL, Dixon JB. Night eating syndrome: impact on bariatric surgery. Obes Surg. 2006;16:811–20.
5. Stunkard AJ, Allison KC, Geliebter A, Lundgren JD, Gluck ME, O'Reardon JP. Development of criteria for a diagnosis: lessons from the night eating syndrome. Compr Psychiatry. 2009;50:391–9.
6. Vander Wal JS. Night eating syndrome: a critical review of the literature. Clin Psychol Rev. 2012;32: 49–59.
7. Parker K, Brennan L. Measurement of disordered eating in bariatric surgery candidates: a systematic review of the literature. Obes Res Clin Pract. 2015;9:12–25.
8. Colles SL, Dixon JB, O'Brien PE. Night eating syndrome and nocturnal snacking: association with obesity, binge eating and psychological distress. Int J Obes. 2007;31:1722–30.
9. Sarach O, Atasoy N, Akdemir A, et al. The prevalence and clinical features of the night eating syndrome in psychiatric out-patient population. Compr Psychiatry. 2015;57:79–84.
10. Amianto F, Ottone L, Abbate Daga G, Fassino S. Binge-eating disorder diagnosis and treatment: a recap in front of DSM-5. BMC Psychiatry. 2015; 15:70.
11. Stice E, Marti CN, Rohde P. Prevalence, incidence, impairment, and course of the proposed DSM-5 eating disorder diagnoses in an 8-year prospective community study of young women. J Abnorm Psychol. 2013;122(2):445–57.
12. Lydecker JA, Grilo CM. Different yet similar: examining race and ethnicity in treatment-seeking adults with binge eating disorder. J Consult Clin Psych. 2016;84(1):88–94.
13. Hoek HW. Epidemiology of eating disorders in persons other than the high-risk group of young western females. Curr Opin Psychiatry. 2014;27:423–5.
14. Agh T, Kovacs G, Pawaskar M, Supina D, Inotai A, Voko Z. Epidemiology, health-related quality of life and economic burden of binge eating disorder: a systematic review of the literature. Eat Weight Disord. 2015;20:1–12.
15. Calugi S, Dalle Grave R, Marchesini G. Night eating syndrome in class II–III obesity: metabolic and psychopathological features. Int J Obes. 2009;33: 899–904.
16. Grilo CM, Masheb RM. Night-time eating in men and women with binge eating disorder. Behav Res Ther. 2004;42:397–407.
17. Shingleton RM, Thompson-Brenner H, Thompson DR, Pratt EM, Franko DL. Gender differences in clinical trials of binge eating disorder: an analysis of aggregated data. J Consult Clin Psych. 2015;83(2): 382–6.
18. Striegel-Moore RH, Franko DL, Thompson D, Affenito S, Kraemer HC. Night eating: prevalence and demographic correlates. Obesity. 2006;14(1): 139–47.

19. Franko DL, Thompson-Brenner H, Thompson DR, et al. Racial/ethnic differences in adults in randomized clinical trials of binge eating disorder. J Consult Clin Psych. 2012;80(2):186–95.
20. Brownley KA, Peat CM, La Via M, Bulik CM. Pharmacological approaches to the management of binge eating disorder. Drugs. 2015;75:9–32.
21. Alfonsson S, Parling T, Ghaderi A. Group behavioral activation for patients with severe obesity and binge eating disorder: a randomized controlled trial. Behav Modif. 2015;39(2):270–94.
22. De Zwaan M, Hilbert A, Swan-Kremeier L, et al. Comprehensive interview assessment of eating behavior 18–35 months after gastric bypass surgery for morbid obesity. Surg Obes Relat Dis. 2010;6: 79–87.
23. Gallant AR, Lundgren J, Drapeau V. The night-eating syndrome and obesity. Obes Rev. 2012;13: 528–36.
24. Grucza RA, Przybeck TR, Cloninger CR. Prevalence and correlates of binge eating disorder in a community sample. Compr Psychiatry. 2007;48:124–31.
25. Hudson JI, Coit CE, Lalonde JK, Pope HG. By how much will the proposed new DSM-5 criteria increase the prevalence of binge eating disorder? Int J Eat Disord. 2012;45:139–41.
26. Castellini G, Godini L, Gorini Amedei S, et al. Psychopathological similarities and differences between obese patients seeking surgical and non-surgical overweight treatments. Eat Weight Disord. 2014;19:95–102.
27. Lundgren JD, Allison KC, Crow S, et al. Prevalence of the night eating syndrome in a psychiatric population. Am J Psychiatry. 2006;163(1):156–8.
28. Allison KC, Lundgren JD, O'Reardon JP, et al. Proposed diagnostic criteria for night eating syndrome. Int J Eat Disord. 2010;43:241–7.
29. Aronoff NJ, Geliebter A, Zammit G. Gender and body mass index as related to the night-eating syndrome in obese outpatients. J Am Diet Assoc. 2001;101:102–4.
30. Rand CSW, Macgregor AMC, Stunkard AJ. The night eating syndrome in the general population and among postoperative obesity surgery patients. Int J Eat Disord. 1997;22:65–9.
31. Goldschmidt AB, Le Grange D, Powers P, et al. Eating disorder symptomatology in normal-weight vs. obese individuals with binge eating disorder. Obesity. 2011;19:1515–8.
32. Dingemans AE, van Furth EF. Binge eating disorder psychopathology in normal weight and obese individuals. Int J Eat Disord. 2012;45:135–8.
33. Marshall HM, Allison KC, O'Reardon JP, Birketvedt G, Stunkard AJ. Night eating syndrome among non-obese persons. Int J Eat Disord. 2004;35:217–22.
34. Carrard I, Van der Linden M, Golay A. Comparison of obese and nonobese individuals with binge eating disorder: delicate boundary between binge eating disorder and non-purging bulimia nervosa. Eur Eat Disord Rev. 2012;20:350–4.
35. Lundgren JD, Rempfer MV, Brown CE, Goetz J, Hamera E. The prevalence of night eating syndrome and binge eating disorder among overweight and obese individuals with serious mental illness. Psychiatry Res. 2010;175:233–6.
36. Lundgren JD, Allison KC, O'Reardon JP, Stunkard AJ. A descriptive study of non-obese persons with night eating syndrome and a weight-matched comparison group. Eat Behav. 2008;9:343–51.
37. Allison KC, Grilo CM, Masheb RM, Stunkard AJ. Binge eating disorder and night eating syndrome: a comparative study of disordered eating. J Consult Clin Psych. 2005;73(6):1107–15.
38. Grilo CM, White MA, Barnes RD, Masheb RM. Psychiatric disorder co-morbidity and correlates in an ethnically diverse sample of obese patients with binge eating disorder in primary care settings. Compr Psychiatry. 2013;54:209–16.
39. de Zwaan M, Roerig DB, Crosby RD, Karaz S, Mitchell JE. Nighttime eating: a descriptive study. Int J Eat Disord. 2006;39:224–32.
40. Stunkard AJ. Eating disorders and obesity. Psychiatr Clin North Am. 2011;34:765–71.
41. Picot AK, Lilenfeld LRR. The relationship among binge severity, personality psychopathology, and body mass index. Int J Eat Disord. 2003;34:98–107.
42. Mitchell JE, Selzer F, Kalarchian MA, et al. Psychopathology before surgery in the Longitudinal Assessment of Bariatric Surgery-3 (LABS-3) Psychosocial Study. Surg Obes Relat Dis. 2012; 8:533–41.
43. Jones-Corneille LR, Wadden TA, Sarwer DB, et al. Axis I psychopathology in bariatric surgery candidates with and without binge eating disorder: results of structured clinical interviews. Obes Surg. 2012; 22(3):389–97.
44. Becker DF, Grilo CM. Comorbidity of mood and substance use disorders in patients with binge-eating disorder: associations with personality disorder and eating disorder pathology. J Psychosom Res. 2015; 79:159–64.
45. Rieger E, Wilfley DE, Stein RI, Marino V, Crow SJ. A comparison of quality of life in obese individuals with and without binge eating disorder. Int J Eat Disord. 2005;37:234–40.
46. Gluck ME, Geliebter A, Satov T. Night eating syndrome is associated with depression, low self-esteem, reduced daytime hunger, and less weight loss in obese outpatients. Obes Res. 2001;9(4): 264–7.
47. Perez M, Warren CS. The relationship between quality of life, binge-eating disorder, and obesity status in an ethnically diverse sample. Obesity. 2012;20(4): 879–85.
48. Vinai P, Ferri R, Ferrini-Strambi L, et al. Defining the borders between sleep-related eating disorder

and night eating syndrome. Sleep Med. 2012;13: 686–90.
49. De Zwaan M, Mitchell JE, Howell LM, et al. Characteristics of morbidly obese patients before gastric bypass surgery. Compr Psychiatry. 2003; 44(5):428–34.
50. Mitchell JE, King WC, Pories W, et al. Binge eating disorder and medical comorbidities in bariatric surgery candidates. Int J Eat Disord. 2015;48:471–6.
51. Kalarchian MA, Marcus MD, Levine MD, et al. Psychiatric disorders among bariatric surgery candidates: relationship to obesity and functional health status. Am J Psychiatry. 2007;164(2):328–74.
52. Fairburn CG, Cooper Z. The eating disorder examination. In: Fairburn CG, Wilson GT, editors. Binge eating: nature, assessment, and treatment. 12th ed. New York: The Guilford Press; 1993. p. 317–60.
53. Masheb RM, Grilo CM, Whites MA. An examination of eating patterns in community women with bulimia nervosa and binge eating disorder. Int J Eat Disord. 2011;44(7):618–24. doi:10.1002/eat.20853.
54. Birgegard A, Clinton D, Norring C. Diagnostic issues of binge eating in eating disorders. Eur Eat Disord Rev. 2013;21:175–83.
55. Fairburn CG, Cooper Z, Doll HA, Norman P, O'Connor M. The natural course of bulimia nervosa and binge eating disorder in young women. Arch Gen Psychiatry. 2000;57:659–65.
56. O'Reardon JP, Ringel BL, Dinges DF, Allison KC, Rogers NL, Martino NS, Stunkard AJ. Circadian eating and sleeping patterns of the night eating syndrome. Obes Res. 2004;12:1789–96.
57. Stunkard AJ, Grace WJ, Wolff HG. The night-eating syndrome: a pattern of food intake among certain obese patients. Am J Med. 1955;19:78–86.
58. Berner LA, Allison KC. Behavioral management of night eating disorders. Psychol Res Behav Manag. 2013;6:1–8.
59. Birketvedt GS, Florholmen J, Sundsfjord J, et al. Behavioral and neuroendocrine characteristics of the night-eating syndrome. JAMA. 1999;282:657–63.
60. Napolitano MA, Head S, Babyak MA, Blumenthal JA. Binge eating disorder and night eating syndrome: psychological and behavioral characteristics. Int J Eat Disord. 2001;30:193–203.
61. Fairburn CG, Beglin SJ. Assessment of eating disorders: interview or self-report questionnaire? Int J Eat Disord. 1994;16(4):363–70.
62. American Psychiatric Association. Diagnostic and statistical manual of mental disorders. 5th ed. Washington, DC: American Psychiatric Association; 2013.
63. Marino JM, Ertelt TW, Lancaster K, Steffen K, Peterson L, de Zwaan M, Mitchell JE. The emergence of eating pathology after bariatric surgery: a rare outcome with important clinical implications. Int J Eat Disord. 2012;45:179–84.
64. Pazeres de Assis P, Alves da Silva S, Vieira de Melo CYS, de Arruda MM. Eating habits, nutritional status and quality of life in late postoperative gastric bypass Roux-Y. Nutr Hosp. 2013;28(3):637–42.
65. Rusch MD, Andris D. Maladaptive eating patterns after weight-loss surgery. Nutr Clin Pract. 2007;22: 41–9.
66. Segal A, Kinoshita Kussunoki D, Larino MA. Postsurgical refusal to eat: anorexia nervosa, bulimia nervosa or a new eating disorder? A case series. Obes Surg. 2004;14:353–60.
67. Sousa Novais PF, Rasera Junior I, Shiraga EC, Marques de Oliveira MR. Food aversions in women during the 2 years after Roux-En-Y gastric bypass. Obes Surg. 2011;21:1921–7.
68. Allison KC, Wadden TA, Sarwer DB, Fabricatore AN, Crerand CE, Gibbons LM, et al. Night eating syndrome and binge eating disorder among persons seeking bariatric surgery: prevalence and related features. Obesity. 2006;14(S3):77S–82.
69. Dymek-Valentine M, Rienecke-Hoste R, Alverdy J. Assessment of binge eating disorder in morbidly obese patients evaluated for gastric bypass: SCID versus QEWP-R. Eat Weight Disord. 2004;9(3): 211–6.
70. Elder KA, Grilo CM, Masheb RM, Rothschild BS, Burke-Martindale CH, Brody ML. Comparison of two self-report instruments for assessing binge eating in bariatric surgery candidates. Behav Res Ther. 2006;44(4):545–60.
71. Kalarchian MA, Marcus MD, Wilson GT, Labouvie EW, Brolin RE, LaMarca LB. Binge eating among gastric bypass patients at long-term follow-up. Obes Surg. 2002;12:270–5.
72. Fairburn CG, Cooper Z, O'Connor M. Eating disorder examination. In: Fairburn CG, editor. Cognitive behavior therapy and eating disorders. New York: Guilford Press; 2008. p. 315–8.
73. First MB, Spitzer RL, Gibbon M, Williams JBW. Structured clinical interview for DSM-IV-TR Axis I disorders, clinician version. Arlington, VA: American Psychiatric Association; 2007.
74. Sheehan DV, Lecrubier Y, Harnett-Sheehan K, Janavs J, Weiller E, Bonara LI, Keskiner A, Schinka J, Knapp E, Sheehan MF, Dunbar GC. Reliability and validity of the M.I.N.I. International neuropsychiatric interview (M.I.N.I.): according to the SCID-P. Eur Psychiat. 1997;12:232–41.
75. Allison KC, Crow SJ, Reeves RR, West DS, Foreyt JP, DiLillo VG, Wadden TA, Jeffrey RW, Van Dorsten B, Stunkard AJ, The Eating Disorders Subgroup of the Look AHEAD Reearch Group. Binge eating disorder and night eating syndrome in adults with type 2 diabetes. Obesity. 2007;15(5):1287–93.
76. Elder KA, Grilo CM. The Spanish language version of the Eating Disorder Examination Questionnaire: comparison with the Spanish language version of the eating disorder examination and test-retest reliability. Behav Res Ther. 2007;45(6):1369–77.
77. Grilo CM, Masheb RM, Wilson GT. Different methods for assessing the features of eating disorders in

patients with binge eating disorder: a replication. Obes Res. 2001;9(7):418–22.
78. Kalarchian MA, Wilson GT, Brolin RE, Bradley L. Assessment of eating disorders in bariatric surgery candidates: self-report questionnaire versus interview. Int J Eat Disord. 2000;28:465–9.
79. Wilfley DE, Schwartz MB, Spurrell EB, Fairburn CG. Assessing the specific psychopathology of binge eating disorder patients: interview or self-report? Behav Res Ther. 1997;35:1151–9.
80. de Zwaan M, Mitchell JE, Specker SM, Pyle RL, Mussell MP, Seim HC. Diagnosing binge eating disorder: level of agreement between self-report and expert-rating. Int J Eat Disord. 1993;14(3):289–95.
81. Barnes RD, Masheb RM, White MA, Grilo CM. Comparison of methods for identifying and assessing obese patients with binge eating disorder in primary care settings. Int J Eat Disord. 2011;44: 157–63.
82. Taylor VH, Stonehocker B, Steele M, Sharma AM. An overview of treatments for obesity in a population with mental illness. Can J Psychiatry. 2012; 57:13–20.
83. National Task Force on the Prevention and Treatment of Obesity. Dieting and the development of eating disorders in overweight and obese adults. Arch Intern Med. 2000;160:2581–9.
84. Alexandraki I, Palacio C, Mooradian AD. Relative merits of low-carbohydrate versus low-fat diet in managing obesity. South Med J. 2015;108(7): 401–16.
85. Dubnov-Raz G, Berry EM. Dietary approaches to obesity. Mt Sinai J Med. 2010;77:488–98.
86. Jain A. Treating obesity in individuals and populations. BMJ. 2005;331:1387–90.
87. Johns DA, Hartmann-Boyce J, Jebb SA. Diet or exercise interventions vs combined behavioral weight management programs: a systematic review and meta-analysis of direct comparisons. J Acad Nutr Diet. 2014;114:1557–68.
88. Williams RL, Wood LG, Collins CE, Callister R. Effectiveness of weight loss interventions—is there a difference between men and women: a systematic review. Obes Rev. 2015;16:171–86.
89. Elfhag K, Rossner S. Who succeeds in maintaining weight loss? A conceptual review of factors associated with weight loss maintenance and weight regain. Obes Rev. 2005;6:67–85.
90. Wing RR, Phelan S. Long-term weight loss maintenance. Am J Clin Nutr. 2005;82(suppl):222S–5.
91. da Luz FQ, Hay P, Gibson AA, et al. Does severe dietary energy restriction increase binge eating in overweight or obese individuals? A systematic review. Obes Rev. 2015;16:652–65.
92. Wonderlich SA, de Zwaan M, Mitchell JE, Peterson C, Crow S. Psychological and dietary treatments of binge eating disorder: conceptual implications. Int J Eat Disord. 2003;34:S58–73.
93. Murphy R, Straebler S, Basden S, Cooper Z, Fairburn CG. Interpersonal psychotherapy for eating disorders. Clin Psychol Psychother. 2012;19(2):150–8.
94. Telch CF, Agras S, Linehan MM. Dialectical behavior therapy for binge eating disorder. J Consult Clin Psych. 2001;69(6):1061–5.
95. Cassin SE, von Ranson KM, Heng K, Brar J, Wojtowicz AE. Adapted motivational interviewing for women with binge eating disorder: a randomized controlled trial. Psychol Addict Behav. 2008;15:364–75.
96. Kristeller JL, Wolever RQ, Sheets V. Mindfulness-based eating awareness training (MB-EAT) for binge eating disorder: a randomized clinical trial. Mindfulness. 2012;3(4).
97. Grilo CM, White MA, Masheb RM, et al. Predicting meaningful outcomes to medication and self-help treatments for binge-eating disorder in primary care: the significance of early rapid response. J Consult Clin Psych. 2015;83:387–94.
98. Pawlow LA, O'Neil PM, Malcolm RJ. Night eating syndrome: effects of brief relaxation training on stress, mood, hunger, and eating patterns. Int J Obes Relat Metab Disord. 2003;27:970–8.
99. Smink FRE, van Hoeken D, Hoek HW. Epidemiology, course and outcome. Curr Opin Psychiatry. 2013; 26:543–8.
100. McElroy SL, Hudson J, Ferreira-Cornwell MC, Radewonuk J, Whitaker T, Gasior M. Lisdexamfetamine Dimesylate for adults with moderate to severe binge eating disorder: results of two pivotal phase 3 randomized controlled trials. Neuropsychopharmacology. 2016;41(5):1251–60.
101. McElroy SL, Hudson J, Mitchell JE, Wilfley D, Ferreira-Cornwell MC, Joseph Gao J, Wang J, Whitaker T, Jonas J, Gasior M. Efficacy and safety of lisdexamfetamine for treatment of adults with moderate to severe binge-eating disorder. JAMA Psychiatry. 2015;72(3):235–46.
102. Stefano SC, Bacaltchuk J, Blay SL, Appolinário JC. Antidepressants in the short-term treatment of binge eating disorder: systematic review and meta-analysis. Eat Behav. 2008;9:129–36 (Abstract).
103. White MA, Grilo CM. Bupropion for overweight women with binge-eating disorder: a randomized, double-blind, placebo-controlled trial. J Clin Psychiatry. 2013;74:400–6 (Abstract).
104. Guerdjikova AI, McElroy SL, Winstanley EL, et al. Duloxetine in the treatment of binge eating disorder with depressive disorders: a placebo-controlled trial. Int J Eat Disord. 2012;45:281–9.
105. McElroy SL, Arnold LM, Shapira NA, et al. Topiramate in the treatment of binge eating disorder associated with obesity: a randomized, placebo-controlled trial. Am J Psychiatry. 2003;160:255–61.
106. McElroy SL, Hudson JI, Capece JA, et al. Topiramate for the treatment of binge eating disorder associated with obesity: a placebo-controlled study. Biol Psychiatry. 2007;61:1039–48.

107. McElroy SL, Kotwal R, Guerdjikova AI, et al. Zonisamide in the treatment of binge eating disorder with obesity: a randomized, controlled trial. J Clin Psychiatry. 2006;67:1897–906.
108. O'Reardon JP, Allison KC, Martino NS, Lundgren JD, Heo M, Stunkard AJ. A randomized, placebo-controlled trial of sertraline in the treatment of night eating syndrome. Am J Psychiatry. 2006;163(5):893–8.
109. Vander Wal JS, Gang CH, Griffing GT, Gadde KM. Escitalopram for treatment of night eating syndrome: a 12-week, randomized, placebo-controlled trial. J Clin Psychopharmacol. 2012;32(3):341–5.
110. O'Reardon JP, Stunkard AJ, Allison KC. Clinical trial of sertraline in the treatment of night eating syndrome. Int J Eat Disord. 2004;35(1):16–26.
111. Allison KC, Studt SK, Berkowitz RI, et al. An open-label efficacy trial of escitalopram for night eating syndrome. Eat Behav. 2013;14(2):199–203.
112. Milano W, De Rosa M, Milano L, Capasso A. Agomelatine efficacy in the night eating syndrome. Case Rep Med. 2013;2013:867650. doi:10.1155/2013/867650.
113. Milano W, De Rosa M, Milano L, Riccio A, Sanseverino B, Capasso A. Successful treatment with agomelatine in NES: a series of five cases. Open Neurol J. 2013;7:32–7.
114. Winkelman JW. Treatment of nocturnal eating syndrome and sleep-related eating disorder with topiramate. Sleep Med. 2003;4(3):243–6.
115. Tucker P, Masters B, Nawar O. Topiramate in the treatment of comorbid night eating syndrome and PTSD: a case study. Eat Disord. 2004;12(1):75–8.
116. Cooper-Kazaz R. Treatment of night eating syndrome with topiramate: dawn of a new day. J Clin Psychopharmacol. 2012;32(1):143–5.
117. Friedman S, Even C, Dardennes R, Guelfi JD. Light therapy, obesity, and night-eating syndrome. Am J Psychiatry. 2002;159(5):875–6.
118. Friedman S, Even C, Dardennes R, Guelfi JD. Light therapy, non- seasonal depression, and night eating syndrome. Can J Psychiatry. 2004;49(11):790.
119. Sorensen KW, Herrington H, Kushner RF. Nutrition and weight regain in the bariatric surgical patient. In: Kushner RF, Still CD, editors. Nutrition and bariatric surgery. Boca Raton, FL: Taylor & Francis Group, LLC; 2015. p. 265–79.
120. Chesler BE. Emotional eating: a virtually untreated risk factor for outcome following bariatric surgery. Scientific World Journal. 2012;2012:365961.
121. Sheets CS, Peat CM, Berg KC, et al. Post-operative psychosocial predictors of outcome in bariatric surgery. Obes Surg. 2015;25:330–45.
122. Konttinen H, Peltonen M, Sjostrom L, Carlsson L, Karlsson J. Psychological aspects of eating behavior as predictors of 10 year weight changes after surgical and conventional treatment of severe obesity: results from the Swedish obese subjects intervention study. Am J Clin Nutr. 2015;101:16–24.
123. White MA, Kalarchian MA, Levine MD, Masheb RM, Marcus MD, Grilo CM. Prognostic significance of depressive symptoms on weight loss and psychosocial outcomes following gastric bypass surgery: a prospective 24-month follow-up study. Obes Surg. 2015;25:1909–16.
124. Gormally J, Black S, Daston S, et al. The assessment of binge eating severity among obese persons. Addict Behav. 1982;7:47–55.
125. van Strien T, Frijters JE, Bergers GP, Defares PB. The Dutch Eating Behavior Questionnaire (DEBQ) for assessment of restrained, emotional and external eating behavior. Int J Eat Disord. 1986;5:295–315.
126. Garner DM. Eating Disorder Inventory-3. Professional manual. Lutz, FL: Psychological Assessment Resources; 2004.
127. Mintz LB, O'Halloran MS, Mulholland AM, Schneider PA. Questionnaire for eating disorder diagnoses: reliability and validity of operationalizing DSM-IV criteria into a self-report format. J Couns Psychol. 1997;44(1):63–79.
128. Spitzer RL, Devlin M, Walsh BT, Wing R, Marcus M, Stunkard A, Wadden T, Yanovski S, Agreas S, Mitchell J, Nonas C. Binge eating disorder: a multisite field trial of the diagnostic criteria. Int J Eat Disord. 1992;11:203.
129. Allison KC, Stunkard AJ, Thier SL. Overcoming night eating syndrome. Oakland, CA: New Harbinger; 2004.
130. Stunkard AJ, Messick S. The three-factor eating questionnaire to measure dietary restraint, disinhibition and hunger. J Psychosom Res. 1985;29(1):71–83.
131. Grupski AE, Hood MM, Hall BJ, Azarbad L, Fitzpatrick SL. Examining the Binge Eating Scale in screening for binge eating disorder in bariatric surgery candidates. Obes Surg. 2013;23:1–6.
132. Marcus MD, Wing RR, Hopkins J. Obese binge eaters: Affect, cognitions, and response to behavioral weight control. J Consult Clin Psychol. 1988;3:433–439.

11 Addictive Disorders in Severe Obesity and After Bariatric Surgery

Carrol Zhou and Sanjeev Sockalingam

11.1 Introduction

In this chapter, we discuss addictive disorders in severe obesity, a very important clinical consideration in this patient population. The chapter begins with an overview of the prevalence of substance use disorders in severely obese and bariatric surgery patient populations, followed by a discussion of the neurobiological and physiological correlates of addiction and obesity. We discuss tools for addiction screening and summarize the various forms of psychosocial and pharmacological treatment options for addiction in the context of severe obesity. We finish the chapter with a vignette to help integrate the information learned in this chapter into a clinical scenario.

C. Zhou, M.D.
Department of Psychiatry, University of Toronto, 250 College Street, 8th floor, Toronto, ON, Canada M5T 1R8
e-mail: carrol.zhou@mail.utoronto.ca

S. Sockalingam (✉)
Toronto Western Hospital Bariatric Surgery Program, Centre for Mental Health, University Health Network, 200 Elizabeth Street, Toronto, ON, Canada M5G 2C4

Department of Psychiatry, University of Toronto, Toronto, ON, Canada
e-mail: sanjeev.sockalingam@uhn.ca

11.2 Prevalence of Substance Use Disorders

11.2.1 Substance Use Disorders in Bariatric Surgery Candidates

Past research has shown that a higher body mass index (BMI) is associated with higher rates of substance use and substance use disorders [1, 2]. The lifetime prevalence of a substance use disorder in bariatric surgery candidates ranges between 24 and 35 % [3–5]. The rate of current substance use disorders at the time of surgery is significantly lower, ranging from 1 to 7.6 % [3, 6]. In a recent meta-analysis of all studies examining psychiatric disorder prevalence rates in bariatric surgery candidates, the current rates for any substance use disorder were 3 % [7]. Although the low rates of current substance use disorders in bariatric surgery candidates could represent true remission, patients may also be underreporting current substance use due to concerns about delays in surgery, a result of an active substance use disorder.

Alcohol use disorder (AUD) is the most studied substance use disorder in the bariatric surgery patient population. Data from bariatric surgery candidates suggests that the prevalence of AUDs is similar to that of the general population (7.6 % versus 8.5 %) [4]. Although additional research

S. Sockalingam, R. Hawa (eds.), *Psychiatric Care in Severe Obesity*,
DOI 10.1007/978-3-319-42536-8_11

suggests that the prevalence of lifetime AUDs is higher among candidates for bariatric surgery compared to the general population in North America, some studies have not replicated this finding [3, 8–10].

Prevalence rates for cigarette smoking in bariatric surgery candidates have been as high as 38 % in the literature, with more than half of these patients reporting heavy smoking [11]. Moreover, several studies suggest that rates of cigarette smoking in bariatric surgery candidates do not significantly change pre- and post-bariatric surgery [12, 13]. Older adults undergoing bariatric surgery are more likely to reduce cigarette smoking after surgery compared to young adult patients [12]. Despite these trends, some patients may experience new-onset cigarette smoking after surgery, with reported rates ranging from 9.6 to 12.1 % in small studies [11, 13]. Large prospective studies are needed to clearly elucidate trends in cigarette smoking after bariatric surgery.

Data on prevalence rates of other substance use disorders has been limited due to a paucity of literature. One study showed that 8 % of bariatric patients were chronic opioid users preoperatively, which is higher than the 3 % prevalence rate in the general population [14]. This study contrasts data from the Longitudinal Assessment of Bariatric Surgery-2 (LABS-2) study, which showed that 1.5 % of pre-bariatric surgery patients had a lifetime history of an opioid use disorder [6]. Additional presurgery lifetime substance use disorder rates from the LABS-2 study for cannabis, stimulants, cocaine, and polysubstances were 7.5 %, 3.5 %, 2 %, and 1 %, respectively [15]. Moreover, it appears that benzodiazepine and opioid use disorders among bariatric surgery patients is more likely to be an issue after bariatric surgery [16].

In addition to substance use disorders, the concept of "addiction transfer" (defined as patients moving from an addiction to food to other types of addiction) after bariatric surgery has generated interest in determining prevalence rates of non-substance-related addictive issues, such as compulsive shopping and problem gambling. In a study using structured clinical interviews conducted by telephone, rates of current nondrug-related addictive behaviors in bariatric surgery candidates were 11.5 % [15]. Specific addictive behaviors with the highest current preoperative prevalence included compulsive buying (8.5 %), followed by kleptomania (1 %), pathological gambling (1 %), impulsive–compulsive non-paraphilic sexual behavior (1 %), and exercise dependence (1 %). It should be noted that these behaviors, if present prior to bariatric surgery, were no longer present at 3 years post-bariatric surgery in nearly half of patients (10 of 23 patients in this study) [15]. Therefore, nonalcohol addictive behaviors are not uncommon in severely obese patient populations and warrant exploration prior to bariatric surgery to clearly outline their course after weight loss surgery.

11.2.2 Prevalence of Substance Use Post-bariatric Surgery

Trends from several research studies suggest that addictive behaviors are more likely to increase post-bariatric surgery. Longitudinal observational studies have shown that patients report significant increases in the frequency of composite addictive behaviors (combination of alcohol use, recreational drug use, cigarette smoking, shopping, gambling, sexual activity, internet use, and exercise) 24 months after surgery when compared to their presurgical baseline [17]. Long-term data from the Swedish Obesity Study suggests that these increases in AUD diagnoses and self-reported alcohol problems can persist up to 15 years post-surgery [18].

In a large multicentre longitudinal observational study of bariatric surgical patients, frequency of alcohol consumption and AUDs significantly increased in the second postoperative year compared with the year prior to surgery or the first postoperative year [4]. Notably, 7.9 % of participants not reporting an AUD in the preoperative assessment developed a postoperative AUD, making up more than half of the postoperative AUD patients [4].

Male sex, family history of substance use (especially multiple members of the family with AUD),

Table 11.1 Risk factors of developing a substance use disorder after RYGB surgery

Patient demographic and social factors	Substance use related factors
Males[a]	Family history of a substance use disorder[a]
Younger age	Presurgery nicotine use[a]
Lower interpersonal support presurgery	Post-surgery recreational drug use[a]
Presurgery food addiction	Regular alcohol consumption before surgery[a] (two or more alcoholic drinks per week)
Intake of high glycemic index and high sugar/low fat foods	History of an alcohol use disorder in the 12 months prior to surgery[a]

[a]Only identified as a risk factor for alcohol misuse after bariatric surgery

younger age at time of surgery, smoking, regular alcohol consumption, preoperative AUD, postoperative smoking or recreational drug use, a lower sense of social belonging, and postoperative treatment of mental health and emotional issues were all independently related to an increased likelihood of AUD after surgery [4]. Several of these predictors of AUD (specifically, male sex, younger age, smoking, recreational drug use) are also risk factors for AUD in the general population [19, 20]. Additional risk factors for developing substance use disorders post-bariatric surgery include presurgery "food addiction" (measured by the Yale Food Addiction Scale) and consumption of high glycemic or high sugar/high fat foods [21, 22]. Table 11.1 summarizes potential risk factors for post-surgery substance use disorders.

Interestingly, multiple studies have shown that compared to other surgical procedures, those who underwent the Roux-en Y gastric bypass (RYGB) surgery had an increased risk of developing AUDs after surgery [4, 17, 23]. In the Swedish Obesity Study, patients who underwent RYGB had a higher risk of medium alcohol use consumption, self-reported alcohol use problems, and alcohol use diagnoses compared to vertical banded gastroplasty and gastric banding [18]. Additional studies have shown that the sleeve gastrectomy and laparoscopic gastric-banding procedures do not result in significant changes in alcohol metabolism [24, 25]. RYGB has not been linked in any published studies to an increased risk of other addictive disorders other than alcohol.

As previously mentioned, there are currently few papers that studied the prevalence of other substance use disorders. One study stated that 77 % of chronic opioid users continued to use opioids at 1 year post-surgery follow-up, and they also used a significantly higher amount of opioids than prior to surgery [14]. A retrospective cohort study identified the following risk factors for postoperative chronic opioid use: presurgery opioid use, presurgery use of nonnarcotic analgesics, presurgery antianxiety agents, and cigarette smoking [26]. A case report of a patient who developed narcotic addiction post-bariatric surgery highlights how difficulties detecting substance use can lead to poor patient outcomes [27]. The patient had frequent complaints of vague abdominal pain, which resulted in high doses of prescribed opioids, multiple exploratory laparoscopies, and one laparotomy procedure before a substance use disorder was considered. This case underscores the importance of having awareness of potential postoperative substance dependence, which can assist in earlier identification of potential substance use issues leading to improved care and outcomes for affected patients.

11.2.3 Addiction Transfer After Bariatric Surgery

A controversial topic in the scientific literature today is the concept of "addiction transfer," which describes the replacement of one addictive behavior for another. In brief, some researchers postulate that after bariatric surgery, an individual may shift from overeating, their original form of addictive behavior, to a different substance use disorder. This concept is derived from the observation that patients use binge eating to ameliorate negative emotional states [28]. After surgery, binge eating is no longer a viable alternative for patients, and the notion of addiction transfer suggests that patients turn to other behaviors to alleviate negative emotions. Limited data is available on actual prevalence rates of new-onset addictive behaviors after surgery; however, a study following 201 patients post-bariatric surgery identified a 3 % rate for new-onset addictive behaviors after surgery [15]. Nonetheless, the available evidence is still preliminary, and further research is needed to validate this purported model.

11.3 Neurobiological and Physiological Correlates of Substance Use in Severe Obesity

11.3.1 Background on Addiction Pathways

The pathway responsible for the most reinforcing characteristics of addictive substances, in both the general and bariatric patient population, is the mesolimbic dopamine system [29, 30]. This pathway includes dopaminergic neurons in the ventral tegmental area (VTA) of the midbrain and their targets in the limbic forebrain, especially the nucleus accumbens (NAc). Eventually, neuronal signaling from the NAc reaches the frontal cortex, which is heavily involved in the decision-making process. Various drugs of addiction, regardless of its distinct mechanism of action, converge on the mesolimbic pathway and increase dopaminergic transmission to the NAc after acute administration. They can do so either directly, like cocaine, or indirectly, in the case of opioids [29].

In addiction to drugs of abuse, the rewarding effects of food have also been associated with dopamine (DA) release [31]. The mesolimbic pathway, specifically DA effects in the NAc, has been associated with the motivational processes related to appetite [32] and the drive to eat [33, 34]. The role of DA regulation in obesity is evident through research demonstrating an association between the Taq I A allele and reduced DA dopamine-2 (D2) receptors in brain regions [35]. Based on these findings, researchers purport that obese patients with the Taq I A allele may be predisposed to using food to compensate for this reduction in DA D2 receptors and to stimulate DA activity.

Additional important brain regions that interact with the mesolimbic pathway in substance use disorders include the amygdala, hippocampus, and hypothalamus, among many others. In contrast to drugs of abuse, the relationship between the mesolimbic pathway and hypothalamus in food consumption is mediated through several peripheral signaling pathways involving peptides and hormones, such as leptin, insulin, and cholecystokinin [36]. These peripheral signaling pathways are more specific to obesity and food regulation, whereas drugs of abuse rely on direct effects on mesolimbic structures and the reward system [36, 37].

Moreover, chronic drug use is associated with additional adaptations in dopamine function via both dopamine dependent and independent circuits. Chronic exposure of many addictive substances causes an impaired dopamine signaling system due to the body's attempt to adapt to repeated drug activation (i.e., drug tolerance). Specifically, baseline levels of dopamine are reduced, and normal rewarding stimuli may be less effective at eliciting typical increases in DA transmission. When the person with addiction discontinues substance use, the body can no longer maintain homeostasis, thus resulting in symptoms of withdrawal. Additional disruptions in the corticotropin-releasing factor (CRF) system can also contribute to the negative affective symptoms during substance withdrawal [29].

11.3.2 Now vs. Later Brain Structures in Drug Addiction and Obesity

Balancing behaviors that provide a reward immediately versus behaviors that can provide an advantage later is critical for human adaptive functioning. The "now versus later" model has been used to describe how both addictions and obesity are based on an excessive emphasis of obtaining immediate reward in lieu of choosing actions that promote long-term gains. The circuit responsible for now versus later decision-making involves many of the same anatomical structures of the mesolimbic pathway [37]. According to this model, different signaling patterns of DA can favor the now versus later processes. Specifically, phasic signaling of dopamine in the reward pathway signals "now," whereas tonic signaling in control circuits connected to the reward pathways favors "later." Areas of the brain that mediate "now" signaling include the ventromedial prefrontal cortex and the NAc. Areas of the brain that mediate the "later" signaling include the medial prefrontal cortex, dorsolateral prefrontal cortex (DLPFC), anterior cingulate cortex (ACC), and the caudate [37]. Interestingly, these areas reduce their baseline activity to the body's attempt to adapt to chronic drug exposure. This results in a dysfunctional decision-making circuit in individuals with addictions leading to "hypofrontality," defined by impulsive and compulsive substance use behaviors.

This "now versus later" model and resulting impulsive and compulsive behaviors are applicable to obesity. Studies showing reductions in D2 receptor in the striatum (including the NAc) in obese animal models and associated decreases in activity in various regions of the frontal lobe provide further support for the impulsivity and compulsivity observed in eating in some obese patients [38, 39]. The result of these shared pathways between obesity and drug addiction has generated much discussion on the conceptualizing of obesity as "food addiction"; however, much of the evidence for food addiction is based on rat models, and we have yet to identify specific food substances or molecules that cause addiction to date [40]. Despite these parallels between drug addiction and obesity neurobiological pathways, clinicians should not be preoccupied with justifying food addiction nomenclature and should instead be using the understanding of these shared pathways to develop potential therapeutic alternatives for both substance use and obesity.

11.3.3 The Role of Adipokines on Neurobiological Pathways Related to Addictive Disorders

Ghrelin is an endogenous molecule that plays an important role in long-term weight regulation. Through several pathways, ghrelin can bind to growth hormone secretagogue receptors in the hypothalamus, which leads to signaling cascades leading to increased food intake [41]. Although plasma ghrelin is elevated in individuals undergoing long-term diets, plasma ghrelin is markedly suppressed following bariatric surgery, and this change in ghrelin is hypothesized to contribute to sustaining weight loss after bariatric surgery [42, 43].

Interestingly, there is some research that ghrelin could also impact the reward system pathways. It is suggested that ghrelin acts on the mesolimbic reward circuit via cholinergic afferents extending to the VTA and enhancing dopamine effects in the brain [44, 45]. Moreover, data from animal models has not shown reproducible results regarding the effects of ghrelin on post-surgery alcohol use [46–48]. Therefore, it is unclear whether decreases in ghrelin post-bariatric surgery could impact the frequency of addictive behavior and substance use in post-bariatric surgery patients.

Leptin, an appetite regulating peptide responsible for satiety, is produced by adipocytes and regulates energy balance by suppressing hunger [49]. Patients with obesity can develop leptin resistance over time, which impairs satiety signaling in response to high-energy stores [50]. Few studies have identified a positive correlation between leptin levels and food-cued brain activations in the mesolimbic area [51, 52]. Thus, the creation of a leptin-resistant state may result in elevations in leptin resulting in altered homeostatic regulation of reward pathways related to food [52].

11.4 Altered Substance Use Metabolism with Bariatric Surgery

11.4.1 Altered Alcohol Metabolism After Bariatric Surgery

As noted earlier in this chapter, RYGB has been associated with increased rates of alcohol use disorders post-bariatric surgery [18]. Researchers postulate that increases in alcohol sensitivity and a change in ethanol pharmacodynamics following RYGB may increase alcohol's reinforcing effects, resulting in the observed increase in AUD rates after bariatric surgery [53].

Post-RYGB patients reach higher peak blood alcohol levels more rapidly than age- and BMI-matched controls ingesting the same amount of ethanol and take longer to return to baseline [54]. There are two potential reasons for this phenomenon. Firstly, post-RYGB patients have rapid emptying of liquids from the gastric pouch into the jejunum, thus resulting in faster speed of absorption. Secondly, the portion of the stomach that secretes alcohol dehydrogenase, which metabolizes alcohol, is bypassed by RYGB [55]. The changes of the effect of alcohol on post-RYGB individuals could make alcohol more reinforcing and an individual more susceptible to AUD post-bariatric surgery.

11.4.2 Altered Metabolism of Other Substances After Bariatric Surgery

Data on metabolism of other substances is lacking; however, there is some evidence that these substances can be metabolized in a way that enhances abuse liability in the postoperative phase. Recent data suggests that the propensity for substance abuse may be increased with two substances, namely, opioid pain medications and benzodiazepines [16]. Opioids may also provide benefits to RYGB patients post-surgery because of their effects on the gastrointestinal (GI) tract. Specifically, opioids decrease gastric motility and increase intestinal transit time, which could mitigate adverse effects associated with "dumping syndrome," a post-RYGB condition characterized by dizziness, nausea, cramps, bloating, diarrhea, chills, and hot flashes, particularly following consumption of sweet foods. Benzodiazepines may have abuse liability because they are rapidly absorbed in the GI tract; the exact nature of benzodiazepine absorption among RYGB patients is unknown [16].

11.4.3 Impact of Substance Use on Bariatric Surgery Outcomes

There is conflicting evidence regarding substance use and its impact on weight loss after bariatric surgery [56]. There is some evidence that post-bariatric surgery patients meeting criteria for substance use disorders experienced a lower percentage of total weight loss than those who did not have substance use disorders [23]. Studies have also shown that patients with presurgery substance use who participated in substance use treatment programs before surgery were more likely than patients without substance use disorders to have sustained weight loss postoperatively [57, 58]. It should be noted that patients participating in substance use disorder programs presurgery were more likely to have higher depressive symptoms post-surgery compared to controls [57]. Despite this conflicting data on postoperative substance use and weight loss, the onset of substance use disorders after surgery has been linked to worse mental health outcomes, such as depression and eating psychopathology [59].

In addition to the impact of substance use disorders on patients' quality of life and mental health, certain substances can have detrimental effects on surgical outcomes. Both nicotine use, specifically cigarette smoking, and alcohol use perioperatively have been associated with increased risk of postoperative ulcers in gastric bypass patients [60]. Moreover, cigarette smoking has been associated with increased incidence of prolonged intubation, re-intubation, sepsis, shock, and length of stay after laparoscopic bariatric surgery [61].

After bariatric surgery, patients who experience substance use relapse can suffer additional medical complications. Given that post-bariatric surgery patients are already at risk of thiamine deficiency and in severe cases, Wernicke encephalopathy, independent of alcohol use, patients who experience a relapse of their alcohol use disorder after surgery are likely to be at increased risks of these nutritional complications [62, 63].

Moreover, opioid use after bariatric surgery can exacerbate constipation immediately after surgery, resulting in increased pain and discomfort. Therefore, knowledge regarding substance-related bariatric surgery complications is essential in effectively counseling patients on potential risks of substance use postoperatively.

11.5 Risk Assessment Tools for Substance Use Disorders

Current assessment tools for addictions in patients with severe obesity are the same as those utilized for the general population; however, it should be noted that these self-report and screening tools should not replace more detailed clinical interviews and substance use assessments once a patient is determined to be at risk [15]. Moreover, the use of specific substance use assessment tools as part of the bariatric surgery assessment process can assist clinicians in assessing patient readiness for these weight loss procedures. It is possible to observe changes in biological markers of heavy alcohol consumption, such as elevated liver enzymes (e.g., gamma glutamyl-transferase (GGT), serum aspartate aminotransferase (AST), and alanine aminotransferase (ALT)), which may provide some insight into alcohol use; however, the sensitivity of these markers is variable, and these markers are not specific for the detection of problem drinking [64]. Therefore, clinical interviews and questionnaires are the mainstay of substance use assessment in this patient population.

Given that alcohol use disorders are a well-studied substance use disorder after bariatric surgery, assessment tools for alcohol use disorders have been a focus for bariatric clinicians. These tools are summarized below.

11.5.1 CAGE Questionnaire

The CAGE is a brief questionnaire that was developed by Dr. John A. Ewing in 1970 as a short clinical tool to screen for problem drinking in a patient. It consists of four simple questions [65] (see Table 11.2). Two “yes” responses indicate that the possibility of alcoholism should be investigated further. There have been many studies that validated its use [65–67]. Some studies suggest that positive CAGE testing is associated with a 91–93 % sensitivity for identification of excessive drinking and alcoholism [66, 67]. The advantages of the CAGE are that it is a simple screening tool that is easy to administer even in time-constrained settings. However, other studies suggest that the CAGE is more suitable for screening for advanced alcoholism but are less sensitive in detecting those with mild drinking problems, who actually form a larger proportion of the general population [68].

Table 11.2 CAGE questionnaire [65]

Questions	Yes	No
Have you ever felt you needed to **C**ut down on your drinking?		
Have people **A**nnoyed you by criticizing your drinking?		
Have you ever felt **G**uilty about drinking?		
Have you ever felt you needed a drink first thing in the morning (**E**ye-opener) to steady your nerves or to get rid of a hangover?		

Note: Two or more positive responses considered clinically significant

11.5.2 The Alcohol Use Disorders Identification Test (AUDIT)

The AUDIT is a 10-item instrument developed by a six country collaborative project led by the World Health Organization (WHO) to assess alcohol use and alcohol-related consequences and has well-established validity and reliability [68, 69]. A total score (range: 0–40) is calculated using this 10-item questionnaire, each of which is scored from 0 to 4 points, with a higher score reflecting greater severity of AUD (please see the appendix for the copy of an AUDIT questionnaire). Additionally, subsets of items cover different domains of consumption, such as consumption at a hazardous level, symptoms of alcohol dependence, and alcohol-related harm to self and others. These questions were selected from a larger 150-item assessment schedule, which was administered to 1888 persons attending various primary care facilities. They were selected on the basis of their representativeness for these conceptual domains and their perceived usefulness for intervention. Among those diagnosed as having hazardous or harmful alcohol use, 92% had an AUDIT of 8 or more and 94% of those with nonhazardous drinking behaviors had scores of less than 8. AUDIT is also a simple method of early detection of harmful drinking behaviors meant for the primary health care setting. A study comparing the AUDIT and the CAGE suggests that AUDIT was superior to the CAGE in the identification of patients with heavy drinking or active alcohol abuse or dependence [70].

The AUDIT has been used to stratify patients in terms of risk in bariatric surgery programs [71]. Positive AUDIT scales for hazardous alcohol use have been used to prompt further investigation, such as additional toxicology screening for additional substances. Studies comparing the AUDIT to structured psychiatric interview have also shown that the AUDIT results in higher rates of alcohol use problems and underscores the need for further clinical assessment to elucidate the presence of an AUD [15].

11.6 Treatment of Addictive Behaviors Before and After Bariatric Surgery

Patients undergoing bariatric screening undergo psychological or psychiatric evaluations, which include an assessment of substance use disorders. Presurgery assessment should consist of identification of risk factors for postoperative substance use (Table 11.1). Individuals with multiple risk factors should be referred to addictions services and receive multimodal treatments for addiction to minimize risk post-surgery.

Post-surgery screening and evaluation for substance use disorders should involve an interprofessional team and assessments longitudinally. Given the increased prevalence of postsurgical alcohol use problems over time, bariatric surgery and primary care teams should work collaborative to continue to screening for substance use issues and to appropriately refer or provide addictions interventions to mitigate long-term risks of substance use disorders postoperatively (Fig. 11.1). Specific interventions for substance use disorders are predominantly based on evidence from general addictions intervention

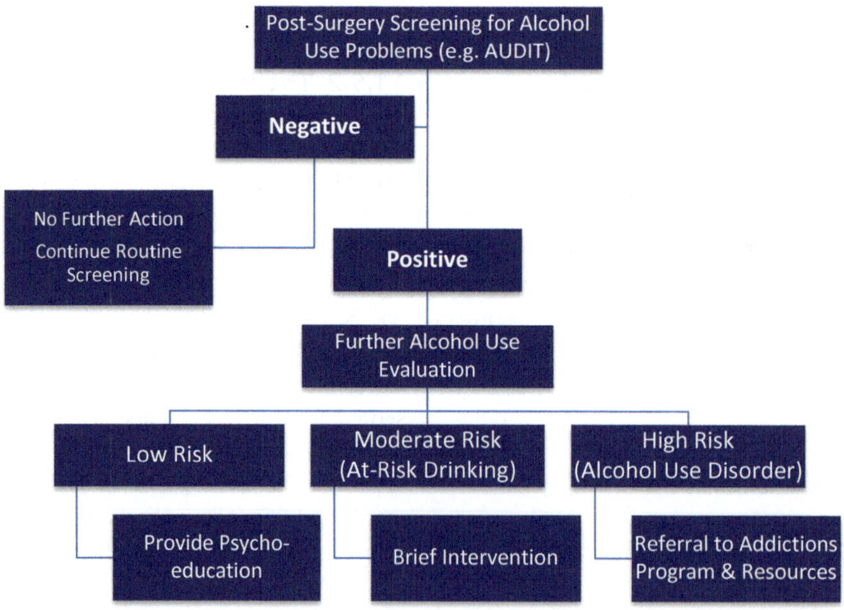

Fig. 11.1 Post-bariatric surgery screening and intervention for alcohol use

literature due to limited studies in bariatric surgery populations. Psychosocial and pharmacological approaches are summarized below.

11.6.1 Psychoeducation

Due to concerning data regarding the increased risk of developing substance use disorders, namely, alcohol use disorder, after surgery, it is important to discuss these risks and addiction prevention with bariatric surgery candidates early in the presurgery assessment process [71].

Patient education regarding alcohol use after bariatric surgery should include specific information regarding changes in alcohol pharmacokinetics. For example, specific to alcohol, patients should be given information that alcohol might be much more intoxicating after surgery and that a single glass of wine could potentially make the serum alcohol concentration above the legal driving limit in a post-bariatric patient [72]. As well, some bariatric patients can show atypical symptoms of intoxication (e.g., dizziness), and it can take a much longer time for a post-bariatric surgery patient to return to sobriety. The adverse effects of alcohol and other substances of abuse also need to be included in the discussion, as well as the fact that bariatric surgery patients might be at increased risk of alcohol-related problems after surgery. Both patients and families should be given information on available community resources should they feel they need help with addiction after bariatric surgery.

Ashton and colleagues reported the benefit of their alcohol use patient education groups in bariatric surgery candidates [73]. In their study, patients with a history of a substance use disorder or at-risk substance use were referred to a single 90-min group education session. After attending this session, patients reported improved knowledge regarding the negative effects of substance use post-surgery and increased healthy coping strategies. Furthermore, patients reported being more likely to stop drinking after the education group intervention. Therefore, early identification of at risk patients for alcohol use problems presurgery can facilitate patient engagement in presurgery alcohol use interventions; however, further research is needed to determine long-term efficacy of these programs in supporting sustained weight loss in patients with severe obesity.

11.6.2 Motivational Interviewing

Motivational interviewing (MI) is both a mindset and a treatment philosophy used to help people evoke their own intrinsic motivation when they experience ambivalence about changing a particular behavior [74]. The theoretical underpinning of MI is such that without motivation, knowledge provided to the patient alone will not generate a change in behavior. As well, only when individuals believe they have a problem, will they be motivated to change more effectively [75, 76]. Motivational interviewing as an intervention for severe obesity management is summarized in a chapter later in this book (see Chap. 20). A large body of research has demonstrated the efficacy of motivational interviewing in reducing drug use and other addictive behaviors including risky sexual behaviors and diet/exercise [77, 78]. Treatment with motivational interviewing both during the pre- and post-bariatric surgery should be offered if available to patients who are identified as being at risk for alcohol or other substance-related disorders.

11.6.3 Cognitive Behavioral Therapy (CBT)/Relapse Prevention

CBT/relapse prevention is a therapeutic method based on the approach of CBT, which are grounded in the principles of operant conditioning and social learning theories. The goals of CBT/relapse prevention include the identification of drug use within the context of its antecedents and consequences and the generation of effective behavioral alternatives that facilitate one's ability to stay away from the substance. This therapeutic intervention includes and is not limited to relapse analysis (analyzing high-risk situations for relapse and early warning signs of relapse), drug refusal skill development, affect management skill enhancement, and the identification of cognitive distortions towards the substance of use. There is a large amount of evidence to support the use of cognitive behavioral therapy in the treatment of alcohol use disorders and other substance use disorders [79–81].

11.6.4 12-Step Programs

A 12-step program is a set of spiritual principles outlining the method to overcome addictive behaviors and originated as alcoholics anonymous (AA) for alcohol use problems. Currently, 12-step programs exist for multiple substances including overeaters anonymous for obesity [82]. Approximately, 9 % of the US general population has attended an AA meeting in their lifetime [83].

The original 12 steps focused on the admission of having a substance use problem and surrendering the hope for recovery through the recognition of the loss of control. It frequently made references to a greater power that could restore balance in the person's lives and also contained action items to be completed by the recovering participant, such as making amends to friends and family that may have been previously hurt [84]. Since then, the wording of these steps has been altered to remove gender-biased language, and there are secular groups that omit references to a deity or deities. Auxiliary groups to AA, such as Al-Anon and Nar-Anon, are available for the family and caregivers of people suffering from substance use disorders.

11.6.5 Other Treatment Options

There are a variety of other psychosocial treatment modalities, including brief intervention, contingency management/community reinforcement, psychodynamic/interpersonal therapy, drug counseling, family therapy, network therapy, and residential treatment. These modalities should be considered based on weight loss and bariatric surgery program's availability of such interventions and resources. Ideally, a combination of multiple modalities can support patients in managing addictive disorders in the context of severe obesity.

11.6.6 Comparison of Psychosocial Treatment Modalities for Addictive Disorders

Limited literature on the efficacy of psychosocial interventions for addictive disorders exists in patients with severe obesity or undergoing bariatric surgery. As a result, current psychosocial management of addictive disorders is extrapolated from literature from general addiction literature.

Evidence from the treatment of alcohol use disorders in Project MATCH, a landmark study led by the US National Institute on Alcohol Abuse and Alcoholism (NIAAA), was a multisite client-treatment matching study examining efficacy of psychosocial treatments for alcohol use disorders [85]. This project attempted to utilize different client attributes to match them to either motivational enhancement therapy (MET, involving principles of MI), CBT, or a 12-step program (Twelve Step Facilitation treatment, also known as TSF) in outpatient or aftercare settings. This study found that all three interventions produced significant reductions in drinking that were sustained over the 3-year follow-up period and that matching specific client characteristics to a particular therapeutic modality did not generally result in significant differences in outcomes. However, when conducting subgroup analyses, the authors found that clients that had higher levels of anger had better outcomes in MET, and those with lower levels of anger benefited from a more structured program such as a 12-step program and CBT more than MET [85]. Furthermore, patients with more supportive social networks benefitted more from the 12-step program than

MET [85]. Self-efficacy (i.e., measured confidence to stop drinking in relation to one's temptation to drink) was the strongest predictor of outcome in both the outpatient and aftercare population. Therefore, these factors can be considered when recommending substance use treatment to patients undergoing severe obesity management. Additional research is needed to identify the efficacy of specific psychosocial interventions for addictive disorders post-bariatric surgery.

11.7 Pharmacology for Addictive Disorders in Obesity

We will offer an overview on the various pharmacological agents available to treat different substance use disorders, even though evidence on efficacy specifically in the bariatric surgery population is lacking. Special attention will be paid to the medications' potential effect on a patient's weight and potential impact on bariatric surgery outcomes.

11.7.1 Alcohol

The three medications on the market with United States Food and Drug Administration approval of use in alcohol disorder include disulfiram, naltrexone, and acamprosate. It should be noted that there is growing evidence for a number of other drugs including gabapentin, topiramate, and baclofen. Interestingly, some drugs that have potential to treat addiction have also shown to produce weight loss. Naltrexone has been shown to cause weight loss and has been studied for its weight loss effects in combination with bupropion [86]. It is hypothesized that naltrexone impacts the two key systems that regulate food intake and bodyweight in the central nervous system: the mesolimbic dopaminergic pathway, as discussed previously, and the hypothalamic melanocortin system [86]. Topiramate has also been shown to cause weight loss due to the loss of appetite [87]. Interestingly, both naltrexone and topiramate are associated with GI side effects such as nausea and appetite suppression, which could also contribute to weight loss. There is no evidence that disulfiram and acamprosate impact weight. One of baclofen's side effects is dysgeusia, an unpleasant taste sensation that persists in the patient's mouth after medication administration. It has been postulated that this could cause involuntary weight loss, although there is sparse evidence on this subject [88]. Moreover, this side effect may reduce diet adherence post-surgery.

11.7.2 Nicotine

Nicotine replacement therapy, bupropion, and varenicline are the mainstay treatment for nicotine use disorder. Bupropion has been shown in clinical trials to also produce weight loss [86]. However, smoking cessation, whether treated with therapy or not, is associated with a mean increase of 4–5 kg in body weight after 12 months of abstinence and does not differ between different pharmacotherapies used to support cessation [89]. Variations between individuals are large; however, 16 % of quitters can lose weight, while 13 % gaining more than 10 kg [89]. Unlike cigarette smoking, nicotine replacement therapy has not been shown to affect wound healing after surgery [90].

11.7.3 Medication Treatment for Other Substances

There is limited evidence on the pharmacological treatment of cocaine use disorder, with some emerging literature on the possible use of topiramate in cocaine dependence [91]. For opioid use disorders, there are two maintenance therapies currently available for the long-term management of opioid withdrawal symptoms: methadone and buprenorphine/naloxone. Methadone initiation has been associated with increases in BMI [92]. There is currently no clear literature on the effect of buprenorphine/naloxone on weight.

Case Vignette

The following case vignette will illustrate the management of a bariatric surgery candidate with multiple risk factors for post-surgery alcohol use. The case will provide a framework to reinforce substance use risk factors and potential interventions for addictive disorders in patients undergoing bariatric surgery.

Presurgery: Mary is a 35-year-old female who has lived with obesity for most of her life. She has hyperlipidemia, diabetes mellitus type 2, and knee pain, which has limited her mobility. She has been referred for bariatric surgery and is motivated for this procedure to lose weight and improve her health. Mary has no children and is in a 4-year common-law relationship. Both Mary and her partner have had challenges with alcohol use and her partner continues to drink on weekends. Mary states she underwent substance use treatment in an addictions program and completed two past 30-day inpatient alcohol treatment programs. In addition to alcohol use, she has a history of major depression, which has been stable for 2 years.

Mary has a family history of alcohol use disorders including both of her parents. She states she has been "pretty good" and initially indicates that alcohol is not an issue for the last 2 years after her last outpatient treatment program. However, at her second appointment with the dietitian in the bariatric surgery program, Mary reports alcohol use on the weekend in her food records. Upon further exploration, she discloses that she usually drinks 4–5 drinks per day on the weekend with her husband and her neighbors. She does not feel this is an issue given how much she consumed in the past. She also has been taking her husband's oxycodone for her knee pain. In addition to her partner, she has minimal social supports except for a few friends and endorses feeling alone at home at times.

Risk Stratification and Perioperative Management: Due to Mary's alcohol use risk factors, including her current binges, family history of alcohol use disorders, and self-reported isolation, her surgery was deferred until she addressed these modifiable risk factors. She received motivational interviewing and psychoeducation in the bariatric surgery program. The team facilitated a referral to the partner outpatient addictions program for further support and to assist Mary in achieving alcohol use abstinence. Mary was able to engage in these treatments due to alignment of her alcohol use cessation with her goal of having bariatric surgery to improve her overall health.

Postoperative Management: Mary is seen at 6 months post-surgery and reports trying a couple of drinks and feeling "slammed" by the drinks, which is unusual for her. She reports conflict with her partner after surgery and a related decline in her depression. She does not feel she needs help at this time and receives support and education about the risks of resuming alcohol post-surgery in her case. She is screened with the AUDIT and does not meet the threshold for hazardous alcohol use.

At 18 months post-surgery, Mary schedules an urgent follow-up with the social worker in the bariatric surgery program after missing her follow-up appointments. She reports a relapse in her alcohol use and is consuming 3–4 drinks of alcohol most days of the week. She has not experienced any complicated alcohol withdrawal symptoms. Her partner urged her to see someone in the program and she obliged after several months. A bariatric psychiatrist reassesses Mary and she scores in the hazardous level

(continued)

(continued)

on the AUDIT. She received psychoeducation and motivational interviewing and agrees to work with the psychiatrist. She has experienced a depression relapse, and she is eventually restarted on an antidepressant after reducing her alcohol use. She reengages with her community alcohol treatment program and is started on naltrexone in addition to ongoing psychological treatment. She is able to achieve abstinence from alcohol use and joins a 12-step program as well as part of her recovery. These interventions have improved her social isolation, and she is able to continue to work on lifestyle changes and self-care after bariatric surgery. Her primary care team is involved and continues to monitor her substance use using the AUD screening instruments and questions.

11.8 Summary and Take Home Points

This chapter has outlined several common pathways of substance use disorders, especially AUDs, and severe obesity. There are several key points to consider when treating patients with severe obesity and addictions both before and after bariatric surgery:

- Patients with severe obesity have higher rates of some addictive disorders compared to the general population, specifically AUD.
- Additional non-alcohol-related addictive behaviors are present before massive weight loss interventions, and these conditions should be included as part of initial psychosocial assessments.
- Evidence suggests that there is a small but increased risk of new-onset alcohol use disorders after bariatric surgery, and this risk may be higher for patients undergoing RYGB.
- Patients should be educated on postoperative changes with alcohol absorption and metabolism following RYGB. Additional education on potential shared pathways for addictive behaviors and obesity should be discussed including clarification of the concept of addiction transfer.
- Pre- and postoperative screening and appropriate substance use treatments should be provided to patients undergoing bariatric surgery and should follow a stepped-care approach. These interventions should include appropriate pharmacological interventions, psychological treatments (such as motivational interviewing), and referral for more intense programs.

References

1. Farhat T, Iannotti RJ, Simons-Morton BG. Overweight, obesity, youth, and health-risk behaviors. Am J Prev Med. 2010;38(3):258–67.
2. McLaren L, Beck CA, Patten SB, Fick GH, Adair CE. The relationship between body mass index and mental health. A population-based study of the effects of the definition of mental health. Soc Psychiatry Psychiatr Epidemiol. 2008;43(1):63–71.
3. Kalarchian MA, Marcus MD, Levine MD, Courcoulas AP, Pilkonis PA, Ringham RM, et al. Psychiatric disorders among bariatric surgery candidates: relationship to obesity and functional health status. Am J Psychiatry. 2007;164(2):328–34. quiz 74.
4. King WC, Chen JY, Mitchell JE, Kalarchian MA, Steffen KJ, Engel SG, et al. Prevalence of alcohol use disorders before and after bariatric surgery. JAMA. 2012;307(23):2516–25.
5. Suzuki J, Haimovici F, Chang G. Alcohol use disorders after bariatric surgery. Obes Surg. 2012;22(2): 201–7.
6. Mitchell JE, Selzer F, Kalarchian MA, Devlin MJ, Strain GW, Elder KA, et al. Psychopathology before surgery in the longitudinal assessment of bariatric surgery-3 (LABS-3) psychosocial study. Surg Obes Relat Dis. 2012;8(5):533–41.
7. Dawes AJ, Maggard-Gibbons M, Maher AR, Booth MJ, Miake-Lye I, Beroes JM, et al. Mental health conditions among patients seeking and undergoing bariatric surgery: a meta-analysis. JAMA. 2016;315(2):150–63.
8. Black DW, Goldstein RB, Mason EE. Psychiatric diagnosis and weight loss following gastric surgery for obesity. Obes Surg. 2003;13(5):746–51.
9. Rosenberger PH, Henderson KE, Grilo CM. Psychiatric disorder comorbidity and association with eating disorders in bariatric surgery patients: a cross-

sectional study using structured interview-based diagnosis. J Clin Psychiatry. 2006;67(7):1080–5.
10. Sarwer DB, Cohn NI, Gibbons LM, Magee L, Crerand CE, Raper SE, et al. Psychiatric diagnoses and psychiatric treatment among bariatric surgery candidates. Obes Surg. 2004;14(9):1148–56.
11. Grace DM, Pederson L, Speechley KN, McAlpine D. A longitudinal study of smoking status and weight loss following gastroplasty in a group of morbidly obese patients. Int J Obes. 1990;14(4):311–7.
12. Lent MR, Hayes SM, Wood GC, Napolitano MA, Argyropoulos G, Gerhard GS, et al. Smoking and alcohol use in gastric bypass patients. Eat Behav. 2013;14(4):460–3.
13. Tae B, Pelaggi ER, Moreira JG, Waisberg J, de Matos LL, D'Elia G. Impact of bariatric surgery on depression and anxiety symptoms, bulimic behaviors and quality of life. Rev Col Bras Cir. 2014;41(3):155–60.
14. Raebel MA, Newcomer SR, Reifler LM, Boudreau D, Elliott TE, DeBar L, et al. Chronic use of opioid medications before and after bariatric surgery. JAMA. 2013;310(13):1369–76.
15. Mitchell JE, Steffen K, Engel S, King WC, Chen JY, Winters K, et al. Addictive disorders after Roux-en-Y gastric bypass. Surg Obes Relat Dis. 2015;11(4): 897–905.
16. Wiedemann AA. Differences between post-bariatric patients and controls in a substance abuse rehabilitation program: Implications for treatment. Eastern Michigan University; 2012.
17. Conason A, Teixeira J, Hsu CH, Puma L, Knafo D, Geliebter A. Substance use following bariatric weight loss surgery. JAMA Surg. 2013;148(2):145–50.
18. Svensson PA, Anveden A, Romeo S, Peltonen M, Ahlin S, Burza MA, et al. Alcohol consumption and alcohol problems after bariatric surgery in the Swedish obese subjects study. Obesity (Silver Spring). 2013;21(12):2444–51.
19. Substance Abuse and Mental Health Services Administration. Results from the 2013 national survey on drug use and health: summary of national findings. Rockville, MD: Mental Health Services Administration (SAMHSA); 2014. NSDUH Series H-48, HHS Publication No. (SMA) 14-4863.
20. Hasin DS, Stinson FS, Ogburn E, Grant BF. Prevalence, correlates, disability, and comorbidity of DSM-IV alcohol abuse and dependence in the United States: results from the National Epidemiologic Survey on Alcohol and Related Conditions. Arch Gen Psychiatry. 2007;64(7):830–42.
21. Fowler L, Ivezaj V, Saules KK. Problematic intake of high-sugar/low-fat and high glycemic index foods by bariatric patients is associated with development of post-surgical new onset substance use disorders. Eat Behav. 2014;15(3):505–8.
22. Ivezaj V, Saules KK, Schuh LM. New-onset substance use disorder after gastric bypass surgery: rates and associated characteristics. Obes Surg. 2014;24(11): 1975–80.
23. Reslan S, Saules KK, Greenwald MK, Schuh LM. Substance misuse following Roux-en-Y gastric bypass surgery. Subst Use Misuse. 2014;49(4): 405–17.
24. Changchien EM, Woodard GA, Hernandez-Boussard T, Morton JM. Normal alcohol metabolism after gastric banding and sleeve gastrectomy: a case-crossover trial. J Am Coll Surg. 2012;215(4):475–9.
25. Gallo AS, Berducci MA, Nijhawan S, Nino DF, Broderick RC, Harnsberger CR, et al. Alcohol metabolism is not affected by sleeve gastrectomy. Surg Endosc. 2015;29(5):1088–93.
26. Raebel MA, Newcomer SR, Bayliss EA, Boudreau D, DeBar L, Elliott TE, et al. Chronic opioid use emerging after bariatric surgery. Pharmacoepidemiol Drug Saf. 2014;23(12):1247–57.
27. Wendling A, Wudyka A. Narcotic addiction following gastric bypass surgery—a case study. Obes Surg. 2011;21(5):680–3.
28. Engel SG, Kahler KA, Lystad CM, Crosby RD, Simonich HK, Wonderlich SA, et al. Eating behavior in obese BED, obese non-BED, and non-obese control participants: a naturalistic study. Behav Res Ther. 2009;47(10):897–900.
29. Nestler EJ. Is there a common molecular pathway for addiction? Nat Neurosci. 2005;8(11):1445–9.
30. Salamone JD, Correa M, Farrar A, Mingote SM. Effort-related functions of nucleus accumbens dopamine and associated forebrain circuits. Psychopharmacology (Berl). 2007;191(3):461–82.
31. Salamone JD, Cousins MS, Snyder BJ. Behavioral functions of nucleus accumbens dopamine: empirical and conceptual problems with the anhedonia hypothesis. Neurosci Biobehav Rev. 1997;21(3):341–59.
32. Bassareo V, Di Chiara G. Modulation of feeding-induced activation of mesolimbic dopamine transmission by appetitive stimuli and its relation to motivational state. Eur J Neurosci. 1999;11(12):4389–97.
33. Martel P, Fantino M. Mesolimbic dopaminergic system activity as a function of food reward: a microdialysis study. Pharmacol Biochem Behav. 1996;53(1): 221–6.
34. Berridge KC, Robinson TE. What is the role of dopamine in reward: hedonic impact, reward learning, or incentive salience? Brain Res Brain Res Rev. 1998; 28(3):309–69.
35. Noble EP, Gottschalk LA, Fallon JH, Ritchie TL, Wu JC. D2 dopamine receptor polymorphism and brain regional glucose metabolism. Am J Med Genet. 1997;74(2):162–6.
36. Volkow ND, Wang GJ, Tomasi D, Baler RD. Obesity and addiction: neurobiological overlaps. Obes Rev. 2013;14(1):2–18.
37. Volkow ND, Baler RD. NOW vs LATER brain circuits: implications for obesity and addiction. Trends Neurosci. 2015;38(6):345–52.
38. Fineberg NA, Potenza MN, Chamberlain SR, Berlin HA, Menzies L, Bechara A, et al. Probing compulsive and impulsive behaviors, from animal models to

endophenotypes: a narrative review. Neuropsychopharmacology. 2010;35(3):591–604.
39. Johnson PM, Kenny PJ. Dopamine D2 receptors in addiction-like reward dysfunction and compulsive eating in obese rats. Nat Neurosci. 2010;13(5):635–41.
40. Hebebrand J, Albayrak O, Adan R, Antel J, Dieguez C, de Jong J, et al. "Eating addiction", rather than "food addiction", better captures addictive-like eating behavior. Neurosci Biobehav Rev. 2014;47:295–306.
41. Klok MD, Jakobsdottir S, Drent ML. The role of leptin and ghrelin in the regulation of food intake and body weight in humans: a review. Obes Rev. 2007;8(1):21–34.
42. Cummings DE, Weigle DS, Frayo RS, Breen PA, Ma MK, Dellinger EP, et al. Plasma ghrelin levels after diet-induced weight loss or gastric bypass surgery. N Engl J Med. 2002;346(21):1623–30.
43. Karamanakos SN, Vagenas K, Kalfarentzos F, Alexandrides TK. Weight loss, appetite suppression, and changes in fasting and postprandial ghrelin and peptide-YY levels after Roux-en-Y gastric bypass and sleeve gastrectomy: a prospective, double blind study. Ann Surg. 2008;247(3):401–7.
44. Jerlhag E, Egecioglu E, Dickson SL, Andersson M, Svensson L, Engel JA. Ghrelin stimulates locomotor activity and accumbal dopamine-overflow via central cholinergic systems in mice: implications for its involvement in brain reward. Addict Biol. 2006;11(1):45–54.
45. Skibicka KP, Hansson C, Egecioglu E, Dickson SL. Role of ghrelin in food reward: impact of ghrelin on sucrose self-administration and mesolimbic dopamine and acetylcholine receptor gene expression. Addict Biol. 2012;17(1):95–107.
46. Davis JF, Schurdak JD, Magrisso IJ, Mul JD, Grayson BE, Pfluger PT, et al. Gastric bypass surgery attenuates ethanol consumption in ethanol-preferring rats. Biol Psychiatry. 2012;72(5):354–60.
47. Davis JF, Tracy AL, Schurdak JD, Magrisso IJ, Grayson BE, Seeley RJ, et al. Roux en Y gastric bypass increases ethanol intake in the rat. Obes Surg. 2013;23(7):920–30.
48. Hajnal A, Zharikov A, Polston JE, Fields MR, Tomasko J, Rogers AM, et al. Alcohol reward is increased after Roux-en-Y gastric bypass in dietary obese rats with differential effects following ghrelin antagonism. PLoS One. 2012;7(11), e49121.
49. Munzberg H. Leptin-signaling pathways and leptin resistance. Forum Nutr. 2010;63:123–32.
50. Pan H, Guo J, Su Z. Advances in understanding the interrelations between leptin resistance and obesity. Physiol Behav. 2014;130:157–69.
51. Grosshans M, Vollmert C, Vollstadt-Klein S, Tost H, Leber S, Bach P, et al. Association of leptin with food cue-induced activation in human reward pathways. Arch Gen Psychiatry. 2012;69(5):529–37.
52. Simon JJ, Skunde M, Hamze Sinno M, Brockmeyer T, Herpertz SC, Bendszus M, et al. Impaired cross-talk between mesolimbic food reward processing and metabolic signaling predicts body mass index. Front Behav Neurosci. 2014;8:359.
53. Steffen KJ, Engel SG, Wonderlich JA, Pollert GA, Sondag C. Alcohol and other addictive disorders following bariatric surgery: prevalence, risk factors and possible etiologies. Eur Eat Disord Rev. 2015;23(6):442–50.
54. Hagedorn JC, Encarnacion B, Brat GA, Morton JM. Does gastric bypass alter alcohol metabolism? Surg Obes Relat Dis. 2007;3(5):543–8. discussion 8.
55. Lee SL, Chau GY, Yao CT, Wu CW, Yin SJ. Functional assessment of human alcohol dehydrogenase family in ethanol metabolism: significance of first-pass metabolism. Alcohol Clin Exp Res. 2006;30(7):1132–42.
56. Heinberg LJ, Ashton K. History of substance abuse relates to improved postbariatric body mass index outcomes. Surg Obes Relat Dis. 2010;6(4):417–21.
57. Pulcini ME, Saules KK, Schuh LM. Roux-en-Y gastric bypass patients hospitalized for substance use disorders achieve successful weight loss despite poor psychosocial outcomes. Clin Obes. 2013;3(3–4):95–102.
58. Clark MM, Balsiger BM, Sletten CD, Dahlman KL, Ames G, Williams DE, et al. Psychosocial factors and 2-year outcome following bariatric surgery for weight loss. Obes Surg. 2003;13(5):739–45.
59. Yanos BR, Saules KK, Schuh LM, Sogg S. Predictors of lowest weight and long-term weight regain among Roux-en-Y gastric bypass patients. Obes Surg. 2015;25(8):1364–70.
60. Scheffel O, Daskalakis M, Weiner RA. Two important criteria for reducing the risk of postoperative ulcers at the gastrojejunostomy site after gastric bypass: patient compliance and type of gastric bypass. Obes Facts. 2011;4 Suppl 1:39–41.
61. Haskins IN, Amdur R, Vaziri K. The effect of smoking on bariatric surgical outcomes. Surg Endosc. 2014;28(11):3074–80.
62. Stroh C, Meyer F, Manger T. Beriberi, a severe complication after metabolic surgery—review of the literature. Obes Facts. 2014;7(4):246–52.
63. Aasheim ET. Wernicke encephalopathy after bariatric surgery: a systematic review. Ann Surg. 2008;248(5):714–20.
64. Saunders JB, Aasland OG, Amundsen A, Grant M. Alcohol consumption and related problems among primary health care patients: WHO collaborative project on early detection of persons with harmful alcohol consumption—I. Addiction. 1993;88(3):349–62.
65. Ewing JA. Detecting alcoholism. The CAGE questionnaire. JAMA. 1984;252(14):1905–7.
66. Bernadt MW, Mumford J, Taylor C, Smith B, Murray RM. Comparison of questionnaire and laboratory tests in the detection of excessive drinking and alcoholism. Lancet. 1982;1(8267):325–8.
67. Kitchens JM. Does this patient have an alcohol problem? JAMA. 1994;272(22):1782–7.
68. Saunders JB, Aasland OG, Babor TF, de la Fuente JR, Grant M. Development of the Alcohol Use Disorders

Identification Test (AUDIT): WHO collaborative project on early detection of persons with harmful alcohol consumption—II. Addiction. 1993;88(6): 791–804.
69. Babor TF, Higgins-Biddle JC, Saunders JB, Monteiro MG. The Alcohol Use Disorders Identification Test: guidelines for use in primary care. Geneva: World Health Organization; 2001.
70. Bradley KA, Bush KR, McDonell MB, Malone T, Fihn SD. Screening for problem drinking: comparison of CAGE and AUDIT. Ambulatory Care Quality Improvement Project (ACQUIP). Alcohol Use Disorders Identification Test. J Gen Intern Med. 1998;13(6):379–88.
71. Heinberg LJ, Ashton K, Coughlin J. Alcohol and bariatric surgery: review and suggested recommendations for assessment and management. Surg Obes Relat Dis. 2012;8(3):357–63.
72. Woodard GA, Downey J, Hernandez-Boussard T, Morton JM. Impaired alcohol metabolism after gastric bypass surgery: a case-crossover trial. J Am Coll Surg. 2011;212(2):209–14.
73. Ashton K, Heinberg L, Merrell J, Lavery M, Windover A, Alcorn K. Pilot evaluation of a substance abuse prevention group intervention for at-risk bariatric surgery candidates. Surg Obes Relat Dis. 2013;9(3):462–7.
74. Miller WR, Rollnick S. Talking oneself into change: motivational interviewing, stages of change, and therapeutic process. J Cogn Psychother. 2004;18(4):299–308.
75. DiClemente CC, Prochaska JO, Fairhurst SK, Velicer WF, Velasquez MM, Rossi JS. The process of smoking cessation: an analysis of precontemplation, contemplation, and preparation stages of change. J Consult Clin Psychol. 1991;59(2):295–304.
76. Ockene JK, Quirk ME, Goldberg RJ, Kristeller JL, Donnelly G, Kalan KL, et al. A residents' training program for the development of smoking intervention skills. Arch Intern Med. 1988;148(5):1039–45.
77. Lundahl B, Burke BL. The effectiveness and applicability of motivational interviewing: a practice-friendly review of four meta-analyses. J Clin Psychol. 2009;65(11):1232–45.
78. Burke BL, Arkowitz H, Menchola M. The efficacy of motivational interviewing: a meta-analysis of controlled clinical trials. J Consult Clin Psychol. 2003; 71(5):843–61.
79. Irvin JE, Bowers CA, Dunn ME, Wang MC. Efficacy of relapse prevention: a meta-analytic review. J Consult Clin Psychol. 1999;67(4):563–70.
80. Miller WR, Wilbourne PL. Mesa Grande: a methodological analysis of clinical trials of treatments for alcohol use disorders. Addiction. 2002;97(3):265–77.
81. Miller W, Brown J, Simpson T, Handmaker N, Bien T, Luckie L, et al. What works? A methodological analysis of the alcohol treatment outcome literature. In: Hester RK, Miller WR, editors. Handbook of alcoholism treatment approaches: effective alternatives. Boston, MA: Allyn and Bacon; 1995. p. 12–44.
82. Yeary J. The use of overeaters anonymous in the treatment of eating disorders. J Psychoactive Drugs. 1987;19(3):303–9.
83. Room R, Greenfield T. Alcoholics anonymous, other 12-step movements and psychotherapy in the US population, 1990. Addiction. 1993;88(4):555–62.
84. Twelve steps and twelve traditions. New York: Alcoholics Anonymous World Services, Inc.; 2005.
85. Project MATCH secondary a priori hypotheses. Project MATCH Research Group. Addiction. 1997;92(12):1671–98.
86. Greenway FL, Fujioka K, Plodkowski RA, Mudaliar S, Guttadauria M, Erickson J, et al. Effect of naltrexone plus bupropion on weight loss in overweight and obese adults (COR-I): a multicentre, randomised, double-blind, placebo-controlled, phase 3 trial. Lancet. 2010;376(9741):595–605.
87. Bray GA, Hollander P, Klein S, Kushner R, Levy B, Fitchet M, et al. A 6-month randomized, placebo-controlled, dose-ranging trial of topiramate for weight loss in obesity. Obes Res. 2003;11(6):722–33.
88. Moriguti JC, Moriguti EK, Ferriolli E, de Castilho Cacao J, Iucif Jr N, Marchini JS. Involuntary weight loss in elderly individuals: assessment and treatment. Sao Paulo Med J. 2001;119(2):72–7.
89. Aubin HJ, Farley A, Lycett D, Lahmek P, Aveyard P. Weight gain in smokers after quitting cigarettes: meta-analysis. BMJ. 2012;345, e4439.
90. Nolan MB, Warner DO. Safety and efficacy of nicotine replacement therapy in the perioperative period: a narrative review. Mayo Clin Proc. 2015;90(11): 1553–61.
91. Kampman KM, Pettinati H, Lynch KG, Dackis C, Sparkman T, Weigley C, et al. A pilot trial of topiramate for the treatment of cocaine dependence. Drug Alcohol Depend. 2004;75(3):233–40.
92. Fenn JM, Laurent JS, Sigmon SC. Increases in body mass index following initiation of methadone treatment. J Subst Abuse Treat. 2015;51:59–63.

12 Sleep and Severe Obesity

Elliott Kyung Lee and Raed Hawa

12.1 Introduction

This chapter briefly outlines normal sleep architecture and the important elements needed for sleep to function adequately and is followed by characteristics of sleep (quantity, quality, and duration) that have been related to obesity. Treatment options that are available for obstructive sleep apnea and obesity hypoventilation syndrome (the two commonest sleep disorders associated with obesity) are explored.

Case Vignette

Janet is a 42-year-old married female with a long-standing history of obesity. She is 5′3″ and 235 lb (BMI = 41.6 kg/m^2). She has hypertension and type II diabetes. She has constantly felt tired during the day. Because of concerns about her weight contributing to her health problems, she was referred to a weight loss clinic. Initially, she tried a behavioral approach of dieting combined with some aqua fitness, but found that she could only lose a modest amount of weight. Consequently, she was referred to a surgeon for possible consideration of bariatric surgery. Before considering surgery, her surgeon wanted her to be screened for obstructive sleep apnea.

In her sleep assessment, she stated that her sleep quality has always been poor, but she has never been a good sleeper. She usually goes to bed around 10 PM, and although she can fall asleep quickly, she wakes up 4–5 times per night on average. She goes to the bathroom at least twice at night. Her husband reported that she snores loudly, and sometimes she looks like she is either choking at night, or sometimes not breathing at all. She wakes up around 8 AM typically and needs two alarms to awaken. There is a glass of water by the bedside, because her throat is always dry and sore in the mornings. She wakes up with headaches every morning. She would like to arrive at work before 0930h, but is unable to do so, due to difficulty waking in the mornings. During the day, she frequently feels sleepy, but combats this with

(continued)

E.K. Lee, M.D., F.R.C.P.(C.), D. A.B.S.N. (✉)
Department of Psychiatry and Institute for Mental Health Research (IMHR), Royal Ottawa Mental Health Center (ROMHC), University of Ottawa, Ottawa, ON, Canada
e-mail: Elliott.Lee@theroyal.ca

R. Hawa
Toronto Western Hospital Bariatric Surgery Program, University Health Network, 399 Bathurst Street, Toronto, ON, Canada M5T 2S8

Department of Psychiatry, University of Toronto, Toronto, ON, Canada
e-mail: Raed.Hawa@uhn.ca

S. Sockalingam, R. Hawa (eds.), *Psychiatric Care in Severe Obesity*,
DOI 10.1007/978-3-319-42536-8_12

(continued)
4–5 cups of coffee throughout the day. She has frequent feelings of shortness of breath, but wonders if she is just stressed. On her way home from work, she sometimes finds that she can doze off occasionally at a stop sign. Her Epworth Sleepiness Score was 17. She was scheduled for a sleep study.

Sleep is a reversible behavioral state of perceptual disengagement from and unresponsiveness to the environment [1]. Although sleep is an important part of life, the precise function of sleep is unclear. In 2015, the National Sleep Foundation, the American Academy of Sleep Medicine, and the Sleep Research Society suggested that the appropriate amount of nightly sleep for healthy adults should be 7–9 h [2, 3]. Although most people should be spending approximately one-third of their life sleeping, population estimates from the United States National Health and Nutrition Examination Survey (NHANES) from 2007 to 2010 suggest that almost 40 % of adults over the age of 20 are sleeping less than 6 h a night [4]. According to Statistics Canada in their 2010 General Social Survey, 46 % of Canadians choose to cut back on their sleep to add more time to their day [5]. Obesity has become an increasing public health concern where over 1 in 3 people in the United States according to the NHANES data (2007–2012) are obese [6]. Recent evidence has linked sleep disturbances with the pathogenesis of obesity, through a variety of mechanisms.

12.2 Normal Sleep Architecture and Sleep Control

Sleep is currently divided into two main stages: rapid eye movement (REM) sleep and non-REM (NREM) sleep. NREM sleep is normally divided into three stages: N1 sleep is a light stage of sleep; N2 is a slightly deeper stage of sleep; and N3 is the deepest, most physically and cerebrally restorative stage of sleep. During N3 sleep, the body is least responsive to external stimuli. N3 sleep is also called deep sleep, or delta sleep (referring to the frequency of the EEG) or slow wave sleep (SWS). REM sleep is often referred to as the dreaming sleep, as most dreaming occurs in REM sleep. Muscle atonia and rapid eye movements characterize REM sleep. Normal healthy nighttime sleep sees 4–6 cycles of NREM followed by REM sleep in a given night, with a preponderance for NREM sleep in the first half of the night, and REM sleep in the second half of the night [7]. Under normal circumstances, healthy sleep is controlled by two regulatory processes—process “S” and process “C”. Process “S” refers to a homeostatic drive to sleep, positing that the longer the period of wakefulness, the greater the drive for sleep that will accumulate. The second process, Process “C,” refers to a circadian drive that follows a daily (“circadian”) rhythm, which is responsible for instance, for an increasing sleepiness in the mid afternoon for most people. The degree of daytime sleepiness experienced by a person is largely determined by three dimensions of the previous night’s sleep—sleep quantity, sleep quality, and sleep timing. When one or more of these variables of sleep are compromised, several problems can occur.

12.2.1 Connection of Sleep Duration to Obesity: Possible Underlying Mechanisms

Numerous epidemiological studies have demonstrated a link between short sleep duration, particularly less than 7 h a night, and metabolic consequences including diabetes and cardiovascular disease [8–10]. Numerous studies from around the world have shown an association between short sleep duration and obesity including Australia [11], Canada [12], the United States [13], Japan [14], and Korea. Several meta-analyses have also found an association between short sleep duration (generally under 7 h) and obesity with higher risk for obesity with increasing sleep deprivation [15–18]. Although the precise mechanism behind the relationship between sleep deprivation and obesity is not clear, growing evidence is implicating leptin and ghrelin. Leptin is a cytokine produced by adipocytes (i.e., an adipokine) that inhibits appetite. Ghrelin is a hormone released by the stomach that stimulates appetite. Leptin and ghrelin both act on hypothalamic nuclei to regulate energy balance [19]. Several studies have demonstrated that short sleep duration is associated with reductions in leptin and increases in ghrelin, with accompanying increases in subjective feelings of hunger [20–22], though not all studies [23]. These studies have been reviewed elsewhere [24, 25]. Further studies have implicated sleep restriction to impairments in glucose metabolism consequently increasing the risk for type II diabetes mellitus [26–28]. Additional studies examining caloric intake following sleep deprivation show that caloric intake nearly doubles in sleep deprived states compared to baseline, with sleep deprived individuals being more likely to choose foods with a high fat content over fruits and vegetables, along with a tendency toward increased snacking [24, 25]. Studies evaluating energy expenditure following sleep deprivation have been less consistent owing to several methodological issues. Some investigators have found total or partial sleep deprivation reduces energy expenditure [23, 29] while others have not [30–32]. As a result, several reviews posit that energy expenditure does not change much in response to sleep deprivation. Consequently, accumulating evidence suggests a causal role for sleep deprivation and subsequent obesity, which may be mediated through a variety of mechanisms. Sleep deprivation and its effects on subsequent increased caloric intake have produced the most consistent results, with the effects of sleep deprivation on leptin and ghrelin as well as energy expenditure being less uniform. These effects may also be modified by other factors such as age, gender, and physical fitness and have as yet to be adequately explored [24].

12.2.2 Connection of Sleep Quality to Obesity: Possible Underlying Mechanisms

Thus far, most studies evaluating a connection between sleep and obesity have focused on sleep quantity and effects on obesity. Separating the effects of sleep quality to sleep quantity can be challenging from an experimental standpoint. An initial investigation by Gonnissen and colleagues [33] compared two randomized groups of men who had either uninterrupted sleep or sleep interrupted every 90 min. These interruptions did not affect sleep quantity. Those in the fragmented sleep group reported feeling less full and had a stronger desire to eat after dinner compared to the nonsleep fragmented group. This process may be mediated by changes in insulin sensitivity. The sleep fragmented group had a shift in insulin secretion without changes in glucose secretion, with decreased insulin concentrations seen in the morning, and higher insulin levels in the afternoon. Elevated evening cortisol was also seen, which may have mediated these insulin effects. Further evidence comes from Stamatakis and Punjabi, who showed that excess sleep fragmentation has been associated with a decrease in insulin sensitivity and glucose effectiveness [34]. Such findings have significant implications for sleep disorders such as obstructive sleep apnea (OSA), which is associated with decreased sleep quantity, decreased sleep quality (frequent interruptions in sleep due to sleep-disordered breathing events), and intermittent hypoxemia. OSA has been associated with a higher risk of diabetes and increases in insulin resistance [35].

12.2.3 Connection of Sleep Timing to Obesity: Possible Underlying Mechanisms

Circadian misalignment has also been linked to several neuroendocrine changes that may lead to obesity and type II diabetes [25]. This has been most commonly observed in shift workers, a population in which an increased risk of diabetes [36] and obesity [37–39] is seen. In modern society, this can also be seen when biological preferences for sleep wake rhythms become misaligned with social (e.g., school, work) obligations. The subsequent desynchrony results in not only a misalignment of optimal timing of sleep relative to sleep timing preference (i.e., chronotype) but also a secondary sleep deprivation and has been termed social jetlag [40]. Social jetlag, or "living against our internal clock" has also increasingly been found to be associated with obesity [41, 42]. The mechanisms by which circadian misalignment may contribute to the development of obesity are largely similar to those mechanisms that are thought to connect sleep deprivation to obesity, i.e., alterations in leptin, ghrelin, and glucose regulation [25]. Circadian misalignment has been associated with alterations in glucose metabolism and insulin sensitivity [43, 44], even when controlling for sleep duration. In addition to glucose metabolism, decreases in leptin levels with ongoing circadian misalignment have also been seen [43, 44].

Melatonin has also been investigated for a potential link with obesity. Melatonin is hormone normally produced by the pineal gland during nighttime hours (in the absence of light) to help regulate circadian rhythms. It is tightly synchronized to the light/dark cycle, under the control of a "master biological clock" within the hypothalamus called the suprachiasmatic nucleus (SCN) [45]. A growing body of literature suggests melatonin deficiency may be linked to obesity, and that melatonin administration may have a role in obesity prevention [46]. The precise nature of this relationship of melatonin to obesity is complex, as diet, timing, and pattern of melatonin administration may influence this hormone's actions on various hormones that influence energy intake and expenditure, including insulin, leptin, and adiponectin [46].

Consequently, the relationship between sleep and obesity is complex, with several potential mechanisms being involved to connect sleep to obesity. Alterations in the quantity, quality, and timing of sleep all have the potential to increase the risk of developing excessive daytime sleepiness and subsequent obesity, which may be mediated through a variety of mechanisms including alterations in glucose metabolism, insulin sensitivity, leptin and ghrelin levels, caloric intake, and energy expenditure. Even in the absence of sleep problems or sleep disorders, patients with obesity can still suffer from significant daytime sleepiness. Several hypotheses have been proposed to explain these symptoms. One hypothesis has suggested that adipose tissue may release soporific substances into the blood stream, including tumor necrosis factor alpha and other somnogenic cytokines such as interleukin-6 (IL-6) [47, 48]. Significant research is needed to better understand these mechanisms and to understand how other factors such as age, gender, and baseline physical fitness may alter the connection between sleep, sleepiness, and obesity.

12.2.4 Sleep Disorders and Obesity

The two commonest sleep disorders associated with obesity are sleep-disordered breathing, particularly obstructive sleep apnea/hypopnea syndrome and obesity hypoventilation syndrome (OHS) [49]. Obstructive sleep apnea (OSA) is characterized by repetitive episodes of full (apnea) or partial (hypopnea) collapse of the upper airway during sleep. The severity of this is measured by the apnea hypopnea index (AHI) which is the frequency of apneas and hypopneas per hour of sleep. Events may also include "respiratory effort-related arousals" (RERAs), a form of hypopnea without significant hypoxemia. OSA has routinely been defined as an AHI $\geq$ 5/h, while the diagnosis of OSA *syndrome* typically requires a complaint of excessive daytime sleepiness with the AHI criterion [50]. The respiratory disturbance index (RDI) is the AHI added to the RERA index (frequency of RERAS per hour of sleep) and is also commonly used in clinical practice. Earlier epidemiologic data by Young and colleagues in 1993 estimated the prevalence of OSA syndrome to be 4 % in men and 2 % in women, with male sex and obesity being highlighted as major risk factors for OSA syndrome [51]. According to a 2015 review of epidemiologic studies, prevalence estimates suggest sleep-disordered breathing (defined as an apnea hypopnea index (AHI $\geq$ 5) is present in 22 % of men (range 9–37 %) and 17 % of women (range 4–50 %) [52]. While advances in diagnostic equipment along with changes in definitions of sleep-disordered breathing have contributed to changes in prevalence estimates of OSA syndrome, a leading contributing factor to the increase in prevalence of sleep-disordered breathing is the obesity epidemic [52]. The prevalence of OSA rises to 50 % in obese subjects (25). Moreover, 60–90 % of OSA patients are obese [25, 49, 53].

12.3 Mechanisms by Which Obesity and Sleep-Disordered Breathing Are Connected

There are several mechanisms by which obesity contributes to sleep-disordered breathing. Increased obesity may lead to increased adipose deposition in pharyngeal walls, leading to a decreased cross sectional area of the oropharynx [54]. Additionally, increased abdominal fat decreases lung volumes and lung capacity, including functional residual capacity, which can alter upper airway mechanics, specifically reducing the size and stiffness of the upper airway and thus increasing collapsibility [55]. Moreover, obesity is associated with central leptin resistance. Leptin, normally produced in adipose tissue, typically increases respiratory drive but in obesity, leptin resistance is seen, i.e., there is a higher serum leptin level but decreased respiratory drive and ventilation response to carbon dioxide retention (i.e. hypercapnic response) [56].

12.4 OSA: Clinical Features

Common clinical features of obstructive sleep apnea include snoring, witnessed apneas (pauses in breathing) during sleep, nocturnal choking or gasping for breath, insomnia, and unexplained excessive daytime sleepiness [57, 58]. Other symptoms may include frequent difficulties with concentration, irritability, poor libido, nighttime urination, and morning headaches [57]. The presence of OSA is frequently accompanied by several medical and psychiatric complications including cardiovascular disease, hypertension, diabetes, major depressive disorder, gastroesophageal reflux disease, and major neurocognitive disorders [52, 57–59]. Left untreated, OSA can lead to a higher risk of motor vehicle accidents, pulmonary hypertension, stroke, and cardiac arrhythmias including atrial fibrillation [57]. Despite that OSA is a common disease associated with a significant health problems, 75–80 % of OSA patients remain undiagnosed [60]. Consequently, untreated OSA represents a large public health burden [60]. OSA has also been linked to disturbances in glucose regulation, lipid metabolism, and fatty liver disease, consequently leading many to suggest OSA should be considered part of metabolic syndrome [61, 62].

12.5 OSA: Risk Factors, Diagnosis

Although several risk factors have been connected to OSA including alcohol use, nasal congestion, increasing age, craniofacial anatomy, polycystic ovarian syndrome, and menopause, obesity ranks as the most pressing risk factor given the obesity epidemic in North America [63]. Several indirect measures of obesity are associated with a higher risk of sleep-disordered breathing including body mass index, waist-to-hip ratio, and increased neck circumference (>17 in. in men, >16 in. in women) [64, 65]. These factors, however, become less significant in predicting sleep-disordered breathing in adults over 60 years old [65].

The gold standard test for obstructive sleep apnea is the nocturnal polysomnogram or overnight sleep study. Several physiologic recordings occur in the polysomnogram, including electroencephalogram, electrooculogram, electrocardiogram, electromyogram (chin and leg), as well as pulse oximetry (to measure oxygen saturation in the blood). Additionally, there are several measures of respiration, including respiratory inductance plethysmography bands around the chest and abdomen, and a nasal pressure transducer and oral thermistor to measure airflow through the oronasal passages. While the gold standard polysomnogram is a level I greater than or equal to sign (7 channel) polysomnogram that is done in a laboratory setting, newer technologies have been increasingly used due to the high cost and inconvenience of the laboratory study. One option is a level III polysomnogram, which generally has fewer leads (for instance, in many cases no EEG leads, but measures of oxygen saturation, breathing, snoring, and electrocardiogram) and can be done in the patient's home (i.e. a "home sleep study"). Other devices have also been developed to assess for OSA such as Watch PAT (a device that measures peripheral arterial tonometry (PAT) as a surrogate test for the presence of sleep-disordered breathing). Although considered less accurate than the level I study, the reasonable accuracy with noncomplicated patients, coupled with the convenience and relative low cost of these tests make them a viable alternative to consider in select cases.

Due to the expense and inconvenience with the aforementioned investigations, several screening questionnaires have also been developed in an attempt to screen for sleep disorders including obstructive sleep apnea. While such questionnaires can be useful in identifying patients who are at high risk for having OSA, none of these is an adequate surrogate for polysomnography, the gold standard for diagnosis of OSA. Consequently, all patients who are assessed to be at high risk for OSA by questionnaire data should have their diagnosis confirmed with polysomnography. Some of the more commonly used questionnaires include the Berlin Questionnaire, The Epworth Sleepiness Score, and the STOP-BANG questionnaire. The Berlin questionnaire is a self-filled questionnaire that is divided into three sections, the first is on breathing problems in sleep such as snoring and witnessed apneas, the second section probes symptoms of daytime sleepiness, and the third section can be filled out by the physician which includes blood pressure and body mass index [66]. The Epworth Sleepiness Score is a simple self-filled questionnaire consisting of eight questions assessing the propensity to doze in several situations [67]. This test is aimed at measuring levels of daytime sleepiness, which may not necessarily be adequate for screening for sleep-disordered breathing, since OSA severity does not always correlate with daytime sleepiness [68]. The STOP-BANG questionnaire is an 8-item questionnaire designed to screen for OSA. It consists of eight questions practitioners can ask patients to assess for the likelihood of sleep-disordered breathing being present [69]. Questions include (a) do you (S)nore loudly—loud enough to be heard through closed doors or your bed partner elbows you for snoring at night; (b) are you (T)ired, fatigued, or sleepy during the daytime; (c) anyone (O)bserved you stop breathing or choking or gasping during your sleep?; (d) do you have or are you being treated for high blood (P) ressure; (e) (B)MI ≥ 35 kg/m^2; (f) (A)ge older than 50 years old?; (g) (N)eck size large? (Circumference ≥ 17 in. for men or ≥ 16 in. for women); (h) (G)ender—male. Three to four out of eight positive answers suggest an intermediate risk for having OSA, while 5–8 positive answers are associated with a high risk of having OSA, with higher scores or certain combinations of points having a higher likelihood for having OSA [70, 71]. The predictive performance of the STOP-BANG questionnaire for identifying OSA in obese patients and morbidly obese patients is significantly improved, with a score of 4 having a sensitivity of 88 % for severe OSA in this population [72]. A finding of serum bicarbonate (HCO_3^-) ≥ 28 mmol/L in addition to a score of ≥ 3 from the STOP-BANG significantly improves the specificity for moderate and severe OSA [73]. As a result of the relative convenience and ease of use of this screening tool, the STOP-BANG questionnaire is frequently used to screen for OSA in community as well as preoperative settings.

12.6 OSA Treatment Options

12.6.1 Continuous Positive Airway Pressure (CPAP) Therapy

CPAP therapy is the gold standard for treatment of OSA. This consists of a mask connected to a flow generator that blows room air at a specified pressure to splint the airway open. A large Cochrane review demonstrated that CPAP use in OSA patients is associated with improvements in subjective and objective sleepiness, quality of life, cognitive function, and blood pressure [74]. CPAP therapy has also been shown to be helpful for reducing cardiovascular morbidity and mortality in patients with OSA in long-term follow-up studies [59]. Other studies have shown CPAP use to be associated with reductions in motor vehicle accidents, health care utilization, and even marital conflict [75–77]. Studies regarding the efficacy of CPAP therapy for subsequent weight loss have produced inconsistent results. Although some studies have shown CPAP therapy to be associated with weight loss [78, 79], others have found no effect [80] or even weight gain [81] following CPAP therapy administration. CPAP adherence is a common struggle for patients and a common clinical challenge. Nasal and skin irritation, abdominal bloating, and pressure marks on the face are common complaints associated with CPAP use. Mask fit can be problematic, leading to excessive leak and compromised efficacy of CPAP use. CPAP use can also interfere with intimacy, which can be another barrier to treatment [82]. Minimal reasonable use of CPAP has been classically defined as at least 4 h of use on 70 % of nights [83, 84], but for adequate benefits including improvements in alertness, daytime functioning, and memory to be realized, other investigators suggest at least 6 h of nightly use [85].

12.6.2 Weight Loss

Weight loss has also been shown to be helpful for OSA, with the reduction in AHI seen being proportional to the degree of weight loss in two randomized controlled trials utilizing nonsurgical interventions for weight loss [86, 87]. Bariatric surgery has been shown to be helpful for weight loss with proportionate decreases in AHI seen in a large meta-analysis by Greenburg and colleagues evaluating studies with pre and postpolysomnographic data available [88]. Several other studies have also suggested improvement in sleep-disordered breathing with surgical interventions for weight loss [89–91]. Greenburg's study was the only study that had inclusion criteria that included pre/post-AHI measurements. Weight loss may be therapeutic for sleep apnea through a number of mechanisms. For instance, the loss of both visceral and subcutaneous fat may relieve pressure on the neck, upper airway, and even diaphragm to assist with respiration [89].

12.6.3 Other Options

Other conventional treatment options for OSA include surgical options, with the goal being to widen the airway. A conventional procedure that can be used for mild OSA is a uvulopalatopharyngoplasty (UPPP) procedure, where the uvula is excised along with possible palatal resection. While success rates can be quite variable, ranging from 16 to 83 %, the quality of evidence for efficacy of this procedure is relatively weak [92, 93]. Radiofrequency ablation can also be used for mild OSA in select circumstances. This consists of a temperature-controlled radiofrequency probe inserted in the tongue or soft palate to stiffen tissues to open the airway, but evidence for efficacy of this procedure is also weak [92]. Maxillomandibular advancement is a facial surgery in which the maxilla and mandible are simultaneously excised and advanced forward before being reattached to the skull to increase retroglossal and retropalatal space. This procedure has demonstrated significant efficacy (67–100 %) for treatment of severe OSA, but with the exception of select cases in which there can be significant cosmetic benefit due to craniofacial abnormalities, this procedure often is considered a last resort due to the invasiveness and time necessary for completion [92, 93]. Success rates in the morbidly obese population were found to be lower compared to all OSA patients in a meta-analysis performed by Camacho and colleagues [94]. Adenotonsillectomy is generally considered the treatment of choice in pediatric OSA [95, 96], but benefits in the adult population are less clear [92].

Mandibular advancement devices or oral appliances are devices fabricated by specially trained dentists to attach to the jaw, but protrude the mandible forward to increase retropalatal space. These devices have generally been accepted as reasonable treatment options for mild to moderate sleep-disordered breathing but efficacy rates decrease with more severe sleep-disordered breathing [97]. Compared with CPAP, these devices may not be as effective, but they are often more acceptable than CPAP therapy for patients [98]. A more recent nasal expiratory positive airway pressure (EPAP) device has been developed for treatment of sleep-disordered breathing. This device, called Provent, is a disposable device attached to the nostrils with an adhesive. It has a one-way valve that utilizes a patient's own expiration to generate nasal EPAP to splint the airway open. A 2015 meta-analysis suggests the use of this device may help in cases of mild and position-related apnea and has efficacy comparable to oral appliances [99]. Another novel treatment being investigated for treatment of OSA involves a neurostimulator implanted in the upper chest. Once initiated by a handheld remote, this *hypoglossal nerve* stimulator stimulates key muscles of the upper airway during respiration to reduce sleep-disordered breathing [100]. Early results showed significant efficacy for moderate to severe OSA and consequently the Food And Drug Administration (FDA) in the United States has approved the clinical use of this device. It is not currently recommended for use in patients with a BMI above 32 kg/m^2 since it has not been adequately evaluated in obese patients though this may change as new data become available [101].

12.7 Obesity Hypoventilation Syndrome (OHS)

Obesity hypoventilation syndrome (OHS) refers to a disorder where there is evidence of hypoventilation with persistent hypercapnia ($PaCO_2 > 45$ mmHg) during wakefulness, in patients with obesity (BMI >30 kg/m^2), and other disorders of respiratory function have been excluded (e.g., neuromuscular disorders, chest wall disorders, etc.) [102]. Consequently, a physical finding of obesity alone with a suggestive history is not sufficient to make a diagnosis of OHS; as an arterial blood gas is needed to confirm the presence of hypercapnia. This disorder is a chronic condition associated with significant medical morbidities including diabetes, respiratory failure, cardiovascular disease, and hormonal changes, as well as psychosocial sequelae including high rates of unemployment, social isolation, and impaired activities of daily living [103]. Without treatment, there is a significant mortality risk associated with this condition [104]. Population estimates of the prevalence of this disorder are generally lacking, likely owing to under recognition and diagnosis, but estimates suggest approximately 0.15–0.6 % of the US population is afflicted with this condition [105, 106]. Prevalence rates rise sharply, however, with increasing obesity, as the prevalence in patients with a BMI over 35 kg/m^2 is 9–20 %, and is up to 50 % in hospitalized patients with a BMI of >50 kg/m^2 [107, 108]. Up to 90 % of patients with OHS have OSA [105], but this leaves 10 % of OHS patients without OSA. These patients develop sleep-related hypoventilation that is particularly evident in REM sleep [105].

12.8 Clinical Features of OHS

Typically these patients come to the attention of respiratory and/or sleep specialists after symptoms of right-sided heart failure (cor pulmonale) become evident [105]. Early symptoms of OHS can include poor quality sleep, daytime sleepiness, lack of energy, and shortness of breath at nighttime. Patients may even suffer from symptoms of depression during the day [102]. Many of these symptoms can be caused or exacerbated by comorbid sleep-disordered breathing, with early symptoms being indistinguishable. Shortness of breath (dyspnea), however, is usually more prominent in OHS patients. When OHS is more severe, other findings may include significant peripheral edema and congestive heart failure. OHS patients are more likely to have diabetes mellitus and hypertension [102]. These problems often contribute to poor exercise tolerance and significant social consequences including decreased interest in daily activities and withdrawal from social obligations because of significant physical symptoms [103]. Left unrecognized, untreated OHS patients have significantly higher rates of hospitalization and mortality [102].

12.9 Treatment Options for OHS

12.9.1 CPAP Therapy

Positive Airway Pressure (PAP) therapy is the mainstay of treatment [109–111]. Improvements have been seen in PCO_2 levels, sleep quality, mortality, and quality of life (reviewed in [111]). CPAP introduces a positive end expiratory pressure (PEEP) to maintain upper airway patency. Conventionally, CPAP is initiated to treat both comorbid sleep-disordered breathing if present, as well as associated hypoventilation. CPAP therapy may be helpful for OHS through a variety of mechanisms besides maintaining airway patency. CPAP therapy may play a role in reducing atelectasis and maintaining small airway patency to decrease ventilation perfusion mismatch to improve subsequent oxygenation [111]. The volume inflating effect of CPAP will also increase functional residual capacity, which can be helpful for OHS [110]. A 2015 study by Masa and colleagues suggests that noninvasive ventilation (NIV; see later) and CPAP therapy have superior benefits for OHS clinical symptoms and sleep variables compared to interventions limited to lifestyle modifications [112]. Studies suggest at least 4.5 h of CPAP use a night is necessary to see benefits in $PaCO_2$ and PaO_2 for hypercapnic patients with OSA, with benefits possibly plateauing at 5–7 h of therapy [113]. It can be tempting to consider adding nocturnal oxygen therapy for these patients within the CPAP device, but overoxygenation at night can actually exacerbate hypercapnia by suppressing ventilation [114].

12.9.2 Noninvasive Positive Pressure Ventilation (NIPPV—BIPAP and Other Ventilatory Support Therapies)

Bilevel therapy introduces an inspiratory positive airway pressure (IPAP) in addition to an expiratory positive airway pressure (EPAP). This inspiratory support increases tidal volume when patients inhale, and the device can be triggered spontaneously by patients (S-mode) to deliver this pressure, or a timed breath may be delivered according to a specific backup rate if patients are unable to trigger the device within a specified time period (Spontaneous/timed, or S/T mode). There is also a timed mode, where the device delivers pressurizations at a preset respiratory rate regardless of patient respiratory efforts. Hence these devices are considered a form of assisted ventilation, since they are now providing some respiratory support. There is a paucity of evidence regarding recommending one form of PAP therapy over another for OHS (e.g., Bilevel Spontaneous mode, Bilevel with backup rate, or CPAP therapy) though one study by Piper and colleagues suggests that in OHS patients without severe nocturnal hypoxemia, use of BIPAP therapy may be more comfortable and produce improvements in daytime psychomotor vigilance compared to CPAP therapy [115]. Consequently, while evidence is limited, there is general consensus that if CPAP therapy fails to adequately address hypoxemia and hypercapnia associated with OHS, then some form of NIPPV such as BiPAP therapy should be strongly considered [111]. Newer PAP modalities are being evaluated for treatment of OHS, such as AVAPS (average volume assured pressure support) with comparable daytime benefits to BiPAP use (e.g., for daytime hypercapnia, sleep architecture/efficiency) and some evidence of additional benefits particularly for patient adherence, but long-term data are lacking at this time [111].

12.9.3 Weight Loss

Weight loss can offer substantial benefit to sleep-related hypoventilation, though significant weight loss is needed to see these benefits realized. Not only can weight loss be beneficial for sleep-disordered breathing, but benefits can also be seen in respiratory drive, gas exchange, pulmonary function tests, and respiratory muscle strength [111]. There is a much higher likelihood of such weight loss being achieved with bariatric surgery compared to conventional nonsurgical weight loss measures such as behavioral management, dietary changes, physical activity, and medication management [116].

12.9.4 Tracheostomy

Although tracheostomy can be an effective treatment for sleep-disordered breathing, it is now offered in only a minority of patients in which conventional treatments for sleep-disordered breathing have failed. Prior to the advent of CPAP therapy introduced by Sullivan and colleagues in 1981 [117], tracheostomy was the treatment of choice for sleep-disordered breathing. Further research suggests patients with morbid obesity ($BMI > 40\ kg/m^2$) are at significant risk for tracheostomy complications, most commonly related to tube obstruction or malpositioning of the tracheostomy tube after being dislodged [118].

12.9.5 Pharmacotherapy

Acetazolamide, a carbonic anhydrase inhibitor, decreases serum bicarbonate levels and thus induces a metabolic acidosis which subsequently stimulates ventilation [119]. This medication has been suggested to be helpful in stimulating ventilation in OHS patients with hypercapnic respiratory failure [120] but will not adequately treat OHS patients with OSA in the absence of PAP therapy [121]. Side effects can include dizziness, paresthesias, and electrolyte imbalance [110]. Long-term data are lacking, consequently limiting the use of this treatment option. In post menopausal women, the use of medroxyprogesterone has been shown to have some benefit in reducing hypercapnia and increasing nocturnal oxygenation, but was not accompanied by benefits in the frequency of sleep-disordered breathing events or sleep quality [122]. As with acetazolamide, long-term data are lacking; consequently caution is warranted, especially given the risk of thromboembolism associated with this medication [110].

12.9.6 Insomnia and Obesity

This topic has received relatively little attention, though an association has been recognized between obesity and insomnia, independent of other potential mediating covariates such as physical and mental health as well as social background [123]. At least one study has suggested obesity is a risk factor for the development of chronic insomnia independent of sleep-disordered breathing [124]. Insomnia has been associated with unhealthy behaviors such as physical inactivity and heavy alcohol use [125], which could play a role in mediating a relationship between obesity and insomnia. Further work is needed to elucidate the nature of these associations.

Case Vignette: Postsleep Study

Janet completed an overnight polysomnogram that showed an AHI of 85/h, with oxygen saturation dropping to a minimum of 68 % during a total sleep time of 5 h and 49 min. Mean oxygen saturation was 85 % (normal is >90 %). Events were more severe in REM sleep. Due to concerns about her low baseline oxygen saturation, an arterial blood gas (ABG) on room air was drawn in the morning. This showed a PaO_2 of 54 mmHG, a $PaCO_2$ of 61 mmHG, and a bicarbonate (HCO_3-) of 34 mmol/L. Based on her polysomnography results, she was diagnosed with severe OSA that was REM related. Based on her ABG results and her clinical assessment she was diagnosed with obesity hypoventilation syndrome (OHS). Followup investigations including blood tests and a computerized tomography (CT) of her chest did not reveal any evidence of other cardiorespiratory or endocrinologic (e.g. thyroid) problems. After discussing these results with her sleep specialist, she was subsequently started on a trial of autotitrating CPAP (APAP) minimum 5 maximum 20 cm of water pressure. In reviewing the compliance data, this showed that she was able to use the APAP every night after a 2-week acclimatization period, and she was able to sleep through the night on most nights, and consequently got up earlier, and had more energy during the day. She no longer dozed at the wheel at stop signs, and even seemed to be in a better mood with people, being more patient and upbeat. She was no longer waking up with headaches (which likely were caused by daytime hypercapnia). Her shortness of breath during the day also improved markedly. Follow up ABG showed normalization of PaO_2, $PaCO_2$ and bicaronate.While the APAP was helping significantly, she was still interested in proceeding with bariatric surgery to lose weight.

After having bariatric surgery and adjusting her diet, she went on to lose 90 lb over the next year, bringing her weight to 145 lb with a BMI of 25.7 kg/m^2. At times, she felt the APAP machine was getting cumbersome and was blowing too much air for her, so she stopped using it 10 months postoperatively. At the advice of her family doctor, she visited the sleep specialist again, and he recommended repeating a diagnostic polysomnography study. This time her AHI was 4/h with oxygen saturation dropping to a minimum of 91 %, and mean oxygen saturation stayed at 95 % during a total sleep time of 6 h and 53 min. ABG on room air was also drawn and all values were within normal limits. She was relieved to hear that her sleep-disordered breathing and OHS were cured.

12.10 Summary and Take Home Messages

- Recent evidence has linked sleep disturbances with the pathogenesis of obesity, through a variety of mechanisms.
- Alterations in the quantity, quality, and timing of sleep all have the potential to increase the risk of developing excessive daytime sleepiness and subsequent obesity, which may be mediated through a variety of mechanisms including alterations in glucose metabolism, insulin sensitivity, leptin and ghrelin levels, caloric intake, and energy expenditure (Fig. 12.1)
- The two commonest sleep disorders associated with obesity are obstructive sleep apnea/hypopnea syndrome (OSAS) and obesity hypoventilation syndrome (OHS).
- Treatment options are available to help with the obesity-related sleep disorders in terms of CPAP, BIPAP, mandibular advancement device, and surgical interventions (Table 12.1).

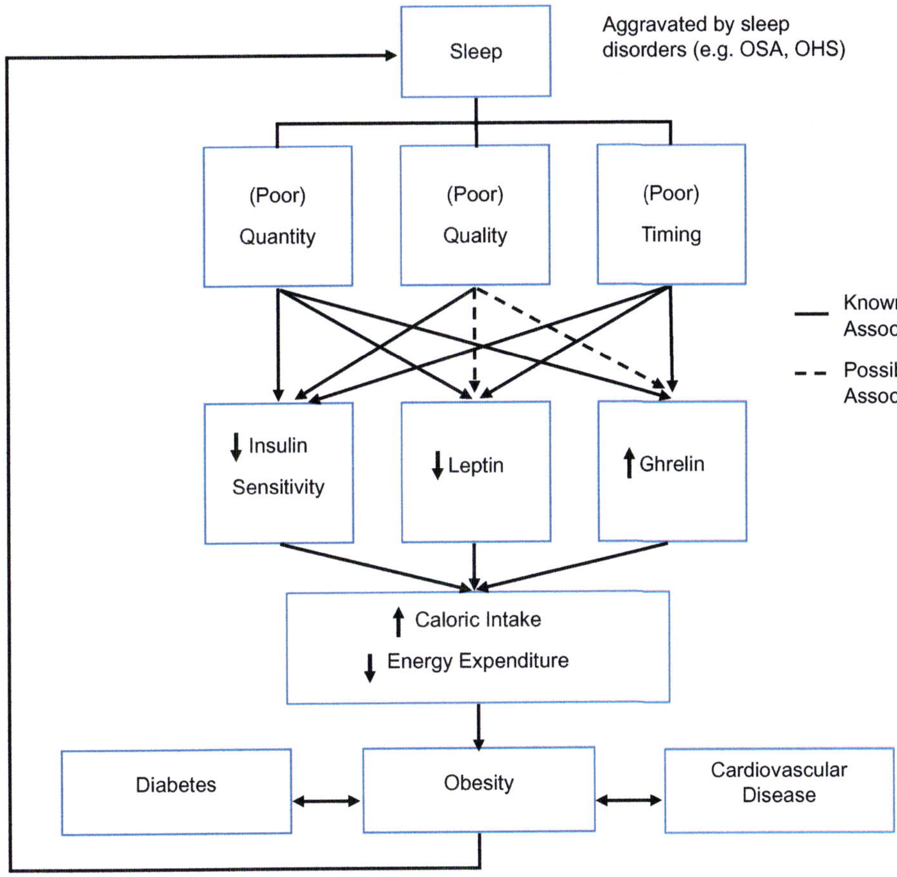

Fig. 12.1 Sleep mechanisms and their connections to obesity

Table 12.1 Comparison of various apnea treatment modalities in terms of advantages, drawbacks, and cost

Treatments for OSA	Description	Advantages	Drawbacks	Cost	Comments
CPAP therapy	Mask connected to device on nightstand, blows room air into airway to splint airway open. Used to treat all severities of OSA (mild, moderate, severe)	Very effective for mild to severe OSA; robust benefits seen in cardiovascular health, mood symptoms, and numerous other benefits	Inconvenient—e.g. maintenance issues, wearing a mask every night, may induce claustrophobia. Travelling with the device may be inconvenient	$$$ (insurances may cover)	Gold Standard for treatment of OSA. If not effective or not tolerated, APAP or BiPAP can also be tried
Uvulopalatopharyngoplasty (UPPP), tonsillectomy	Surgical procedure to extract uvula and/or tonsils if obstructing airway. May be helpful for mild to moderate OSA	If effective, may be a cure for OSA. Higher likelihood of success in pediatric population (particularly tonsillectomy) and mild OSA; lower success rate with increasing severity of OSA	Can be painful; high failure rate	$ (often covered by health plans)	Tonsillectomy is often considered the treatment of choice for the pediatric population
Mandibular advancement device (MAD)	Oral appliance worn at night to protrude lower jaw forward to open airway. Indicated for mild to moderate OSA routinely	Convenient to use, moderate success rate for mild to moderate OSA	Not as effective for treating severe OSA; may damage teeth, aggravate temporomandibular joint problems. Patients can break these devices overnight	$$$ (may or may not be covered by health plans)	Higher efficacy rate in women, patients with positional OSA. Lower efficacy rate in obese patients
Weight loss	Can be helpful for all severities of OSA, if the patient is overweight	If effective, may be a cure for OSA	Maintenance of weight loss can be challenging	Variable, by mechanism (e.g., surgery, diet, etc.)	
Maxillomandibular advancement (MMA)	Bilateral osteotomy of upper and lower jaw to open airway	If effective, may be a cure for OSA. High success rate in appropriately selected candidates	May be painful, time consuming, complicated (may require multiple specialists—e.g., orthodontists to align teeth, surgeon, etc.)	$$$$$	Considered when additional cosmetic benefits are expected, and/or when other options have failed
Provent	Disposable nasal device worn over nostrils; uses nasal EPAP to maintain airway patency	If effective, can be convenient to treat OSA (e.g., for travel)	High failure rate; expensive with daily use; may be difficult to tolerate particularly in acclimatization period	$ (but cumulative cost can be significant)	Can be combined with modalities (e.g., use CPAP at home, provent for travelling)
Neurostimulator (hypoglossal nerve stimulator)	Device implanted in upper chest; when stimulated activates key muscles of upper airway to maintain airway patency	If effective, can be convenient to use	Very costly; more research needed to assess optimal patients for this procedure	$$$$$$$$ ($15–30 K, variable)	

OSA obstructive sleep apnea, *CPAP* continuous positive airway pressure, *APAP* autotitrating CPAP, *BiPAP* bilevel positive airway pressure, *EPAP* expiratory positive airway pressure

Acknowledgement The authors would like to thank Dr. Judith Leech, Dr. Naomi Spitale and Dr. Sanjeev Chander for their suggested edits and review of this chapter.

References

1. Carskadon MA, Dement WC. Normal human sleep: an overview. In: Kryger MH, Roth T, Dement WC, editors. Principles and practice of sleep medicine. 5th ed. St. Louis: Elsevier; 2011. p. 16–26.
2. Hirshkowitz M, Whiton K, Albert SM, et al. National Sleep Foundation's sleep time duration recommendations: methodology and results summary. Sleep Health. 2015;1:40–3.
3. Consensus Conference Panel, Watson NF, Badr MS, et al. Joint consensus statement of the American Academy of Sleep Medicine and Sleep Research Society on the recommended amount of sleep for a healthy adult: methodology and discussion. J Clin Sleep Med. 2015;11:931–52.
4. Dashti HS, Scheer FA, Jacques PF, Lamon-Fava S, Ordovas JM. Short sleep duration and dietary intake: epidemiologic evidence, mechanisms, and health implications. Adv Nutr. 2015;6:648–59.
5. Statistics Canada. General social survey: overview of the time use of Canadians; 2011.
6. Yang L, Colditz GA. Prevalence of overweight and obesity in the United States, 2007–2012. JAMA Intern Med. 2015;175:1412–3.
7. Silber MH, Ancoli-Israel S, Bonnet MH, et al. The visual scoring of sleep in adults. J Clin Sleep Med. 2007;3:121–31.
8. Hasler G, Buysse DJ, Klaghofer R, et al. The association between short sleep duration and obesity in young adults: a 13-year prospective study. Sleep. 2004;27:661–6.
9. Marshall NS, Glozier N, Grunstein RR. Is sleep duration related to obesity? A critical review of the epidemiological evidence. Sleep Med Rev. 2008;12:289–98.
10. Patel SR. Reduced sleep as an obesity risk factor. Obes Rev. 2009;10 Suppl 2:61–8.
11. Magee CA, Iverson DC, Caputi P. Sleep duration and obesity in middle-aged Australian adults. Obesity (Silver Spring). 2010;18:420–1.
12. Chaput JP, Lambert M, Gray-Donald K, et al. Short sleep duration is independently associated with overweight and obesity in Quebec children. Can J Public Health. 2011;102:369–74.
13. Anic GM, Titus-Ernstoff L, Newcomb PA, Trentham-Dietz A, Egan KM. Sleep duration and obesity in a population-based study. Sleep Med. 2010;11:447–51.
14. Hsieh SD, Muto T, Murase T, Tsuji H, Arase Y. Association of short sleep duration with obesity, diabetes, fatty liver and behavioral factors in Japanese men. Intern Med. 2011;50:2499–502.
15. Cappuccio FP, Taggart FM, Kandala NB, et al. Meta-analysis of short sleep duration and obesity in children and adults. Sleep. 2008;31:619–26.
16. Chen X, Beydoun MA, Wang Y. Is sleep duration associated with childhood obesity? A systematic review and meta-analysis. Obesity (Silver Spring). 2008;16:265–74.
17. Patel SR, Blackwell T, Redline S, et al. The association between sleep duration and obesity in older adults. Int J Obes (Lond). 2008;32:1825–34.
18. St-Onge MP, Shechter A. Sleep disturbances, body fat distribution, food intake and/or energy expenditure: pathophysiological aspects. Horm Mol Biol Clin Investig. 2014;17:29–37.
19. Bayon V, Leger D, Gomez-Merino D, Vecchierini MF, Chennaoui M. Sleep debt and obesity. Ann Med. 2014;46:264–72.
20. Spiegel K, Tasali E, Penev P, Van Cauter E. Brief communication: sleep curtailment in healthy young men is associated with decreased leptin levels, elevated ghrelin levels, and increased hunger and appetite. Ann Intern Med. 2004;141:846–50.
21. Mullington JM, Chan JL, Van Dongen HP, et al. Sleep loss reduces diurnal rhythm amplitude of leptin in healthy men. J Neuroendocrinol. 2003;15:851–4.
22. Spiegel K, Leproult R, Van Cauter E. Impact of sleep debt on metabolic and endocrine function. Lancet. 1999;354:1435–9.
23. Benedict C, Hallschmid M, Lassen A, et al. Acute sleep deprivation reduces energy expenditure in healthy men. Am J Clin Nutr. 2011;93:1229–36.
24. St-Onge MP. The role of sleep duration in the regulation of energy balance: effects on energy intakes and expenditure. J Clin Sleep Med. 2013;9:73–80.
25. Depner CM, Stothard ER, Wright Jr KP. Metabolic consequences of sleep and circadian disorders. Curr Diab Rep. 2014;14:507.
26. Spiegel K, Knutson K, Leproult R, Tasali E, Van Cauter E. Sleep loss: a novel risk factor for insulin resistance and Type 2 diabetes. J Appl Physiol. 2005;99:2008–19.
27. Nedeltcheva AV, Kessler L, Imperial J, Penev PD. Exposure to recurrent sleep restriction in the setting of high caloric intake and physical inactivity results in increased insulin resistance and reduced glucose tolerance. J Clin Endocrinol Metab. 2009;94:3242–50.
28. Buxton OM, Pavlova M, Reid EW, Wang W, Simonson DC, Adler GK. Sleep restriction for 1 week reduces insulin sensitivity in healthy men. Diabetes. 2010;59:2126–33.
29. Schmid SM, Hallschmid M, Jauch-Chara K, et al. Short-term sleep loss decreases physical activity under free-living conditions but does not increase food intake under time-deprived laboratory conditions in healthy men. Am J Clin Nutr. 2009;90:1476–82.
30. Jung CM, Melanson EL, Frydendall EJ, Perreault L, Eckel RH, Wright KP. Energy expenditure during

sleep, sleep deprivation and sleep following sleep deprivation in adult humans. J Physiol. 2011;589:235–44.
31. St-Onge MP, Roberts AL, Chen J, et al. Short sleep duration increases energy intakes but does not change energy expenditure in normal-weight individuals. Am J Clin Nutr. 2011;94:410–6.
32. Calvin AD, Carter RE, Adachi T, et al. Effects of experimental sleep restriction on caloric intake and activity energy expenditure. Chest. 2013;144:79–86.
33. Gonnissen HK, Hursel R, Rutters F, Martens EA, Westerterp-Plantenga MS. Effects of sleep fragmentation on appetite and related hormone concentrations over 24 h in healthy men. Br J Nutr. 2013;109:748–56.
34. Stamatakis KA, Punjabi NM. Effects of sleep fragmentation on glucose metabolism in normal subjects. Chest. 2010;137:95–101.
35. Mesarwi O, Polak J, Jun J, Polotsky VY. Sleep disorders and the development of insulin resistance and obesity. Endocrinol Metab Clin North Am. 2013;42:617–34.
36. Kivimaki M, Batty GD, Hublin C. Shift work as a risk factor for future type 2 diabetes: evidence, mechanisms, implications, and future research directions. PLoS Med. 2011;8, e1001138.
37. Karlsson B, Knutsson A, Lindahl B. Is there an association between shift work and having a metabolic syndrome? Results from a population based study of 27,485 people. Occup Environ Med. 2001;58:747–52.
38. Morikawa Y, Nakagawa H, Miura K, et al. Effect of shift work on body mass index and metabolic parameters. Scand J Work Environ Health. 2007;33:45–50.
39. van Amelsvoort LG, Schouten EG, Kok FJ. Duration of shiftwork related to body mass index and waist to hip ratio. Int J Obes Relat Metab Disord. 1999;23:973–8.
40. Wittmann M, Dinich J, Merrow M, Roenneberg T. Social jetlag: misalignment of biological and social time. Chronobiol Int. 2006;23:497–509.
41. Parsons MJ, Moffitt TE, Gregory AM, et al. Social jetlag, obesity and metabolic disorder: investigation in a cohort study. Int J Obes (Lond). 2015;39:842–8.
42. Roenneberg T, Allebrandt KV, Merrow M, Vetter C. Social jetlag and obesity. Curr Biol. 2012;22:939–43.
43. Scheer FA, Hilton MF, Mantzoros CS, Shea SA. Adverse metabolic and cardiovascular consequences of circadian misalignment. Proc Natl Acad Sci U S A. 2009;106:4453–8.
44. Buxton OM, Cain SW, O'Connor SP, et al. Adverse metabolic consequences in humans of prolonged sleep restriction combined with circadian disruption. Sci Transl Med. 2012;4:129ra43.
45. Cajochen C, Krauchi K, Wirz-Justice A. Role of melatonin in the regulation of human circadian rhythms and sleep. J Neuroendocrinol. 2003;15:432–7.
46. Szewczyk-Golec K, Wozniak A, Reiter RJ. Inter-relationships of the chronobiotic, melatonin, with leptin and adiponectin: implications for obesity. J Pineal Res. 2015;59:277–91.
47. Vgontzas AN, Papanicolaou DA, Bixler EO, Kales A, Tyson K, Chrousos GP. Elevation of plasma cytokines in disorders of excessive daytime sleepiness: role of sleep disturbance and obesity. J Clin Endocrinol Metab. 1997;82:1313–6.
48. Vgontzas AN, Bixler EO, Tan TL, Kantner D, Martin LF, Kales A. Obesity without sleep apnea is associated with daytime sleepiness. Arch Intern Med. 1998;158:1333–7.
49. Ryan S, Crinion SJ, McNicholas WT. Obesity and sleep-disordered breathing—when two 'bad guys' meet. QJM. 2014;107:949–54.
50. Sleep-related breathing disorders in adults: recommendations for syndrome definition and measurement techniques in clinical research. The report of an American Academy of Sleep Medicine Task Force. Sleep. 1999;22:667–89.
51. Young T, Palta M, Dempsey J, Skatrud J, Weber S, Badr S. The occurrence of sleep-disordered breathing among middle-aged adults. N Engl J Med. 1993;328:1230–5.
52. Franklin KA, Lindberg E. Obstructive sleep apnea is a common disorder in the population—a review on the epidemiology of sleep apnea. J Thorac Dis. 2015;7:1311–22.
53. Peppard PE, Young T, Palta M, Dempsey J, Skatrud J. Longitudinal study of moderate weight change and sleep-disordered breathing. JAMA. 2000;284: 3015–21.
54. Shelton KE, Woodson H, Gay S, Suratt PM. Pharyngeal fat in obstructive sleep apnea. Am Rev Respir Dis. 1993;148:462–6.
55. Gifford AH, Leiter JC, Manning HL. Respiratory function in an obese patient with sleep-disordered breathing. Chest. 2010;138:704–15.
56. Campo A, Fruhbeck G, Zulueta JJ, et al. Hyperleptinaemia, respiratory drive and hypercapnic response in obese patients. Eur Respir J. 2007;30: 223–31.
57. Epstein LJ, Kristo D, Strollo Jr PJ, et al. Clinical guideline for the evaluation, management and long-term care of obstructive sleep apnea in adults. J Clin Sleep Med. 2009;5:263–76.
58. Miller JN, Berger AM. Screening and assessment for obstructive sleep apnea in primary care. Sleep Med Rev. 2015;29:41–51.
59. Marin JM, Carrizo SJ, Vicente E, Agusti AG. Long-term cardiovascular outcomes in men with obstructive sleep apnoea-hypopnoea with or without treatment with continuous positive airway pressure: an observational study. Lancet. 2005;365: 1046–53.
60. Aurora RN, Collop NA, Jacobowitz O, Thomas SM, Quan SF, Aronsky AJ. Quality measures for the care of adult patients with obstructive sleep apnea. J Clin Sleep Med. 2015;11:357–83.
61. Bonsignore MR, Borel AL, Machan E, Grunstein R. Sleep apnoea and metabolic dysfunction. Eur Respir Rev. 2013;22:353–64.
62. Stansbury RC, Strollo PJ. Clinical manifestations of sleep apnea. J Thorac Dis. 2015;7:E298–310.
63. Young T, Peppard PE, Gottlieb DJ. Epidemiology of obstructive sleep apnea: a population health perspec-

tive. Am J Respir Crit Care Med. 2002;165: 1217–39.
64. Tishler PV, Larkin EK, Schluchter MD, Redline S. Incidence of sleep-disordered breathing in an urban adult population: the relative importance of risk factors in the development of sleep-disordered breathing. JAMA. 2003;289:2230–7.
65. Young T, Shahar E, Nieto FJ, et al. Predictors of sleep-disordered breathing in community-dwelling adults: the Sleep Heart Health Study. Arch Intern Med. 2002;162:893–900.
66. Netzer NC, Stoohs RA, Netzer CM, Clark K, Strohl KP. Using the Berlin Questionnaire to identify patients at risk for the sleep apnea syndrome. Ann Intern Med. 1999;131:485–91.
67. Johns MW. A new method for measuring daytime sleepiness: the Epworth sleepiness scale. Sleep. 1991;14:540–5.
68. Ramachandran SK, Josephs LA. A meta-analysis of clinical screening tests for obstructive sleep apnea. Anesthesiology. 2009;110:928–39.
69. Chung F, Yegneswaran B, Liao P, et al. STOP questionnaire: a tool to screen patients for obstructive sleep apnea. Anesthesiology. 2008;108:812–21.
70. Chung F, Subramanyam R, Liao P, Sasaki E, Shapiro C, Sun Y. High STOP-Bang score indicates a high probability of obstructive sleep apnoea. Br J Anaesth. 2012;108:768–75.
71. Chung F, Yang Y, Brown R, Liao P. Alternative scoring models of STOP-bang questionnaire improve specificity to detect undiagnosed obstructive sleep apnea. J Clin Sleep Med. 2014;10:951–8.
72. Chung F, Yang Y, Liao P. Predictive performance of the STOP-Bang score for identifying obstructive sleep apnea in obese patients. Obes Surg. 2013;23:2050–7.
73. Chung F, Chau E, Yang Y, Liao P, Hall R, Mokhlesi B. Serum bicarbonate level improves specificity of STOP-Bang screening for obstructive sleep apnea. Chest. 2013;143:1284–93.
74. Giles TL, Lasserson TJ, Smith BH, White J, Wright J, Cates CJ. Continuous positive airways pressure for obstructive sleep apnoea in adults. Cochrane Database Syst Rev. 2006;(1):CD001106.
75. Sassani A, Findley LJ, Kryger M, Goldlust E, George C, Davidson TM. Reducing motor-vehicle collisions, costs, and fatalities by treating obstructive sleep apnea syndrome. Sleep. 2004;27:453–8.
76. Baron KG, Smith TW, Czajkowski LA, Gunn HE, Jones CR. Relationship quality and CPAP adherence in patients with obstructive sleep apnea. Behav Sleep Med. 2009;7:22–36.
77. Albarrak M, Banno K, Sabbagh AA, et al. Utilization of healthcare resources in obstructive sleep apnea syndrome: a 5-year follow-up study in men using CPAP. Sleep. 2005;28:1306–11.
78. Loube DI, Loube AA, Erman MK. Continuous positive airway pressure treatment results in weight less in obese and overweight patients with obstructive sleep apnea. J Am Diet Assoc. 1997;97: 896–7.
79. Saito T, Saito T, Sugiyama S, Asai K, Yasutake M, Mizuno K. Effects of long-term treatment for obstructive sleep apnea on pulse wave velocity. Hypertens Res. 2010;33:844–9.
80. Sivam S, Phillips CL, Trenell MI, et al. Effects of 8 weeks of continuous positive airway pressure on abdominal adiposity in obstructive sleep apnoea. Eur Respir J. 2012;40:913–8.
81. Redenius R, Murphy C, O'Neill E, Al-Hamwi M, Zallek SN. Does CPAP lead to change in BMI? J Clin Sleep Med. 2008;4:205–9.
82. Ye L, Pack AI, Maislin G, et al. Predictors of continuous positive airway pressure use during the first week of treatment. J Sleep Res. 2012;21:419–26.
83. Kribbs NB, Pack AI, Kline LR, et al. Objective measurement of patterns of nasal CPAP use by patients with obstructive sleep apnea. Am Rev Respir Dis. 1993;147:887–95.
84. Pepin JL, Krieger J, Rodenstein D, et al. Effective compliance during the first 3 months of continuous positive airway pressure. A European prospective study of 121 patients. Am J Respir Crit Care Med. 1999;160:1124–9.
85. Weaver TE, Grunstein RR. Adherence to continuous positive airway pressure therapy: the challenge to effective treatment. Proc Am Thorac Soc. 2008;5:173–8.
86. Tuomilehto HP, Seppa JM, Partinen MM, et al. Lifestyle intervention with weight reduction: first-line treatment in mild obstructive sleep apnea. Am J Respir Crit Care Med. 2009;179:320–7.
87. Foster GD, Borradaile KE, Sanders MH, et al. A randomized study on the effect of weight loss on obstructive sleep apnea among obese patients with type 2 diabetes: the Sleep AHEAD study. Arch Intern Med. 2009;169:1619–26.
88. Greenburg DL, Lettieri CJ, Eliasson AH. Effects of surgical weight loss on measures of obstructive sleep apnea: a meta-analysis. Am J Med. 2009;122: 535–42.
89. Ashrafian H, le Roux CW, Rowland SP, et al. Metabolic surgery and obstructive sleep apnoea: the protective effects of bariatric procedures. Thorax. 2012;67:442–9.
90. Haines KL, Nelson LG, Gonzalez R, et al. Objective evidence that bariatric surgery improves obesity-related obstructive sleep apnea. Surgery. 2007;141:354–8.
91. Buchwald H, Avidor Y, Braunwald E, et al. Bariatric surgery: a systematic review and meta-analysis. JAMA. 2004;292:1724–37.
92. Aurora RN, Casey KR, Kristo D, et al. Practice parameters for the surgical modifications of the upper airway for obstructive sleep apnea in adults. Sleep. 2010;33:1408–13.
93. Smith DF, Cohen AP, Ishman SL. Surgical management of OSA in adults. Chest. 2015;147:1681–90.
94. Camacho M, Teixeira J, Abdullatif J, et al. Maxillomandibular advancement and tracheostomy for morbidly obese obstructive sleep apnea: a systematic review and meta-analysis. Otolaryngol Head Neck Surg. 2015;152:619–30.

95. Baugh RF, Archer SM, Mitchell RB, et al. Clinical practice guideline: tonsillectomy in children. Otolaryngol Head Neck Surg. 2011;144:S1–30.
96. Ishman SL. Evidence-based practice: pediatric obstructive sleep apnea. Otolaryngol Clin North Am. 2012;45:1055–69.
97. Ramar K, Dort LC, Katz SG, et al. Clinical practice guideline for the treatment of obstructive sleep apnea and snoring with oral appliance therapy: an update for 2015. J Clin Sleep Med. 2015;11:773–827.
98. Okuno K, Pliska BT, Hamoda M, Lowe AA, Almeida FR. Prediction of oral appliance treatment outcomes in obstructive sleep apnea: a systematic review. Sleep Med Rev. 2015;30:25–33.
99. Riaz M, Certal V, Nigam G, et al. Nasal expiratory positive airway pressure devices (Provent) for OSA: a systematic review and meta-analysis. Sleep Disord. 2015;2015:734798.
100. Strollo Jr PJ, Soose RJ, Maurer JT, et al. Upper-airway stimulation for obstructive sleep apnea. N Engl J Med. 2014;370:139–49.
101. Wolski CA. Which Patients Are Good Candidates For Inspire Upper Airway Stimulation? Sleep Review: The Journal for Sleep Specialists 2016 February 16, 2016.
102. Piper AJ, Grunstein RR. Obesity hypoventilation syndrome: mechanisms and management. Am J Respir Crit Care Med. 2011;183:292–8.
103. Borel JC, Borel AL, Monneret D, Tamisier R, Levy P, Pepin JL. Obesity hypoventilation syndrome: from sleep-disordered breathing to systemic comorbidities and the need to offer combined treatment strategies. Respirology. 2012;17:601–10.
104. Nowbar S, Burkart KM, Gonzales R, et al. Obesity-associated hypoventilation in hospitalized patients: prevalence, effects, and outcome. Am J Med. 2004;116:1–7.
105. Balachandran JS, Masa JF, Mokhlesi B. Obesity hypoventilation syndrome epidemiology and diagnosis. Sleep Med Clin. 2014;9:341–7.
106. Mokhlesi B, Saager L, Kaw R. Q: should we routinely screen for hypercapnia in sleep apnea patients before elective noncardiac surgery? Cleve Clin J Med. 2010;77:60–1.
107. Yap JC, Watson RA, Gilbey S, Pride NB. Effects of posture on respiratory mechanics in obesity. J Appl Physiol. 1995;79:1199–205.
108. Pierce AM, Brown LK. Obesity hypoventilation syndrome: current theories of pathogenesis. Curr Opin Pulm Med. 2015;21:557–62.
109. Palen BN, Kapur VK. Tailoring therapy for obesity hypoventilation syndrome. Am J Respir Crit Care Med. 2015;192:8–10.
110. Piper A. Obesity hypoventilation syndrome: weighing in on therapy options. Chest. 2016;149(3): 856–68.
111. Shetty S, Parthasarathy S. Obesity hypoventilation syndrome. Curr Pulmonol Rep. 2015;4:42–55.
112. Masa JF, Corral J, Alonso ML, et al. Efficacy of different treatment alternatives for obesity hypoventilation syndrome. Pickwick study. Am J Respir Crit Care Med. 2015;192:86–95.
113. Mokhlesi B, Tulaimat A, Evans AT, et al. Impact of adherence with positive airway pressure therapy on hypercapnia in obstructive sleep apnea. J Clin Sleep Med. 2006;2:57–62.
114. Manthous CA, Mokhlesi B. Avoiding management errors in patients with obesity hypoventilation syndrome. Ann Am Thorac Soc. 2016;13:109–14.
115. Piper AJ, Wang D, Yee BJ, Barnes DJ, Grunstein RR. Randomised trial of CPAP vs bilevel support in the treatment of obesity hypoventilation syndrome without severe nocturnal desaturation. Thorax. 2008;63:395–401.
116. Gloy VL, Briel M, Bhatt DL, et al. Bariatric surgery versus non-surgical treatment for obesity: a systematic review and meta-analysis of randomised controlled trials. BMJ. 2013;347:f5934.
117. Sullivan CE, Issa FG, Berthon-Jones M, Eves L. Reversal of obstructive sleep apnoea by continuous positive airway pressure applied through the nares. Lancet. 1981;1:862–5.
118. El Solh AA, Jaafar W. A comparative study of the complications of surgical tracheostomy in morbidly obese critically ill patients. Crit Care. 2007;11:R3.
119. Teppema LJ, Dahan A. Acetazolamide and breathing. Does a clinical dose alter peripheral and central CO(2) sensitivity? Am J Respir Crit Care Med. 1999;160:1592–7.
120. Raurich JM, Rialp G, Ibanez J, Llompart-Pou JA, Ayestaran I. Hypercapnic respiratory failure in obesity-hypoventilation syndrome: CO(2) response and acetazolamide treatment effects. Respir Care. 2010;55:1442–8.
121. Powers MA. Obesity hypoventilation syndrome: bicarbonate concentration and acetazolamide. Respir Care. 2010;55:1504–5.
122. Anttalainen U, Saaresranta T, Vahlberg T, Polo O. Short-term medroxyprogesterone acetate in postmenopausal women with sleep-disordered breathing: a placebo-controlled, randomized, double-blind, parallel-group study. Menopause. 2014; 21:361–8.
123. Lallukka T, Haario P, Lahelma E, Rahkonen O. Associations of relative weight with subsequent changes over time in insomnia symptoms: a follow-up study among middle-aged women and men. Sleep Med. 2012;13:1271–9.
124. Singareddy R, Vgontzas AN, Fernandez-Mendoza J, et al. Risk factors for incident chronic insomnia: a general population prospective study. Sleep Med. 2012;13:346–53.
125. Haario P, Rahkonen O, Laaksonen M, Lahelma E, Lallukka T. Bidirectional associations between insomnia symptoms and unhealthy behaviours. J Sleep Res. 2013;22:89–95.

13 Psychiatric Suitability Assessment for Bariatric Surgery

Weronika Gondek

13.1 Introduction

The aim of this chapter is to review the current evidence base for a psychosocial assessment of bariatric surgery candidates and provide recommendations for providers who evaluate weight-loss surgery patients preoperatively. The purpose is to equip practitioners working with bariatric surgery candidates with the tools to help perform evaluation and make appropriate recommendations to patients and surgical teams. Two case vignettes of common clinical presentations will be used to illustrate the assessment process and highlight possible challenges. Recent recommendations and guidelines for the aims of the evaluation, the key elements of the assessment, psychosocial contraindications, and the most common outcomes of the evaluation will be summarized. Finally, the need for a standardized assessment tool as well as multidisciplinary and collaborative approach to bariatric candidates will be highlighted.

Case Vignettes

Case Vignette 1: Andrea

Andrea is a 41-year-old divorced female who self-referred to the bariatric program. Her body mass index (BMI) was 42 kg/m^2. Her past medical history was significant for gastroesophageal reflux and hypertension as well as obstructive sleep apnea. Her primary care physician recently told her that she was prediabetic. Her past psychiatric history was significant for a long history of Bipolar II disorder and posttraumatic stress disorder related to childhood sexual trauma, as well as a history of cocaine abuse. She was hospitalized psychiatrically 5 years ago for severe depression with suicidal thoughts. Her medication regimen included Lamotrigine 200 mg daily, Bupropion XL 300 mg daily, and Trazodone 100 mg at bedtime as needed for sleep. The surgical team contacted the psychiatrist directly before Andrea's visit for her evaluation. Both the surgeon and the program coordinator were extremely concerned about Andrea's psychiatric history and reluctant to consider her a surgical candidate despite patient's unparalleled enthusiasm and perfect adherence with nutritionist's recommendations.

(continued)

W. Gondek, M.D. (✉)
Department of Psychiatry and Behavioral Sciences, Johns Hopkins University School of Medicine, 600 North Wolfe Street, Meyer 101, Baltimore, MD 21287-7101, USA
e-mail: wmicula1@jhmi.edu

S. Sockalingam, R. Hawa (eds.), *Psychiatric Care in Severe Obesity*, DOI 10.1007/978-3-319-42536-8_13

(continued)

Case Vignette 2: Peggy

Peggy is a 50-year-old widowed female who was referred to the bariatric program by her primary care physician. Her BMI was 47 kg/m^2. Her past medical history was significant for diabetes, osteoarthritis, and fibromyalgia. She had a past psychiatric history of anxiety and mild depression but was never treated with any psychotropic medications or hospitalized psychiatrically. She had no substance use history. The bariatric team had no concerns about her candidacy, but noticed that she missed 3 out of 5 required weight-loss support groups as well as the scheduled appointment with the program's nutritionist.

13.2 Background

As described earlier in this book, obesity has reached epidemic proportions in the United States and worldwide [1]. Most conventional treatments for those with severe obesity have a modest and often short-lived effect in terms of weight loss and improvements in obesity-related disorders. Bariatric surgery is the only procedure that has been consistently shown to result in sustainable long-term weight loss and significant improvement in medical comorbidity [2]. Bariatric surgery is recommended for well-informed and motivated patients with a Body Mass Index (BMI) ≥40 kg/m^2 or for individuals with a BMI ≥35 kg/m^2 and one or more severe obesity-related comorbidities, such as type II diabetes, hypertension, hyperlipidemia, obstructive sleep apnea, nonalcoholic fatty liver disease, and gastroesophageal reflux disease [3]. Patients with a BMI of 30–34.9 kg/m^2 with diabetes or metabolic syndrome may also be offered a bariatric procedure, although currently there is a lack of long-term data demonstrating net benefit [4].

13.3 Psychopathology in Bariatric Candidates

The current and lifetime rates of psychopathology in bariatric surgery candidates are very high. About one-third of patients presenting for a preoperative evaluation have at least one current Axis I diagnosis and over two-thirds have a lifetime history of any psychiatric diagnosis [5]. Recent meta-analysis of 59 published papers estimated that 23 % of bariatric candidates suffer from current mood disorder and about 17 % present with current eating disorder. The most common psychiatric disorders are depression (19 %), binge eating disorder (17 %), and anxiety (12 %) [6]. In addition, prevalence estimates are 9 % for history of suicidal ideations, 3 % for substance use disorders, and 1 % for Post-traumatic Stress Disorder [6]. While presurgical psychological evaluations may be helpful in identifying psychopathology, in prospective studies, preoperative psychiatric diagnoses have not been consistently linked to suboptimal weight loss, weight regain, or redevelopment of maladaptive behaviors [7]. A substantial proportion of bariatric candidates present themselves in an overly favorable light during the psychological evaluation, and there is low congruence between clinically derived and research-based diagnoses, which may impact accurate assessment.

Depression. As outlined earlier, depression is a significant comorbidity in obese individuals. Preoperative depression may impede postoperative weight loss, and higher depression scores after the surgery have been associated with less weight loss. However, some studies have reported that depression improves significantly after the surgery, but the improvement may begin to decline over time [2]. Dawes et al. [6] found that there is no clear evidence that preoperative depression affects weight loss. In addition, moderate-quality evidence supports findings that weight-loss surgery is associated with reduction in prevalence, frequency, and severity of depressive symptoms. This can be potentially related to improvement in body image and interpersonal relationships after massive weight loss, as well as possible alteration in brain biochemical signaling.

Self-harm and suicide. Existing evidence has identified an increased rate of suicide after bariatric surgery, as well as an increased rate of self-harm emergencies [8]. A systematic review of 30 studies suggested that suicide risk for patients undergoing bariatric surgery was four times higher than in the general population [9]. While the exact reasons for an increased risk of suicide in this population are unknown, several factors have been postulated, including possible depression and difficulty adjusting to changes in lifestyle and eating behavior [10], increased prevalence of a past history of suicide attempts (73 times higher than in the normal population) [11], disappointment with inadequate weight loss or subsequent weight regain [12], increased alcohol abuse after the surgery [6], or the lack of an antidepressant effect of ghrelin leading to depression and suicidal tendencies [13]. In addition, Bhatti et al. [8] recently reported that self-harm emergencies in bariatric patients (primarily medication overdose) increased by approximately 50 % in the 3 years after the surgery.

Eating disorders. The most common eating disorder in the presurgical candidates is binge eating disorder (BED), and it is the second most common psychiatric disorder in this population, following major depressive disorder. Its rates vary from 4 to 49 % and are difficult to estimate primarily due to classification problems because the actual diagnostic criteria were not developed until the publication of DSM-5. Some studies suggest a relationship between preoperative BED and poorer outcomes, yet the majority of studies have not found this association. The impact of the development of BED postoperatively or the continuation of preexisting BED on bariatric surgery outcomes is another important issue and it is affected by surgical alterations causing inability to ingest large amounts of food. Therefore, some authors have proposed that the experience of loss of control over eating even small amounts of food should define binge eating in postsurgical population [14]. Very little is known about the prevalence of bulimia nervosa prior to bariatric surgery, perhaps due to denial or minimization of purging symptoms out of concern for surgical eligibility, as bulimia nervosa is considered a contraindication for bariatric surgery [4]. There have been reports of development of bulimia nervosa postoperatively; however, the actual rates are unknown. There is also a dearth of information about a lifetime history of anorexia nervosa in patients seeking bariatric procedures. Anorexia nervosa-like presentation appears to be quite frequent among patients receiving specialized care for eating disorders after the surgery and includes patients with significant weight loss, fear of weight gain, dietary restriction, and disturbances in self-perception of shape and weight [15]. In addition, it is important to remember certain behaviors after gastric bypass surgery that can be easily confused with disordered eating, such as vomiting, which frequently occurs in the short term after bypass surgery as patients adjust to their diminished intake capacity. It can also present in response to "plugging" when they experience the sensation of food being stuck in the stomach pouch, and it typically decreases as patients adjust and learn how to eat appropriately. However, these behaviors should be monitored as some patients will self-induce them as a means of weight loss or to prevent weight gain after the surgery [14].

Anxiety disorders. Prevalence estimates for anxiety disorders (including generalized anxiety disorder and social phobia) in bariatric population vary from 12 to 24 % at the time or presurgical evaluation, and are even up to 37.5 % for a lifetime diagnosis of anxiety disorder [7]. In addition, the rates seem to remain the same after the surgery [16]. Studies of association of anxiety and postoperative outcomes have yielded inconsistent findings, and most recent meta-analysis of available research evidence reported no association between anxiety and postsurgical weight loss [6].

Substance use disorders. A lifetime history of substance use disorder is more likely in bariatric surgery candidates compared with general population [17]. About one-third of patients have a lifetime history of alcohol use disorder [7]. In contrast, current rates of alcohol and substance use are only around 3 % and are much lower than in general population [4]. Following RYGB there are certain changes in pharmacokinetics of alcohol, including accelerated alcohol absorption, higher maximum alcohol concentration, and a longer time to eliminate alcohol. Similar changes have been demonstrated in patients following sleeve gastrectomy. These alterations have been postulated to cause increase in alcohol consumption and increased rates of alcohol use disorders after the weight-loss surgery [6]. Overall, the literature regarding the impact of alcohol and substance use disorders on weight-loss outcomes is mixed. It has been suggested that the patients who fail to make lifestyle changes in regards to their substance use may fail to make other changes (including dietary) and it could impact their outcomes long term. There is a general consensus that patients with current substance use disorders should delay surgery until their problem is addressed [18]. It may be useful for patients to agree to toxicology screening as a part of their treatment plan. Bariatric candidates should be warned about increased risk for alcohol use disorders after the surgery and may be advised to avoid all alcohol after the procedure [19]. According to national statistics, cannabis (marijuana) is the most commonly used illicit drug in the USA, and its use among young people has been increasing since 2007. However, no empirical research has examined the effects of cannabis use after the weight-loss surgery. A review of the obesity surgery literature revealed that many practitioners generalize from data regarding alcohol abuse to all substances, and for the majority of the programs cannabis use remains a contraindication to bariatric surgery [20].

Thought disorders. There is a very limited research that has examined whether bariatric surgery can be safe and effective in patients diagnosed with thought disorders, including schizophrenia. As discussed in contraindications section of this chapter, these patients are typically denied the surgery despite overall lack of research to support this recommendation. Patients with thought disorders exhibit deficits in memory, attention, and executive functioning and similar cognitive deficits are associated with obesity across the lifespan and can be further exacerbated by medical comorbidities such as sleep apnea and type II diabetes [7]. It has been reported that patients with thought disorders have similar weight-loss outcomes as matched controls; however, their underlying psychopathology may worsen following the surgery [21].

Psychotropic medications use in bariatric population. Almost half of individuals seeking bariatric surgery report current use of psychotropic medications, which is more than six times higher than in general population. Overwhelming majority reports taking antidepressants (87.7 %), followed by anxiolytics (9.6 %) and mood stabilizers (2.7 %) [22]. In addition, most patients continue using antidepressant medications after the surgery [23]. Current research supports the need for careful monitoring of psychiatric medication use and ongoing monitoring of patients' psychiatric symptoms after the surgery, especially in malabsorptive procedures. Reduced antidepressant levels can occur immediately postsurgery, leading to discontinuation syndrome and adverse effects, and they can remain decreased up to 1 year after the procedure [24]. Alterations in pharmacokinetics of psychotropic medications are not very well understood and can be affected by the type of surgical procedure, the changes in the gastrointestinal tract milieu, and medication solubility and availability (see Chap. 20 for further details). It is important to remember that the vast majority of patients prescribed medications receive them from their primary care physician and they may benefit from referral to a mental health professional that is familiar with taking care of bariatric surgery patients [25].

13.4 Mental Health Evaluation

Unlike many other surgical and medical procedures, both short-term and long-term outcomes associated with weight-loss surgery are dependent on psychological and behavioral factors present before and after the surgery. Successful bariatric outcomes are not only dependent on the surgical procedures but also require significant and lifelong changes in eating patterns and physical activity. At the same time, weight-loss surgery has wide-ranging and profound psychosocial effects. Thorough and specialized preoperative psychosocial assessment is an important part of a comprehensive bariatric treatment protocol [26]. This is endorsed in the 2013 update for the clinical practice guidelines for the preoperative nutritional, metabolic, and nonsurgical support of bariatric candidates [4]. Based on the survey of present practices, preoperative psychosocial assessment has become the standard of care in about 90 % of centers offering weight-loss surgery [27], and it is required for bariatric surgery centers to be nationally accredited by the American College of Surgeons and the American Society for Metabolic and Bariatric Surgery. There is a growing emphasis that the preoperative psychosocial assessment at the very minimum should be used to identify possible contraindications for surgery, such as uncontrolled substance use or poorly controlled mental illness [4]. More comprehensive evaluation can provide information that can guide treatment planning and provide recommendations to both the patient and surgical team that are aimed at facilitating the best possible outcomes [28]. While there may be psychological reasons for denying clearance for surgery, it has been stressed that the evaluation is not only diagnostic and that it should not be seen as a gatekeeper, but as an opportunity to provide support and education. It can be an intervention preparing the candidates for required postsurgical behavioral changes and it can help challenge unrealistic weight-loss expectations that patients may have [29]. The psychosocial evaluation of weight-loss surgery candidates should be a multifaceted process that can serve many functions. On one hand, it can help enhance the patient's readiness for weight-loss procedure through increasing knowledge of surgery and postoperative behavioral regimen. On the other hand, it can help minimize the barriers to optimal weight-loss outcomes through identifying and addressing potential postoperative challenges and establishing ongoing connection with behavioral health providers [30]. In addition, it can be an invaluable contribution to the interdisciplinary bariatric team, through reducing clinic burden, helping managing risk and liability, and providing comprehensive guidance [26].

13.4.1 Process of the Evaluation

Psychosocial evaluation, as well as pre- and postoperative support are essential in the process of weight-loss surgery, but are not recognized as a formal area of specialization.

Specific testing methods, evaluator credentials, and the degree to which results of the assessment influence surgical decision making vary among bariatric programs and might be influenced by local or national quality criteria to which particular center adheres [31]. According to the best practice update of evidence-based guidelines for psychosocial evaluation and treatment of weight-loss surgery patients, assessment should be performed by a social worker, psychologist, or psychiatrist with a background and at least some experience in pre- and postoperative assessment of bariatric candidates [17]. Most mental health professionals involved with bariatric programs report approximately a 4-year experience performing presurgical evaluations [32]. Based on the survey of 103 psychologists who indicated that they provided presurgical evaluations, about one-third of them (34 %) reported having done 101–500 evaluations, and 19 % of responders reported having completed over 500 evaluations. The amount of experience required to establish competence in this task remains unknown [33]. It has been stressed however, that because of special requirements of the bariatric population, and the need to prepare patients for variety of lifestyle changes, as well as the need to detect and treat disordered relationship with food, mental health providers should be familiar with medical psychology [27]. About 26 % of the weight-loss surgery programs in the US have their own mental health professional on staff, and 65 % refer patients to mental health providers in their community.

Only 6 % allow patients choose their own provider for the evaluation. Most frequently the professional conducting evaluation is a clinical psychologist, followed by psychiatrist and master level professional [27]. While there is a considerable variability in the content of presurgical psychosocial assessment across different bariatric centers, information is typically gathered via a clinical interview and administration of self-report questionnaires [2]. More than half of the programs use formal psychological testing as a part of the assessment. Despite the frequency of use of psychological testing, there are little guidelines available on which tests should be utilized to assess patient suitability for surgery. Commonly used symptom inventories or screening instruments assess symptoms of depression, eating disorders, and anxiety disorders. They include the Beck Depression Inventory (BDI-II), which has demonstrated satisfactory internal consistency and validity in bariatric surgery population [31], and Minnesota Multiphasic Personality Inventory (MMPI-2) which assesses psychiatric and personality traits and has been found reliable and valid to use in this population [34]. The Symptom Checklist-90-Revised (SCL-90-R) has also been validated in bariatric surgery patients and its hostility scale was predictive to the adherence to treatment plans [35]. Other tests used in the process of evaluation of bariatric candidates include Eating Disorder Inventory-2, Beck Anxiety Inventory, Eating Disorders Examination (EDE-Q), Binge Eating Scale, and cognitive measures, such as Mini Mental Status Exam [27, 32, 33].

13.4.2 Psychosocial Contraindications for Weight-Loss Surgery

While there is a growing emphasis on preoperative psychosocial assessment, ineligibility criteria are discussed infrequently in the literature. To this date research has not identified consistent contraindications to weight-loss surgery. This may be because mental heath professionals may have different approach and may use different criteria when evaluating bariatric candidates for distinctive weigh-loss surgical procedures, as gastric bypass (RYGB) and laparoscopic adjustable gastric banding (LAGB) carry different risks, produce different mean weight loss, and have different postsurgical requirements [32]. In addition, ethical concerns are raised whether psychosocial characteristics should disqualify patients from the most effective weight loss and potentially a lifesaving treatment [31]. Clinical practice guidelines published in 2013 list only substance abuse, poorly controlled psychiatric illness, and bulimia as clear contraindications to the surgery [4]. There is a general consensus that a psychiatric disorder per se should not be an exclusion criterion for bariatric surgery. Nevertheless, there may be psychiatric reasons to delay or deny surgery [36]. Based on the survey of present practices in 2005, the most commonly endorsed definite psychosocial contraindications for surgery included: current illicit drug use (88.9 %), active and uncontrolled symptoms of schizophrenia (86.4 %), severe developmental disability with IQ below 50 (81.5 %), heavy alcohol drinking (77.8 %). Most frequently reported possible contraindications included presence of an eating disorder, symptoms of bipolar disorder, and history of suicide attempts [27]. The survey of mental health professionals performing bariatric evaluations by Fabricatore in 2007 yielded similar results, with substance abuse or dependence, eating disorders, psychotic disorders, depression, suicidal ideations, and suicide attempts being cited as most common psychiatric contraindications [32]. To summarize, the most common reasons for deferring bariatric surgery are significant psychopathology such as active psychosis (including thought disorder symptoms), current substance dependence, untreated eating disorders (specifically anorexia nervosa or bulimia nervosa), untreated depression, and/or active suicidal ideation [2]. In addition, inadequate knowledge about the surgery resulting in inability to provide informed consent, unrealistic expectations for weight loss, and lack of social support have most frequently been reported as nonpsychiatric contraindications [2, 27, 32, 33, 36].

13.4.3 Key Elements of the Evaluation

The American Society for Metabolic and Bariatric Surgery divided the key elements of the assessment into four main categories, as outlined in the guidelines published in 2004: behavioral, cognitive and emotional, psychiatric, and current life situation. One of the first published clinical psychosocial assessment tools—the Boston Interview for Bariatric Surgery provided a standardized approach to interviewing patients for bariatric surgery. It has been widely used since its publication in 2004; however, procedures for psychosocial evaluations have remained quite varied across different bariatric programs [37]. Wadden and Sarwer [38] published the model of assessment that incorporated a self-report instrument called WALI—the Weight and Lifestyle Inventory. It is focused on the same areas of evaluation, with emphasis on patient-oriented approach. Recently, Thiara et al. [39] developed a comprehensive tool called the Toronto Bariatric Interprofessional Psychosocial Assessment of Suitability Scale (BIPASS) and assessed its reliability and validity using retrospective patient data in a multiprofessional clinical setting (see Appendices). The significance of the BIPASS lies in its ability to standardize the psychosocial assessment process and increase the rigor in identifying psychosocial risks that warrant further intervention before the surgery. The use of clinical assessment tools such as the BIPASS could streamline the decision-making process when determining surgical candidacy by reducing clinician bias and presenting pertinent psychosocial information in a succinct and reliable manner. It could also help standardize the psychosocial assessment process across the bariatric centers, guide future research directions, and improve clinical outcomes. Although to this date a standardized protocol for preoperative psychological evaluation does not exist, there is a general consensus among bariatric surgery centers, that the domains that should be assessed include: weight history, current and past weight-loss attempts, eating and diet behavior, eating pathology, current and past psychiatric functioning, substance use, medical history, understanding and knowledge about the surgery and pre- and postsurgical behavioral change requirements, motivation and expectations about surgery, physical activity, and relationships and support system [4, 17, 18, 29, 31, 38].

It has been proposed that the interview should begin with an open-ended question about the ways the weight has affected patient's life, which can provide valuable information about patient's reasons for losing weight and helps build rapport [29]. A vast majority of bariatric candidates present themselves in a very positive light during the psychological evaluation and it may cause problems with accuracy of the assessment [4]. Mental health clinicians should emphasize that the evaluation is to help facilitate favorable surgical outcome and is a standard part of surgical preparation. Some authors suggested that using statements like "we want to help you decide if the bariatric surgery is the right choice for you" could ease patients' concerns and foster honest responding [31].

Weight history. It should be viewed as a "weight autobiography," a narrative account of weight changes over the years with attention to associated biological, developmental, or environmental factors. Age of onset of obesity can frequently provide insight into genetic influences in a particular patient. Many of bariatric candidates blame themselves for being obese and it is helpful to discuss how genetic factors can play a role in their obesity [38]. On the other hand, there are patients who experience rapid weight gain following a traumatic or difficult experience. Ability to correlate their weight changes with stressful factors can help appreciate what role food plays in their life and yield insight into their coping mechanisms [40].

Current and past weight-loss attempts. Patients should be asked what weight-loss methods they have tried in the past and with what results. The National Institute of Health guidelines for bariatric surgery stipulate that surgery should be considered only for patients who failed conservative weight-loss methods in the long term. In addition, insurance companies frequently require documentation of participation in at least 6 month-long medically supervised weight-loss regimens to consider providing coverage for a bariatric procedure [41]. A great majority of bariatric candidates have made significant efforts and had many previous unsuccessful attempts at weight loss. They are often ashamed of inability to control their weight [42]. Information about their efforts can help clinicians to ascertain more about the types of interventions to which they might be most responsive and help facilitate the formulation of recommendations that are individually tailored to the patients' strengths and areas of vulnerability [37].

Eating and diet behaviors. This section examines several aspects of patient's current eating behaviors such as food preferences, typical portion sizes, and structure of daily meals and snacks. Inquiring about food preferences and sources sheds light on potential contributors to weight gain such as frequent consumption of convenience foods or overconsumption of high-calorie items such as sweets, sodas, or alcohol. The typical pattern of daily meals and snacks is also important to assess, because patients will need to maintain a pattern of frequent, structured, healthy meals and snacks after surgery [37]. It is not uncommon for patients to remark, "I don't know why I'm so overweight; I only eat once a day." Patients often eat with less than optimal frequency, skip breakfast, or go long periods without eating, only to overeat later due to hunger. This part of the assessment also yields important information about the patient's ability to adhere to a consistent routine and to meet his or her own nutritional needs [29]. It is important to remember and convey to the patients that diet after bariatric surgery is based upon a staged approach. In general, it starts with clear and full liquids which are maintained for anywhere from 1 to 2 days up to 2 weeks after operation. Subsequently, soft, moist foods are introduced with an emphasis on protein sources, fruits, and vegetables. Gradually, as the gastrointestinal tract heals and patients are able to tolerate more volume, the diet is advanced to solid foods. Throughout all of the diet stages, patients should consume adequate fluids to prevent dehydration [4]. Postoperative diet plans are generally surgeon or institution specific; however, patients are advised to eat slowly, chew food extensively, to stop eating as soon as they reach satiety, and to avoid taking food and beverages at the same time (patients should wait 30 min after a meal before consuming liquids) [43].

Eating pathology. In addition to probing into the presence of formal eating disorders, binging, and purging, it is important to assess possible other problematic eating patterns that might contribute to obesity or affect surgical outcomes, such as grazing, emotional, and night eating. Grazing is described as continuous, unstructured eating that may or may not reach binge proportions. Ongoing problems with grazing after the weight-loss surgery put patients at risk of a suboptimal weight-loss outcome [44]. Night eating syndrome is characterized by evening hyperphagia (eating more than a quarter of daily calories after the evening meal), poor sleep onset, or maintenance and morning anorexia [45]. Emotional eating refers to eating in response to negative emotions, such as stress, anxiety, or loneliness. It is particularly important to assess whether eating is the patient's primary way of coping with negative emotions, because for the first several months after surgery, patients will be limited in relying on eating as a coping strategy. When this is identified during the presurgical assessment, it is important to educate patients about the challenges that may arise after the surgery and problem solve about how to develop alternative coping mechanisms [29].

Current and past psychiatric functioning. A brief psychiatric history and mental status, as well as evaluation of substance use should be performed. This is intended more for screening rather than diagnostic purposes as presurgical assessment should not be aimed solely at diagnosing psychopathology. Rather, it is essential to perform psychiatric review of systems, screen for active symptoms of mood, psychosis, active substance use, or suicidality, as those can be potential contraindications for the surgery [32]. In addition, it is important to ask about history of trauma. Some authors have suggested that the excess weight may serve as a "shield" that protects patients from anxiety-provoking romantic or sexual attention and that those patients may feel vulnerable with significant weight loss [46].

Medical history. This portion of the interview assesses the degree to which the patients are informed about their medical conditions and treatment and provides information about their potential for adherence to postoperative care and guidelines. Patients' ability to be compliant with care is reflected in how they manage their current medical conditions (e.g., consistently taking medications, or checking blood glucose levels according to provider's recommendations) [29]. In situations where patient's adherence and ability to make significant behavioral changes is questionable, the evaluating clinician may request that patient returns in 1 month with a log of daily blood glucose readings or demonstrate the ability to keep scheduled appointments with his treatment providers [37].

Understanding and knowledge about the surgery and pre- and postsurgical behavioral change requirements. It is important to ensure that patients are making a well-informed decision to pursue bariatric surgery by assessing their knowledge about the surgery, possible risks and complications, and the postsurgical regimen. The complexity of the information provided during the informed consent for bariatric surgery can be overwhelming and difficult to comprehend. The mental health clinician should collaborate with other members of the team to assure that information is provided using simple language, multiple formats, and that the patients are encouraged to ask questions [31]. In addition, patients' decision making may be influenced by different misconceptions about various procedures, for example, some patients perceive laparoscopic adjustable gastric banding as virtually risk free, easily reversible, and equally effective procedure to Roux-en-Y gastric bypass [37].

Motivation and expectations about surgery. In general, patients may expect to lose about 60–85 % of their excess body weight within 12–18 months following the RYGB surgery or 40–50 % excess body weight following LAGB. Thus, most patients will remain overweight or even obese following the procedure [37]. It is not unusual for candidates to overestimate the amount of weight loss expected after the surgery and underestimate the intensity of recovery process. Unrealistic weight-loss expectations may lead patients to take greater surgical risks than they would otherwise [47]. Challenging those unlikely expectations at the start of treatment may serve to protect against feelings of dissatisfaction with weight-loss outcomes after the surgery.[26] In addition, it is also important to examine patients' preconceptions about postoperative behavioral changes. Patients should be educated about the importance of maintaining a planned, structured eating schedule, adequate hydration, avoiding calorie-dense foods and beverages, slowing the pace of eating, taking vitamins and supplements, limiting alcohol consumption, and maintaining a consistent exercise regimen. They must be aware that these changes ought to be permanent if they want to achieve the best weight-loss outcomes [48].

Relationships and support system. Patients should be asked whether the members of their support network endorse their decision to pursue weight-loss surgery. In some cases loved ones think that the surgery is "the easy way out" or that patients should lose weight on their own. Although many patients report that their relationships will be unaffected or positively affected by the weight loss, it is important to know and convey to the candidates that some partners may feel threatened by patients' increased activity level, attractiveness, and improved self-esteem following a weight-loss transformation [49].

Physical activity. Generally speaking, individuals seeking weight-loss surgery are not very active physically. The evaluation should yield information about potential barriers to increasing physical activity, such as pain or self-consciousness about exercising in public, to help facilitate consistent physical activity before and after surgery. It has been documented that increase in postsurgery activity level is related to improved weight-loss outcomes [30].

13.4.4 Results of the Evaluation

In most of the cases the results of mental health evaluation are summarized in the medical record (if the mental health professional and bariatric providers use the same medical record system) or are used to generate a letter to the treating surgeon that summarizes the biological, environmental, social and psychological factors associated with patient's obesity and documents formal psychiatric diagnoses established at the time of evaluation. In addition, most mental health professionals make explicit recommendations about candidate's appropriateness for bariatric surgery [32]. Typically one of three recommendations is provided: the patient is unconditionally "cleared" for bariatric surgery and there appear to be no psychosocial concerns; the patient is appropriate for surgery contingent upon receiving psychiatric and/or nutritional counseling prior to surgery; or the patient is deemed "unready" for the surgery at this time [25]. Available research in this area suggests that the vast majority of programs unconditionally recommend most of the candidates. Pawlow et al. [22] found that 81.5 % of patients have no psychological contraindications for surgery. Other studies indicated that approximately 60–75 % candidates received an unconditional recommendation to proceed with the weight-loss procedure [50]. Only a small percentage of presurgical mental health evaluations result in denial of bariatric surgery for psychological reasons. Reported rates of psychological ineligibility seem to be very similar across the studies and have been estimated at about 3–4 % [22, 25, 27, 51]. As discussed in the contraindications section of this chapter, the most common mental health reasons for surgical ineligibility are significant psychopathology (psychosis, thought disorder, current substance dependence, suicidality, untreated eating disorders) and inability to provide informed consent. Another recommendation that frequently follows a psychosocial evaluation is temporary deferral of the surgery until candidates receive treatment for their current psychological condition. These rates are more varied; some studies reported that approximately 15 % of patients were deferred [22, 33], while others reported rates as high as 31 %. Some programs recommend postponing surgery for anywhere from 6 weeks to 6 months if the patients are judged to have poorly controlled psychopathology or little knowledge about the surgery or postoperative dietary changes [25]. However, findings of several recent studies suggest that deferring surgery greatly diminishes the chances that patients will subsequently return to have the procedure [29]. Only 16 % of patients who were deferred after initial evaluation because of underlying eating pathology followed through with treatment, and 12 % of patients never returned for surgery [52]. Pawlow et al. [22] reported that only 10 % of those candidates who were deferred returned to the clinic and were cleared for surgery within 2 years. The remainder either did not undergo weight-loss surgery or did so at a center where their psychosocial problems were not detected or were not viewed as a barrier to treatment. Almost all mental health providers make recommendations for the candidates that include attending support group meetings and increase the knowledge about the surgery [27]. Other recommendations that should be communicated to the rest of the bariatric team that can help facilitate optimal patient care include suggestions about information being explained to patients in concrete ways, both verbally and in writing to ensure that they are well educated about surgery and requisite lifestyle changes [25]. In addition, it is important to remember that many of those patients who were psychologically cleared do not have the surgery for various reasons, including medical exclusion, personal decision, lack of third-party coverage, and inability to pay [22]. Merrell et al. [50] reported that the most common reasons for not reaching surgery included withdrawal from the program, outstanding program requirements, self-canceled surgery, insurance denial, or switching to nonsurgical weight management. It is common for insurance companies to have demands beyond requirements maintained by bariatric programs. Sadhasivam et al. [51] found that 30 % patients who did not undergo surgery despite being deemed suitable candidates by the bariatric team had insurance-related reasons. The most common requirement in the United States is completion of medically supervised weight-loss program for at least 6 months in order to document inability to lose weight via traditional methods [41], even though recent studies documented no difference in weight-loss outcomes after the surgery [53].

Case Vignettes Revisited

Case Vignette 1: Andrea

Andrea presented in a timely manner for her psychiatric appointment. She was pleasant and engaging. She reported a steady weight gain over the years that started after her first pregnancy 25 years ago. She described herself as an emotional eater and admitted to having a habit of grazing on snacks throughout the day. She reported that she is not good about planning ahead and oftentimes grabs a quick fast-food lunch while at work. Recently, she started a pre-op nutritional program and was able to lose 8 lbs in 3 weeks. She reported that she was hospitalized psychiatrically 5 years ago for severe depression with suicidal thoughts but has been stable since. She has been seeing her psychiatrist monthly and her therapist weekly. She has been attending a support group for trauma survivors and has a perfect compliance with her appointments and psychotropic medications. The psychiatrist was able to obtain collateral from Andrea's mental health providers and they confirmed both her stability as well as her perfect adherence to treatment. Andrea reported that she has not used any cocaine in over 5 years and has been active in NA (Narcotics Anonymous). Her toxicology screen at the time of her initial appointment was negative for any substances. She reported that she'd been thinking of the weight-loss surgery for many years, especially in the context of having tried numerous diets and weight-loss programs without much success. She knew that she would prefer a gastric band procedure, so that it does not interfere with her psychotropic medications. She thought that she would lose about 100 lbs over 12 months following her procedure and was hoping that her health and mobility will improve significantly. Two of her family members had a weight-loss surgery in the past and they had very good outcomes. In fact, Andrea's entire family was extremely supportive of her decision to have surgery. Despite initial concerns primarily related to Andrea's chronic mental illness, the evaluation revealed that she is a very well informed and highly motivated surgical candidate with extensive mental health and social support. She was deemed to be a suitable candidate from psychiatric perspective. The evaluating psychiatrist recommended that she continues her regular mental health treatment and recommended that her providers remain in contact with the bariatric program to assure stability during not only pre- but also postoperative phase of her surgery.

Case Vignette 2: Peggy

Peggy presented 40 min late for her presurgical evaluation. She was relatively cooperative but seemed tired and disengaged. She reported that her primary care physician had urged her to lose weight for years and that she was never able to comply with any dietary suggestions. She reported that she struggles with immobility and chronic fibromyalgia pain and this is why she came late to the appointment. She also remarked that her primary care physician "hasn't been happy" about her ongoing and escalating use of opioid pain medications. She reported that she reluctantly decided to pursue the surgery upon prompting of her son, whom she described as a "health freak." In fact, she wasn't sure whether the weight-loss surgery was the best option for her, as she never had any surgical procedures before and did not like the idea of "being cut on." At the same time she reported feeling like she has "no other option" because of the pressure that

(continued)

(continued)
she felt from her son and her doctor. She reported that she was always of normal weight until her early forties when the husband left her for another woman and she gained 100 lbs over the course of 1 year. She admitted to eating a lot of fast and convenience foods due to her mobility limitations. She reported that she lives by herself, her son lives out of state, and she has no other family members or friends in the area because "they all abandoned her when the husband left." In addition, when the recommendations of regular attendance of weight-loss support groups and nutritional appointments were discussed, she told the evaluator that she lives far from the bariatric center and doesn't think that she would be able to get there more often. Furthermore, she remarked that she really does not understand the rationale behind frequent visits, as the surgery will "take care of all her weight problems." Based on the evaluation the psychiatrist had serious concerns about Jane's candidacy. It was recommended that in order to keep moving forward with the program she needs to adhere with recommendations to keep all of her appointments with a nutritionist and attend at least one weight-loss support group per month to help improve her knowledge about required dietary and lifestyle changes. In addition, she was referred to a health psychologist to help work on her chronic pain issues and motivation for making lifelong changes to her diet and physical activity. She was asked to return to the clinic for a reevaluation in 3 months. The surgical team was supportive of psychiatrist's recommendations and agreed to defer the surgery until Peggy is able to demonstrate improved motivation, compliance, and interest in necessary behavioral and dietary changes. Peggy continued to miss her appointments and eventually withdrew from the program several weeks later.

13.5 Summary and Recommendations

- Presurgical psychosocial assessment is not a diagnostic interview, rather a screening that helps identify poorly controlled mental illness or substance use disorders. It offers a unique opportunity to identify potential barriers to weight loss and an opportunity for education and support to help facilitate the best possible surgical outcome.
- Presence of a psychiatric disorder should not automatically exclude patient's candidacy for bariatric surgery.
- Mental health providers play an integral role in facilitating communication between the candidates and bariatric teams, providing guidance to multidisciplinary teams and managing risk and liability.
- There is a need for a standardized psychosocial assessment process across the bariatric centers, which can help guide future research directions and improve clinical outcomes.

References

1. Flegal KM, Carroll MD, Kit BK, Ogden CL. Prevalence of obesity and trends in the distribution of body mass index among US adults, 1999–2010. JAMA. 2012;307(5):491–7.
2. Muller A, Mitchell JE, Sondag C, de Zwaan M. Psychiatric aspects of bariatric surgery. Curr Psychiatry Rep. 2013;15(10):397.
3. NIH conference. Gastrointestinal surgery for severe obesity. Consensus Development Conference Panel. Ann Intern Med. 1991;115(12):956–61.
4. Mechanick JI, Youdim A, Jones DB, Garvey WT, Hurley DL, McMahon MM, et al. Clinical practice guidelines for the perioperative nutritional, metabolic, and nonsurgical support of the bariatric surgery patient—2013 update: cosponsored by American Association of Clinical Endocrinologists, the Obesity Society, and American Society for Metabolic & Bariatric Surgery. Endocr Pract. 2013;19(2):337–72.
5. Mitchell JE, Selzer F, Kalarchian MA, Devlin MJ, Strain GW, Elder KA, et al. Psychopathology before surgery in the longitudinal assessment of bariatric surgery-3 (LABS-3) psychosocial study. Surg Obes Relat Dis. 2012;8(5):533–41.
6. Dawes AJ, Maggard-Gibbons M, Maher AR, Booth MJ, Miake-Lye I, Beroes JM, et al. Mental health conditions among patients seeking and undergoing bariat-

ric surgery: a meta-analysis. JAMA. 2016;315(2):150–63.
7. Marek RJ, Ben-Porath YS, Heinberg LJ. Understanding the role of psychopathology in bariatric surgery outcomes. Obes Rev. 2016;17(2):126–41.
8. Bhatti JA, Nathens AB, Thiruchelvam D, Grantcharov T, Goldstein BI, Redelmeier DA. Self-harm emergencies after bariatric surgery: a population-based cohort study. JAMA Surg. 2016;151(3):226–32.
9. Peterhansel C, Petroff D, Klinitzke G, Kersting A, Wagner B. Risk of completed suicide after bariatric surgery: a systematic review. Obes Rev. 2013;14(5):369–82.
10. Pories WJ, Caro JF, Flickinger EG, Meelheim HD, Swanson MS. The control of diabetes mellitus (NIDDM) in the morbidly obese with the Greenville Gastric Bypass. Ann Surg. 1987;206(3):316–23.
11. Windover AK, Merrell J, Ashton K, Heinberg LJ. Prevalence and psychosocial correlates of self-reported past suicide attempts among bariatric surgery candidates. Surg Obes Relat Dis. 2010;6(6):702–6.
12. Hsu LK, Benotti PN, Dwyer J, Roberts SB, Saltzman E, Shikora S, et al. Nonsurgical factors that influence the outcome of bariatric surgery: a review. Psychosom Med. 1998;60(3):338–46.
13. Kluge M, Schussler P, Dresler M, Schmidt D, Yassouridis A, Uhr M, et al. Effects of ghrelin on psychopathology, sleep and secretion of cortisol and growth hormone in patients with major depression. J Psychiatr Res. 2011;45(3):421–6.
14. Conceicao EM, Utzinger LM, Pisetsky EM. Eating disorders and problematic eating behaviours before and after bariatric surgery: characterization, assessment and association with treatment outcomes. Eur Eat Disord Rev. 2015;23(6):417–25.
15. Marino JM, Ertelt TW, Lancaster K, Steffen K, Peterson L, de Zwaan M, et al. The emergence of eating pathology after bariatric surgery: a rare outcome with important clinical implications. Int J Eat Disord. 2012;45(2):179–84.
16. de Zwaan M, Enderle J, Wagner S, Muhlhans B, Ditzen B, Gefeller O, et al. Anxiety and depression in bariatric surgery patients: a prospective, follow-up study using structured clinical interviews. J Affect Disord. 2011;133(1–2):61–8.
17. Greenberg I, Sogg S, Perna FM. Behavioral and psychological care in weight loss surgery: best practice update. Obesity (Silver Spring). 2009;17(5):880–4.
18. Edwards-Hampton SA, Wedin S. Preoperative psychological assessment of patients seeking weight-loss surgery: identifying challenges and solutions. Psychol Res Behav Manage. 2015;8:263–72.
19. Heinberg LJ, Ashton K, Coughlin J. Alcohol and bariatric surgery: review and suggested recommendations for assessment and management. Surg Obes Relat Dis. 2012;8(3):357–63.
20. Rummell CM, Heinberg LJ. Assessing marijuana use in bariatric surgery candidates: should it be a contraindication? Obes Surg. 2014;24(10):1764–70.
21. Shelby SR, Labott S, Stout RA. Bariatric surgery: a viable treatment option for patients with severe mental illness. Surg Obes Relat Dis. 2015;11(6):1342–8.
22. Pawlow LA, O'Neil PM, White MA, Byrne TK. Findings and outcomes of psychological evaluations of gastric bypass applicants. Surg Obes Relat Dis. 2005;1(6):523–7. discussion 8–9.
23. Cunningham JL, Merrell CC, Sarr M, Somers KJ, McAlpine D, Reese M, et al. Investigation of antidepressant medication usage after bariatric surgery. Obes Surg. 2012;22(4):530–5.
24. Hamad GG, Helsel JC, Perel JM, Kozak GM, McShea MC, Hughes C, et al. The effect of gastric bypass on the pharmacokinetics of serotonin reuptake inhibitors. Am J Psychiatry. 2012;169(3):256–63.
25. Sarwer DB, Cohn NI, Gibbons LM, Magee L, Crerand CE, Raper SE, et al. Psychiatric diagnoses and psychiatric treatment among bariatric surgery candidates. Obes Surg. 2004;14(9):1148–56.
26. Sogg S, Friedman KE. Getting off on the right foot: the many roles of the psychosocial evaluation in the bariatric surgery practice. Eur Eat Disord Rev. 2015;23(6):451–6.
27. Bauchowitz AU, Gonder-Frederick LA, Olbrisch ME, Azarbad L, Ryee MY, Woodson M, et al. Psychosocial evaluation of bariatric surgery candidates: a survey of present practices. Psychosom Med. 2005;67(5):825–32.
28. Ghaferi AA, Lindsay-Westphal C. Bariatric surgery—more than just an operation. JAMA Surg. 2016;151:232–3.
29. Sogg S, Mori DL. Psychosocial evaluation for bariatric surgery: the Boston interview and opportunities for intervention. Obes Surg. 2009;19(3):369–77.
30. Ratcliffe D, Sogg S, Friedman KE. Letter to the editor: a comparative study of three-year weight loss and outcomes after laparoscopic gastric bypass in patients with "yellow light" psychological clearance. Obes Surg. 2015;25(3):539–40.
31. Rouleau CR, Rash JA, Mothersill KJ. Ethical issues in the psychosocial assessment of bariatric surgery candidates. J Health Psychol. 2014;21(7):1457–71.
32. Fabricatore AN, Crerand CE, Wadden TA, Sarwer DB, Krasucki JL. How do mental health professionals evaluate candidates for bariatric surgery? Survey results. Obes Surg. 2006;16(5):567–73.
33. Walfish S, Vance D, Fabricatore AN. Psychological evaluation of bariatric surgery applicants: procedures and reasons for delay or denial of surgery. Obes Surg. 2007;17(12):1578–83.
34. Marek RJ, Ben-Porath YS, Ashton K, Heinberg LJ. Minnesota multiphasic personality inventory-2 restructured form (MMPI-2-RF) scale score differences in bariatric surgery candidates diagnosed with binge eating disorder versus BMI-matched controls. Int J Eat Disord. 2014;47(3):315–9.
35. Friedman KE, Applegate KL, Grant J. Who is adherent with preoperative psychological treatment recommendations among weight loss surgery candidates? Surg Obes Relat Dis. 2007;3(3):376–82.

36. Marcus MD, Kalarchian MA, Courcoulas AP. Psychiatric evaluation and follow-up of bariatric surgery patients. Am J Psychiatry. 2009;166(3):285–91.
37. Sogg S, Mori DL. Revising the Boston interview: incorporating new knowledge and experience. Surg Obes Relat Dis. 2008;4(3):455–63.
38. Wadden TA, Sarwer DB. Behavioral assessment of candidates for bariatric surgery: a patient-oriented approach. Surg Obes Relat Dis. 2006;2(2):171–9.
39. Thiara G, Yanofksy R, Abdul-Kader S, Santiago VA, Cassin S, Okrainec A, et al. Toronto bariatric interprofessional psychosocial assessment suitability scale: evaluating a new clinical assessment tool for bariatric surgery candidates. Psychosomatics. 2016;57(2):165–73.
40. D'Argenio A, Mazzi C, Pecchioli L, Di Lorenzo G, Siracusano A, Troisi A. Early trauma and adult obesity: is psychological dysfunction the mediating mechanism? Physiol Behav. 2009;98(5):543–6.
41. Frezza EE. Six steps to fast-track insurance approval for bariatric surgery. Obes Surg. 2006;16(5):659–63.
42. Gibbons LM, Sarwer DB, Crerand CE, Fabricatore AN, Kuehnel RH, Lipschutz PE, et al. Previous weight loss experiences of bariatric surgery candidates: how much have patients dieted prior to surgery? Surg Obes Relat Dis. 2006;2(2):159–64.
43. Bloomberg RD, Fleishman A, Nalle JE, Herron DM, Kini S. Nutritional deficiencies following bariatric surgery: what have we learned? Obes Surg. 2005; 15(2):145–54.
44. Saunders R. "Grazing": a high-risk behavior. Obes Surg. 2004;14(1):98–102.
45. Colles SL, Dixon JB. Night eating syndrome: impact on bariatric surgery. Obes Surg. 2006;16(7):811–20.
46. Kalarchian MA, Marcus MD, Levine MD, Courcoulas AP, Pilkonis PA, Ringham RM, et al. Psychiatric disorders among bariatric surgery candidates: relationship to obesity and functional health status. Am J Psychiatry. 2007;164(2):328–34. quiz 74.
47. Wee CC, Jones DB, Davis RB, Bourland AC, Hamel MB. Understanding patients' value of weight loss and expectations for bariatric surgery. Obes Surg. 2006;16(4):496–500.
48. Sheets CS, Peat CM, Berg KC, White EK, Bocchieri-Ricciardi L, Chen EY, et al. Post-operative psychosocial predictors of outcome in bariatric surgery. Obes Surg. 2015;25(2):330–45.
49. Bocchieri LE, Meana M, Fisher BL. Perceived psychosocial outcomes of gastric bypass surgery: a qualitative study. Obes Surg. 2002;12(6):781–8.
50. Merrell J, Ashton K, Windover A, Heinberg L. Psychological risk may influence drop-out prior to bariatric surgery. Surg Obes Relat Dis. 2012;8(4): 463–9.
51. Sadhasivam S, Larson CJ, Lambert PJ, Mathiason MA, Kothari SN. Refusals, denials, and patient choice: reasons prospective patients do not undergo bariatric surgery. Surg Obes Relat Dis. 2007;3(5):531–5. discussion 5–6.
52. Devlin MJ, Goldfein JA, Flancbaum L, Bessler M, Eisenstadt R. Surgical management of obese patients with eating disorders: a survey of current practice. Obes Surg. 2004;14(9):1252–7.
53. Horwitz D, Saunders JK, Ude-Welcome A, Parikh M. Insurance-mandated medical weight management before bariatric surgery. Surg Obes Relat Dis. 2016; 12(3):496–9.

Part IV

Nutrition and Psychotherapeutic Treatments in Obesity

14 Nutrition Management of Severe Obesity

Katie Warwick and Lorraine Gougeon

In this chapter we discuss the nutritional management of the severely obese patient. Section 14.1 begins with an overview of the non-surgical nutrition management of obesity including how to talk to your patients about their weight, what types of diets work and what don't, the role of meal timing, physical activity and how the Registered Dietician (RD) is your best resource for weight management. This is followed by an overview of the nutritional management of the bariatric surgery patient. Section 14.2 will include pre- and post-surgery dietary guidelines, nutrition-related complications including weight regain and the role of the RD on the Bariatric Surgery Team. Both sections will include information on prevalence, diagnosis and treatment of micronutrient deficiencies. We finish the chapter with a case to help integrate the information learned into a clinical scenario.

K. Warwick, R.D. (✉) • L. Gougeon, R.D.
Toronto Western Hospital Bariatric Surgery Program, University Health Network, 399 Bathurst Street, 4th Floor, East Wing, Room 460, Toronto, ON, Canada M5T 2S8
e-mail: Katie.warwick@uhn.ca; Lorraine.Gougeon@uhn.ca

14.1 Nutrition Interventions for the Non-surgical Treatment of Obesity

14.1.1 How to Talk About Weight

Obesity is a chronic disease. One with physical, psychological and societal implications. One that cannot be cured, but managed. As a mental health practitioner you may encounter patients who come to you for various reasons. Some issues may be related to excess weight, some may be a result of excess weight. Either way it is important to have an understanding of how to have appropriate and productive conversations with your patients that will help them to improve their health.

When discussing weight, finding the right wording can be difficult. A study performed by Wadden and Diddie involved surveying 167 obese women to determine the preferred term for describing obesity [1]. Of all the terms suggested the only one that was seen favourably was the term "weight". Some that were seen most negatively included "fatness", "excess fat" and "obesity" [1]. Therefore, it would be appropriate to ask a patient "if they are interested in talking about their weight", not as appropriate to ask if you can talk about their obesity. This is not to say that you cannot use the term obesity in medical settings or in research; however, it is impor-

S. Sockalingam, R. Hawa (eds.), *Psychiatric Care in Severe Obesity*,
DOI 10.1007/978-3-319-42536-8_14

tant to use people's most preferred term. Obesity was officially classified as a chronic disease by the American Medical Association in 2013 and by the Canadian Medical Association in 2015 [2, 3]. Therefore, it is more appropriate to say that a person *has obesity*, rather than to say that person *is obese*.

Always approach conversations about weight with your patients from a place of empathy and support [4]. Avoid using catch phrases like "nothing tastes as good as slim feels". These can come across as patronizing and quickly break your therapeutic alliance [4].

It is also important to follow the patient's lead in terms of how much they want to discuss their weight. Help them to clarify their motivations for weight loss. If they want to lose weight only for reasons of aesthetics and not for health, it may be helpful to work though the underlying issues that are contributing to their desire for thinness [4]. If their motivation is for health, steering them towards a comprehensive weight management programme that seems like a good fit for them may be more appropriate. Timing is also important. Help your patients to determine whether or not now is the ideal time to undergo major changes to their diet and activity level [4]. By helping patients to identify other competing priorities they can anticipate roadblocks in their journey towards weight management and start to strategize ways around them.

When directing patients towards weight management programmes it is important to become aware of what proven treatments exist and how to help your patient's navigate the world of food and nutrition without wasting their time and energy on the latest fad. In today's society we are bombarded with messages about food and nutrition. We are told what to eat, what not to eat, how much to eat, when we should eat, what will make us fat, what will make us slim, what to eat more of, less of and everything in between. As health professionals we can guide our patients towards a diet that will work for them and not harm their health. The Canadian Obesity Network has outlined the following recommendations [5].

Avoid diets that contain the following:

1.	A one size fits all approach—meaning that the diet doesn't require any personalized information such as height, weight or personal goals
2.	Nutrition advice given by somebody who has minimal or no formal training in nutrition. It is important to explore the practitioners' educational background
3.	Exercise is recommended as the *main proponent* of weight loss
4.	The programme promotes or implies dramatic, rapid weight loss at a pace of greater than 3 lb per week
5.	The programme requires a client to spend large sums of money at the start, or commit to paying for services over a certain period of time with no policy for withdrawing from the programme and getting partial or complete refunds
6.	The programme recommends consuming less than 800 kcal per day
7.	The programme requires the use of several expensive supplements, injections or herbal remedies
8.	The programme makes specific and unrealistic claims about losing a certain type of weight (e.g. fat) or losing weight from a specific area of your body (e.g. Lose belly fat now!)
9.	The programme is of short duration (weeks or months) and has no long-term maintenance plan
10.	The programme provides you with none or few statistics on success rates and has unrealistic claims such as "proven effective for 95 % of people"

There is a commonly held belief that diets don't work and that the only way to lose weight permanently is to undergo bariatric surgery. This is however a myth. Certain diets can work for certain people. A recent longitudinal randomized control study the Look AHEAD (Action for Health in Diabetes) [6] trial has proven otherwise. Of over 5000 participating adults with diabetes mellitus, the 825 who received lifestyle intervention consisting of reduced energy dietary and physical activity prescription with cognitive behavioural counselling lost at least 10 % of their body weight and maintained that loss for the length of the 8 year trial [7]. While 10 % may not sound like a lot, this amount has been proven to be adequate to significantly improve the co-morbidities of obesity. In fact, weight loss of only 3–5 % when maintained has been proven to reduce triglycerides, blood glucose and the risk of diabetes mellitus. Sustained weight loss of 5 % or more reduced additional risk factors such as that for cardiovascular disease [7]. These numbers are useful for health professionals to use when helping patients to determine a realistic weight loss goal. The pace of weight loss that is typically recommended is 0.5–2.0 lb/week [8].

Example of how to calculate a realistic weight loss goal:

Sally is 5 ft 2″ and 190 lbs.

3–5 % of 190 lb = 5.7–9.5 lb.

Because the total weight loss goal is less than 10 lb it makes sense to go at a more moderate pace of 0.5–1.0 lb per week. If Sally had more than 10 lbs to lose then it would be appropriate to go at a slightly faster pace of 2-3 lbs/week.

14.1.2 What Diets Work

When it comes to diets there is no one size fits all. Low fat, low carb, high protein or low calorie can all work for some people and not for others. Weight is a numbers game, and kilocalories or "calories" are the currency of weight [4]. Therefore, all effective diets include some form of calorie reduction. What's more important than the type diet is whether or not people can stick with it in the long term. In the following we will outline the most common weight loss programmes and the supporting evidence for their effectiveness. Small manageable changes may be more realistic for most people rather than jumping in and changing the entire diet at once. This will all depend on the person's level of nutrition knowledge and their motivation to change.

14.1.3 Energy-Focused Diets

Very Low Calories Diets (VLCDs) are less than 800–900 kcal/day and are very structured typically using meal replacement bars or shakes. These diets are only considered helpful for those who have a body mass index of 30 or greater and are often used in preparation for abdominal surgery including weight loss surgery (Academy of nutrition and dietetics 2016). This diet has proven to be effective for short-term weight loss with an average weight loss of 16.1 ± 1. 6 % at 4 months and 6.3 ± 3.2 % by 1 year (Academy of nutrition and dietetics 2016). Maintenance and long-term health outcomes beyond 1 year have not been studied as this diet is not considered to be sustainable.

Low Calorie Diets (LCDs) have greater than 800 kcal/day but less than 1600 kcal/day [7]. They can be highly structured, like VLCDs, and include the use of meal replacement bars or shakes or they can be semi-structured using meal plans. Research suggests that the greater the structure of the diet the more likely one is to adhere to it [7]. A meta-analysis of six studies comparing LCDs with or without meal replacements found that the meal replacement group lost 2.43 kg more weight after 1 year than the non-meal replacement VLC dieters [7].

14.1.4 Macronutrient-Focused Diets

Macronutrients (Carbohydrates, Fat and Protein) have long been investigated for their effects on weight loss. In the 1980s the low fat diet was all the rage but was quickly followed by the low carb diets of Dr. Atkins and South Beach. When considering a macronutrient-focused diet it is important to realize that you cannot change the amount of one nutrient in the diet without inadvertently changing the amount of the other nutrients [7]. For example, if someone chooses to follow a low-fat diet then they will end up either consuming more protein or more carbohydrates. Depending on what macronutrient you are limiting or having more of you can see various health effects. However, it is important to note that no one macronutrient-focused diet has proven to be any more effective than any other for weight loss [7]. It is instead more important to determine what diet would work best given a patient's food preference, dieting history and level of nutrition knowledge.

A diet is considered low-carbohydrate if it recommends consuming no more than 20 g of carbohydrate per day during the period of weight loss and no more than 50 g of carbohydrate per day once one's weight loss goal is achieved [7]. Low-carbohydrate diets with no limit on fat or protein intake produce an increase in high-density lipoproteins and a reduction in triglycerides while combined low-carbohydrate, low-fat diets promote a greater reduction in low-density lipoprotein. Depending on the person's cardiometabolic profile they may want to chose one diet over the other for this reason [7].

High-protein diets recommend consuming at least 20 % of daily calories from protein [7]. Sometimes these diets use meal replacement bars or shakes and are often combined with an energy restriction to promote weight loss [7].

Dietary pattern focused and the portfolio diet do not put restrictions on or promote particular macronutrients. Instead they focus on the diet as a whole to promote overall health [7]. Adding more fruits and vegetables to your diet by having one serving at each meal or snack is an example of this type of diet. These types of diets have not been proven to be more or less effective than any other [7].

Both the DASH and Mediterranean diet have been proven to be effective for managing cardiovascular risk factors such as high blood pressure. In terms of weight loss, neither has been shown to cause weight loss on their own; however, both can be effective when combined with a calorie restriction [7].

14.1.5 Meal Timing

Research on the impact of the timing of meals, how much is consumed at various times of the day, eating frequency and breakfast consumption is limited [7].

One RCT that examined the timing of energy intake and weight loss found that women who consumed more of their energy earlier in the day lost more weight than those who did not [7]. Jacubowicz et al. also found that eating a larger percentage of calories earlier in the day equated to a greater reduction in waist circumference and fasting glucose levels [9]. Those randomized to the breakfast group also reported higher feelings of satiety and lower levels of hunger throughout the day. For this reason, it may be beneficial to encourage those struggling with their weight to shift more of their calories to earlier in the day [9]. Breakfast, however, because it is not consistently defined as a certain amount of calories or as being eaten at a certain time, has not been adequately researched and therefore not definitely proven to assist with weight management.

14.1.6 Food Logging

Food logging is an important self-management strategy that is part of most weight loss programmes. This is because it is an effective tool for bringing one's awareness to food and eating challenges while also providing a way to reflect on progress made.

Logging the traditional way, using pen and paper, or a food logging notebook is however very time consuming and requires a high level of commitment from the patient. In order for paper food records to be effective they should be reviewed weekly or biweekly with a RD or RDN so that she can assess the macronutrient and calorie intake of logged foods and can work collaboratively with the patient to provide education around what foods are better choices and to set up a plan for changes moving forward. Because this can often be a tedious and time-consuming process both for the patient and the RD or RDN, electronic food logging has become more prevalent. Many free websites and applications are available for most portable electronic devices. The benefit of electronic food logging is that it provides real-time feedback on the calorie and nutrient content of the food at the time the food is logged. For example, if when a patient logs their morning coffee with two cream and two sugar they instantly see that this is over 200 kcal, this alone may work as a deterrent for ordering it either in the moment or in the future. While still time consuming to initiate, most electronic food logging programmes have time saving functions including being able to save frequent meals to prevent people from having to enter all the ingredients of a meal each time, as well as an import recipe function that allows for the instant nutrient analysis of any recipe found online. Unfortunately research on stand-alone electronic weight loss programmes is still in its infancy; however, some short trials how proven that they are more effective than minimal interventions [7]. That being said, there is consensus that comprehensive weight loss programmes that include both electronic self-monitoring strategies as well as counselling by a trained clinician produce greater and longer-lasting results [7]. RDs and RDNs will often also use "food and mood" logs as a CBT tool to help patients deconstruct and problem solve strategies for overcoming emotional eating.

14.1.7 Physical Activity

While physical activity alone has not been proven to be an effective weight management strategy we would be remiss if we didn't talk about the way that it can augment any diet programme. In a recent meta-analysis it was shown that a combined programme of diet and exercise produced slightly more (1.7 kg) weight loss at 12 months than diet alone [7]. One might argue that this is a very modest difference for the amount of effort it takes to incorporate physical activity into a lifestyle; however, we cannot overlook the other health benefits that come with physical activity. These include improved cardiometabolic health, improved mood and decreased risk of certain cancers [10]. Physical activity has also been proven to play a more important role in weight maintenance after weight loss. The National Weight Control Registry reports that 90 % of participants (members have lost an average of 66 lb and maintained it for 5.5 years) report that they exercise on average 1 hour per day [11]. Currently, Health Canada and the US Department of Health and Human Services both recommend 150 minutes of moderate intensity activity per week or 30 minutes per day most days of the week. Ideally, moderate intensity is accumulated in occasions that are at least 10 minutes in length [7].

14.1.8 Micronutrient Deficiencies of Obesity

Since obesity is often considered to be a disease of overconsumption, nutritional deficiencies may not be expected. They are however shockingly prevalent. Those who eat an abundance of highly processed convenience foods of low nutritional quality are particularly at risk of nutrient deficiencies. There are also underlying mechanisms associated with obesity such as chronic inflammation that can impact the transportation of certain micronutrients e.g. iron, and changes in intestinal microflora which can impact vitamin absorption [12]. Micronutrient deficiencies are often diagnosed when patients are being assessed for bariatric surgery. A Spanish study performed in 2011 by Moize et al. revealed that of 231 patients studied prior to bariatric surgery, only 25 % did not present with nutritional deficiencies. 38.2 % presented with at least one, 22 % presented with two and 11.4 % presented with three nutritional deficiencies [13]. Deficiencies included vitamin D (67 %) iron deficiency anaemia (22.2 %); and deficiencies of vitamin A, B1 and B6 were present in 10.2 %, 7.2 % and 15.9 %, respectively. Vitamin and mineral deficiencies can not only cause long-term health issues such as blindness and osteoarthritis but can also have a significant impact on a person's current quality of life. Iron deficiency, for example, can have an impact on mood, energy levels and sleep (related to restless leg syndrome). If these underlying deficiencies are not treated as part of a comprehensive weight management programme then they could potentially impact a person's chance of successfully losing weight. Therefore, it is recommended that screening for micronutrient deficiencies and treatment of said deficiencies should be an integral part of any weight management programme.

14.1.9 Why a Registered Dietician Is Your Greatest Ally in Weight Management

Registered Dietician (RD) in Canada and Registered Dietician Nutritionist RDN in the United States are regulated professional designations that are only used for those who have completed an appropriate undergraduate degree in science majoring in dietetics followed by a accredited Dietetic Internship or Masters Degree. Anyone can call themselves a "nutritionist", but you have to have completed the above-mentioned education and belong to a regulatory college of dietetics to call yourself an RD or an RDN. The reason why the RD or RDN is your greatest ally when it comes to helping your patients achieve weight management is because they are not only experts in food and nutrition but they are governed by a regulatory college that ensures that the advice they give is evidence based. RDs and RDNs will never promote products or diets that are based on anecdotal evidence. They will however help clients to determine what type of programme would be a good fit for them. Many RDs and RDNs have done extensive additional training in Motivational Interviewing, Cognitive Behavioural Therapy (CBT), Acceptance and Commitment Therapy and Mindfulness-based meditation. CBT has been shown in both the Look AHEAD study and the Diabetes Prevention Program to assist patients to achieve significant sustainable weight loss as compared to education alone [7].

14.2 Nutrition Interventions in Bariatric Surgery

Bariatric surgery is a proven option for successful weight loss and resolution of obesity-related co-morbidities. The Roux-en-Y gastric bypass (RYGB) and the sleeve gastrectomy (SG) are the most common weight loss surgery procedures performed in North America [14, 15]. RYGB is a restrictive and metabolic procedure and the SG is a restrictive procedure where 80 % of the stomach is removed providing early satiety and resulting in smaller food portions. Both procedures require significant lifestyle changes including dietary modifications and lifelong commitment to taking vitamin and mineral supplements. Nutrition concerns following other less common procedures such as laparoscopic gastric banding, vertical banded gastroplasty and bilopancreatic diversion, with or without duodenal switch, will not be discussed in this chapter and are summarized in other reviews [16].

Expected weight loss after bariatric surgery is dependent upon the type of surgical procedure. A meta-analysis by Buchwald et al. [17] showed that the overall percentage of excess weight loss (%EWL) for all surgery types was 61.2 % (95 % CI, 58.1–64.4 %). There is considerable inter-individual variation in weight loss response to the RYGB and SG as described by de Hollanda et al. [18]. They found that older age, male gender, presence of pre-surgery T2DM and higher pre-surgery BMI were characteristics of poor weight loss outcomes. Li et al. [19] conducted a recent review of 62 studies published after 2008 that included 18,449 patients in which %EWL was reported in 20 studies. They reported significantly higher excess weight loss in patients undergoing a RYGB compared to those receiving a SG.

The success of bariatric surgery is also dependent upon many non-surgical factors; patient education and willingness to make permanent lifestyle changes are critical. Patients must be prepared from a physical, psychological and knowledge perspective. They should be able to demonstrate their readiness by making changes to their diet before surgery. These changes involve following a regular meal pattern and making nutritious food choices. Recommended dietary changes prior to surgery are shown in Fig. 14.1.

There is debate as to the need to demonstrate weight loss prior to surgery [20]. In some bariatric programmes this is mandatory in order to qualify for surgery, to prevent post-op complications or to optimize post-op weight loss.

14.2.1 Nutrition Assessment

Assessment by an RD is important to determine a patient's readiness and suitability for surgery. The RD reviews the patient's lifetime weight history with particular attention to causes of weight gain and previous weight loss attempts. Weight loss expectations and realistic weight loss goals are also discussed. Current diet is assessed using food logs or 24 h recall to determine typical meal patterns; food preparation and shopping skills; frequency of eating out and evidence of disordered eating such as night eating, binging or grazing.

Recommended Dietary Change in Preparation for Bariatric Surgery

- Follow a regular meal pattern; have 3 meals and 1-3 snacks per day
- Drink 6-8 cups of fluid per day; choose mostly non calorie drinks, avoid carbonated beverages and reduce caffeine intake
- Choose a variety of nutritious foods including lean proteins, whole grains, vegetables, fruit and dairy products
- Use portion control
- Practice the eating techniques required after surgery including eating slowly and chewing well
- Keep a food journal

Fig. 14.1 Recommended dietary change in preparation for bariatric surgery

The RD assesses the patient's knowledge of nutrition and bariatric surgery and addresses any specific learning needs as required. Readiness to change is addressed throughout the assessment process and the patient should be able to demonstrate this by making changes to their current diet.

14.2.2 Nutrition Education

Bariatric surgery candidates present with varying levels of nutrition knowledge. The RD plays an important role in assessing knowledge and providing the necessary nutrition education to optimize the patients understanding of the role nutrition plays in maintaining health and achieving weight loss after surgery. Nutrition education includes a review of the process of digestion before and after surgery, post-surgery diet progression, supplement requirements, nutritious food choices and proper eating and drinking techniques after surgery. In addition, nutrition complications such as nausea and vomiting, dehydration, food intolerance, constipation, hair loss, reactive hypoglycaemia and dumping syndrome should be reviewed and prevention strategies discussed. Finally, weight loss expectations and strategies for long-term weight loss are important for bariatric surgery candidates to understand.

Learning about the role of nutrition and eating for health continues after surgery when patients return for follow-up visits. Taube-Schiff et al. [21] looked at nutrition knowledge of bariatric surgery candidates before and 1 month after surgery. They found that knowledge significantly increased after surgery in most study participants. In those subjects whose knowledge decreased over time, depression and anxiety scores, older age, male gender and time between education and surgery were contributing factors.

The RD provides detailed, written information that can be referred to before and after surgery. This includes general nutrition principles, a description of the normal digestive process, how digestion changes after bariatric surgery, protein and vitamin and mineral recommendations, eating technique, diet progression, portion sizes, product information and sample menus. Written materials also review nutrition complications, mindful eating techniques and ways to prevent weight regain and strategies for lifelong healthy eating.

14.2.3 Post-surgery Diet

Progression of food texture and measured portion sizes are recommended after bariatric surgery. To allow the gastrointestinal tract to heal the diet is advanced slowly from a period of liquids only to smooth or pureed foods, then soft moist foods and finally regular textured foods [22]. Individual tolerance of food texture and type varies considerably and it may take 3–6 months to be able to tolerate most foods. Portions sizes are also gradually increased from ¼ to ½ cup early post-surgery to a meal size of one to two cups. Patients are encouraged to limit portion sizes over the long term.

The technique of eating changes after bariatric surgery. Foods must be eaten slowly and chewed very well to help aid digestion, to avoid over filling the smaller stomach and to prevent foods from obstructing the gastrojejunal anastomosis. Eating slowly also allows the patient to recognize when their stomach is full. Poor eating technique may cause vomiting, nausea and pain.

Liquids should be sipped slowly and separated from solid foods to prevent solids from moving too quickly through the stomach pouch which may cause dumping syndrome in RYGB patients. With both RYGB and SG surgeries eating and drinking at the same time is discouraged as this can fill the stomach too quickly causing discomfort and limiting food intake making it difficult to meet nutrient requirements.

Eating at regular intervals is important after surgery. Without internal hunger cues patients could go long periods without eating making it difficult to meet their nutrition needs. A meal or snack every 3–4 h is recommended and patients may require reminders to maintain this regular eating pattern.

Table 14.1 Micronutrient supplementation recommendations after Roux en Y gastric bypass and sleeve gastrectomy

Supplements	Recommendations
Multivitamin/mineral	• 2 per day each providing 100 % DRI for vitamins and minerals
	• Each pill should have a minimum
	– 1.2 mg Thiamine (vitamin B1)
	– Less than 500 μg folate
	– 7.5–15 mg Zinc
	– 1 mg Copper
Vitamin B12	• 350–500 μg/day oral or sublingual or
	• 1000 μg/month intramuscularly
Calcium	• Calcium citrate preferred for RYGB
	• 1200–1500 mg per day in 500 mg divided doses
	• Avoid taking within 2 h of multivitamin or iron supplements
Vitamin D	• 3000 IU/day from all sources
Iron	• 45–60 mg per day via multivitamins and additional supplements
	• Vitamin C may be added to enhance the absorption of iron salts used as an additional supplement

14.2.4 Nutrition Complications

Non-adherence to post-surgery diet guidelines may lead to nutrition complications that impact long-term health and successful weight maintenance. Following we review common nutrition-related concerns after bariatric surgery.

Vitamins and minerals: Because bariatric surgery restricts food portions and with the RYGB reduces the absorptive surface of the small bowel, vitamin and mineral supplements are required to prevent micronutrient deficiencies [23, 24]. Nutrients at risk include but are not limited to iron, calcium, vitamin D, folate and Vitamin B12. Taking vitamins and minerals is a lifelong commitment for all patients undergoing bariatric surgery. Table 14.1 outlines the recommended vitamin and mineral supplements after RYGB and SG.

Vitamin and mineral deficiencies can occur months or years after bariatric surgery. Many believe that since the SG is not a malabsorptive procedure supplements are not necessary but Moize et al. [25] in a 5-year follow-up study showed that nutrition deficiencies occurred in both RYGB and SG patients demonstrating the need for vitamin mineral supplementation for both types of surgery. Table 14.2 shows common vitamin and mineral deficiencies after bariatric surgery including symptoms and treatment recommendations. These deficiencies can be managed by taking supplements as recommended, having regular laboratory monitoring and attending regular follow-up appointments with health care providers who will assess nutrition status and make recommendations to correct deficiencies.

Table 14.2 Common nutrient deficiencies after bariatric surgery

Nutrient	Deficiency symptoms	Treatment	Food sources
Vitamin A	Night blindness, xerosis, Bitot's spots, poor wound healing	10,000–2500 IU/day for 1–2 weeks	Orange or dark green vegetables and fruit, liver, fortified dairy products, fish
Vitamin D	Osteomalacia	50,000 IU/week ergocalciferol (D2) orally for 8 weeks	Fortified dairy products, fatty fish, eggs, fortified cereals
	Disorders of calcium deficiency		
Vitamin B12 (Cobolamin)	Pernicious anaemia	1000 μg/week IM for 8 weeks, then 1000 μg/month IM for life or 350–500 m μg/day orally	Meat, fish, poultry, and eggs
	Pale, fatigue, short of breath		Milk and milk products, fortified soy and rice beverages
	Tingling or numbness in extremities		
	Sore, red tongue		
	Irritability, forgetfulness		
Thiamine (Vitamin B1)	Anorexia	With hyperemesis: parenteral dose of 100 mg per day for 7 days followed by 50 g orally per day until complete recovery	Pork, enriched whole grains, nuts and seeds, legumes
	Gait ataxia		
	Paraesthesia		
	Muscle cramps		
	Irritability		
	Advanced: Wernicke–Korsakoff Syndrome		
Folate	Glossitis, mouth ulcers	1000 μg/day orally; up to 5 mg/day if severe	Dark green vegetables, legumes, beans and lentils,
	Macrocytic anaemia	>1000 μg/day can mask hematologic effects of B12 deficiency	Enriched flour and grain products
	Diarrhoea	Avoid alcohol	
Calcium	Leg cramping	Ensure adequate calcium intake in divided doses	Milk, cheese, yogurt, kefir
	Hypocalcaemia and tetany		Leafy green vegetables, legumes and almonds
	Neuromuscular hyperexcitability		Canned fish with bones
	Osteoporosis		Fortified soy and rice beverages
Zinc	Altered taste sensations, poor appetite, changes in sense of smell	60 mg elemental zinc twice daily for 8 weeks	Seafood, meat, seeds, dried peas and beans
	Poor wound healing, hair loss, muscle wasting		
	Diarrhoea		

14.2.5 Protein

A minimum of 60 g of protein per day or up to 1.5 g/kg body weight should be adequate for the post-surgery patient [24]. Protein requirements are difficult to meet after bariatric surgery especially during the early post-operative period due to the small size of the stomach pouch and the possible development of intolerance or aversion to high protein foods, particularly meat, eggs and dairy. Modular protein supplements made from high quality protein sources such as whey, casein, eggs and soy are recommended for 1–2 months after surgery or until protein requirements can be met through food sources. Inadequate protein intake may result in inadequate energy intake, reduction in lean body mass, excessive weight loss and micronutrient deficiencies. Patients who do not follow the recommended guidelines for eating technique such as eating slowly, taking small bites and chewing thoroughly could experience nausea, vomiting and early satiety which may further limit their protein intake.

14.2.6 Fluids

Adequate hydration is challenging for the bariatric surgery patient. A goal of at least 1.5 L of fluids per day is recommended. Since liquids should be sipped slowly and separated from solid food it may be difficult to meet this recommendation especially during high-risk periods such as increased exercise or episodes of vomiting. Non-calorie fluids are recommended and patients are usually cautioned against having carbonated drinks and the excessive use of caffeinated beverages though the evidence for this is limited [24].

14.2.7 Gastroenterological Concerns

Food intolerances are common after bariatric surgery; however, the extent of this problem is variable. Patients may experience pain, discomfort or bloating after eating certain foods. Meat, dairy, bread, rice and pasta are common problem foods. Vomiting due to the limited stomach capacity after restrictive bariatric procedures occurs most often in the early months after surgery as the patient is adapting to the eating techniques and food volume restrictions. If vomiting persists or is accompanied by abdominal pain, bloating or diarrhoea surgical complications such as stricture, bowel obstruction or ulcer should be investigated.

14.2.8 Dumping Syndrome

Associated with many types of gastric surgery, dumping syndrome (DS) is common after bariatric surgery occurring in 40–76 % of patients after RYGB [26]. DS after RYGB is due to the small gastric pouch and gastrojejunostomy which allow rapid movement of energy-dense food into the small bowel. This is accompanied by a release of gastrointestinal (GI) and pancreatic hormones and a rapid fluid shift from the general circulation to the GI circulation.

Since the SG is a restrictive procedure DS seems unlikely to occur but there have been reports of symptoms of DS in 30–40 % of SG patients [27, 28]. DS presents with a number of vasomotor and GI symptoms that occur after eating caused by rapid gastric emptying. Dumping syndrome is usually described as either early DS, occurring within 30 min of eating or late DS, within 1–4 h after a meal. Symptoms of early DS include feeling full quickly, abdominal cramps, nausea, diarrhoea, dizziness, fatigue and heart palpitations. Late DS is characterized by symptoms related to hypoglycaemia such as sweating, shakiness, hunger, decreased concentration and fainting.

To prevent DS bariatric surgery patients are counselled to eat small frequent meals, avoid drinking liquids with meals (separate by at least 30 min) and choose complex carbohydrates rather than refined sugars. Adding fibre and protein to meals and snacks may help slow gastric emptying and digestion. There are pharmacological options available for the treatment of DS when dietary measures fail [27].

14.2.9 Reactive Hypoglycaemia

Rapid absorption of concentrated carbohydrates can lead to hyperinsulinaemia and result in low blood glucose or hypoglycaemia. Symptoms include sweating, palpitations, shaking, weakness, confusion and hunger. Reactive hypoglycaemia can occur after RYGP due to dumping syndrome, beta cell hyper function, hyperinsulinaemia or beta cell mass. Nutrition intervention to prevent hypoglycaemia includes eating small, frequent meals, having protein and complex or high fibre carbohydrate foods at each meal and snack, avoiding foods and beverages that contain simple carbohydrates and avoiding fluids with or immediately after eating. In severe cases pharmacological or surgical treatment may be required.

14.2.10 Weight Regain

Weight recidivism may occur after bariatric surgery regardless of surgery type. A review study by Karmali et al. [29] estimated that 10–20 % of patients regain a significant amount of weight in 10 years of follow up. As a result of this obesity-related co-morbidities may reoccur. Causes of weight regain may be related to patient behaviour such as non-adherence to diet and exercise recommendations or to surgical factors such as dilation of the pouch or sleeve or dilation of the stoma (RYGB). Hormonal imbalances may also contribute to weight gain. It is possible that patients with higher levels of ghrelin and lower levels of peptide YY may be more likely to regain weight. Recurrent reactive hypoglycaemia causing increased hunger may also be a contributor. See Fig. 14.2 for an overview of causes of weight regain. Patients who are non-compliant to nutrition guidelines including making poor food choices and increasing portion sizes will have increased energy intake and weight gain over time. Loss of control leading to binge eating or grazing may also be a significant contributor to weight regain. Follow up with the multidisci-

Fig. 14.2 What causes weight regain after bariatric surgery?

What Causes Weight Regain After Bariatric Surgery?

Causes associated with the patient

Non adherence to dietary recommendations

- poor diet quality
- inappropriate food choices
- increasing food portions sizes
- lack of nutrition follow up counselling

Mental health conditions

- binge eating
- grazing

Physical inactivity

Causes associated with the surgery

Hormonal changes

- ↑ghrelin ↓peptide YY
- reactive hypoglycemia

RYGB

- pouch and/or stoma dilation
- gastro-gastric fistula

SG

- sleeve dilation

plinary team for nutritional and psychological support is essential for the treatment of suboptimal weight loss or weight regain. Nutrition strategies for encouraging long-term weight loss and preventing weight regain are summarized in Table 14.3.

Table 14.3 Nutrition strategies for long-term weight maintenance and prevention of weight regain

Nutrition recommendations	How to
Follow a regular meal pattern. Eat at regular times, avoid skipping meals	Have three meals and 1–3 snacks per day
	Eat every 3–4 h
Plan balanced meals including nutrient-dense foods	Choose lean proteins, whole grains, lower fat dairy foods and a variety of vegetables and fruit
Avoid energy-dense, nutrient-poor food choices	Replace foods such as chips, sweets, pastries, fried foods with more nutritious choices such as fruit, low fat cheese, yogurt, nuts and seeds, bean dips and vegetables
Avoid calorie-containing beverages	Choose water in place of fruit juice, soft drinks, sports drinks and sweetened coffee or tea beverages. Limit or avoid alcoholic beverages
Eat mindfully	Learn ways to manage emotional eating or to prevent slipping back into old habits such as eating rapidly, distracted eating and grazing
Take supplements as recommended	Plan to take vitamins and minerals at regular times throughout the day
	Follow up with laboratory testing as recommended by your health care provider
Exercise	Be more active. Aim for 30 min of moderate exercise five times a week. Exercise according to your ability
Know your weight	Once a week check your weight to limit relapse
	Ask for help to manage weight regain
Follow up	Keep appointments with RD as recommended by your bariatric centre

14.2.11 Role of the RD in Post-op Care

Follow up with an RD is recommended at 1, 3, 6 and 12 months post-surgery and annually thereafter [24]. Endevelt and colleagues showed that counselling by a dietician as little as one time post-surgery resulted in a BMI reduction of 5 % more than those with no post-surgery nutrition follow up [30].

The RD will assess protein, fluid and energy intake and will review any food tolerance issues as well as adherence to supplement recommendations. Laboratory findings will be used by the RD to assess nutrient inadequacies or deficiencies. The RD also works on goal setting with the patient, gives practical strategies for achieving and maintaining weight loss, and provides encouragement to engage in lifelong healthy eating behaviours and physical activity [24].

A Case Vignette

Linda is a 45-year-old woman who has been referred by her family physician for bariatric surgery. She lives with her husband and two children and works full time as a school teacher. Linda has struggled with her weight since her pregnancies at ages 30 and 32 and currently weighs 123.6 kg, her height is 1.66 m and her BMI is 44.82. She does not have a lot of insight into the causes of continued weight gain in recent years but does admit to some emotional eating when feeling stressed. She also reports having a poor diet from an early age as her mother disliked cooking so the family ate a lot of fast foods and pre-packaged meals. Linda has diabetes mellitus that is currently being managed with metformin. Other obesity-related co-morbidities include obstructive sleep apnoea (OSA), stress urinary incontinence and back pain. Her prescription medications also include thyroid hormone replacement and an antidepressant.

(continued)

(continued)

Linda reports a history of depression and has taken antidepressants on and off for the past 15 years. Although she tried psychotherapy a few times Linda has never attended more than three or four sessions each time. She also has social anxiety disorder and reports worrying about what other people think of her as well as feeling self-conscious about her weight. She has no history of smoking or drug use. She is a current drinker consuming 1–2 alcoholic drinks per week. At the bariatric programme nursing assessment she was also found to have iron deficiency anaemia.

Linda is eligible for bariatric surgery based on BMI and obesity-related comorbidities but a full assessment by a multidisciplinary team will determine her suitability, commitment and readiness for surgery and the lifestyle changes required.

Pre-surgery nutrition assessment: At her individual nutrition assessment appointment Linda demonstrated good knowledge of bariatric surgery as well as the diet progression and supplement requirements post-op but her overall nutrition knowledge was lacking. She often chooses high fat, high sugar beverages and snacks stating she was unaware that these were nutrient-poor options.

A review of previous diet attempts showed that Linda has not tried any commercial or medically supervised weight loss programmes. She has tried several times to eat healthier but could not identify what that meant or why she was not successful. Linda has an unrealistic weight loss goal of 64 kg. The RD reviewed weight loss expectations and encouraged her to also consider non-scale goals. Linda acknowledged that her main reason for pursuing bariatric surgery is to improve her health, mobility and energy level.

A diet history using a 3-day food diary showed an irregular eating pattern, often skipping breakfast, daily intake of high fat sugary beverages and inadequate intake of protein foods, fruits, vegetables and whole grains. Portion sizes are reported as large. Linda often makes poor snack choices relying on chips, candy bars, baked goods and ice cream if she is hungry in the late afternoon. She eats fast food at dinner once or twice a week when the family is in a rush to get to evening activities. In preparation for bariatric surgery Linda states that she has changed her diet by cutting down her intake of carbonated beverages and drinking more water, paying more attention to food choices by reading food labels and trying to eat breakfast more often. However, a 24 h recall did not reflect these changes.

From a nutrition perspective Linda is not ready for bariatric surgery as her nutrition knowledge is inadequate; she has not made changes to her current intake and has had no formal diet attempts in the past. Linda was referred to a non-surgical weight loss programme for education and treatment.

Upon arriving to the non-surgical weight loss programme Linda met with an RD. A thorough assessment of her current eating habits was performed which involved exploring not only what she was eating, but how she was eating, and when. Her weight loss goal was also reviewed and she was encouraged to set a goal weight loss of 3–5 % to start. This equated to 3.7–6.2 kg (8–14 lb) at a rate of 0.5 kg or 1 lb per week. Linda did not feel this was fast enough so the evidence around realistic weight loss was reviewed and she was educated about the impact that this amount of weight loss could have for her diabetes, OSA, urinary stress incontinence and back pain. The RD communicated Linda's vitamin deficiencies to her general practitioner who prescribed a high dose vitamin D3 supplement that Linda was to take once/week for 8 weeks as well as an iron supplement to take daily. Because it was evident through the assessment that

(continued)

(continued)

Linda had little awareness as to where her extra calories were coming from she was encouraged to start logging her food intake daily. She was shown a mobile application that she could download to her phone for free and the RD demonstrated how to use it. Linda seemed confident that this was something she could do so she was asked to log her food intake for 2 weeks and return to the see the RD. Upon her next visit to the clinic Linda was weighed at 119.5 kg. She was happy with her progress. Linda also reported that logging her food intake made her realize how many calories were in some of the foods and drinks she was consuming that she was unaware off. She was shocked that her morning glass of 100 % real fruit juice intake added 130 calories and 22 grams of sugar to her day. Linda targeted this as the next area for her to change. She also noticed that her calorie intake was much higher on the days when she didn't pack a lunch and bought something out. This was also something she felt she could work on. The RD provided her with some healthy meal options for lunch and some accompanying recipes. Linda continued to return for follow-up biweekly for 3 months. During this time she identified that she is an emotional eater and that this is most likely to occur in the evening when she is lonely. The RD utilized some CBT strategies with her such as "thought stopping" and helped her come up with alternate ways of coping with loneliness. Most of the time Linda came with 80 % of her food records complete; however, 1 week she stopped logging all together. At this point the RD used motivational interviewing to help Linda to get back on track. They used a decisional balance worksheet. Linda identified that her biggest barrier to logging her food intake was when she ate something bad she felt guilty about it and didn't want to record it. The RD discussed the principle of eating healthy 80 % of the time and eating less healthy 20 % of the time rather than expecting perfection. Linda reported that she thought this would help her to feel less guilty and log her intake even when she did indulge in higher calorie foods. Over the following weeks Linda logged her intake more successfully and lost a total of 14 kg, exceeding her goal. Her dose of metformin was decreased and she reported feeling less back pain. Linda however felt that she had hit a stall. She didn't feel that there was much more she could change about her eating without feeling hungry all the time. For this reason Linda was re-referred for bariatric surgery.

Although Linda had lost 14 kg and was feeling better her health issues were not improving and she felt surgery was still her best option long term.

Linda's diet has improved as she is now eating breakfast regularly and she is making it a priority to have fruit and vegetables at each meal. She is making more nutritious choices and aiming to have balanced meals. She has stopped purchasing energy-dense coffee drinks and fruit juices and is drinking more water, herbal teas and unsweetened iced tea. Her snack choices include cheese and fruit, low fat low sugar yogurt, low fat crackers with nut butter or raw vegetables with hummus or bean dip.

Linda is planning her meals and grocery shopping with these menus in mind. She is using a grocery list and reading food labels more carefully. She also finds that batch cooking has provided her with options rather than choosing fast foods when her family needs quick meals. She is now monitoring her intake using a mobile application that she finds easy to use. She feels that this has helped her food knowledge and has often influenced her food choices. Linda is also applying some techniques of mindful eating knowing that eating slowly and thoughtfully will be important after surgery.

(continued)

(continued)

Her overall understanding of general nutrition principles has been enhanced by her education at the non-surgical programme and she is much more prepared for the challenges of lifelong dietary change required after bariatric surgery.

Post-surgery nutrition follow up: Linda had an uneventful stay in hospital after a RYGB and was provided with follow-up appointments in the bariatric clinic on discharge. Her nutrition appointments with an RD were made for 1, 3, 6 and 12 months and then at 1-year post-op.

One-month follow up: Linda reported feeling tired and struggling with fluids; water "feels heavy" in her stomach and doesn't taste the same. She was taking all of her protein and vitamin mineral supplements as recommended. The RD reassured her that her struggle with water was common and suggested varying the temperature or to try adding flavourings or very dilute fruit juice to it. Drinking technique was also reinforced to ensure slow sips of fluids. Recovery from surgery and a low energy intake were the likely causes of her fatigue. This was reviewed with Linda and she was advised that she should see a gradual improvement in energy level.

Month three follow up: Linda reported feeling well but that she is "never hungry" and sometimes forgets to eat. She has discontinued her protein supplements but does take all of the recommended vitamins and minerals. Linda was struggling with protein foods especially red meat, chicken and eggs. These foods hurt her stomach so she avoids them. The RD recommended using a clock or timer to remind Linda to eat as skipping meals can lead to inadequate intake and protein energy malnutrition. Due to her protein aversion it is also important Linda look for alternatives to meat such as dairy foods, beans and legumes, soy foods and fish. The RD provided a list of high protein snack options and recommended she go back to having one protein supplement per day. This would ensure an adequate intake until she is able to tolerate more food sources of protein. Laboratory values were reviewed by the RD and were found to be in normal range.

Month six follow up: Linda missed this appointment due to work commitments.

One-year follow up: Linda is very pleased with the results of surgery; she no longer has diabetes mellitus, her sleep apnoea is improved to the point that she will be having another sleep study to determine if she still needs CPAP. She is enjoying activities with her family such as bike riding, swimming and weekend hiking. Linda has lost 70 % of her excess weight but reports weight loss has stopped and she very concerned about gaining weight as she feels she can eat all foods again. She reports her anxiety about this has occasionally led to extra snacking or grazing in the evenings.

The RD suggested going back to the principles of long-term weight management after bariatric surgery. Linda felt that she should measure and track her intake again to be sure she is maintaining portion control and making nutritious food choices most of the time. The RD also suggested some strategies for behaviour change such as alternative activities in the evenings to help manage snacking and suggested that Linda consider enrolling in a mindful eating group. Linda will also discuss her anxiety with the psychologist and ask for help to deal with her symptoms.

14.3 Summary and Take Home Points

This chapter has outlined the nutritional management of severe obesity, including both non-surgical and surgical interventions. The management of obesity from a nutrition perspective is complicated and it is important to consider all variables that can impact the patient's success in achieving weight loss.

- When talking to your patients about their weight, avoid using words such as fatness and obesity. Simply use the word "weight" and always approach the conversation from a place of empathy and understanding.
- Help your patients to avoid fad diets by referring to the checklist provided.
- Any type of diet that involves calorie reduction can work. What is more important than the type of diet is whether or not someone can stick to it in the long term.
- Micronutrient deficiencies are prevalent in the obese population (both pursuing surgery and post-surgery). These should be screened for as part of any weight management programme and treated in order to maximize the patient's wellness and chance of success.
- Physical activity is important for weight maintenance but not an effective stand-alone strategy for weight loss.
- Bariatric surgery has been proven to be the most effective weight loss strategy for severe obesity.
- The success of the bariatric surgery patient is dependant on changes to the patient's lifestyle including diet, exercise, emotional well-being and adherence to supplement recommendations.
- There is a risk of nutrition-related complications after bariatric surgery including dumping syndrome, vomiting, dehydration, protein malnutrition and weight regain.
- The RD is your greatest ally in helping your patients achieve weight loss. They can provide education and counselling that has been proven to help patients achieve success.

References

1. Wadden TA, Didie E. What's in a name? Patients' preferred terms for describing obesity. Obes Res [Internet]. 2003;11(9):1140–6. doi:10.1038/oby.2003.155. [cited Sep 2003].
2. American Medical Association. AMA adopts new policies on second day of voting at annual meeting [Internet]. Chicago: AMA; 2013. http://www.ama-assn.org/ama/pub/news/news/2013/2013-06-18-new-ama-policies-annual-meeting.page
3. Canadian Medical Association. CMA recognizes obesity as a disease [Internet]. Ottawa: CMA; 2015. [cited 14 Apr 2016]; [about 1 screen]. https://www.cma.ca/En/Pages/cma-recognizes-obesity-as-a--disease.aspx
4. Freedhoff Y, Sharma AM. Best weight: a practical guide to office-based obesity management. La Vergne: Lightning Source; 2013.
5. Canadian Obesity Network. The 10 checks of a healthy weight-management program. Edmonton: CON; 2016. [cited 14 Apr 2016]; [about 1 screen]. http://www.obesitynetwork.ca/managing-obesity. Accessed 14 Apr 2016.
6. Wadden TA. Eight-year weight losses with an intensive lifestyle intervention: the look AHEAD study. Obesity [Internet]. 2014;22(1):5–13. doi:10.1002/oby.20662.
7. Raynor HA, Champagne CM. Position of the academy of nutrition and dietetics: interventions for the treatment of overweight and obesity in adults. J Acad Nutr Diet [Internet]. 2016;116(1):129–47. doi:10.1016/j.jand.2015.10.031. [cited Jan 2016].
8. Mayo Clinics. Weight loss: strategies for success [Internet]. Rochester: Mayo Clinics; 2016. [cited 14 Apr 2016]; [about 1 screen]. http://www.mayoclinic.org/healthy-lifestyle/weight-loss/in-depth/weight-loss/art-20047752. Accessed 14 Apr 2016.
9. Jakubowicz D, Barnea M, Wainstein J, Froy O. High caloric intake at breakfast vs. dinner differentially influences weight loss of overweight and obese women. Obesity [Internet]. 2013;21(12):2504–12. doi:10.1002/oby.20460.
10. Centers for Disease Control and Prevention. Division of Nutrition, Physical Activity, and Obesity. The benefits of physical activity [Internet]. Atlanta: Centers for Disease Control and Prevention; 2015. [cited 14 Apr 2016]; [about 1 screen]. http://www.cdc.gov/physlactivity/basics/pa-health/index.htm.
11. The National Weighr Control Registry. NWCR facts [Internet]. Providence: The National Weigh Control Registry; 2016. [cited 14 Apr 2016]; [about 1 screen]. www.nwcr.ws/Research/default.htm.
12. Stein J, Stier C, Raab H, Weiner R. Review article: the nutritional and pharmacological consequences of obesity surgery. Aliment Pharmacol Ther [Internet]. 2014;40(6):582–609. doi:10.1111/apt.12872. [cited Sep 2014].
13. Moize V, Deulofeu R, Torres F, de Osaba JM, Vidal J. Nutritional intake and prevalence of nutritional deficiencies prior to surgery in a Spanish morbidly obese population. Obes Surg [Internet]. 2011;21(9):1382–8. doi:10.1007/s11695-011-0360-y. [cited Sep 2011].
14. Canadian Institute for Health Information. Bariatric surgery in Canada report. Ottawa: CIHI; 2014. 34p. [cited 5 Apr 2016]. https://secure.cihi.ca/free_products/Bariatric_Surgery_in_Canada_EN.pdf.
15. Esteban Varela J, Nguyen NT. Laparoscopic sleeve gastrectomy leads the U.S. utilization of bariatric surgery at academic medical centers. Surg Obes Relat Dis. 2015;11(5):987–90.

16. Bloomberg RD, Fleishman A, Nalle JE, Herron DM, Kini S. Nutritional deficiencies following bariatric surgery: what have we learned? Obes Surg. 2005;15(2):145–54.
17. Buchwald H, Avidor Y, Braunwald E, Jensen MD, Pories W, Fahrbach K, Schoelles K. Bariatric surgery: a systematic review and meta-analysis. J Am Med Assoc [Internet]. 2004;292(14):1724–37. doi:10.1001/jama.2014.10706.
18. de Hollanda A, Ruiz T, Jimenez A, Flores L, Lacy A, Vidal J. Patterns of weight loss response following gastric bypass and sleeve gastrectomy. Obes Surg [Internet]. 2014;25(7):1177–83. doi:10.1007/s11695-014-1512-7.
19. Li J, Lai D, Wu D. Laparoscopic Roux-en-Y gastric bypass versus laparoscopic sleeve gastrectomy to treat morbid obesity-related comorbidities: a systematic review and meta-analysis. Obes Surg [Internet]. 2016;26(2):429–42. doi:10.1007/s11695-015-1996-9. [cited Feb 2016].
20. Gerber P, Anderin C, Thorell A. Weight loss prior to bariatric surgery: an updated review of the literature. Scand J Surg [Internet]. 2015;104(1):33–9. doi:10.1016/j.appet.2014.06.009.
21. Taube-Schiff M, Chapparo M, Gougeon L, Warwick K, Weiland M, Plummer C, Shakory S, Sockalingam S. Examining nutrition knowledge of bariatric surgery patients: what happens to dietary knowledge over time? Obes Surg [Internet]. 2014;24(8):1138–9. doi:10.1007/s11695-015-1846-9.
22. Isom K. Standardizing the evolution of the postoperative bariatric diet. Diabetes Spectr [Serial on the Internet]. 2012;25(4):222–8. doi:10.2337/diaspect.25.4.222. [cited 4 Apr 2016].
23. Aills L, Blankenship J, Buffington C, Furtado M, Parrott J. ASMBS allied health nutritional guidelines for the surgical weight loss patient. Surg Obes Relat Dis [Internet]. 2008;4(5 Suppl):S73–108. doi:10.1016/j.soard.2008.03.002.
24. Mechanick JI, Youdim A, Jones DB, Garvey WT, Hurley DL, McMahon MM, Heinberg LJ, Kushner R, Adams TD, Shikora S, Dixon JB, Brethauer S, American Association of Clinical Endocrinologists, Obesity Society, American Society for Metabolic & Bariatric Surgery. Clinical practice guidelines for the perioperative nutritional, metabolic, and nonsurgical support of the bariatric surgery patient—2013 update: cosponsored by American Association of Clinical Endocrinologists, the Obesity Society, and American Society for Metabolic & Bariatric Surgery. Endocr Pract [Internet]. 2013;19(2):337–72. doi:10.1002/oby.20662. [cited Mar–Apr 2013].
25. Moize V, Andreu A, Flores L, Torres F, Ibarzabal A, Delgado S, Lacy A, Rodriguez L, Vidal J. Long-term dietary intake and nutritional deficiencies following sleeve gastrectomy or Roux-en-Y gastric bypass in a Mediterranean population. J Acad Nutri Diet [Internet]. 2013;113(3):400–10. doi:10.1016/j.jand.2012.11.013. http://ovidsp.ovid.com/ovidweb.cgi?T=JS&PAGE=reference&D=emed11&NEWS=N&AN=23438491 (Embase).
26. Handzlik-Orlik G, Holecki M, Orlik B, Wylelol M, Dulawa J. Nutrition management of the post-bariatric surgery patient. Nutr Clin Prac [Internet]. 2015;30(3):383–92. doi:10.1177/0884533614564995.
27. Berg P, McCallum R. Dumping syndrome: a review of the current concepts of pathophysiology, diagnosis, and treatment. Dig Dis Sci [Internet]. 2016;61(1):11–8. doi:10.1007/s10620-015-3839-x.
28. Tack J, Deloose E. Complications of bariatric surgery: dumping syndrome, reflux and vitamin deficiencies. Best Pract Res Clin Gastroenterol [Internet]. 2014;28(4):741–9. doi:10.1016/j.bpg.2014.07.010.
29. Karmali S, Brar B, Shi X, Sharma AM, De Gara C, Birch DW. Weight recidivism post-bariatric surgery: a systematic review. Obes Surg [Internet]. 2013;23(11):1922–33. doi:10.1007/s11695-013-1070-4.
30. Endevelt R, Ben-Assuli O, Klain E, Zelber-Sagi S. The role of dietician follow-up in the success of bariatric surgery. Surg Obes Relat Dis [Internet]. 2013;9(6):963–8. doi:10.1016/j.soard.2013.01.006.

The Role of Social Support in Weight Loss Management for Morbidly Obese Individuals

15

Anna Wallwork and Lynn Tremblay

This chapter will discuss the role of social support on the treatment and weight loss outcomes of individuals with morbid obesity and those pursing bariatric surgery. Sources and functions of social support will be defined, with the roles of significant others and peers/similar others being explored in more detail. Literature on how these sources of support incite motivation for behaviour change will be provided. The chapter will proceed with suggestions and considerations for clinical practice and these will be demonstrated within a concluding case-based scenario.

Case Vignette

Pre-surgery: Brian is a 42-year-old married man who attended the clinic by himself for his initial social work appointment. He has been married for 12 years and reports that although his wife also struggles with her weight, she does not completely support his decision to seek bariatric surgery and thinks that he can lose weight on his own if he wanted though she believes he does not need to lose very much. He informs the social worker that his wife appears confident about her body size and has expressed no desire to lose weight, change how she eats or cooks, or conform to societal standards. Brian reports that he has a brother who is athletic, has never struggled with his weight, and does not understand how Brian "got to be this size". His brother is often encouraging Brian to join the gym and eat well. Brian also reports that he has informed two of his closest friends of his desire to lose weight/have bariatric surgery and that they have expressed mixed feelings. Much of their social activities involve pub food and beer and they are uncertain how this will impact their relationship with Brian after surgery. Brian expressed how his motivation for surgery has waned since sharing his intentions with his close family and friends and not receiving the support he anticipated he would. He is wondering if surgery is the right choice for him and whether he can be successful in his efforts.

Post-surgery: After significant weight loss, Brian attended the clinic to see the social worker for a follow-up appointment. He reports that it has been a challenge to

(continued)

A. Wallwork, M.A., M.S.W. (✉)
L. Tremblay, M.S.W., R.S.W.
Toronto Western Hospital Bariatric Surgery Program, University Health Network, 4E-460, 399 Bathurst Street, Toronto, ON, Canada M5T 2S8
e-mail: anna.wallwork@uhn.ca; lynn.tremblay@uhn.ca

S. Sockalingam, R. Hawa (eds.), *Psychiatric Care in Severe Obesity*, DOI 10.1007/978-3-319-42536-8_15

(continued)
routinely eat healthy and be physically active as his partner has no desire to join him in implementing these changes. He misses time with his wife which was usually spent sitting on the sofa watching television or going out to eat. Furthermore, he reports that his wife will often bring unhealthy foods into the home which he struggles with as he finds it easy to give in to temptations. His brother has been involved in his journey and encourages Brian to reach for goals that Brian does not feel he is capable of accomplishing at this time. Specifically, Brian reports that his brother wants him to do a 10 km race with him and has become a food police on the occasions that he sees Brian indulging in some of his favourite foods. As for his friends, Brian shared that they often continue to invite him to their regular outing of wings and beer, but he often declines. At times, Brian has suggested to do other activities to which his friends have been reluctant to agree to, but have on a few occasions.

15.1 Literature Review

The impact of embarking on a significant weight loss journey, via bariatric surgery or otherwise, extends well beyond an individual's weight in pounds; it requires extensive behavioural modification and lifestyle adjustments in order to maintain resultant health improvements and long-term weight loss success. Bariatric surgery specifically is considered a life-altering procedure that requires a lifelong commitment from the individual undergoing surgery. The pre- and post-surgical timeframe has been associated with high levels of stress and anxiety often concerning interpersonal relationships, life and social events, work, general health [1, 2], and body image [3]. The possibility of significant physical and mental impairment has also been noted in patients 2 years post-surgery [4]. Modifying personal habits while adjusting to the psychosocial stresses of surgery can prove challenging. While the bariatric clinician plays a key role in the provision of psychoeducation, advice, support, encouragement, and positive reinforcement for the patient, the majority of behavioural change processes occur in patients' home and professional work environments. Therefore, one's social support network plays a pertinent role in the weight loss journey.

15.1.1 Social Support

Thoits [5] delineates *social support* as a coping resource, or a social "fund", from which people may draw when handling stressors. It has been broadly defined as those functions performed by important others, such as partners, family members, friends, and colleagues, to assist a person in achieving personal goals or to meet the demands of a particular situation [6] with the most cited supportive functions including emotional/affective, informational, and instrumental assistance [7] as well as companionship [8]. Emotional/affective support refers to expressions of love, caring, esteem, value, encouragement, sympathy, concern, and empathy [9, 10]. Informational assistance includes the provision of facts, advice, or guidance that may help a person deepen his or her own understanding of the presenting issue and/or contribute to problem-solving [8, 10]. Instrumental support consists of offering material or behavioural assistance with practical tasks or problems [10]. Finally, companionship support has been referred to as the sharing of daily activities and ideas with others [8].

In the context of health, and in this case, weight management for severe obesity, support persons may trigger positive behavioural changes by providing reassurance around commitment and progress, offering information about nutrition and physical activity, or through the accompanying adoption of healthy changes to support the client's adherence to treatment. It has been argued that one's access to functions of support depend on his/her immediate social network and quality of

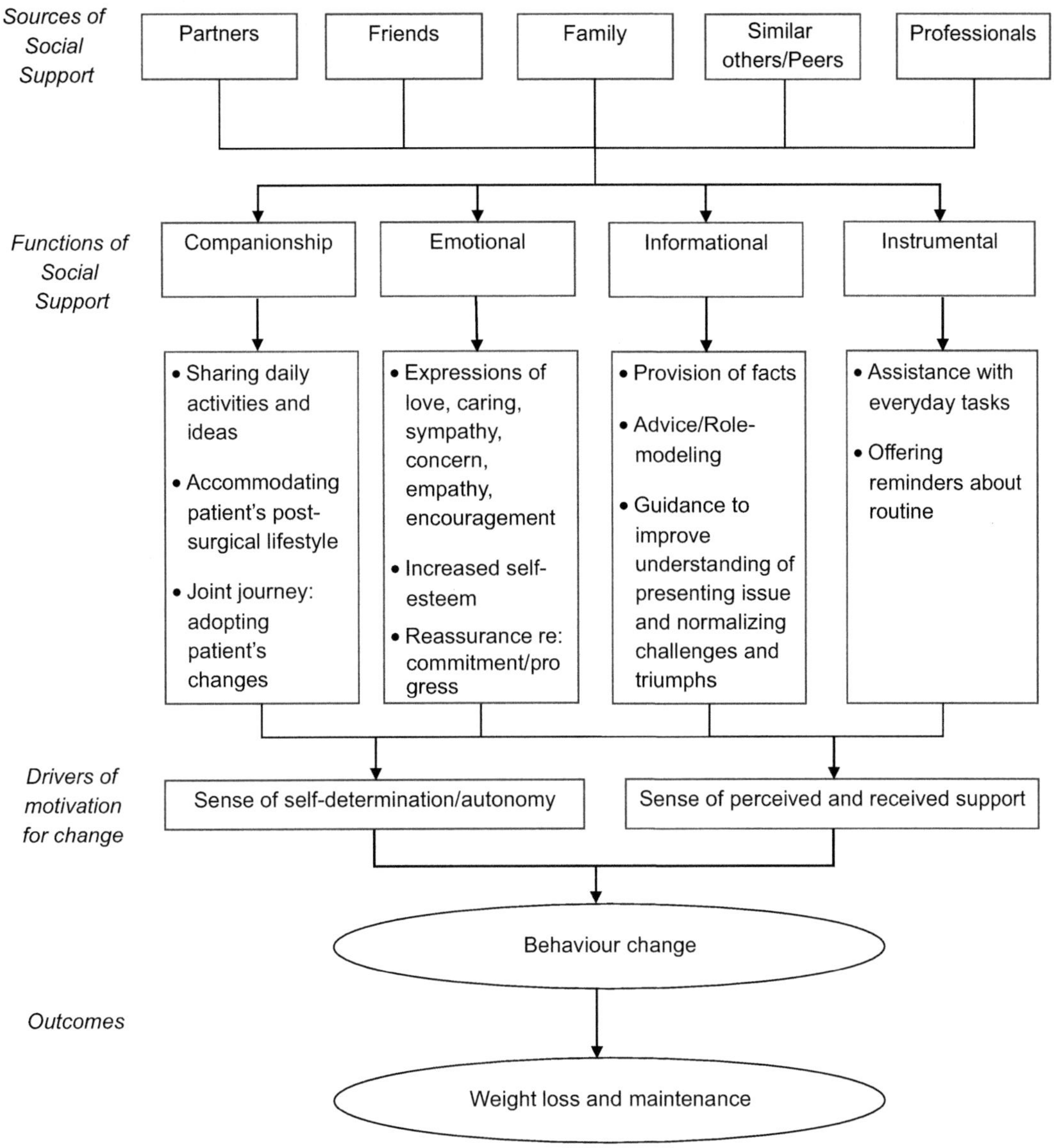

Fig. 15.1 The role of social support on weight loss outcomes

relationships to both primary group members, or "significant others" (relations of informal, intimate, and enduring quality with those who do not possess firsthand experience with the stressor confronting the individual), and secondary group members, or "similar others"/"peers" (relations more formal and less personal in nature with those who *do* have prior personal experience with the given stressor) [10, 11].

Deci and Ryan [12] also offer self-determination theory as a way to examine interpersonal support and the motivation for health behaviour change. The theory suggests that any behaviour varies by the degree to which is it experienced as autonomously supported (support that nurtures and promotes one's sense of self-determination) or controlled (support that aims to induce change by applying pressure or contingent rewards/punishments). Autonomy supportive environments and interventions are linked with better goal functioning as it pertains to weight management [13, 14]. *Perceived* autonomous support from one's important others has also been found to be associated with higher need satisfaction and greater autonomous motivation, in turn, manifesting in increased physical activity and healthier eating behaviours [15]; as well, *perceived* autonomous support from health care clinicians has predicted self-regulation and subsequent greater initial and long-term weight loss [16].

It is also important to note that while being positively correlated with health, social support can also work against healthy behavioural modification. Relationships may involve interpersonal strain or be sources of stress which can counteract the mitigating effects of the availability of social support [10]. Additionally, one's peers may provide ill-informed informational support that clients rely on, or may remain actively engaged in the negative health behaviours that clients are trying to change, such as heavy alcohol consumption and excessive indulgent eating, which can impact the likelihood of success for morbidly obese clients attempting weight loss.

All in all, the support provided to individuals pursuing weight loss should fit the identified need [17]. Making behavioural changes is a complex process and using various modes of intervention is advocated [18] while also recognizing the fluctuating degrees of support required at different stages of the change process [19].

15.1.2 Role of Support from Family/Friend/Close Others

Generally, individuals attempting weight loss identify their spouse, a relative, or a friend as their strongest supporter, though they may also receive support from various other individuals in their lives [11]. Family and friends are considered an "organic" source of support and are viewed "as more enduring" relationships that are vital in the weight loss process ([20], p. 66). There is little research, however, to distinguish how support from family members is similar to or different than support from friends; as well, overall impact of support and what types of support are most beneficial remain unclear [21]. What we do know is that, as per Christakis and Fowler [22] who argue that one's risk of obesity is influenced by associating with other obese individuals, so too does weight loss appear to be socially contagious with greater weight loss being achieved by an individual when their partner also participates in a weight loss programme [23] and/or who also loses weight [24]. Related to this is the idea that when negative reactions occur and a lack of support from family and friends exists, individuals have reported that their attempts at weight loss or maintenance are challenged and more difficult to achieve articulating that this experience undermines their sense of belonging to, and feeling valued by, important others subsequently leading to negative poor emotional consequences. Such psychological impact has occurred even when individuals do successfully lose weight, due to perceptions that their lifestyle changes were not accepted by their support system [25].

The literature has established that support from significant others plays a vital role in the success of the individual attempting weight loss. Significant others, and families in general, are often the providers of instrumental support, and when they are unable to fulfil this role, friends often step in to assist the individual in their weight loss journey. Ogle and colleagues [11] outline two forms of instrumental support provided by family: one is assisting with daily tasks such as food preparation, shopping, and transportation to appointments to allow the individual to focus on weight loss/maintenance; the second is helping individuals adhere to the dietary regimen by offering assistance with and "gentle reminders" about the routine. This is often enacted by role modelling desirable behaviours to assist the individual attempting to lose or maintain weight loss. It is also provided through acting as a "joint" collaborator [11, 26] on the weight loss journey with the individual; that is, family members often make adjustments in their own eating patterns, avoid certain foods that are problematic for the client, modify meal plans, only buy healthy groceries to bring into the home, and elicit input and negotiate on where to dine out. Ogle and colleagues' [11] research also identified close others as supporters in altering the focus of social events around things that do not involve food, acting as exercise partners, and in attending patient and family support groups. Essentially, supportive family and close others have been shown to make the behavioural changes part of their lifestyle as well.

Lewis and colleagues [27] have also suggested that when couples interdependently ascribe a health threat as meaningful for one of the partners or for the relationship, it transforms one's motivation from being self-centred to that of relationship centred, in turn enhancing motivation for the couple to act cooperatively in the adoption of health-promoting behaviour change and to cope communally. Individuals attempting to lose weight have reported being grateful for their supportive others' encouragement, understanding, flexibility, and inspiration towards their health and fitness goals and in some cases, they reported the collaboration as a method of holding them accountable to their changes as opposed to making the changes independently [11].

Primarily, however, family and friends are providers of emotional/affective and companionship support. They provide empathy, compassion, and the emotional support needed to sustain those embarking on a weight loss journey during difficult times [10] as well as motivation and encouragement [11, 28]. They also provide verbal appraisals on appearance, which may be perceived by the client as admiration and pride, may help increase self-esteem and confidence, and may provide incentive to continue with the lifestyle changes. This has been especially helpful for those who underwent bariatric surgery as it recognizes their efforts towards weight loss. Partners also offer verbal feedback on any behavioural or personality changes they observe in the individual along their weight loss journey or use "healthy" humour to comment on certain body changes (i.e. bust size). For someone pursuing weight loss, these can all contribute to the development of an emergent new self and is said to reinforce and enhance confidence in the changes occurring [11].

Ng and colleagues [15] discuss the difference between significant others providing more autonomy-promoting support versus more coercive and guilt-promoting methods of support, which have been shown to produce poorer long-term outcomes and impede weight loss attempts overall. Better weight loss outcomes occur when an individual chooses to make the behavioural changes needed in relation to their meaning and importance, as well as believing that they can accomplish their goals and are supported by others [25]. Essentially, support systems involving a controlling interpersonal style are related to lower levels of change implementation or adherence to lifestyle changes within individuals attempting weight loss. Controlling supportive behaviours, such as contingent rewards or intimidation tactics, need thwarting and should be addressed within the clinical setting. Some individuals possess a greater predisposition towards autonomy and are able to motivate themselves towards change [16]. In these instances, even supportive attempts by close others to help monitor food intake or provide gentle reminders could be seen as challenging their autonomy and their ability to implement the changes required. Therefore, the interpersonal styles of the support system should be taken into account; the provision of psychoeducation for significant others may help them better understand what kinds of supports are beneficial and detrimental to their loved one attempting weight loss.

From a systems theory point of view, changes in one family member mutually influence and is influenced by other members within the family unit, which implies that a person can be better understood within the context of his/her familial support system. Characteristics such as family structure, communication, problem-solving abilities, and the various roles family members play are impacted when one member is making significant changes [29]. In the treatment of obese adolescents, clinical practice guidelines recommend the inclusion of family throughout the process to determine family unit competency, stability, level of support for the obese patient, their comprehension of medical complications related to surgical treatments, and the need for lifelong investment in lifestyle changes [30]. This suggests the importance of forming partnerships within the family in the pursuit of weight loss management for enhancing chances of success [31] regardless of the age of identified client.

With respect to support from friends specifically, changes in interpersonal dynamics have also been noted after bariatric surgery when significant weight loss occurs in one member of the friendship dyad. Challenges experienced may include jealousy or dissatisfaction in the change to routine social endeavours that typically revolve around food and drink. The opposite has also been noted where relationships can alternatively thrive after surgery. The impact of the surgery is "multifaceted and highly dependent on each individual's set of circumstances and experiences" ([20], p. 69). Interestingly, friendship networks are said to incur the most restructuring and changes as a result of bariatric surgery [32].

15.1.3 Role of Peer Support

The role of peer support is often crucial to morbidly obese individuals pursing weight loss management as the genuine feeling of being empathically understood by someone, particularly if one does not perceive this from their significant others, provides therapeutic relief in the face of the ongoing stressor. Thoits [10] provides that a peer's "direct experiential knowledge is the key to their provisions of effective emotional sustenance as well as active coping assistance" (p. 154). Individuals pursuing weight loss management programmes, and bariatric surgery specifically, receive a great deal of support from "similar others" frequently within the context of both face-to-face support groups and online support forums. In addition to the provision of empathic understanding, "like others" provide informational support to weight management patients, serve to normalize the challenges and triumphs across the weight loss journey, validate concerns and feelings, and can serve as aspirational role models for newer participants [10, 11]. Support group environments offer opportunities for facilitated discussions related to emotional eating and other disordered eating behaviours, relationship issues, body image and excess skin concerns, dietary changes, exercise, and stress management. Additionally, the mere existence of similar others who have effectively coped and achieved success generates hope in individuals pursing similar feats; one can envision a desired self in their future, thus motivating them towards that goal [33].

Evidence provides that support groups after weight loss surgery are a valuable component of continuing follow-up care. In their systematic review, Livhits and colleagues [34] illustrated that all studies found a positive association between post-operative support groups and weight loss. Additionally, Beck and colleagues' [35] meta-analysis also supported the finding that patients attending psychotherapeutic interventions or support groups in combination with bariatric surgery appeared to have greater weight loss as compared to those treated with bariatric surgery alone. Significant differences in excess weight loss 1 year after surgery have been noted in patients who have attended support group as compared to those who have not [36, 37].

In addition to face-to-face support, online support forums, most commonly in the form of message boards and chat rooms, are becoming increasingly popular in the current digital age and rise of social media. The interactions occurring within these mediums can be similar to those that take place in person, however have been shown to be especially valued for being readily available as needed and for the immediacy of feedback that can be obtained [11]. With respect to online bariatric forums specifically, individuals have been shown to actively engage in an effort to give back to other newly post-operative clients as well as to keep themselves accountable throughout their own continued weight loss journey [20]. For those unable to attend support groups in person due to proximity of location, transportation limitations, or social anxieties, online forums provide a comparable platform for accruing similar benefits. Social media may also fill a gap for those with a limited social network, satisfying the need for support and connectedness. Though the isolated benefits of participating in online support platforms is still unclear, social media appears to play a role in retaining and engaging participants in the pursuit of weight loss management [38]. Given that patients will often not recall advice provided to them preoperatively [39], online and in-person support groups can aid in providing continuing education and factual reminders on an ongoing basis, supplementing clinical appointments with health professionals.

The role of peer mentors and coaches for weight loss management has also been preliminarily studied as a supplement to clinical care with the argument that between treatment appointments, mentors, and coaches can provide ongoing support, accountability, information to support behavioural change, and effective role modelling of optimal health behaviour typically by phone or online [40]. Appropriately trained individuals, without any formal professional health care education, who have previously achieved their own significant weight loss through lifestyle modification, may be perceived as more accessible to clients and more familiar with their lived experiences than health care providers [41]. Though social influence can occur among peer dyads, the proven efficacy of such mentors and coaches remains unclear and requires further research.

15.1.4 Professional Support

Though falling outside of Thoit's [10] primary/secondary supportive others distinction, health care providers also play a unique role in providing social support to individuals pursuing weight loss management, surgically or otherwise, though this relationship may have more limited impact in comparison to patients' natural support networks [19]. Due to the nonreciprocal relationship, and the limits to accessibility and proximity inherent between patients and providers contributing to weaker social ties, health professionals draw from their collective professional experience and expertise to help individuals navigate their weight loss journey mainly through the provision of informational support related to best practices, self-management tools, and resources to support weight loss goals and maintenance. In general, patients tend to perceive health professionals as credible and trustworthy experts in the field thereby accepting the medically based information provided to them. Additionally, health professionals are sources of empathy, acknowledge struggles, provide encouragement, serve as advocates, and empower patients to make decisions for themselves even when patients' close others may not agree [10, 11].

Ogle and colleagues [11] has identified that having significant experience working with morbidly obese individuals allows clinicians to understand a client's history of weight loss struggle and thus are able to provide an approach that conveys a genuine appreciation for their patient's experience, even though they have not similarly shared the experience firsthand. In addition to the provision of informational support to assist with weight loss and maintenance in the physical sense, health professionals also address the accompanying psychosocial issues that often arise and which may impede success (including but not limited to the risk of cross addictions, interpersonal strain, social withdrawal or isolation, and mental health challenges). Facilitating discussions that lead clients to anticipate potential personal and relationship challenges they may encounter on their weight loss journey, aiding in their preparation to address such challenges, and helping them problem-solve when issues arise, are important aspects of the supportive role played by clinicians. Individuals who have undergone weight loss surgery have also identified health professionals as providers of emotional/affective support in the sense of offering praise for their progress and reigniting motivation during times of struggle (see Fig. 15.1) [11].

15.2 Clinical Implications

15.2.1 Involving Significant Others

Support vs. sabotage: The importance of social support in achieving lifestyle changes for weight loss management in morbidly obese individuals has been acknowledged in the literature. Shared family dynamics among those in the same home can commonly lead to shared negative health behaviours (including poor eating and lifestyle habits, substance use, and other high-risk health behaviours) highlighting the importance of targeting the family unit for obesity treatment and intervention. Of particular importance is the role of significant others throughout all stages of the weight loss journey. In bariatric clinics, it is helpful for psychosocial clinicians to have clients reflect on whether or not they would anticipate a significant weight loss negatively affecting any of their important relationships. This may allow the client to work with the clinician in identifying potential challenges and problem-solve around preventing interpersonal strain. Additionally, if a client identifies one of his/her primary supporters as being a potential saboteur in his/her weight loss journey, it is recommended that, at a minimum, an opportunity be provided by the clinician for the client to be seen with this significant other prior to weight loss surgery or treatment in order to facilitate a discussion around helpful versus unhelpful support for the individual [42]. It has also been suggested to overtly include the potential saboteur in the entire treatment process as much as is possible by encouraging their participation in clinical consultations, educations sessions, and support groups. At all of these encounters, benefits and stressors to the relationship subsequent to weight loss intervention/bariatric surgery can be explored and brainstorming strategies to cope with identified stressors can be collaboratively negotiated [43]. As such, empowering significant others of morbidly obese patients to serve as effective supporters may also indirectly help the patient towards successful adherence to lifestyle changes. It should be recognized that clinicians may encounter individuals who engage in self-sabotaging behaviours themselves based on their own rational of a perceived lack of social support [24].

Perception plays a role in effecting change in individuals pursuing weight loss and therefore the perceptions of support or sabotage within different support systems is an important area to address clinically. Exploring clients' perception of support, as compared to what their family and friends believe is supportive behaviour, will help clinicians better understand the social environments of their patients in order to more accurately provide them with what they need to be successful in their weight loss journey. It may simply be the case that support systems may not know the right things to do or say for fear of doing the wrong thing. Perceived support is a subjective measure and should be bolstered as best as possible within the clinical setting although it should be recognized that this can be more challenging than helping patients obtain the provision of practical/structural support [19].

Helping significant others adjust to client changes: Although significant others are generally welcomed and encouraged to attend appointments with individuals pursuing surgical and behavioural weight loss management treatments, there is no official forum for them to explore their own perspectives and experiences and to elicit their support despite the known impact on patients' lifestyle modifications. This is especially crucial for significant others who also battle their own weight and who struggle with adapting to the changes. Providing psychoeducation to both clients and their significant others on the potential impacts of lifestyle modification and/or surgery on family members, or for what may be experienced as a couple, is also of benefit to ensure that a more thorough understanding is gained by all those closely involved, as well as to manage significant others' expectations following surgery. This could be done verbally through one-on-one individual appointments, through a group session, or conveyed in writing in an informational handout provided to clients at their appointments.

Helping support persons understand the change process can aid in decreasing any uncertainty they may feel and help them to better prepare for upcoming changes. Resistance from family members in adjusting to lifestyle changes required after bariatric surgery has been noted [11, 20, 44] and adjustment challenges with respect to a partner's lifestyle changes post-surgery has reportedly disturbed the balance within relationships [43], at times leading to spousal conflict and even divorce [45].

Changes in family dynamics serve to highlight both strengths and weaknesses during a difficult time. Research by Chi and colleagues [46] found that how couples experienced and coped with the stressor of bariatric surgery was related to relationship dynamics that were present prior to the surgery; that is, positively functioning couples continued to work collaboratively to navigate the changes brought on by one partner undergoing surgery while interpersonally strained couples demonstrated difficulty in coming together throughout the change process. The lifestyle change process was, for most couples, one that led to a new, more harmonious, "normal". It was also noted that supporting partners who struggled with their own weight were more likely to be challenged in making lifestyle changes alongside the patient though these support persons did demonstrate greater empathy towards their partner's weight struggles due to sharing a similar experience.

Related to bariatric surgery specifically, significant others should be informed to recognize that there is a transitional stage right after surgery wherein they may have a tendency to gain weight (e.g. "the garbage can effect" or "clean your plate syndrome") and in turn should be provided with the appropriate education to help them avoid the potential pitfall of possible weight gain in the first place. Also, providing education and supporting significant others in adopting the lifestyle changes of bariatric patients, which have been shown in some studies to result in collateral weight loss effects [31], may provide significant others with the motivation to implement these changes. Due to the significant impact of bariatric surgery specifically on the family unit, it has been argued that health care professionals should shift their focus from client-centred practice to family-centred practice in order to target all individuals involved/affected by surgery which can contribute to enhanced family functioning as a whole and better success overall [44].

15.2.2 Promoting the Role of Support Groups

Given the salient role of peer support groups in the success of individuals pursuing weight loss management, it is important for clinicians to encourage their patients to be a part of bariatric communities, both in person and online. If providing a support group through a professional clinic, factors that may contribute to increased attendance and engagement include offering flexible meeting times or weekend meetings for better accommodation, and structuring the provision of new information related to topics of interest [34]. Desired topics identified by bariatric patients include: adjustment and difficulties following surgery, best foods to eat for individual needs, nutrition, exercise, helpful tips after surgery, how to deal with weight loss plateaus, life-altering changes, societal changes, and plastic surgery [47].

Offering a support group for preoperative and newly post-operative patients separate from longer term post-operative patients (e.g. 1-year post-surgery and greater) is a way to better cater to all individuals as the experiences, concerns, and challenges of these groups usually differ [20]. This can help prevent patients feeling alienated by ongoing discussion and provide more opportunities for greater coverage of pertinent topics by weight loss journey stage.

Additionally, opening up bariatric patient support groups to include family and friends can offer significant others the opportunity to share and receive information pertaining to their concerns, increase their understanding of the surgical and medical treatment processes from the patient perspective, receive guidance on how best to provide support to their loved ones, and may incite motivation towards making lifestyle modifications themselves.

15.2.3 Challenges Providing Professional Support

Clinically in practice, patients have at times expressed concern over a lack of comprehension and sensitivity from their "normal sized" health care practitioners. It is not unusual for a patient to present their motivations for wanting to lose weight and accentuate their perspective by providing the clinician, "wouldn't understand", or at a minimum thinking this without overtly vocalizing it. In bariatric clinical settings specifically,

Role of Social Worker or Other Psychosocial Health Care Professionals in Case Vignette

Pre-surgery: After the initial meeting between social work staff and Brian, several recommendations were made. He was encouraged to connect with a peer support group, either formally through the clinical programme or through online groups or forums, as this can provide him an opportunity to discuss his ongoing challenges, discover others who have experienced and navigated similar situations, and to elicit positive forms of support which he has identified as missing in his close knit social support network. Having the chance to hear from others who have had bariatric surgery and the impact it has had on their lives may positively influence Brian's waning feelings of motivation to pursue surgery himself.

The social worker also highlighted the importance of support within his home environment for weight loss success and offered to meet with Brian and his wife to discuss Brian's goals and his wife's concerns. This is a good opportunity to explore strategies and collaboration that meets both of their needs. A dialogue can be facilitated that would support Brian in expressing his reasons for seeking surgical weight loss and how his partner can best support him towards that goal. The social worker can also provide some psychoeducation to his wife with respect to potential benefits and challenges on their relationship as a result of the stress of surgery. Brian's wife would also be encouraged to attend a patient and family support group as a means to enhance her own understanding of the weight loss expectations and behavioural modifications related to bariatric surgery, as well as to hear the perspectives and experiences of other partners of bariatric patients.

Post-surgery: When Brian attends the clinic again after experiencing significant weight loss, the social worker acknowledges Brian's achievements and efforts in maintaining behavioural changes the majority of the time despite the interpersonal challenges he has faced. Using strength-based intervention, the social worker explores what Brian identifies as being the things that are most helpful to him in being able to focus and adhere to the recommended lifestyle changes after surgery despite the challenges. Together, clinician and patient can brainstorm ways to further enhance those factors identified by Brian that better promote long-term maintenance.

The social worker also explores with Brian any attempts he has made to communicate with his loved ones regarding the behaviours he identifies as difficult and impeding on his success and he would be encouraged to communicate to them the particular behaviours they exhibit that he perceives as barriers to him in achieving and maintaining long-term weight loss. If necessary, the social worker offers to facilitate a family meeting to discuss his important others' willingness to make changes or alter their communication style to better support Brian, and what that would look like. Promoting communication with loved ones to reach certain agreements and/or brainstorming ideas of activities they can share would be addressed with Brian in clinic.

Brian would be further encouraged to maintain support through various support group formats, and attend regular appointments at the clinic to encourage his maintenance of the lifestyle changes and promote accountability. If necessary, additional appointments and counselling can be offered to Brian should communication with loved ones not reach any agreeable solutions.

health professionals may also at times sense that patients provide calculated answers to assessment questions in order to demonstrate themselves as "suitable" surgical candidates. There is also the concern that weight loss management clinicians are professionally and financially motivated to provide unquestioning support to their patients [11] although this may be of less concern in countries where the weight loss surgery is government funded. Such challenges can prove difficult to navigate when trying to establish a positive therapeutic rapport with clients. The ability of clinicians to draw from their cumulative experiences in working with this population in order to arrive at genuine empathic understanding is something that should be strived for. Interaction should be framed in a manner that assumes the client perspective, conveying appreciation for the affective and cognitive experiences of the client over time (even though he or she has not shared a similar lived experience firsthand), and reflecting back to the client the essence of the personal struggle they have undergone [11, 48]. Arriving at a joint understanding with patients allows them to feel validated, supported, and invested in.

15.3 Summary and Take Home Messages

- Personal support networks play a pertinent role in the behavioural change process for weight loss.
- Functions provided by support networks include: emotional/affective, informational, instrumental, and companionship support.
- Autonomy-promoting environments and *perceived* autonomous support and interventions from others are linked to improved health behaviours, weight management goal functioning, and greater initial and long-term weight loss.
- Social support can work against positive behavioural modification when the relationship is a source of interpersonal strain or when supporters remain engaged in the negative health behaviours the client is attempting to change.
- Weight loss improves when loved ones also participate in the same healthy lifestyle changes and/or also loses weight.
- Differing interpersonal styles of support lead to varied motivating behavioural outcomes, and this should be taken into account in the clinical setting and appropriate psychoeducation provided as needed.
- Significant weight loss promotes changes in interpersonal dynamics, especially within friendship networks.
- Psychotherapy or support groups in combination with bariatric surgery result in greater weight loss than with just surgery alone.
- Clinician identification of potential support network challenges and interpersonal conflicts, and subsequent problem-solving with clients, should occur at the beginning of the weight loss journey.
- Shared family dynamics among those in the same home can lead to shared negative health behaviours highlighting the importance of targeting the family unit for obesity treatment and intervention.
- Meeting with potential saboteurs initially, as well as throughout the weight loss journey, is recommended to discuss helpful versus unhelpful support.
- Primary support persons should be provided with a forum to discuss their challenges, especially if they also struggle with their weight.
- Support groups should be organized for different stages of change and should be open to family and friends.

References

1. Buddeberg-Fischer B, Klaghofer R, Sigrist S, Buddeberg C. Impact of psychosocial stress and symptoms on indication for bariatric surgery and outcome in morbidly obese patients. Obes Surg. 2004;14:361–9.
2. Shiri S, Gurevich T, Feintuch U, Beglaibter N. Positive psychological impact of bariatric surgery. Obes Surg. 2007;17:663–8.
3. Sarwer DB, Fabricatore AN. Psychiatric considerations of the massive weight loss patient. Clin Plast Surg. 2008;35:1–10.

4. Karlsson J, Sjostrom L, Sullivan M. Swedish obese subjects (SOS): an intervention study of obesity: two-year follow-up of health-related quality of life (HRQL) and eating behavior after gastric surgery for severe obesity. Int J Obes. 1998;22:113–26.
5. Thoits PA. Stress, coping, and social support processes: where are we? What next? J Health Soc Behav. 1995;Extra Issue:53–79.
6. Tolsdorf CC. Social networks, support, and coping: exploratory study. Fam Process. 1976;15:407–17.
7. House JS, Kahn RL. Measures and concepts of social support. In: Cohen S, Syme SL, editors. Social support and health. San Diego: Academic; 1985. p. 83–108.
8. Bambina A. Online social support. Youngstown: Cambria Press; 2007.
9. Taylor SE. Social support: a review. In: Friedman HS, editor. The Oxford handbook of health psychology. Oxford: Oxford University Press; 2011. p. 189–214.
10. Thoits PA. Mechanisms linking social ties and support to physical and mental health. J Health Soc Behav. 2011;52:145–61.
11. Ogle JP, Park J, Damhorst ML, Bradley LA. Social support for women who have undergone bariatric surgery. Qual Health Res. 2016;26:176–93.
12. Deci EL, Ryan RM. The "what" and "why" of goal pursuits: human needs and the self-determination of behavior. Psychol Inq. 2000;11:227–68.
13. Powers T, Koestner R, Gorin AA. Autonomy support from family and friends and weight loss in college women. Fam Syst Health. 2008;26:404–16.
14. Silva MN, Vieira PN, Coutinho SR, Minderico CS, Matos MG, Sardinha LB, et al. Using self-determination theory to promote physical activity and weight control: a randomized controlled trial in women. J Behav Med. 2010;33:110–22.
15. Ng JYY, Ntoumanis N, Thøgersen-Ntoumani C. Autonomy support and control in weight management: what important others do and say matters. Br J Health Psychol. 2014;19:540–52.
16. Williams GC, Grow VM, Freedman ZR, Ryan RM, Deci EL. Motivational predictors of weight loss and weight-loss maintenance. J Pers Soc Psychol. 1996;70:115–26.
17. Bianco T. Social support and recovery from sport injury: elite skiers share their experiences. Res Q Exerc Sports. 2001;72:376–88.
18. Calfas KJ, Sallis JF, Zabinski MF, Wilfley DE, Rupp J, Prochaska JJ, et al. Preliminary evaluation of a multicomponent program for nutrition and physical activity change in primary care: PACE+ for adults. Prev Med. 2002;34:153–61.
19. Verheijden MW, Bakx JC, van Weel C, Koelen MA, van Staveren WA. Role of social support in lifestyle-focused weight management interventions. Eur J Clin Nutr. 2005;59 Suppl 1:s179–86.
20. Geraci AA, Brunt AR, Marihart CL. Social support systems: a qualitative analysis of female bariatric patients after the first two years postoperative. Bariatric Surgical Practice and Patient Care. 2014;9:66–71.
21. Vishne TH, Ramadan E, Alper D, Avraham Z, Seror D, Dreznik Z. Long term follow-up and factors influencing success of silastic vertical gastroplasty. Dig Surg. 2004;21:134–41.
22. Christakis NA, Fowler JH. The spread of obesity in a large social network over 32 years. N Engl J Med. 2007;357:370–9.
23. Woodard GA, Encarnacion B, Peraza J, Hernandez-Boussard T. Halo effect for bariatric surgery: collateral weight loss in patients' family members. Ach Surg. 2011;416:1185–90.
24. Kiernan M, Moore SD, Schoffman DE, Lee K, King AC, Taylor C, et al. Social support for healthy behaviors: scale psychometrics and prediction of weight loss among women in a behavioral program. Obes J. 2012;20:756–64.
25. Whale K, Gillison FB, Smith PC. 'Are you still on that stupid diet?': women's experiences of societal pressure and support regarding weight loss, and attitudes towards health policy intervention. J Health Psychol. 2014;19:1536–46.
26. Pories ML, Hodgson J, Rose MA, Pender J, Sira N, Swanson M. Following bariatric surgery: an exploration of the couples' experience. Obes Surg. 2016; 26:54–60.
27. Lewis MA, McBride CM, Pollak KI, Puleo E, Butterfield RM, Emmons KM. Understanding health behavior change among couples: an interdependence and communal coping approach. Soc Sci Med. 2006;62:1369–80.
28. McLean N, Griffin S, Toney K, Hardeman W. Family involvement in weight control, weight maintenance and weight-loss interventions: a systematic review of randomised trials. Int J Obes. 2003;27:987–1005.
29. Smith SR, Hamon RR, Ingoldsby BB, Miller JE, editors. Exploring family theories. 2nd ed. New York: Oxford University Press; 2009. p. 368.
30. Shewsbury VA, Steinbeck KS, Torvaldsen S, Baur LA. The role of parents in pre-adolescent and adolescent overweight and obesity treatment: a systematic review of clinical recommendations. Obes Rev. 2011;12:759–69.
31. Vidot DC, Prado G, De La Cruz-Munoz N, Cuesta M, Spadola C, Messiah SE. Review of family-based approaches to improve postoperative outcomes among bariatric surgery patients. Surg Obes Rel Dis. 2011;11:451–8.
32. Meana M, Ricciardi L. Obesity surgery: stories of altered lives. Reno: University of Nevada Press; 2008.
33. Markus H, Nurius P. Possible selves. Am Psychol. 1986;41:954–69.
34. Livhits M, Mercado C, Yermilov I, Parikh JA, Dutson E, Mehran A, et al. Is social support associated with greater weight loss after bariatric surgery? A systematic review. Obes Rev. 2012;12:142–8.
35. Beck NN, Johannsen M, Stoving RK, Mehlsen M, Zacariae R. Do postoperative psychotherapeutic interventions and support groups influence weight loss following bariatric surgery? A systematic review and

meta-analysis of randomized and nonrandomized trials. Obes Surg. 2012;11:1790–7.
36. McMahon MM, Sarr MG, Clark MM, Gall MM, Knoetgen J 3rd, Service FJ, et al. Clinical management after bariatric surgery: value of a multidisciplinary approach. Mayo Clin Proc. 2006;81:S34–45.
37. Song Z, Reinhardt K, Buzdon M, Liao P. Association between support grop attendance and weight loss after Roux-en-Y gastric bypass. Surg Obes Relat Dis. 2008;4:100–3.
38. Chang T, Chopra V, Zhang C, Woolford SJ. The role of social medial in online weight management: systematic review. J Med Internet Res. 2013;15, e262.
39. Madan AK, Tichansky DS, Taddeucci RJ. Postoperative laparoscopic bariatric surgery patients do not remember potential complications. Obes Surg. 2007;17:885–8.
40. Leahey TM, Wing RR. A randomized controlled pilot study testing three types of health coaches for obesity treatment: professional, peer, and mentor. Obesity (Silver Spring). 2013;21(5):928–34.
41. Dutton GR, Phillips JM, Kukkalla M, Cherrington AL, Safford MM. Pilot study evaluating the feasibility and initial outcomes of a primary care weight loss intervention with peer coaches. Diabetes Educ. 2015;41:361–8.
42. Sogg S, Mori DL. The Boston interview for gastric bypass determining the psychological suitability of surgical candidates. Obes Surg. 2004;14:370–80.
43. Andrews G. Intimate saboteurs. Obes Surg. 1997; 7:445–8.
44. Bylund A, Benzein E, Persson C. Creating a new sense of we-ness: family functioning in relation to gastric bypass surgery. Bariatric Surgical Practice and Patient Care. 2013;8:152–60.
45. Hafner RJ, Roger J. Husband's adjustments to wives' weight loss after gastric restriction for morbid obesity. Int J Obes. 1990;14:1069–78.
46. Chi M, Tremblay L, Wallwork A, Boyce J. Living with bariatric patients: partners' perspectives. Can J Diabetes. 2015;39:S29.
47. Orth WS, Madan AK, Taddeucci RJ, Coday M, Tichansky DS. Support group meeting attendance is associated with better weight loss. Obes Surg. 2008;18:391–4.
48. Bogo M. Social work practice: concepts, processes, and interviewing. New York: Columbia University Press; 2006. p. 311.

16 Motivational Interviewing for Severe Obesity

Marlene Taube-Schiff, Lauren David, and Stephanie E. Cassin

Case Vignette

Mr. Davis is a 52-year-old married accountant with two teenaged children. He has been speaking with his family physician for several months about making changes to his dietary habits. In terms of weight history, he reported struggling with weight management issues for as long as he can remember. He comes from a family of five siblings, all of whom have experienced issues with obesity. Mr. Davis has indicated that family gatherings are often centred on food and that cooking has been considered a way to show love for one another. Growing up, he remembered being bullied at school for struggling in gym and being the largest one in his class.

As he became older, Mr. Davis continued to struggle with his weight and described that his eating frequently became "out of control". Mr. Davis reported that food has always been his "go-to" coping strategy and that he turns to food when feeling sad, frustrated, or bored. A typical example would be using food to provide relief after a stressful day at work. He reported that he has always found food to be comforting, and stated that nothing else has enabled him to feel "instantly calm" in the way food has. Furthermore, Mr. Davis endorsed a lengthy history of binge eating and often dissociates when he binges.

Since his 20s, Mr. Davis has had a string of weight loss attempts, including fad diets, group-oriented weight-loss programmes, and individual nutritional counselling. He described making necessary dietary changes early on in these programmes, including eating smaller portions and making healthier food choices. Once he was able to lose 80 lbs. However, after 6 months,

(continued)

M. Taube-Schiff, Ph.D., C.Psych. (✉)
Department of Psychiatry, Sunnybrook Health Sciences Centre, 2075 Bayview Avenue, Toronto, ON, Canada M4N 3M5

Department of Psychiatry, University of Toronto, Toronto, ON, Canada
e-mail: marlene.taube-schiff@nygh.on.ca

L. David
Department of Psychology, Ryerson University, Toronto, ON, Canada

S.E. Cassin, Ph.D., C.Psych.
Department of Psychology, Ryerson University, Toronto, ON, Canada

Department of Psychiatry, University of Toronto, Toronto, ON, Canada

Centre for Mental Health, University Health Network, Toronto, ON, Canada

S. Sockalingam, R. Hawa (eds.), *Psychiatric Care in Severe Obesity*,
DOI 10.1007/978-3-319-42536-8_16

(continued)
Mr. Davis reported that his cravings would come back and he would gain the weight he had lost, and then some. He believed this pattern of weight loss and weight regain was inevitable for him. As a result, he was left feeling hopeless about taking control of his weight and reluctant to try out any possible strategies. Further, at 350 lbs, Mr. Davis thought he had too much weight to lose. He would often tell his family physician that he was tired of being "set up for failure" when it comes to his eating. Currently, his family physician is feeling quite stuck and does not know what types of interventions would help move Mr. Davis towards making dietary changes that would improve his long-term health and stop using food as his default coping strategy.

16.1 Introduction

In this chapter, we provide an overview of motivational interviewing (MI) and the rationale for integrating it into the management of severe obesity. We then review the empirical evidence supporting the effectiveness of MI in both paediatric and adult populations with obesity. Finally, we provide a dialogue between Mr. Davis and his family physician in order to illustrate the application of MI techniques in clinical practice.

16.2 Overview of Motivational Interviewing

Motivational interviewing is a collaborative, goal-oriented style of therapeutic communication which aims to enhance intrinsic motivation for, and commitment to, a specific goal by eliciting and exploring an individual's personal reasons for change within a nonjudgmental atmosphere [1]. Ambivalence, described as the experience of simultaneously desiring two incompatible things, poses a significant barrier to change. When an individual feels ambivalent about a specific goal, he/she typically voices "change talk" (i.e. self-motivational statements that favour change) and "sustain talk" (i.e. statements that oppose change) within the same conversation, and sometimes even within the same sentence [1]. Sustain talk is often labelled as "resistance"; however, it is a normal and understandable aspect of ambivalence. Within MI practice, people are believed not to be inherently motivated or unmotivated. Rather, motivation is something that can be fostered during a conversation. If a clinician argues for the importance of change, a client who is feeling ambivalent is likely to defend the status quo. Thus, confrontation elicits defensiveness, which in turn reduces likelihood of behavioural change [1]. Given that people become more committed to that which they voice [2], MI seeks to explore and resolve ambivalence by strategically arranging conversations such that people talk *themselves* into change.

16.3 Rationale for Integrating Motivational Interviewing into the Management of Severe Obesity

Maladaptive behaviours often persist because they perform important functions for individuals; thus, it is understandable that people feel ambivalent about changing certain behaviours. For example, people eat to improve mood, reduce boredom, alleviate anxiety, and distract from stressors; thus, changing eating habits would mean having to develop new coping skills. Similarly, physical activity is effortful, and thus sedentary behaviour can feel more pleasurable in the moment if it is associated with relaxing, such as when reading a good book or enjoying a favourite TV show.

According to the Transtheoretical Model, change occurs in sequence through the following five stages: precontemplation, contemplation, determination/preparation, action, and maintenance [3]. Treatments for obesity often assume that people are ready to take action; however, this assumption is unwarranted in many cases. A mismatch between a patient's stage of change and a clinician's chosen strategy can be met with opposition [4]. For example, a well-intentioned health care professional might develop a meal plan or exercise schedule for a client with obesity, or deliver an evidence-based intervention such as a multicomponent lifestyle intervention or cognitive behavioural therapy [5]. However, the client will likely have difficulty adhering to the treatment plan if he/she is still contemplating whether or not to change eating behaviours and/or increase physical activity. As a result, the client may not improve as expected during treatment, may prematurely drop out of treatment, and/or may have difficulty maintaining progress following treatment if the goals were externally motivated. As noted below in the section on empirical support, MI has been used to improve a number of behaviours related to weight management, including increasing physical activity, improving diet, and reducing disordered eating. It has been used to raise the topic of weight management in primary care settings [6], as a stand-alone intervention [7] and as an adjunct to another intervention to increase motivation and treatment adherence [8].

16.4 Motivational Interviewing Skills and Processes

A number of excellent resources exist for learning the core skills and processes of MI [1, 9], and for applying MI in the treatment of disordered eating [10]. Motivational interviewing comprises four therapeutic processes: *engaging* the client in a therapeutic working alliance, *focusing* the direction of the conversation on the topic of change, *evoking* the client's own motivations for change, and *planning* for change by developing a plan for action and solidifying the client's commitment to change [1]. The core skills of MI ("OARS": open-ended questions, affirmations, reflections, summaries) should be used initially to engage the client, but also continued throughout the conversation about change.

It is best to start the conversation by asking an open-ended question (e.g. "Can you tell me a little bit about your current eating habits?"), which serves to open up a dialogue about the client's eating behaviours and potentially elicit self-motivational statements regarding the need to change eating habits [1]. The client can be asked to list any concerns he/she would like to discuss, and the clinician is advised to ask for permission to discuss any additional concerns that are not mentioned spontaneously by the client. Many maladaptive behaviours are not due to knowledge deficits, thus, it is recommended that clinicians assess the client's prior knowledge (e.g. "Tell me what you already know about dietary recommendations for weight loss") or ask permission to provide information (e.g. "Would you like to know about dietary recommendations for weight loss?") to acknowledge the client's right to agree or disagree with the information or advice provided and to inquire about the client's understanding of the information that has been shared (e.g. "What do you make of these dietary recommendations?").

A number of MI strategies can be used to elicit the client's own motivation for change [1]. Please see Table 16.1 for a quick reference of MI tools for obesity management. For example, the clinician can ask *open-ended questions* that are likely to elicit self-motivational statements regarding the client's desire, ability, reasons, and need for change (e.g. "What ideas do you have for how you could lose weight?"). The clinician can also use the "*importance ruler*" to assess the importance of change from the client's perspective on a scale from 1 to 10, and then process the client's response by having him/her elaborate on the reasons change is important. Another useful strategy is to help the client *envision the future* after he/she had successfully made changes (e.g. "If you lose weight, how do you imagine things would be different in the future?"). In addition to eliciting change talk, the clinician should use the core skills of MI ("OARS") to respond to self-motivational statements, such as asking the client to elaborate on a point (e.g. "Can you say a little bit more about the ways in which you imagine your health improving if you were able to lose some weight?"), reflecting the change talk back to the client, and summarizing the client's

Table 16.1 Quick reference for MI tools

MI strategy	Examples
Open-ended questions	How are you feeling about your current dietary habits?
Importance ruler	How important is it to you to make these dietary changes? (on a scale from 1 to 10; change talk is elicited by probing why and individual did not rate themselves lower than number provided)
Confidence ruler	How confident do you feel about making these dietary changes? (on a scale from 1 to 10; change talk is elicited by probing why an individual did not rate themselves lower than number provided)
Looking forward (i.e. envision future)	If you look ahead 5 years, what would you like your eating habits to be like?
Looking back	Can you remember a time in your life when you had less weight management struggles? Or a time when you felt your eating habits were healthier? What was different then as compared to now? What was life like during those periods of time?
Values	Exploring values with a patient can allow for reflection on why change is important to them. For example, people will often know that they need to change to improve their health or spend more time with young children. Spending time exploring these types of values (or others) can allow for a deepening of how change might align with their value system

self-motivational statements, which can then transition nicely into the planning stage.

Many patients with severe obesity understand that their weight has a number of adverse effects, and acknowledge that it is important to lose weight; however, they lack confidence or self-efficacy in their ability to change. Patients' readiness for change is determined *both* by the perceived importance of change *and* their confidence in their ability to change. A number of strategies can be used in MI to enhance the client's confidence for change [1]. Similar to the strategies noted above, the clinician can use a "*confidence ruler*" to assess the client's confidence in his/her ability to lose weight and ask open-ended questions that are likely to elicit statements of confidence (e.g. "What gives you some confidence that you can lose weight?"). The clinician can also elicit some examples of changes that the client has successfully made in the past, and explore whether any of the skills and strategies he/she used back then might generalize to the changes currently being considered. Additionally, it can be helpful for the client to brainstorm various options for making the change (e.g. ideas for improving eating habits, reducing binge eating, or increasing physical activity). If the client requests suggestions from the clinician, it is best to first ask the client for his/her own ideas in order to increase self-efficacy. If he/she is unable to think of any strategies, the clinician is advised to provide a variety of options and emphasize the client's personal autonomy regarding the decision (e.g. "Some clients have found it helpful to …, others have found it helpful to… You are the expert on yourself, and ultimately it's up to you to decide what will work best for you").

In the event that a client voices a lot of sustain talk, and appears to have little desire to change at the current time, the clinician can use reflective listening skills to mirror the sustain talk back to the client, and help the client envision the future if he/she does not make any changes (e.g. "Suppose you choose not to make any changes to your eating, and continue on as you have been. How do you imagine things might be in 5 years?"), and highlight his/her personal autonomy to choose whether or not to make any changes at the present time [1]. Simply knowing that one has the freedom to choose *not* to make any changes sometimes has the paradoxical effect of increasing motivation for change, and the clinician can express a willingness to return to the conversation in the future if the client so desires.

Prior to developing an action plan, clinicians are advised to test out the client's readiness to proceed [1]. This can be accomplished by simply asking the client directly (e.g. "Would it make sense at this point to start developing a meal plan, or would that be rushing into things?") or by summarizing the change talk the client vocalized throughout the conversation and asking an open-ended question that bolsters self-efficacy and autonomy (e.g. "So, what do you think you'll do?"). Clients are most likely to commit to making changes if they develop a specific action plan and vocalize their intention to carry it out. To this end, it can be helpful for the client to complete a worksheet which summarizes some of the main discussion points, including the client's goal, various options for achieving the goal, action plan, potential barriers to achieving the goal, and some proposed solutions to overcome barriers. The clinician can conclude the conversation with an open-ended question designed to strengthen commitment (e.g. "What steps are you ready to take this week?"), and praise the client's openness to discussing his/her plan for losing weight.

16.5 Empirical Evidence for MI in Obesity Management

There is a burgeoning literature supporting the efficacy of MI for obesity management [11–14]. A number of studies that have examined the use of MI for obesity management in paediatric and adult populations are described below.

Evidence supporting MI for paediatric obesity management. Recent research on the use of MI in paediatric populations with obesity has yielded promising results. For example, a recent randomized controlled trial (RCT) demonstrated that obese adolescents (mean age = 13 years, mean BMI = 29.57 kg/m^2) who were exposed to a standard weight loss management programme of physical activity plus a 6 session MI intervention demonstrated greater weight loss, enhanced physical activity, and increased motivation compared to those in the standard weight loss management programme [15]. However, the significant group differences with respect to weight were not observed 6 months later, and it was speculated that this might have been due to small sample sizes in both groups (n = 28 and 26) [15]. Another pilot RCT suggested that MI is a feasible intervention to enhance healthy eating behaviours in African-American adolescents (aged 13–17 years) with obesity [16]. The group that received the MI intervention reduced their consumption of fast food and soft drinks. They also reported an increase in intrinsic motivation regarding physical activity; however, there were no significant group differences in physical activity levels or BMI. However, given the brevity of the intervention (four sessions) the authors indicated that they did not anticipate differences in BMI [16]. Another study with adolescents (aged 13–17 years) reported that a single session MI intervention lead to reductions in the proportion of calories from fat (as a percentage of the total energy intake) and the amount of dietary cholesterol consumed 3 months following the intervention [17]. Overall, these studies suggest that MI can impact motivation, physical activity, and eating behaviours in youth. The studies conducted with adolescents to date do not demonstrate significant BMI changes following MI interventions; however, a limitation of this literature is that most MI interventions are brief in nature and the potential impact of increased dose (e.g. through additional MI sessions or follow-up booster sessions) remains to be tested.

The use of MI for adolescents (ages 14–18 years) with obesity has been found to be more effective when parental support is incorporated as an active ingredient [18]. A prospective RCT compared participants across three conditions: (1) MI plus parental involvement, (2) MI without parental involvement, and (3) a control group. Both MI interventions focused on healthy eating and physical activity. In the parental involvement condition, adolescents received an extra session of MI with their parents in order to aid parental promotion of the adolescents' weight-related goals and focus on their attitudes towards their adolescents with respect to eating behaviours and physical activity. Significant differences between groups were found on a variety of measures at 12-month follow-up. The MI plus parental involvement group demonstrated greater improvements in BMI, exercise, and nutritional habits as compared with the MI without parental involvement group and control group [18]. Furthermore, a recent study that focused solely on BMI outcomes within a paediatric primary care setting found that a brief MI intervention (i.e. four sessions) delivered to parents of overweight children (ages 2–8 years) yielded statistically significant reductions in BMI as compared to a group that only received usual care [19]. Within this study, parents received: (1) usual care from their primary care physician, (2) MI counselling from their primary care physician, or (3) MI counselling from their primary care physician supplemented by dietetic counselling. This latter group was the only intervention that differed significantly from usual care [19]. It was hypothesized that adding more sessions to the primary care MI intervention alone group might have led to significant differences. Once again, dose of treatment and means of administration of MI intervention techniques are queried as possible factors to be manipulated in producing longer term impact on weight management.

In a recent meta-analysis, the use of parental involvement with MI strategies has also been shown to be beneficial for adolescents presenting with other health-related behaviours, including obesity [20]. The interested reader is referred to this meta-analysis for an overview of 12 studies that examined the use of MI for obesity in paediatric healthcare [20]. According to the meta-analysis, several studies suggested that MI as a stand-alone intervention was more successful than when it was combined with another intervention. We now turn to an overview of the recent empirical evidence for MI interventions for adult obesity management.

Evidence supporting MI for adult obesity management. The literature supporting the use of MI in the treatment of adult obesity has grown rapidly over the past decade. Burke and colleagues [21] were the first to publish a meta-analysis investigating the efficacy of MI in controlled trials across health-behaviour domains, including diet and exercise. They included 30 studies examining MI in their analyses. The MI interventions were, on average, 180 min shorter in duration than other active treatments to which MI was compared, and yet it showed comparative efficacy in addressing dietary and exercise problems. Rubak, Sandboek, Lauritzen, and Christensen [22] have since conducted the most comprehensive review of MI, with the inclusion of 72 RCTs of MI in the treatment of several disease indicators, including weight. MI produced a statistically significant effect in almost three quarters (74 %) of the studies reviewed, with a large combined estimate effect size for BMI reduction in particular. These large meta-analyses speak to the potential role of MI in managing obesity for adults.

A more recent systematic review of the literature examined the use of MI interventions in primary care for individuals with obesity. Twenty-four RCTs were examined and most patients were reported to be "obese" or "overweight" although specific BMIs were not reported for every study [23] Results suggested that in over one-third of the studies analysed, patients who received MI interventions experienced greater weight loss than those who received usual care, often consisting of what was referred to as "standard dietary care" [23]. Half of the studies reported that participants lost 5 % of their initial weight. This review suggests that MI strategies can be used effectively within a primary care setting and may begin to aid in dietary changes that could provide initial weight loss [23].

MI has not only shown promise for improving dietary patterns and physical activity levels, but also for affecting change in obesity-associated medical conditions. For example, a recent study examined the long-term impact of a 6-month MI intervention on both behavioural and biomedical risk factors for cardiovascular disease [7]. A physical activity specialist as well as a registered dietitian delivered the intervention and this group was compared to those receiving standard information. At 18-month follow-up, significant improvements were noted in physical activity (walking) and cholesterol levels although initial BMI reductions were not maintained [7]. MI has also been found effective in improving patients' glucose management and physical activity levels both alone and in combination with other interventions [24]. Thus, the use of MI as a clinical intervention appears to have broader applications for obesity management, extending beyond weight and dietary changes.

MI interventions can be flexibly used across health care settings. In this regard, it has been empirically studied not only as a stand-alone intervention for improving BMI, eating patterns, and self-efficacy [12], but also an adjunctive intervention intended to promote adherence to another treatment. For example, adding MI to a standard behavioural programme for individuals with obesity and type 2 diabetes enhanced adherence to programme recommendations, including higher attendance, greater completion of food diaries, and more frequent blood glucose level recordings [8]. In a larger study examining the same outcomes, increased adherence and engagement in a behavioural programme accounted for a significant portion of the enhanced weight loss seen in the MI group at both the 6- and 18-month follow-ups [25]. Taken together, these studies suggest that MI can be used as an adjunct to behavioural weight loss programmes to increase treatment adherence and optimize weight loss outcomes.

Research has also examined the impact of MI in improving eating pathology that can contribute to obesity, such as binge eating disorder (BED). A recent systematic review concluded that MI holds promise in the treatment of BED and binge eating behaviours [26]. The inclusion of one MI session to a self-help programme for binge eating increased an individual's readiness to change, especially for people in the pre-contemplation and contemplation stages of change [27]. Cassin and colleagues [28] conducted the first RCT examining the efficacy of MI for BED. Compared to a control group (self-help handbook only), the MI group (single-session MI intervention plus the self-help handbook) reported increased confidence in their ability to reduce binge eating after the session and reported greater improvements in binge eating, mood, self-esteem, and quality of life 4 months later. A greater proportion of individuals in the MI group abstained from binge eating (27.8 % vs. 11.1 %) and no longer met diagnostic criteria for BED (87.0 % vs. 57.4 %). A recent study compared MI to psychoeducation as a prelude to self-help treatment for binge eating [29]. Participants had a diagnosis of full or subthreshold DSM-IV BED or nonpurging bulimia nervosa. Individuals in both groups reported decreases in eating-related pathology (i.e. attitudes towards eating, binge eating abstinence). The MI group reported greater readiness to change and eating self-efficacy as compared to the psychoeducation group; however, it did not have a significant impact on actual binge eating behaviour [29]. It is possible that a longer follow-up period is required for readiness to change to translate into modifications in eating-relating pathology, such as binge eating.

Findings from both the paediatric and adult obesity management literature suggest that MI can be delivered in a variety of clinical contexts, including primary care settings, allowing for a potentially extensive impact. Future research should examine the key ingredients in MI sessions, the training required to develop competence in MI, and the number of sessions that might afford the best impact of MI for obesity management.

16.6 Application of MI Techniques

Given the reviewed empirical support for the use of MI in the management of obesity, it could potentially be used to enhance Mr. Davis' intrinsic motivation to change his eating behaviours. It appears as though Mr. Davis is "stuck" (as is his family doctor!). He has had multiple past attempts at weight loss with great initial success, followed by long-term disappointment. These past experiences, and the fact that he is currently at his heaviest weight, have understandably caused him to move back towards a *contemplative* stage of change as opposed to being in *action* mode, as he likely was during his past weight loss attempts. Below is an example dialogue between Mr. Davis and his general practitioner (GP) illustrating a few ways in which these issues can be explored using MI.

GP: It makes sense that you would feel ambivalent about trying to lose weight again. It does involve a lot of effort and you mentioned that you've had difficulties keeping the weight off in the past. On the other hand, it sounds like you're also concerned about your health if you do not lose weight. Can you tell me a little bit more about the concerns you have about your health?

Mr. Davis: I worry about how my obesity impacts my risk of getting sick. My family has a long history of heart problems, and at my current weight there is a greater chance that I could have a heart attack in my 50s or 60s. My wife and kids rely on me, and the thought of being gone too soon terrifies me.

GP: So, it sounds like you're really concerned about the ways in which your weight impacts your physical health, and what that means for your family in the future.

Mr. Davis: Exactly. And even now, my weight affects my ability to do things with them. My arthritis is getting worse, and the pain prevents me from going on trips that we used to take together. It's really beginning to affect my quality of life.

GP: So, you are noticing that your weight affects your arthritis, which, in turn, limits your ability to do a lot of activities you used to enjoy. That sounds difficult. Your quality of life is impacted and it sounds like you are concerned for yourself and your children.

Mr. Davis: Yes. My low self-esteem also holds me back. Even if I wasn't in pain, I don't think I would want to do anything because I'm so embarrassed by how I look.

GP: You've raised a number of reasons why it might be helpful to change your eating. What are the three more important ones to you?

Mr. Davis: Well, it would allow me to get back to the activities I used to enjoy, plus give me confidence to try new ones, all of which would help me reconnect with my family. I'd also like to set a good example for my children, and model a healthy lifestyle so that they don't go down the same path that I did.

GP: How important would you say it is for you to change your eating habits on a scale from 0 to 10; where 0 is not at all important, and 10 is extremely important?

Mr. Davis: I'd say a 6.

GP: That's great. You're already above the midpoint. And why are you at a 6 rather than a 5? *(Note to clinicians, in order to try and elicit change talk, it is important to probe why the individual rated themselves at a higher number compared to a lower number)*

Mr. Davis: Well, I know deep down it's important. Especially, as I get older and my health becomes more of a concern. And now that I'm thinking about how this change may affect my children, it really is a priority. It's now or never.

GP: If you did decide to make changes to your eating, what would that look like?

Mr. Davis: I don't know. All I know from past experiences is what didn't work.

GP: Okay, so you have the advantage now of having gone through this process in the past and learning what was and was not helpful for you. How might you go about it this time in order to succeed?

Mr. Davis: Well I remember that journaling my eating helped, but I always forgot to bring the journal around with me. Perhaps I could start tracking it on my phone instead.

GP: That sounds like an excellent idea. How might monitoring your eating be beneficial for you?

Mr. Davis: It forces me to pay attention to what I was eating, and it was good to see when I was eating in response to emotions rather than actual hunger so that I could try something else first. I could also try doing other activities in the evenings when I normally crave snacks. I find I'm most likely to eat when I'm watching television.

GP: Great! What kinds of activities come to mind?

Mr. Davis: I could call a friend, do some rearranging, or go for a walk.

GP: Good ideas. From what I've heard so far, and correct me if I'm wrong, it sounds like there have been a number of times in the past when you've tried to get control over your eating which haven't been successful in the long run, which is a big part of why it has been so difficult to think about changing your eating habits again. And yet, I am also hearing you say that there are a number of reasons you would like to try again, including your physical health, quality of life, and relationship with your family. From your past experiences, it sounds like you have a number of good ideas regarding strategies that could be helpful in losing weight. So, what do you think you'll do?

Mr. Davis: Well, I mean it's tough. When I vocalize all the reasons I want to lose weight, the harm in trying again seems minimal. I know I'll feel disappointed if this change isn't successful, but I already feel like a disappointment at my weight right now. I've gotten so used to convincing myself that I will never do it that I forget all the reasons I wanted to try it in the first place. I think my past attempts have given me some ideas of where I could try to start with this change. I will start journaling my eating on my phone. I can see how it goes and then judge the next step from there.

As illustrated in the example above, MI strategies can be used to elicit change talk and prompt Mr. Davis to generate his own ideas about how he can begin to get back on track. After some of these strategies have been employed, the clinician may then want to create some concrete plans about what Mr. Davis is willing to try out and reassess these plans as he implements them, ensuring he feels confident to make the changes and exploring barriers and challenges as they might emerge along the way.

16.7 Summary and Take Home Messages

- Motivational interviewing (MI) is a collaborative conversation that aims to increase a client's intrinsic motivation to change.
- MI employs techniques that help to resolve a client's ambivalence regarding behaviour change and to bolster his/her self-efficacy for making the change successfully.
- MI has been used effectively as both a standalone and adjunctive intervention to help individuals with obesity improve eating behaviours and enhance weight loss.
- In positively influencing weight loss and dietary patterns, MI also affects improvements on other weight-related psychosocial and medical outcomes.

References

1. Miller WR, Rollnick S. Motivational interviewing: helping people change. 3rd ed. New York: Guilford Press; 2013.
2. Bem DJ. Self-perception: an alternative interpretation of cognitive dissonance phenomena. Psychol Rev. 1967;74(3):183–200. doi:10.1037/h0024835.
3. Prochaska JO, DiClemente CC. The transtheoretical approach: crossing traditional boundaries of change. Homewood, IL: Dow Jones/Irwin; 1983.
4. Prochaska JO. Change at differing stages. In: Snyder CR, Ingram RE, editors. Handbook of psychological change. New York: Wiley; 2000. p. 109–27.
5. National Institute for Health and Care Excellence. Obesity: identification, assessment, and management (NICE clinical guideline 189). London: NICE; 2014.
6. Hardcastle SJ, Taylor AH, Bailey MP, Castle R. A randomised controlled trial on the effectiveness of a primary health care counselling intervention on physical activity, diet, and CHD risk factors. Patient Educ Couns. 2008;70(1):31–9. doi:10.1136/bmj.d5928.
7. Hardcastle SJ, Taylor AH, Bailey MP, Harley RA, Hagger MS. Effectiveness of a motivational interviewing intervention on weight loss, physical activity and cardiovascular disease risk factors: a randomised controlled trial with a 12-month post-intervention follow-up. Int J Behav Nutr Phys Act. 2013;10:40. doi:10.1186/1479-5868-10-40.
8. Smith DE, Heckemeyer C, Kraft PP, Mason DA. Motivational interviewing to improve adherence to a behavioural weight-control program for older obese women with NIDDM. Diabetes Care. 1997;20(1):52–4. doi:10.2337/diacare.20.1.52.
9. Rollnick S, Miller WR, Butler CC. Motivational interviewing in health care: helping patients change behavior. New York: Guilford Press; 2008.
10. Cassin SE, Geller J. Motivational interviewing in the treatment of disordered eating. In: Arkowitz H, Miller WR, Rollnick S, editors. Motivational interviewing in the treatment of psychological problems. 2nd ed. New York: Guilford Press; 2015. p. 344–64.
11. Carels RA, Darby L, Cacciapaglia HM, Konrad K, Coit C, Harper J, et al. Using motivational interviewing as a supplement to obesity treatment: a stepped-care approach. Health Psychol. 2007;26(3):369–74. doi:10.1037/0278-6133.26.3.369.
12. Meybodi FA, Pourshrifi DH, Dastbaravarde ARR, Saeedi Z. The effectiveness of motivational interview on weight reduction and self-efficacy in Iranian overweight and obese women. Procedia Soc Behav Sci. 2011;30:1395–8. doi:10.1016/j.sbspro.2011.10.271.
13. Navidian A, Abedi M, Baghban I, Fatehizadeh M, Poursharifi H, Dehkordi M. Effects of motivational interviewing on weight loss of individuals suffering from hypertension. Iranian J Nutr Sci Food Technol. 2010;5:45–52.
14. Christie D, Channon S. The potential for motivational interviewing to improve outcomes in the management of diabetes and obesity in paediatric and adult populations: a clinical review. Diabetes Obes Metab. 2014;16(5):381–7. doi:10.1111/dom.12195.
15. Gourlan M, Sarrazin P, Trouilloud D. Motivational interviewing as a way to promote physical activity in obese adolescents: a randomised-controlled trial using self-determination theory as an explanatory framework. Psychol Health. 2013;28(11):1265–86. doi:10.1080/08870446.2013.800518.

16. Macdonell K, Brogan K, Naar-King S, Ellis D, Marshall S. A pilot study of motivational interviewing targeting weight-related behaviors in overweight or obese African American adolescents. J Adolesc Health. 2012;50(2):201–3. doi:10.1016/j.jadohealth.2011.04.018.
17. Berg-Smith SM, Stevens VJ, Brown KM, Van Horn L, Gernhofer N, Peters E, et al. A brief motivational intervention to improve dietary adherence in adolescents. The Dietary Intervention Study in Children (DISC) Research Group. Health Educ Res. 1999;14(3):399–410. doi:10.1093/her/14.3.399.
18. Pakpour AH, Gellert P, Dombrowski SU, Fridlund B. Motivational interviewing with parents for obesity: an RCT. Pediatrics. 2015;135(3):e644–52. doi:10.1543/peds.2014-1987.
19. Resnicow K, McMaster F, Bocian A, Harris D, Zhou Y, Snetselaar L, et al. Motivational interviewing and dietary counseling for obesity in primary care: an RCT. Pediatrics. 2015;135(4):649–57. doi:10.1542/peds.2014-1880.
20. Gayes LA, Steele RG. A meta-analysis of motivational interviewing interventions for pediatric health behavior change. J Consult Clin Psychol. 2014;82(3):521–35. doi:10.1037/a0035917.
21. Burke BL, Arkowitz H, Menchola M. The efficacy of motivational interviewing: a meta-analysis of controlled clinical trials. J Consult Clin Psychol. 2003;71(5):843–61. doi:10.1037/0022-006X.71.5.843.
22. Rubak S, Sandboek A, Lauritzen T, Christensen B. Motivational interviewing: a systematic review and meta-analysis. Br J Gen Pract. 2005;55(513):305–12.
23. Barnes RD, Ivezaj V. A systematic review of motivational interviewing for weight loss among adults in primary care. Obes Rev. 2015;16(4):304–18. doi:10.1111/obr.12264.
24. Martins RK, McNeil DW. Review of motivational interviewing in promoting health behaviors. Clin Psychol Rev. 2009;29(4):283–93. doi:10.1016/j.cpr.2009.02.001.
25. West DS, DiLillo V, Bursac Z, Gore SA, Greene PG. Motivational interviewing improves weight loss in women with type 2 diabetes. Diabetes Care. 2007;30(5):1081–7. doi:10.2337/dc06-1966.
26. Macdonald P, Hibbs R, Corfield F, Treasure J. The use of motivational interviewing in eating disorders: a systematic review. Psychiatry Res. 2012;200(1):1–11. doi:10.1016/j.psychres.2012.05.013.
27. Dunn EC, Neighbors C, Larimer ME. Motivational enhancement therapy and self-help for binge eaters. Psychol Addict Behav. 2006;20(1):44–52. doi:10.1037/0893-164X.20.1.44.
28. Cassin SE, von Ranson KM, Heng K, Brar J, Wojtowicz AE. Adapted motivational interviewing for women with binge eating disorder: a randomized controlled trial. Psychol Addict Behav. 2008;22(3):417–25. doi:10.1037/0893-164X.22.3.417.
29. Vella-Zarb RA, Mills JS, Westra HA, Carter JC, Keating L. A randomized controlled trial of motivational interviewing + self-help versus psychoeducation + self-help for binge eating. Int J Eat Disord. 2015;48(3):328–32. doi:10.1002/eat.22242.

17 Mindful Eating for Severe Obesity

Susan Wnuk and Chau Du

17.1 Introduction

The purpose of this chapter is to review mindful eating interventions for adults with severe obesity. Mindfulness interventions that specifically target problematic eating behaviors such as overeating, binge eating, grazing, and emotional eating[1] will be the focus of this chapter rather than mindfulness interventions like mindfulness-based stress reduction [1] or mindfulness-based cognitive therapy [2, 3] that are used with other mental health conditions like depression and anxiety. Also, we will not include integrative interventions such as acceptance and commitment therapy [4] or dialectical behavior therapy [5], which incorporate mindfulness into protocols that are primarily focused on skills and techniques to increase acceptance and skillful regulation of emotion.

> **Case Vignette**
>
> Betty is a 59-year-old, married Caucasian Canadian female with type 2 diabetes, osteoarthritis, obstructive sleep apnea, hypertension, and lower back pain. At a height of 159 cm and a weight of 78.18 kg, her Body Mass Index (BMI) is 30.50. She has struggled with obesity and yo-yo dieting since her mid-twenties. While Betty reported losing weight through various commercial weight-loss programs in the past, she would often regain all the weight back and more. She further endorsed eating large portions and a history of binge eating since her mid-twenties in response to interpersonal stressors. She estimated that her lowest adult weight was 78.38 kg and her highest was 113.4 kg when she was 21 and 45 years old, respectively.
>
> Betty reported losing approximately 15 kg 1 year ago in the span of 4 months by making heathier food choices and exercising three to four times per week, including swimming, strength training, and gentle

(continued)

[1] The term *problem eating* will be used to refer to eating and overeating in response to cues other than physical hunger and past the point of satiety, including painful or aversive emotions, grazing or frequently eating small amounts of food throughout the day, night eating, and dysregulated or chaotic eating patterns characterized by irregular meal times such as eating once per day or an absence of regular meal times.

S. Wnuk, B.A., M.A., Ph.D. (✉) • C. Du
Toronto Western Hospital Bariatric Surgery Program, University Health Network, 399 Bathurst Street, Toronto, ON, Canada M5T 2S8
e-mail: susan.wnuk@gmail.com

S. Sockalingam, R. Hawa (eds.), *Psychiatric Care in Severe Obesity*,
DOI 10.1007/978-3-319-42536-8_17

(continued)
hatha yoga. However, in the past 6 months, she reported engaging in a two binge eating episodes per week to help her cope with her mother's declining health. Furthermore, she has a difficult relationship with her older brother. Her distress over this relationship prompts her to eat to self-soothe, and she tends to eat in secrecy because she is ashamed of overeating. She also stopped exercising and grazed on bread, crackers, or nuts when she was bored, sad, or feeling overwhelmed. She described feeling "out of control" of her eating at times, grazing during the day and going back for additional portions of food at mealtimes even though she was no longer hungry. Betty did not present with extreme dieting behaviors such as vomiting, laxative abuse, fasting, or excessive exercise to compensate for her eating.

Betty currently lives with her husband of 34 years and described their relationship as loving and supportive. She has three adult children who live on their own. Her highest level of education is a university degree in economics. She has been retired for 4 years after working as a senior manager at an insurance brokerage firm for 15 years. Betty noted that she is the primary caregiver to her aging mother who has dementia. Her husband also expressed concern that Betty avoids dinner invitations or gatherings with their friends or extended family for fear of being criticized about her eating or weight.

At intake, Betty reported some anxiety regarding her weight and longevity and she was tearful when talking about her mother and brother. She completed eight sessions of individual psychotherapy 2 years ago. She is currently on escitalopram for anxiety symptoms and trazodone for sleep.

She enrolled in a ten-session Mindfulness Based Eating and Awareness Training (MB-EAT) program. Her goals were to lose an additional 3–5 kg and hopefully improve blood sugar control by controlling emotional eating and overeating.

17.2 The Roots of Mindful Eating Interventions

In recent years, the topic of mindfulness has experienced a surge in publication in both the popular and academic press, particularly in psychotherapy research [6]. While over the past 30 years a significant amount of scientific research has been devoted to examining the efficacy of mindfulness-based interventions (MBIs) and this research is described below, it is important to acknowledge the many mindful eating books and programs for general audiences that have not been evaluated through research. Patients and practitioners may find these selected books helpful as resource guides.

Mindfulness meditation techniques are practices that aim to improve control over one's attention and the ability to focus. This training is done with an attitude of acceptance and without judgment or interpretation of thoughts, feelings, and sensations [7]. Practitioners train by focusing on stimuli like their own breathing, bodily sensations, sights, sounds, thoughts, and emotions [1, 8]. Many mindfulness exercises can be practiced while sitting or lying down in a relaxed posture, or while engaged in routine activities such as walking and, especially important for our purposes, eating. Regular practice of mindfulness facilitates increased self-awareness and self-acceptance and reduced reactivity to passing thoughts and emotions, thereby improving one's ability to make adaptive choices when experiencing painful emotions or difficult situations [5].

Mindfulness is rooted in Eastern contemplative traditions and is the proposed "heart" of Buddhist meditation [9]. In Buddhist traditions, mindful eating is considered a fundamental aspect in a way of living that helps prevent unnecessary harm to one's body and mind [10]. In *Savor: Mindful Eating, Mindful Life*, Zen Master Thich Nhat Hanh and Harvard nutritionist, Dr. Lilian Cheung applies Buddhist teachings on The Four Noble Truths to understanding eating problems, obesity, and the achievement of a healthy weight. The Four Noble Truths are a framework that identifies recurrent dissatisfaction and at times suffering as the primary ailment of the human condition [11]. Suffering, here, is considered noble because it motivates individuals to gently investigate it and to be open to the possibility for change. According to Hanh and Cheung [12], The Four Noble Truths of Healthy Weight are (1) being overweight or obese is suffering; (2) you can identify the roots of your weight problem; (3) reaching a healthy weight is possible and suffering can end; and, (4) you can follow a mindful path to a healthy weight. Furthermore, it is the awareness of the present moment, and the insight that comes from investigating *why, what*, and *how* individuals eat, that make changing problem eating possible. Many Buddhist teachers recommend that individuals integrate mindfulness with eating as a way to become fully present in the moment with all aspects of daily life, including walking, working, sitting, talking, preparing food, serving, and much more [13, 14].

Dr. Jan Chozen Bays is a pediatrician and a Zen Priest who has been teaching meditation since 1985. In her book, *Mindful Eating: A Guide to Rediscovering a Healthy and Joyful Relationship with Food,* Bays [14] describes seven types of hunger: eye hunger, nose hunger, mouth hunger, stomach hunger, cellular hunger, mind hunger, and heart hunger. These concepts are also taught in *Mindful Eating-Conscious Living* (ME-CL), a nine-session program that focuses on helping individuals struggling with disordered eating and body image issues reestablish a healthy and pleasurable relationship with food and eating. Instead of focusing on weight loss and dieting, Bays' approach encourages participants to engage with all of their senses, cultivate awareness, and to bring loving-kindness and compassion to their everyday lives, including suffering (First Noble Truth).

17.3 Rationale for Mindful Eating Interventions

Now that MBSR and MBCT have been evaluated in many clinical settings for over a decade, research aimed at identifying the mechanisms of change in these interventions has been conducted [15]. Consistent evidence has been found that these mechanisms include a decrease in cognitive and emotional reactivity, increased mindfulness and decreased repetitive negative thinking, and increases in self-compassion and psychological flexibility. Moreover, mindfulness and decreased repetitive negative thinking have been found to be significant mediators of the impact of these interventions on clinical outcomes. While this research has not yet been conducted for mindful eating, we can speculate that similar change processes may be at work.

The ability to change habits is key to weight loss, yet this is a surprisingly complex and difficult task that involves becoming aware of and changing many thoughts, beliefs, behaviors, and emotions related to eating and one's self. These include the type of food, when the food is eaten and with whom, and in what setting or situations. Monitoring and changing these behaviors in the face of fatigue, daily stressors, painful emotions, and unexpected events can be extremely challenging, especially long term [16]. The high-calorie, highly palatable processed convenience foods that are easily accessible and heavily advertised in most developed nations makes these tasks even more difficult. The rationale for mindful eating as an intervention for obesity begins with the understanding that mindfulness practice helps develop an awareness of and acceptance of these challenges and one's responses to them, thereby increasing the odds of making skillful decisions. Unlike traditional diets that provide externally imposed rules about what, when, and how to eat, mindful eating is an "inside out" approach that begins with enhancing awareness of one's personal experience with food and eating. Please see Checklist 1 for a summary of mindful eating principles.

In contrast, mindless eating entails eating without awareness and not prompted by physical hunger, in response to food and eating-related cues such as the size, shape, aroma, and color of food or food packaging and situational distractions or pressures such as social events or people [17]. In fact, in a study investigating the impact of environmental cues on eating-related decisions, Wansink and Sobal [17] found that individuals made 227 eating and beverage-related decisions per day but were only aware of 14 of these. Obese participants made more decisions than overweight or normal weight participants though the difference between obese and normal weight participants was not statistically significant. When the size of servings and serving containers was manipulated, participants underestimated how much they actually ate.

While not every person who is obese has an eating disorder, obese individuals have been found to have higher rates of binge eating disorder (BED) and night eating syndrome (NES) in comparison with those who are not obese [18, 19]. The overeating and nocturnal eating characteristic of these disorders or the subclinical versions of these disorders can contribute to weight gain. In the mindful eating approach to obesity, emotion dysregulation is seen as an important underlying cause of binge eating and other types of problem eating: when experiencing painful emotions, individuals with problem eating overeat or eat impulsively, often with disregard to physical hunger, as an emotion avoidance strategy [20]. Excess calories may thus be consumed in an automatic or dissociative manner [21], thus leading to weight gain over time. This eating may occur with or without prior conscious intent and decision-making [22], further strengthening the rationale for improving mindful awareness of eating as a route to improving eating behavior.

A model of emotional schemas proposed by Leahy [23] suggests that individuals who label their emotions as pathological or aversive may attempt to reduce awareness of their emotional states through impulsive behaviors such as substance use, dissociation, or binge eating. Mindfulness practice counters this tendency by facilitating an acceptance and understanding of painful emotions. Because mindfulness training involves purposeful and sustained attention to internal dialogues, emotions, and bodily cues, patients learn to recognize and allow and tolerate aversive affect without engaging in problematic eating. Evidence for this model has been found in the significant relationship between levels of emotional eating and weight loss success: successful weight control was associated with decreases in emotional eating between baseline and a 1-year follow-up and with low levels of emotional eating at both time points. In contrast, unsuccessful weight control was associated with increases in emotional eating between baseline and follow-up and with high levels at both time points [24].

In addition to empirical support for the affect regulation model, research also suggests that individuals with eating disorders have limited interoceptive awareness [24]. Repeated past diets that teach people to rely on external rules for eating may lead to the loss of one's ability to recognize, accept, or respond to internal cues of hunger, taste, satiety, and fullness [25–27]. This is supported by research identifying the environmental cues that contribute to mindless eating and underestimation of portion sizes [17]. On questionnaire measures of external eating (the tendency to eat in response to the taste, sight, or smell of palatable food), a positive relationship has been found between BMI and obesity [24, 28–30]. Such measures have also been associated with retrospective accounts of adult weight gain [31, 32] and to predict weight regain following weight loss [33].

It is possible that these observations are linked [34]: over time, persistent attempts to avoid or reduce emotions may result in a decreased awareness of internal states. Conversely, a low baseline level of interoceptive awareness may result in elevated distress during intense emotions and an increased likelihood of using avoidant coping strategies like binge eating. Regardless of the directionality of the association, increasing interoceptive awareness may be an important component of treatments targeting affect regulation [35–37]. One study which investigated the link between participants' dispositional mindfulness and eating behavior found that dispositional mindfulness was associated with more restrained, and less emotional and external eating behavior in obese outpatients, above and beyond depression and anxiety symptoms [38]. This finding strengthens the premise that increasing mindfulness may lead to decreased problem eating, and thereby weight loss and/or healthier food choices. Please see Kristeller and Epel [39] for a detailed review of

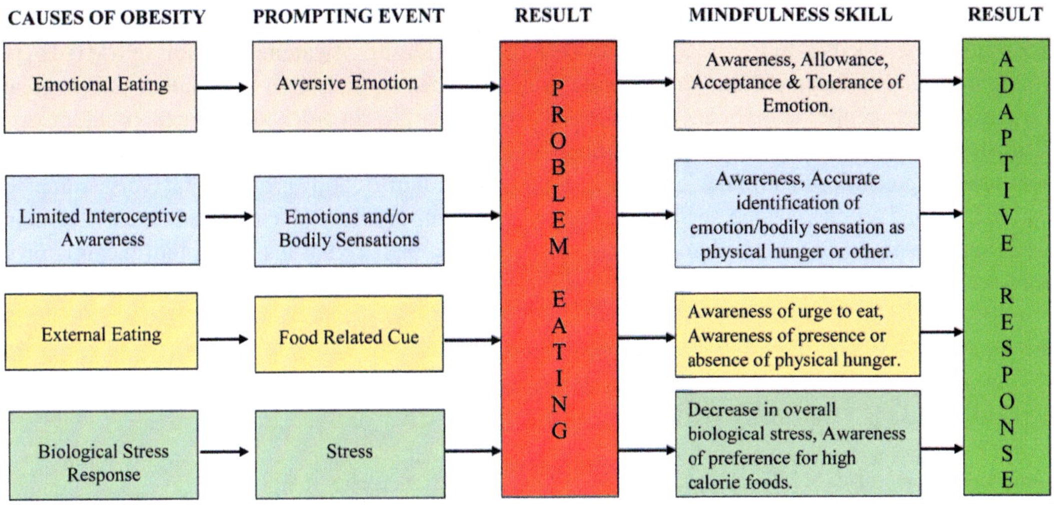

Flow Chart 17.1 Summary of mechanisms of change for mindful eating interventions

the theory and research underpinning the use of mindful eating for individuals who are overweight or obese and struggle with problem eating.

In addition to the links between emotion dysregulation/avoidance and externally cued eating with problem eating, a complementary rationale for mindful eating may be found in our understanding of the body's biological stress response, which has been associated with increased feelings of hunger, preference for high-fat and high-sugar foods, and abdominal fat deposition [40]. Thus, another mechanism for mindfulness meditation's effectiveness may be through its ability to attenuate the biological stress response and improve adaptive responding to stress. Please see Flow Chart 17.1 for an illustration.

17.4 Outcome Research

17.4.1 Overview

Mindfulness approaches have been shown to be effective treatments for psychological and physiological symptoms in patient populations including depression, anxiety, and stress [41, 42] with moderate effectiveness [43] and the body of research evidence for specific mindful eating interventions is preliminary but promising. Mindful eating interventions tend to be modeled after MBSR and MBCT and as such are usually delivered in multi-session closed groups to allow participants to share their experiences and for delivery of the intervention to multiple individuals at one time.

Outcome research that measures change in BMI, eating behaviors, and psychological correlates such as anxiety and depression has been published on several mindfulness-based treatments for eating disorders and problem eating. These are summarized below. Based on the description of treatment in these papers, they appear to share common practice elements such as mindful breathing and eating, body scan meditations, gentle yoga, didactics about healthy eating, and eating-related CBT techniques. Interventions that specifically incorporate mindful eating into all or most sessions should be used with individuals with eating concerns, as compared with mindfulness interventions such MBSR and MBCT that do not have this specific focus [44].

Mindful eating interventions tend to encourage moderation in food choices and the inclusion of small portions of the high-fat, high-sugar, and high-salt foods that individuals typically binge on. These foods are used in mindful eating practice so participants learn to eat them slowly and with full awareness [45]. This is in contrast to typical diets that exclude certain foods or food group and to the food addiction model, which advocates abstaining from "addictive" foods [46].

Mindful eating interventions incorporate a variety of therapeutic components, making it difficult to identify which component or components are responsible for clinical outcomes. So far, dismantling studies, which seek to compare a treatment with and without elements that are purported to be of therapeutic benefit, have not been done. Therefore, it is difficult to establish the superiority of any one treatment protocol in particular, especially without the availability of detailed protocols. The main exception to the lack of protocol availability is Mindfulness-Based Eating Awareness Training (MB-EAT) developed by Kristeller and Hallett [47] to treat binge eating disorder and related problem eating. At this time, MB-EAT is the only research-based mindful eating protocol that is disseminated in its entirety through organized teacher-training courses. MB-EAT is also the mindful eating protocol that has generated the greatest number of publications [21, 47–49]. Please see Table 17.1 for a summary of the components of mindful eating-related mindfulness exercises used in MB-EAT.

Table 17.1 Components of MB-EAT: principles and related exercises (Kristeller & Wolever, 2011)

Concept/principle	Component	Session	Exercise
1. *Cultivating mindfulness*			
(a) Cultivate capacity to direct attention, be aware, disengage reactivity, and be nonjudgmental	(a) Mindfulness meditation practice	1–10	(a) Sitting practice in session. Meditation homework
(b) Cultivate capacity to bring mindfulness into daily experience, including eating	(b) "Mini-meditations." General use of mindfulness	2–10	(b) "Mini-meditation" use. Brief practice in all sessions
(c) Cultivating/engaging inner and outer "wisdom"	(c) Meditation practice/ mindfulness in daily life	All sessions	(c) Encouragement of insight. Wisdom meditation (Session 10)
2. *Cultivating mindful eating*			
(a) Bring mindful attention and awareness to eating experience. Recognizing mindless eating	(a) Meditation practice. Mini-meditations. Chain reaction model	1–10	(a) Wide range of practices (see below for specifics)
(b) Cultivate taste experience/ savoring and enjoying food	(b) Mindfully eating raisins. All mindful eating experiences	1, 2, 4, 6, 7, 9	(b) Raisins: cheese and crackers; chocolate; fruit and veggies; "favorite food"; pot-luck/buffet homework
(c) Cultivate awareness of hunger experience	(c) Hunger awareness	3	(c) Hunger meditation; homework
(d) Awareness and cultivation of sensory-specific satiety/taste satisfaction	(d) Training in sensory-specific satiety, both in and out of session	4, 7	(d) Taste satisfaction "meter"
(e) Making mindful food choices, based on both "liking" and health	(e) "Inner wisdom" and "outer wisdom" in regard to food choice. Mindful decrease in calories	2, 4–6, 7	(e) Choice: chips, cookies, or grapes. Mindful use of nutrition info. 500 Calorie Challenge. Managing social influences
(f) Awareness and cultivation of fullness experience	(f) Mindfully ending a meal	1–6	(f) Fullness awareness/ ratings
(g) Awareness of negative self-judgment regarding eating. Cultivate nonjudgmental awareness of eating experience	(g) Eating challenging foods. Identifying cognitive distortions	2–6, 9, 10	(g) Identifying "black and white" thinking; "surfing the urge"

(continued)

Table 17.1 (continued)

Concept/principle	Component	Session	Exercise
3. *Cultivating emotional balance*			
(a) Cultivate awareness of emotions and emotional reactivity	(a) Learn to identify and tolerate emotional triggers	3–5, 9, 10	(a) Mindfulness practice; chain reaction model; mini-meditations
(b) Meeting emotional needs in healthy ways	(b) Behavior substitution; modifying comfort eating	Most sessions	(b) Emotional eating visualization. Savoring food
4. *Cultivating self-acceptance*			
(a) Acceptance and non-self-judgment of body/self-regulation/gentle exercise	(a) Relationship to the body	1, 3–5, 8	(a) Breath awareness; body scan practice; healing self-touch; chair yoga; pedometers; mindful walking
(b) Recognition of anger at self and others. Acceptance of self/others	(b) Exploring feeling and thoughts toward self and others	4, 5, 10	(b) Loving kindness meditation. Forgiveness meditation. Discussion
(c) Recognizing and engaging capacity for growth. Self-empowerment	(c) Cultivating and honoring wisdom in self	All Sessions	(c) Wisdom meditation. Discussion throughout

17.5 Mindful Eating for Problem Eating

Recent reviews have concluded that mindfulness approaches can improve outcomes in individuals with problem eating [50, 51]. In interventions ranging from 1 to 24 sessions and with 7–150 participants, mindfulness practice effectively decreased binge eating and emotional eating in populations engaging in this behavior. These interventions have been used with both patient and non-patient participants and with overweight and obese participants.

In any early outcome study, Kristeller and Hallett [47] used MB-EAT with 18 overweight/obese women (average BMI = 40) with binge eating disorder. They found a significant improvement in participants' perceived control of eating and awareness of hunger and satiety cues. After the seven session intervention run over 6 weeks, only four participants still met criteria for BED and remaining binges decreased substantially in size. There were no significant changes in weight however, prompting the authors to incorporate more information and skill building regarding nutrition and food choices in future groups. The amount of time participants practiced mindfulness was related to outcomes. Since the publication of this study, several others have been run and disseminated.

For example, Daubenmier et al. [52] investigated the use of a mindful eating intervention with 47 overweight/obese women who were randomly assigned to a 4-month intervention or a wait list group to explore effects of a mindful eating program for stress eating. Participants improved in mindfulness, anxiety, and externally based eating but did not differ on average cortisol awakening response (CAR), weight, or abdominal fat over time. However, obese treatment participants showed significant reductions in CAR and maintained body weight while obese control participants had stable CAR and gained weight. Improvements in mindfulness, chronic stress, and CAR were associated with reductions in abdominal fat.

In a follow-up study, Kristeller et al. [53] conducted an RCT of MB-EAT for 150 individuals with an average BMI of 40.3, 66 % of whom met DSM-IV-TR criteria for BED. The comparison groups were a psychoeducational/cognitive behavior intervention and a wait list control. Weight management was briefly discussed in both the psychoeducation and MB-EAT groups but were not the focus of either treatment. The MB-EAT and psychoeducation participants showed comparable improvement after 1 and 4 months post-intervention on bingeing and depression. At 4 months posttreatment, 5 % of those who had met criteria for BED in the MB-EAT continued to meet criteria for BED, compared with 24 % of those in the psychoeducation group. Amount of mindfulness practice predicted improvement on weight loss and other variables. In terms of weight loss, 29 % in the psychoeducation group and 38 % in the MB-EAT group lost 5 lbs or more during the course of the study. There was an overall pattern of larger effect sizes for the MB-EAT group as compared to the psychoeducation group on measures of reactivity to food including disinhibition and hunger, indicating greater self-regulation and behavioral control in the MB-EAT group.

Bush et al. [54] developed a 10-week group intervention integrating mindfulness and intuitive eating skills for 124 female employees at a university. Participants with anorexia and bulimia were excluded. The goal of the intervention was to reduce body dissatisfaction and decrease problematic eating behaviors. Participants in the treatment condition in comparison to wait list controls reported higher levels of body appreciation and lower levels of problem eating. In addition, mindfulness scores served as a partial mediator of change in outcomes.

Finally, Kidd et al. [55] used an 8-week mindful eating group intervention to investigate changes in mindful eating, self-efficacy for weight loss, depression, weight loss, body fat, and blood pressure in 12 obese women who lived in an urban area. A focus group was conducted afterwards to understand the participants' experiences with mindful eating. The only measured variable that improved statistically was self-efficacy over weight loss. Thematic analyses of the focus group content confirmed increased self-efficacy over weight loss, and the participants described improvements in mood, food choices, and eating behavior. Those who reported applying mindfulness skills reported the greatest change in BMI, mental health, and decreased emotional eating.

17.6 Mindful Eating for Weight Loss

While evidence that mindful eating improves problem eating is consistent across studies and various participant populations, evidence for weight loss is mixed. Mindfulness interventions that do not integrate nutrition information or weight management guidance tend not to produce weight loss. Not surprisingly, of those mindful eating studies that did incorporate weight-loss strategies and where weight loss is a goal, participants lost weight [56, 57].

For example, Dalen et al. [56] developed a 6-week group protocol that combined mindfulness meditation, nutrition information, light yoga, walking meditation, group eating exercises, and group discussion along with brief daily meditation and mindful eating practice for homework. They assessed changes in BMI, eating behavior, psychological distress, and the physiological makers of cardiovascular risk in their ten participants. Post-intervention, participants reported statistically significant increases in mindfulness and cognitive restraint around eating as well as statistically significant decreases in weight, binge eating, depression, and C-reactive protein.

Out of the ten intervention studies on mindful eating reviewed by Katterman et al. [50] that measured weight as an outcome, six provided education on energy balance, nutrition, or exercise, and only one included behavioral weight loss techniques such as problem-solving and encouraging behavioral goal-setting [58]. Among the interventions where weight loss was observed, weight loss served as a primary outcome of the intervention and treatment included either nutrition education alone [56, 57] or nutrition education plus teaching behavioral strategies [58]. Thus, while weight loss may occur when it was a primary outcome, there is no evidence that weight loss occurs in response to mindfulness training in the absence of a specific focus on weight.

17.7 Mindful Eating with Bariatric Surgery Patients

Obese individuals who pursue bariatric surgery report high rates of problem eating including loss of control over eating, binge eating, and chronic overeating [59, 60]. Even when individuals do not meet full criteria for an eating disorder, these disordered eating patterns can prevent optimal adherence to postsurgical eating guidelines, thus contributing to eventual weight regain [61–63]. While the first year after surgery for most patients is characterized by rapid weight loss, once patients transition to weight maintenance, presurgery eating problems may recur. About 20 % of postoperative patients experience insufficient weight loss [64], frequently defined as less than 50 % excess weight loss [65–67].

Given that weight loss with bariatric surgery is associated with the improvement or resolution of medical comorbidities as well as improvements in patient-reported quality of life [68], weight regain is of primary concern for these patients, their families and health care providers. In one study following gastric bypass patients over an average of 28 months, 79 % regained some weight after reaching their lowest weight and 15 % experienced a weight increase of 15 % of more from their lowest weight [69]. Eating-related factors associated with weight regain include binge eating [27], lack of control over food urges, [69] and eating in response to painful affect [70, 71], making mindful eating appropriate for this population too. Indeed, Levin et al. [72] investigated mindfulness and problematic eating in 820 patients seeking bariatric surgery and found that greater mindfulness was related to less binge and emotional eating, as well as less habitual overeating and grazing. Acting with awareness, a facet of mindfulness, was consistently related to eating behavior.

One mindful eating group intervention study has so far been published with post-bariatric surgery patients. The group was conducted in a hospital setting for ten weekly sessions of 75 min each and incorporated CBT strategies such as regular eating, keeping an eating journal that included associated thoughts and feelings, controlling portion sizes, and removing triggering foods from the home. Mindful eating practices were facilitated in each session to improve awareness of reactions to food and eating. The group was composed of seven patients who had either undergone gastric bypass or banding and who reported subjective binges with loss of control and eating to manage emotions. Post-intervention, patients reported improvements in eating, emotion regulation, and depression, changes that theoretically should help patients reduce problem eating and thus prevent weight regain. There was a modest reduction in the participants' overall weight [73].

17.8 Integrating Mindful Eating in Individual Psychotherapy

While the majority of research studies investigating mindful eating have been on group interventions, it is also possible to integrate mindful eating practices into individual therapy sessions. Indeed, Martin [74] proposed that mindfulness is the core of psychotherapy process.

A growing body of literature has examined the benefits [75–77]. In many MBIs, such as MBSR, MBCT and MB-EAT, "The Raisin Exercise" [2] is commonly used to introduce participants to the practice of mindfulness and to engage fully with all of their five senses. Other mindful eating exercises can be incorporated into individual therapy sessions such as rating hunger levels, fullness and taste satiety [21, 48, 78–80]. Please see Script 1 for a mindful eating script that may be used with individuals or groups.

As with the delivery of all MBIs, it is imperative that mindful eating interventions be facilitated by clinicians trained in the principles of mindfulness, specifically mindful eating, and that clinicians develop and maintain a formal and informal mindfulness practice of their own [81]. More importantly, mindfulness can cultivate clinically beneficial qualities in psychotherapists, such as self-attunement, affect tolerance, empathy, openness, acceptance, and compassion [82, 83].

The role of the psychotherapist's mindfulness practice, therefore, would optimize the therapeutic relationship/alliance and produce better outcomes (e.g., symptom reduction) for the client.

17.9 Application of Mindfulness-Based Techniques

Betty attended all ten sessions of MB-EAT and participated well by sharing her mindful eating experiences, insights, and challenges to the bigger group. She completed her homework daily, which included formal (e.g., Body Scan, Sitting) and informal (e.g., Mindful Walking, Eating) mindfulness meditations exercises which lasted between 15 and 30 min and other pleasurable activities that did not involve food.

Betty's binge eating and overall intake of food decreased gradually over the course of the program. Her self-reported frequency of binge eating episodes decreased from eight per month to two per month at 4 months posttreatment. Grazing and emotional eating also declined from 5 times per week to a maximum of 2 per week. She lost 5 kg (to 75.91 kg) within 3 months following posttreatment, bringing her BMI to 29.6 and her diabetes improved.

At 4 months posttreatment, Betty indicated that since participating in MB-EAT she has noticed positive changes in the way she appreciates food. She reported taking the time prior to eating a snack or meal to briefly meditate and attend to her hunger signals. This has helped her to decrease her portion sizes and to savor her meals by slowing down/chewing thoroughly while eating. Betty stated that instead of purchasing foods impulsively at the supermarket, she has developed more awareness and outer wisdom in making healthier nutritional choices. She has also become less critical of herself when she does overeat and takes the time to gently observe her experiences rather than catastrophizing. Her family commented on her ability to be more assertive, calmer, and less reactive in stressful situations. Betty stated, "I used to cry uncontrollably when I was stressed but now I totally bypass the crying fit and just breathe!"

Betty attributed her changes to eating by "being present in the moment," taking the time to pause before eating, paying attention to her hunger signals and practicing mindfulness meditation daily. She further found the group pot-luck to be especially helpful in allowing her to select foods without judgment and "savoring the flavors." She was able to use these new skills when attending dinner gatherings with her friends and family.

17.10 Summary

- The rationale for mindful eating interventions comes from evidence that obesity resulting from problem eating can be caused by emotional eating, lack of interoceptive awareness and externally cued eating. The body's biological stress response may also contribute to obesity and may be modified through mindfulness practice.
- Outcome research on mindful eating is limited but promising. Mindful eating interventions appear effective at treating problem eating associated with weight gain. To facilitate weight loss, information on nutrition and strategies for regulating eating should be incorporated.
- Patients should be educated that while weight loss may result from mindful eating, this is not the only goal of the practice. Rather, it is a means by which to develop a new relationship with food and themselves.
- Mindful eating interventions should be delivered by clinicians trained in the principles of mindfulness, specifically mindful eating. It is also imperative that clinicians develop a formal and informal mindfulness practice of their own.

Appendix

Script 1: Mindful Eating Meditation

This meditation is designed to help you cultivate mindful eating by engaging in all of your five senses while eating. This practice is also a helpful way for you to develop a healthy and pleasurable relationship with food.

Prior to eating a meal or snack, please take a few moments to settle into a relaxed sitting position, with your food placed in front of you, either on a table or on your lap ***(10 s)***.

Allow your back to adopt an erect and comfortable posture ***(5 s)***. If you are sitting on a chair, place your feet flat on the floor, with your legs uncrossed ***(5 s)***. If you feel comfortable, gently close your eyes fully or partially ***(5 s)***.

Take three deep breaths to settle into your body and into this present moment ***(5 s)***.

YOU CAN BEGIN BY NOTICING the way your breath is moving in the body ***(10 s)***. Breathe from your diaphragm, or lower stomach, rather than the chest ***(10 s)***. If you like, you can put your hand on your stomach and feel the way it moves with the breath ***(10 s)***. You may notice that as you breathe in the stomach rises…and as you breathe out it falls ***(5 s)***. Spend a few more moments exploring these breathing sensations ***(5 s)***.

On you next in-breath, focus your attention on your stomach and assess your baseline hunger. Ask yourself: On a scale of 0–10, with 0 being "not hungry at all" and 10 being "extremely hungry," *how hunger am I? And how do I know?*

SIGHT: When you are ready, open your eyes and imagine that you are seeing these food(s) for the first time, being open and curious to whatever arises ***(10 s)***. As you breathe in and out, notice the colors, shapes, and textures of the food in front of you ***(10 s)***.

TOUCH: Breathing in, focus your attention now to your sense of touch. Using utensils or your hands, pick up the food and either feel the texture against your lips or between your fingertips ***(5 s)***. Continue to pay attention to your sensation of touch for the next few moments ***(10 s)***.

SMELLS: On your next in-breath, shift your concentration to noticing the smells of the particular food(s) ***(10 s)***. Bring the food(s) to your nose and inhale deeply. Continue to breathe and focus on the slightest of scents…allowing them to come to you. As best as you can, be aware of any feelings, sensations, or thoughts that are arising and let them be just as they are, without trying to change it ***(10 s)***.

TASTE: When you are ready, shift your attention from awareness of smells to awareness of taste ***(10 s)***. Place the food(s) in your mouth and begin to chew, observing any flavors that arise. Allow yourself to experience and savor the taste. As best as you can, pay attention to how the texture of the food(s) change as you are chewing and breaks down with every bite.

SOUNDS: While you are chewing, notice the sound(s) that the food(s) is making. Be open and receptive to those sounds that may arise while you are eating, without naming or labeling them. Whenever you become aware that the mind has wandered, gently acknowledge where the mind has gone to and as best as you can, return to your practice of eating mindfully. Continue to chew your food(s). When you are ready to swallow, feel the sensation as the food(s) slides down your throat. If you like, you can imagine the food in your stomach.

Now rate your hunger levels on a scale from 0 to 10. Do you notice any changes?

You can continue to eat in this way for another few bites or if you like, until you finish your snack/meal. Remember that you can always return to this mindful eating practice anytime you wish.

Checklist 1: Remember "MANGER" (French = To Eat)

1. <u>M</u>indful check in with one's body, emotions, thoughts, and hunger levels (Scale, 1–10, with 1 being "not hungry" at all and 10 being "starving").
2. <u>A</u>ccess, observe, and savor food with five senses: sight, smell, sound, taste, and touch.
3. <u>N</u>ourish your body with "just enough" food.
4. <u>G</u>ently investigate your hunger throughout eating.
5. <u>E</u>at slowly and chew thoroughly.
6. <u>R</u>ecognize and listen to your inner and outer wisdom.

References

1. Kabat-Zinn J. An outpatient program in behavioral medicine for chronic pain patients based on the practice of mindfulness meditation: theoretical considerations and preliminary results. Gen Hosp Psychiatry. 1982;4:33–47.
2. Segal ZV, Williams JMG, Teasdale JD. Mindfulness-based cognitive therapy for depression: a new approach to preventing relapse. New York: Guilford Press; 2002.
3. Segal ZV, Williams JM, Teasdale J. Mindfulness-based cognitive therapy for depression. 2nd ed. London: Guilford Press; 2013.
4. Hayes SC, Wilson KG, Gifford EV, Follette VM, Strosahl K. Emotional avoidance and behavioral disorders: a functional dimensional approach to diagnosis and treatment. J Consult Clin Psychol. 1996;64:1152–68.
5. Linehan MM. Cognitive-behavioral treatment of borderline personality disorder. New York: Guilford Press; 1993.
6. Shapiro SL, Carlson LE. The art and science of mindfulness: integrating mindfulness into psychology and the helping professions. Washington, DC: American Psychological Association; 2009.
7. Kabat-Zinn J. Wherever you go, there you are: mindfulness meditation in everyday life. New York: Hyperion Books; 1994.
8. Kabat-Zinn J. Full catastrophe living. Using the wisdom of your body and mind to face stress, pain, and illness. New York: Delacorte; 1990.
9. Thera N. The heart of Buddhist meditation. New York: Weiser; 1962.
10. Hanh TH. Creating true peace. New York: Free Press; 2003.
11. Kavatznick R. Zen of eating: Ancient answers to modern weight problems. New York: Berkeley; 1998.
12. Hanh TH, Cheung L. Savor: mindful eating, mindful life. New York: HarperOne; 2010.
13. Hanh TH. How to eat. Berkeley: Parallax Press; 2014.
14. Bays JC. Mindful eating: rediscovering a joyful relationship with food. Boston and London: Shambhala; 2009.
15. Gu J, Strauss C, Bond R, Cavanagh K. How do mindfulness-based cognitive therapy and mindfulness-based stress reduction improve mental health and wellbeing? A systematic review and meta-analysis of mediation studies. Clin Psychol Rev. 2015;37:1–12.
16. Olson KL, Emery CF. Mindfulness and weight loss: a systematic review. Psychosom Med. 2015;77:59–67.
17. Wansink B, Sobal J. Mindless eating. The 200 daily food decisions we overlook. Environ Behav. 2007;39(1):106–23.
18. Urquhart CS, Mihalynuk TV. Disordered eating in women: implications for the obesity pandemic. Can J Diet Pract Res. 2011;72(50):e115–25.
19. Tanofsky-Kraff M, Yanovski SZ. Eating disorder or disordered eating? Non-normative eating patterns in obese individuals. Obes Res. 2004;12(9):1361–6.
20. Heatherton TF, Baumeister RF. Binge eating as escape from self-awareness. Psychol Bull. 1991;110:86–108.
21. Kristeller JL, Baer RA, Quillian-Wolever R. Mindfulness-based approaches to eating disorders. In: Baer RA, editor. Mindfulness-based treatment approaches. Oxford: Academic; 2006.
22. Chesler BE. Emotional eating: a virtually untreated risk factor for outcome following bariatric surgery. Scientific World Journal. 2011;2012:365961. doi:10.1100/2012/365961.
23. Leahy RL. A model of emotional schemas. Cogn Behav Pract. 2002;9(3):177–90.
24. Blair AJ, Lewis VJ, Booth DA. Does emotional eating interfere with success in attempts at weight control? Appetite. 1990;15:151–7.
25. Craighead LW, Allen HN. Appetite awareness training: a cognitive behavioral intervention for binge eating. Cogn Behav Pract. 1995;2:249–70.
26. Ganley RM. Emotion and eating in obesity: a review of the literature. Int J Eat Disord. 1989;8:343–61.
27. Mitchell JE, Lancaster KL, Burgard MA, Howekk M, Krahn DD, Crosby RD, et al. Long-term follow-up of patients' status after gastric bypass. Obes Surg. 2001;11:464–8.
28. Braet C, Van Strien T. Assessment of emotional, externality induced and restrained eating behaviour in nine to twelve-year-old obese and non-obese children. Behav Res Ther. 1997;35:863–73.
29. Delahanty LM, Williamson DA, Meigs JB, Nathan DM, Hayden D. Psychological and behavioral correlates of baseline BMI in the diabetes prevention program (DPP). Diabetes Care. 2002;25:1992–8.
30. Wardle J. Eating style: a validation study of the Dutch eating behaviour questionnaire in normal subjects and women with eating disorders. J Psychosom Res. 1987;31(2):161–9.
31. Hays NP, Bathalon GP, McCrory MA, Roubenoff R, Lipman R, Roberts SB. Eating behaviour correlates of adult weight gain and obesity in healthy women aged 55–65 years. Am J Clin Nutr. 2002;75:476–83.
32. Kayman S, Bruvold W, Stern JS. Maintenance and relapse after weight loss in women: behavioral aspects. Am J Clin Nutr. 1990;52:800–7.
33. McGuire JG, Wing RR, Klem ML, Lang W, Hill JO. What predicts weight regain in a group of successful weight losers? J Consult Clin Psychol. 1999;67:177–85.
34. Fassino S, Piero A, Gramaglia C, Abbate-Daga G. Clinical, psychopathological and personality correlates of interoceptive awareness in anorexia nervosa, bulimia nervosa, and obesity. Psychopathology. 2004; 37:168–74.
35. Leon GR, Fulkerson JA, Perry CL, Early-Zald MB. Prospective analysis of personality and behavioral vulnerabilities and gender influences in the later development of disordered eating. J Abnorm Psychol. 1995;104(1):140–9.
36. Van Strien TV, Engels RCME, Leeuwe JU, Snoek HM. The Stice model of overeating: tests in clinical and non-clinical samples. Appetite. 2005;45(3):205–13.

37. Van Strien T. Ice-cream consumption, tendency toward overeating, and personality. Int J Eat Disord. 2000;28(4):460–4.
38. Ouwens MA, Schiffer AA, Visser LI, Raeijmaekers NJC, Nyklicek I. Mindfulness and eating behaviour styles in morbidly obese males and females. Appetite. 2015;87:62–7.
39. Kristeller JL, Epel E. Mindful eating and mindfulness eating. The science and the practice. Hoboken: Wiley; 2014.
40. Dallman MF. Stress-induced obesity and the emotional nervous system. Trends Endocrinol Metab. 2010;21:159–65.
41. Khoury B, Lecomte T, Fortin G, Masse M, Therien P, Bouchard V, Chapleau MA, Paquin K, Hofman SG. Mindfulness-based therapy: a comprehensive meta-analysis. Clin Psychol Rev. 2013;33:763–71.
42. Gotink RA, Chu P, Busschbach JV, Benson H, Fricchione GL, Hunink MGM. Standardised mindfulness-based interventions in healthcare: an overview of systematic reviews and meta-analyses of RCTs. PLoS One. 2015;10(4):e0124344. http://journals.plos.org/plosone/article?id=10.1371/journal.pone.0124344
43. Goyal M, Sing S, Sibinga EMS, Gould NF, Rowland-Seymour A, Sharma R, Berger Z, Sleicher D, Maron DD, Shihab HM, Ranasinghe PD, Linn S, Saha S, Bass EB, Haythornthwaite JA. Meditation programs for psychological stress and well-being. A systematic review and meta-analysis. JAMA Intern Med. 2014;174(3):257–368.
44. Kearney DJ, Milton ML, Malte CA, McDermott KA, Martinez M, Simpson TL. Participation in mindfulness-based stress reduction is not associated with reductions in emotional eating or uncontrolled eating. Nutr Res. 2012;32:413–20.
45. Wnuk S, Du C, Warwick K, Tremblay L. From mindless to mindful eating: tools to help the bariatric patient succeed. Can J Diabetes. 2015;39 Suppl 1:S14.
46. Ifland JR, Preuss HG, Marcus MT, Rourke KM, Taylor WC, Burau K, Jacobs WS, Kadish W, Manso G. Refined food addiction: a class substance use disorder. Med Hypotheses. 2009;72:518–26.
47. Kristeller JL, Hallett B. Effects of a meditation-based intervention in the treatment of binge eating. J Health Psychol. 1999;4:357–63.
48. Kristeller JL, Wolever RQ. Mindfulness-based eating awareness training for treating binge eating disorder: the conceptual foundation. Eat Disord. 2011;19(1):49–61.
49. Wolever RQ, Best JL. Mindfulness-based approaches to eating disorders. In: Didonna F, editor. Clinical handbook of mindfulness. New York: Springer; 2009. p. 259–88.
50. Katterman SN, Kleinman BM, Hood MM, Nackers LM, Corsica JA. Mindfulness meditation as an intervention for binge eating, emotional eating, and weight loss: a systematic review. Eat Behav. 2014;14:197–204.
51. O'Reilly GA, Cook L, Spruijt-Metz D, Black DS. Mindfulness-based interventions for obesity-related eating behaviors: a literature review. Obes Rev. 2014;15(6):453–61.
52. Daubenmier J, Kristeller J, Hecht FM, Maninger N, Kuwata M, Jhaveri K, Lustig RH, Kemeny M, Karan L, Epel E. Mindfulness intervention for stress eating to reduce cortisol and abdominal fat among overweight obese women: an exploratory randomized controlled study. J Obes. 2011;2011:651936. doi:10.1155/2011/651936.
53. Kristeller JL, Wolever RQ, Sheets V. Mindfulness-Based Eating Awareness Training (MB-EAT) for binge eating disorder: a randomized clinical trial. Mindfulness. 2012;3(4):261–338.
54. Bush HE, Rossy L, Mintz LB, Schopp L. Eat for life: a work site feasibility study of a novel mindfulness-based intuitive eating intervention. Am J Health Promot. 2014;28(6):380–8.
55. Kidd LI, Heifner Graor C, Murrock CJ. A mindful eating group intervention for obese women: a mixed methods feasibility study. Arch Psychiatr Nurs. 2013;27:211–8.
56. Dalen J, Smith BW, Shelley BM, Sloan AL, Leahigh L, Begay D. Pilot study: Mindful Eating and Living (MEAL): weight, eating behavior, and psychological outcomes associated with a mindfulness-based intervention for people with obesity. Complement Ther Med. 2010;18(6):260–4.
57. Miller CK, Kristeller JL, Headings A, Nagaraja H, Miser F. Comparative effectiveness of a mindful eating intervention to a diabetes self-management intervention among adults with type 2 diabetes: a pilot study. J Acad Nutr Diet. 2012;112:1835–42.
58. Timmerman GM, Brown A. The effect of a mindful restaurant eating intervention on weight management in women. J Nutr Educ Behav. 2012;44:22–28. http://dx.doi.org/10.1016/j.jneb.2011.03.143
59. Kalarchian MA, Wilson TG, Brolin RE, Bradley L. Binge eating in bariatric surgery patients. Int J Eat Disord. 1998;23:89–92.
60. Saunders R, Johnson L, Teschner J. Prevalence of eating disorders among bariatric surgery patients. Eat Disord. 1998;6:309–17.
61. Snyder B, Wilson T, Mehta S, et al. Past, present, and future: critical analysis of use of gastric bands in obese patients. Diabetes Metab Syndr Obes. 2010;3:55–65.
62. Toussi R, Fujioka K, Coleman KJ. Pre- and postsurgery behavioral compliance, patient health, and postbariatric surgical weight loss. Obesity. 2009; 17(5):996–1002.
63. Sarwar DB, Dilks RJ, West-Smith L. Dietary intake and eating behavior after bariatric surgery: threats to weight loss maintenance and strategies for success. Surg Obes Relat Dis. 2011;7(5):644–51.
64. Benotti PN, Forse RA. The role of gastric surgery in the multidisciplinary management of severe obesity. Cogn Behav Pract. 1995;169(3):361–7.

65. Junior WS, Do Amaral JL, Nonino-Borges CB. Factors related to weight loss up to 4 years after bariatric surgery. Obes Surg. 2011;21(11): 1724–30.
66. Kruseman M, Leimgruber A, Zumbach F, Golay A. Dietary, weight, and psychological changes among patients with obesity, 8 years after gastric bypass. J Am Diet Assoc. 2010;110(4):527–34.
67. Rawlins ML, Teel II D, Hedgcorth K, Maguire JP. Revision of Roux-en-Y gastric bypass to distal bypass for failed weight loss. Surg Obes Relat Dis. 2011;7:454–9.
68. Herpertz S, Kielmann R, Wolf AM, Langkafel M, Senf W, Hebebrand J. Does obesity surgery improve psychosocial functioning? A systematic review. Int J Obes Relat Metab Disord. 2003;27: 1300–14.
69. Odom J, Zalesin KC, Washington TL, Miller WW, Hakmeh B, Zaremba DL, et al. Behavioral predictors of weight regain after bariatric surgery. Obes Surg. 2010;20(3):349–56.
70. Grothe KB, Dubbert PM, O'Jile JR. Psychological assessment and management of the weight loss surgery patient. Am J Med Sci. 2006;331(4):201–6.
71. Zimmerman M, Francione-Witt C, Chelminski I, et al. Presurgical psychiatric evaluations of candidates for bariatric surgery, part 1: reliability and reasons for and frequency of exclusion. J Clin Psychiatry. 2007;68(10):1557–62.
72. Levin ME, Dalyrymple K, Himes S, Zimmerman M. Which facets of mindfulness are related to problematic eating among patients seeking bariatric surgery? Eat Behav. 2014;15:298–305.
73. Leahey TM, Crowther JH, Irwin SR. A cognitive-behavioral mindfulness group therapy intervention for the treatment of binge eating in bariatric surgery patients. Cogn Behav Pract. 2008;15:364–75.
74. Martin JR. Mindfulness: a proposed common factor. J Psychother Integr. 1997;7:291–312.
75. Cigolla F, Brown D. A way of being: bringing mindfulness into individual therapy. Psychother Res. 2011;21(6):709–21.
76. Gemer CK, Siegel RD, Fulton PR, editors. Mindfulness and psychotherapy. 2nd ed. New York: Guilford Press; 2013.
77. Mace C. Mindfulness in psychotherapy: an introduction. BJPsych Adv. 2007;13:147–54.
78. Boudette R. Integrating mindfulness into the therapy hour. Eat Disord. 2011;19:108–15.
79. Albers S. Using mindful eating to treat food restrictions: a case study. Eat Disord. 2011;19:97–107.
80. Kristeller J, Quillian-Wolever R, Wilkins C, Hallett B. MB-EAT—pre-bariatric surgery: mindfulness based eating awareness training for preparation for bariatric surgery treatment manual. 2010. Unpublished manuscript.
81. Marlatt AG, Bowen S, Chawla N, Witkiewitz K. Mindfulness-based relapse prevention for substance abusers. In: Hink SF, Bien T, editors. Mindfulness and the therapeutic relationship. New York: Guildford Press; 2009.
82. Fulton PR. Mindfulness-based intervention in an individual clinical setting: what difference mindfulness makes behind closed doors. In: Didonna F, editor. Clinical handbook of mindfulness. New York: Springer; 2009. p. 407–16.
83. Bruce NG, Manber R, Shapiro SL, Constantino MJ. Psychotherapist mindfulness and the psychotherapy process. Psychother Theory Res Pract Train. 2010;47(1):83–97.

Cognitive Behavioural Therapy for Severe Obesity

18

Stephanie E. Cassin and Molly Atwood

Case Vignette

Mrs. Jones is a 48-year-old teacher who is married with two children. She was referred by her physician for bariatric surgery, and at the time of the initial assessment, her body mass index (BMI) was 48 kg/m^2. She had a history of depression and occasionally had eating binges. She also had type 2 diabetes and reported significant joint pain. When asked about her expectations regarding the surgery, she hoped that she would lose 100 pounds by the end of the first year (BMI = 32 kg/m^2) and that her diabetes would go into remission. Her surgery went smoothly, and she did not experience dumping syndrome or any other significant complications following the surgery. In fact, she reported that she was able to eat some "junk food" relatively soon after her surgery, as well as larger portion sizes than she had expected. She was disappointed that she was still able to continue some of her old unhealthy eating habits and reported that she wished in some ways that she did experience dumping syndrome to deter her from eating unhealthy foods and large portions.

Although she made some unhealthy food choices and occasionally ate large portions of food, her eating habits had actually improved significantly. In addition, she was working out with a personal trainer once to twice a week plus exercising on her own; her strength and cardiovascular fitness had improved significantly, and she was training for a 5 km race. She lost approximately 70 pounds in the first 8 months following surgery (BMI = 37 kg/m^2), her diabetes went into remission, and her joint pain had reduced significantly. Despite these improvements, she was beginning to give up hope that she would be able to lose 100 pounds in the first year (perhaps even ever) because she was informed prior to surgery that the most drastic weight loss occurs within the first 6–12 months following surgery. In speaking with other bariatric patients, she felt other people were making much greater progress than she was, and this left her feeling

(continued)

S.E. Cassin, Ph.D., C.Psych. (✉)
Department of Psychology, Ryerson University, Toronto, ON, Canada

Department of Psychiatry, University of Toronto, Toronto, ON, Canada

Centre for Mental Health, University Health Network, Toronto, ON, Canada
e-mail: stephanie.cassin@psych.ryerson.ca

M. Atwood
Department of Psychology, Ryerson University, Toronto, ON, Canada

S. Sockalingam, R. Hawa (eds.), *Psychiatric Care in Severe Obesity*, DOI 10.1007/978-3-319-42536-8_18

(continued)
disappointed and discouraged. She began to have thoughts such as "I should have lost more weight by now", "I am never going to reach my goal weight", and "I am going to regain all of my weight and then some." She found this last thought particularly distressing because it made her think, "Why bother continuing to work so hard then?" At her most recent weigh-in at the clinic, her weight loss had plateaued. She reported that she had not been exercising as much the past few weeks and had a few episodes of emotional overeating.

18.1 Introduction

In this chapter, we provide an overview of cognitive behavioural therapy (CBT), the rationale for integrating it into the management of severe obesity, and examples of CBT strategies that can be helpful in working with patients with severe obesity. We then review the empirical evidence supporting the effectiveness of CBT in patients with severe obesity (both surgical and non-surgical populations). Finally, we use a case example to illustrate the application of CBT techniques in clinical practice.

18.2 Overview of Cognitive Behavioural Therapy

Cognitive behavioural therapy (CBT) is a short-term, psychosocial intervention that is based on the premise that thoughts (cognitions), emotions, and behaviours are all interconnected [1]. The way an individual appraises a situation influences his/her emotional response and subsequent behaviour. Conversely, an individual's behavioural response affects his/her cognitions and emotional responses, thus creating a potentially vicious feedback cycle. The cognitive behavioural model posits that "cognitive distortions" (i.e., distorted thoughts) are at the root of psychopathology [1]. For example, having a thought such as "I am never going to lose weight", might lead to feelings of pessimism, helplessness, sadness, and frustration, which in turn lead to withdrawing from social and recreational activities and engaging in emotional overeating or binge eating. This behaviour can then create a self-fulfilling prophecy, such that increased food consumption provides some objective evidence to support the thought, "I am never going to lose weight," which subsequently amplifies negative emotions that further increase vulnerability to maladaptive eating behaviours.

Cognitive behavioural therapy is a skills-based intervention that focuses on the here-and-now. That is, it focuses on the factors that currently maintain problematic thoughts and behaviours to a much greater extent than the issues that originally lead to their development. Given that cognitions, emotions, and behaviours are all interconnected, CBT seeks to disrupt this feedback cycle by teaching clients coping skills to identify and alter maladaptive cognitions and behaviours that perpetuate the cycle of maladaptive eating patterns [1]. Cognitive behavioural therapy is a collaborative treatment approach in that the therapist and client work together to set treatment goals that are mutually agreed upon. The client is expected to actively participate in treatment sessions and practice the coping skills between sessions in order to maximally benefit from treatment and ultimately become his/her *own* therapist.

18.3 Rationale for Integrating CBT into the Management of Severe Obesity

Obesity itself is not a mental disorder; however, individuals with severe obesity have elevated rates of psychopathology, including mood disorders, anxiety disorders, and binge eating disorder (BED) [2–5]. In addition to clinically significant eating disorders, a high percentage of individuals with obesity also endorse maladaptive eating behaviours such as emotional overeating, grazing, and loss of control eating [6, 7].

A proposed mechanism that accounts for this relationship is the tendency for people to eat as a means of coping with emotional difficulties [8–10]. Thus, in order to maintain weight loss, it is important that patients learn coping skills to better manage emotional difficulties. Major clinical guidelines recommend CBT as the gold standard psychosocial treatment for many of the psychological disorders which are prevalent among individuals with severe obesity, including depression [11] and binge eating disorder [12], and as described later in this chapter, empirical research supports the efficacy of CBT for weight management.

18.4 Cognitive Behavioural Therapy for Severe Obesity

A number of excellent resources exist for learning about CBT [1], and applying CBT in the treatment of binge eating [13], and weight management [14–16]. Clinical guidelines for the management of obesity [17] recommend that the following components be included in interventions: goal setting, self-monitoring, physical activity, stimulus control, problem-solving, assertiveness, cognitive restructuring (i.e. modification of distorted thoughts), relapse prevention, and strategies for dealing with weight regain.

18.4.1 Introduction to CBT and Goal Setting

Cognitive behavioural therapy should begin with an introduction to CBT and presentation of a cognitive behavioural model that explains some of the factors that have been implicated in overeating and weight gain [18]. The model should be tailored to the individual client, and focus on the factors that currently maintain his/her maladaptive eating behaviours (e.g., cognitive distortions, negative emotions, high levels of dietary restraint). The CBT model is used to illustrate the feedback cycle that exists, whereby overeating is reinforced by temporary relief or pleasure, but then followed by negative emotions that subsequently increase vulnerability for further overeating. Collaborative goal setting should then be used to develop treatment goals focused on improving eating behaviours. For example, treatment goals might include reducing binge eating or emotional eating, and in order to do so, it would be important to eat healthy meals and snacks at regular time intervals (e.g., self-monitoring using food records, engaging in normalized or "mechanical" eating), schedule pleasurable activities as alternatives to eating (e.g., activity scheduling, self-care), plan for difficult eating situations (e.g., stimulus control, problem-solving, assertiveness training), and reduce susceptibility to overeating by identifying, challenging, and altering maladaptive thoughts (e.g., cognitive restructuring) [14, 18].

18.4.2 Self-Monitoring and Using Food Records to Normalize Eating

Clients begin self-monitoring their eating behaviours using food records early in treatment. Food records are daily journals which are used to monitor the time and location of each episode, the amount and type of food or liquid consumed, the type of eating episode (e.g., snack, meal, binge, graze), and the context of eating episode (e.g., thoughts, emotions, situation). The purpose of the food records is to increase awareness of eating behaviours, identify maladaptive patterns in eating behaviours (e.g., skipping meals which increases vulnerability to subsequent overeating, grazing at home after work in the evening rather than sitting down for a proper meal), change eating behaviours, and monitor progress over time. Some of the recommendations for normalized eating including consuming three meals and two to three snacks per day, consuming something every 3–4 hours, and not grazing in between eating episodes. In addition, to reduce vulnerability to mindless eating, clients are encouraged to eat in a designated eating area (e.g., dining room table) and without distractions (e.g., no television, computer, telephone).

In addition to monitoring their food consumption, clients also begin monitoring their weight. It is not uncommon for individuals with obesity to either avoid the scale altogether or to weigh themselves too frequently, both of which can be maladaptive. Clients are encouraged to weigh themselves once per week at the same day and time so that they have a mechanism in place to receive regular feedback on their eating behaviours. Given that fluctuations can occur for a variety of reasons from week to week, clients are encouraged to plot their weight on a graph and examine monthly trends.

18.4.3 Scheduling Pleasurable and Self-Care Activities

Eating can provide a temporary sense of pleasure and be used to regulate negative emotions, such as depression, anxiety, anger, and boredom [10, 19, 20]. In order to make long-term changes to eating behaviours, it is important to find other pleasurable activities that can be used to ride out urges to overeat, reduce vulnerability to overeating (e.g., by improving mood), and enrich the client's life outside of food. Clients are encouraged to create a list of potentially pleasurable activities, and ideally the list should include a variety of activities that are incompatible with eating, require physical movement, are inexpensive, do not require other people, and can be engaged in at any hour. This is to ensure that the client has some ideas for activities that can be used to ride out a late night urge to overeat while alone.

In addition to regularly engaging in pleasurable activities that do not centre on food, it is important that clients practice good self-care habits to reduce vulnerability to overeating, including exercising regularly, socializing regularly, practicing good sleep hygiene, limiting consumption of alcohol, and avoiding illicit psychoactive substances [14].

18.4.4 Planning for Difficult Eating Situations

As part of treatment, clients identify the places, people, and foods that make it challenging to eat healthy, and learn problem-solving skills to help anticipate and troubleshoot such challenges. For example, a client may identify that he/she will be at greater risk of overeating at an upcoming holiday party. Problem-solving worksheets can be used to brainstorm and evaluate some options for reducing the risk, such as consuming food before the party to reduce hunger, contributing some healthy foods to the party, socializing away from the food table, and enlisting some social support. If a client is concerned that others might put on pressure to overeat during the holidays, assertiveness skills can be used to politely but firmly refuse requests.

Stimulus control refers to a number of strategies designed to reduce temptation to overeating, such as restructuring the environment. For example, a client who has a "junk food" cupboard at home and frequently engages in mindless eating in front of the TV at night could be encouraged to replace the contents of the cupboard with some healthier alternatives, and to meet up with a friend to share a treat at a café after dinner instead. In order to maintain long-term changes to eating habits, it is important to incorporate all foods into a flexible meal plan and not avoid "forbidden foods" altogether. Thus, it is important to develop a plan to enjoy treats in moderation when the temptation to overeat is relatively low.

18.4.5 Using Cognitive Restructuring to Reduce Vulnerability to Overeating

In addition to changing behaviour, CBT focuses on teaching clients skills to identify, evaluate, and challenge negative thoughts that intensify negative emotions and lead to maladaptive behaviours. As mentioned, the cognitive behavioural model assumes that "cognitive distortions" or distorted thoughts are at the root of psychopathology [1]. Below are some examples of cognitive distortions:

- "If I have *one* bad food, I've *totally* blown my diet"—All-or-nothing thinking

- "I *always* blow my diets, *nothing* I try ever works"—Overgeneralizing
- "I've totally blown my diet" (went off track for 1 day, despite eating healthy the rest of the week)—Mental filter, disqualifying the positive
- "No matter what I try, I won't be able to lose weight"—Fortune-teller error
- "If I have *one* bad food, I will regain all my weight and *nothing* else will *ever* work for me"—Catastrophizing
- "I *feel* fat, therefore I must have gained weight"—Emotional reasoning
- "I *should* have lost more weight by now"—Should statement

Patients are taught to use cognitive restructuring worksheets such as "thought records" (adapted from Burns [21] and Greenberger and Padesky [22]) to evaluate the evidence supporting and not supporting their negative thoughts, and to generate more neutral, adaptive, and balanced thoughts that acknowledge the evidence on both sides. The goal of cognitive restructuring is to replace negative thoughts with more benign interpretations in order to reduce the intensity of negative emotions and engage in more adaptive behaviours.

18.4.6 Relapse Prevention

Prior to terminating CBT, clients are taught relapse prevention skills including identifying the progress they have made, identifying triggers for maladaptive eating behaviours and early warning signs that maladaptive eating behaviours are returning, distinguishing between a lapse and a full relapse, reviewing the CBT strategies and handouts, and setting additional goals to continue working on following treatment. The goal of CBT is to teach clients to become their own therapists in order to maintain their progress following treatment, and clients are encouraged to regularly schedule self-therapy sessions following treatment in order to continue the work [1].

18.5 Empirical Evidence for Cognitive Behavioural Therapy in Obesity Management

18.5.1 Cognitive Behavioural Therapy for Individuals with Obesity

Randomized controlled trials (RCTs) examining the efficacy of CBT for individuals with severe obesity demonstrate that CBT is more effective in reducing weight as compared to a wait list control group (WLC). For example, Marchesini and colleagues [23] found that 12 weekly sessions of CBT delivered to 92 patients resulted in an average weight loss of 9.4 kg; in contrast, patients in the WLC group ($n=76$) did not exhibit a significant decrease in weight ($M=0.6$ kg). The CBT group also exhibited significant and superior improvement in health-related quality of life. Stahre and Hällström [24] found comparable results after a 10-week group CBT programme. Specifically, using a completer analysis, they found that patients in the CBT group lost an average of 8.5 kg at post-treatment and 10.4 kg by 1.5-year follow-up. In contrast, patients in the WLC group gained an average of 2.3 kg by 1.5-year follow-up.

Cognitive behavioural therapy has also been shown to be superior to usual care (UC). For example, Munsch, Biedert, and Keller [25] randomized 122 patients to one of two groups: (1) 16 sessions of CBT or (2) usual care consisting of regular contact with their general practitioner and non-specific psychoeducation about weight loss techniques. The CBT group demonstrated weight loss of 4.7 % of their pre-treatment weight, whereas the UC group lost an average of 0.5 % of their pre-treatment weight, and these results were maintained at 1-year follow-up. Eating pathology (as measured by the Three Factor Eating Questionnaire) was significantly improved in the CBT group across the 1-year follow-up period, and positive effects on body image were also reported.

In regard to maintenance of weight loss following treatment, CBT has been shown in some studies to be superior to other established treatments, such as behavioural weight loss therapy (BWL). Sbrocco, Nedegaard, Stone, and Lewis [26] compared group CBT ($n=12$) with group BWL ($n=12$) on weight loss outcomes at post-treatment, and 3-, 6-, and 12-month follow-up. Patients in the BWL group lost significantly more weight ($M=5.6$ kg) than those in the CBT group ($M=2.5$ kg) at post-treatment. At 3-month follow-up, there was no significant difference between groups; however, CBT was found to be superior to BLW at both 6-month follow-up ($M=7.0$ kg vs. $M=4.5$ kg, respectively) and 12-month follow-up ($M=10.1$ kg vs. $M=4.3$ kg). More specifically, those in the BWL group demonstrated weight regain in the follow-up period, whereas those who received CBT continued to lose weight post-treatment. Of note, cognitive therapy alone (i.e. without a behavioural intervention component) appears to be less effective for weight loss than behavioural therapy; however, evidence for durable improvements in psychological correlates of obesity, such as depression, following cognitive therapy are notable even in the absence of significant weight loss [27, 28].

Another line of research has demonstrated that CBT combined with diet and/or physical activity treatment components is superior to CBT alone [29] and diet and physical activity alone [30, 31]. For example, Werrij and colleagues [31] randomized 204 patients to either ten weekly sessions of group CBT plus a dietetic intervention (CDT) or group dietetic intervention plus physical exercise (EDT). Patients were examined on psychological and physiological variables at baseline, post-treatment, and 1-year follow-up. Interestingly, based on an intent-to-treat analysis, at post-treatment both interventions resulted in equivalent, significant improvements in maladaptive cognitions, eating concerns, shape concerns, weight concerns, dietary restraint, eating pathology, depression, and self-esteem. There also was a statistically significant reduction in weight in both groups (4.1 % for CDT vs. 4.3 % for EDT), with no difference between interventions. Most psychological benefits were maintained at 1-year follow-up in both groups, with the exception of dietary restraint and depression. In addition, the CDT intervention was found to be superior in sustaining changes in weight concerns, eating concerns, and weight loss (4.0 % vs. 3.2 %, respectively) as compared to EDT, indicating that the addition of cognitive behavioural strategies to nutritional approaches for weight loss produced superior outcomes.

Taken together, these studies demonstrate that CBT is more effective in facilitating weight loss as compared to WLC (e.g., [23, 24]) and usual care (e.g., [25]) and that adding a dietetic and/or exercise component can enhance weight loss outcomes (e.g., [29, 31]). Further, while BWL may demonstrate superior effects on weight loss in the short term, CBT yields superior results in the longer term [26]. Despite these positive findings, it is important to note that a relatively small proportion of patients achieve clinically significant levels of weight loss (i.e. 5–10% of initial weight) in many studies conducted to date. In addition to weight loss, CBT has also been shown to improve health-related quality of life [23], eating pathology (e.g., [25, 31]), and aspects of general pathology [31] in individuals with severe obesity.

The prevalence of BED in individuals with obesity seeking weight loss treatment is approximately 30 % [32–34]. Individuals with obesity and BED exhibit elevated psychopathology in the form of anxiety, depression, low self-esteem, and poorer quality of life as compared to those without BED [35, 36]. Currently, CBT is the most thoroughly researched and well-supported psychological treatment for this patient population.

Several systematic reviews have reported significantly greater reductions in binge eating frequency following CBT as compared to WLC, BWL, and pharmacotherapy [37–39]. For example, Agras and colleagues [40] reported binge eating remission rates of 55 % following CBT as compared to 9 % in a WLC group. Further, Munsch and colleagues [41] found that CBT was superior to BWL with respect to binge eating abstinence rates (80 % vs. 36 %, respectively) at post-treatment. Additional studies have found similar results at both short-term [42] and longer term follow-up [43, 44].

Binge eating remission rates following CBT typically fall between 40 and 60 % [45]. Although there is some erosion of therapeutic effects in the longer term, remission rates remain high up to 4 years following treatment completion [46]. There appears to be no incremental benefit of the addition of pharmacotherapy to CBT in increasing rates of binge eating remission [42, 47], or in sequencing interpersonal psychotherapy or BWL following CBT in those who show a suboptimal response [38]. There is preliminary evidence that more intensive CBT (i.e. 24 sessions) can increase binge eating remission rates [48] although more research is needed to determine the optimal dose of treatment.

In regard to psychological features of BED, evidence for the efficacy of CBT on certain outcome variables is equivocal. For example, some controlled trials have demonstrated reductions in dietary restraint following CBT [47, 49, 50], whereas others have shown no change [40, 48, 51]. According to one review, it is more clearly established that CBT in individuals with obesity and BED results in improvements in disinhibited eating as well as concerns regarding body shape and weight, even in the absence of weight loss [38]. Furthermore, CBT is associated with improvements in depression, anxiety, self-esteem, interpersonal functioning, and overall quality of life [38]. Studies assessing outcomes up to 1-year following completion of treatment have generally reported maintenance of change in eating-related psychopathology and general psychopathology [38].

Despite notable benefits of CBT on binge eating and associated psychopathology, the vast majority of controlled trials have reported that CBT does not have a significant effect on weight loss in individuals with BED [40, 50, 51]. Studies that have compared CBT to BWL have shown support for the latter in reducing weight, particularly in the short term. For example, Grilo, Masheb, Wilson, Gueorguieva, and White [43] randomized individuals with obesity and BED to either 16 sessions of CBT ($n=45$), BWL ($n=45$), or CBT followed by BWL ($n=35$). The BWL intervention produced statistically greater, although modest, weight loss over the course of treatment (mean BMI loses of −0.9, −2.1, and 1.5 kg/m^2, respectively) and remained superior to CBT in this regard up to 1-year follow-up. Other studies have shown that any short-term advantage of BWL over CBT on weight loss appears to be lost by 2-years following treatment [41, 44].

In addition to the above noted results, Grilo and colleagues [43] found that patients who were abstinent from binge eating following treatment exhibited greater weight loss. Several additional studies have found that patients who experience remission of binge eating following CBT demonstrate superior and sustained weight loss up to 1-year post-treatment (e.g., [50–53]). Thus, cessation of binge eating appears critical to facilitating and maintaining weight loss in individuals with BED.

A separate line of research had demonstrated that adding nutritional education and physical activity to CBT leads to significant reduction in body weight, as compared to CBT alone [29, 54]. For example, Fossati and colleagues [54] reported a mean weight loss of 1.5 kg in patients who received CBT plus nutritional guidance focused mainly on fat restriction, and mean weight loss of 2.8 kg in patients who received CBT plus nutritional guidance and physical activity. In contrast, patients who received CBT alone demonstrated mean weight loss of 0.3 kg.

Collectively, the extant literature indicates that CBT is superior to WLC, pharmacotherapy, and BWL in reducing and eliminating binge eating in individuals with obesity and BED [37–39]. CBT also results in durable improvements in numerous indicators of eating-related and general psychopathology [38]. Although BWL appears to be superior to CBT in facilitating weight loss, actual reported weight loss is minimal [41–43] and is not maintained at longer term follow-up [44]. Lastly, it appears as though suboptimal weight loss following CBT is associated with continuation of binge eating [50–53].

18.5.2 Cognitive Behavioural Therapy for Bariatric Surgery Patients

Over the past several decades, bariatric surgery has emerged as the most effective treatment for severe obesity. However, up to half of patients begin to regain weight within 2 years following surgery, and in almost one-quarter of cases, weight regain is considerable relative to overall weight loss [55, 56]. Outcomes following surgery appear to depend in part on lifestyle changes including adhering to postoperative diet and physical activity guidelines [57]. In addition, several studies have shown that problematic eating patterns (e.g., binge eating, loss of control, emotional eating, grazing) are associated with less weight loss and/or more weight regain following bariatric surgery [58, 59]. Thus, there has been increasing focus in the literature on examining the effectiveness of CBT delivered either pre- or post-operatively in improving psychological factors and difficulties adhering to dietary and physical activity guidelines implicated in poor post-operative outcomes. In comparison to empirical support for CBT in non-surgical obese populations, the literature examining the effectiveness of CBT for bariatric surgery patients is still in its infancy.

Two uncontrolled trials [60, 61] have demonstrated that a group CBT intervention delivered to preoperative bariatric patients results in significant reductions in binge eating frequency and symptomatology (i.e. cognitions, emotions, and behaviours as measured via the binge eating scale [BES]), as well as reported improvements in anxiety, depression, self-esteem, and shape, weight and eating concerns. In addition, Ashton and colleagues [62] found that patients who exhibited a positive response to CBT (i.e., abstinence from binge eating episodes and BES score in the minimal range at post-treatment) demonstrated significantly greater excess weight loss at both 6-months and 12-months post-surgery relative to patients who did not exhibit a positive response to the intervention [62].

Two randomized controlled trials have compared the effectiveness of pre-operative CBT to treatment as usual (TAU). Cassin and colleagues [63] found that a six-session telephone-based CBT intervention improved disordered eating behaviours (i.e., binge eating, emotional eating) and depression immediately post-treatment, whereas the control group reported significant increases in emotional eating and depression over the same time period. Gade and colleagues [64] examined the effectiveness of a ten-session CBT group intervention and found that it improved BMI, disordered eating behaviours (i.e. emotional eating, uncontrolled eating), depression, and anxiety immediately post-treatment. However, at 1-year post-operative follow-up, CBT was no longer superior to TAU [65]. Thus, while CBT demonstrates superior beneficial effects pre-surgery relative to TAU, this does not necessarily translate to improved outcomes in the post-operative period.

Several smaller uncontrolled studies have also examined the effectiveness of CBT for improving psychological factors delivered in the post-operative period. For example, Leahey, Crowther, and Irwin [66] found that ten weekly sessions of group CBT (which incorporated elements of mindfulness-based practice) conducted with seven post-operative bariatric patients resulted in a reduction in binge eating and depressive symptoms, as well as an increase in eating-related self-efficacy and emotional regulation. Although weight loss outcomes varied across patients, overall there was a small improvement in the percentage of weight loss patients achieved from pre to post-intervention. In a small pilot study, Cassin and colleagues [18] found that post-operative patients ($n=6$) who received a six-session CBT intervention reported improvements in binge eating symptomatology (i.e., cognitions, emotions, behaviours), emotional eating, and depressive symptoms.

Cognitive behavioural interventions aimed at optimizing adherence to dietary and physical activity guidelines in bariatric patients are similarly sparse. The limited available evidence to date does not support the notion that targeting adherence to lifestyle guidelines prior to surgery results in beneficial effects following surgery [67, 68]. However, cognitive behavioural interventions targeting dietary and physical activity habits may be particularly helpful when delivered post-operatively, in order to aid patients in enhancing and/or maintaining weight loss following surgery. CBT delivered postoperatively has been shown to produce greater excess weight loss as compared to WLC at both 6- (6.6 % vs. 3.4 %, respectively) and 12-months (5.8 % and 0.9 %) post-treatment [69].

Overall, it is still premature to draw firm conclusions regarding the effectiveness of CBT for bariatric surgery patients given the relatively small literature base. However, the field continues to grow as the potential role of adjunct psychosocial interventions in enhancing bariatric surgery outcomes is increasingly acknowledged. Although no studies have directly compared the effectiveness of a pre-operative and post-operative CBT intervention, a recent review concluded that the evidence is currently strongest for post-operative interventions delivered before significant weight regain occurs [70]. It will be important for future studies to employ larger scale RCTs and examine the durability of treatment improvements and the impact of CBT on long-term weight loss outcomes.

18.6 Application of Cognitive Behavioural Strategies

In working with Mrs. Jones, it would be helpful to first review the CBT model and note the relationship between the trigger (weigh-in), thoughts ("I should have lost more weight by now", "I am never going to reach my goal weight", "I am going to regain all of my weight and then some") and mood (disappointed, discouraged), and the impact these thoughts could potentially have on behaviour (stop exercising and consuming well-balanced meals, therefore becoming a self-fulfilling prophecy).

Next, it would be helpful to review Mrs. Jones' food records and weight graph for any notable changes that might be contributing to her weight plateau. If the food records identify that Mrs. Jones is regularly engaging in maladaptive eating behaviours (e.g., emotional eating, binge eating, loss of control eating, grazing), it is important to focus on behavioural strategies to reduce overeating including developing a plan for normalized eating, scheduling pleasurable activities in the place of overeating, engaging in problem-solving to plan for challenging eating situations, and using stimulus control techniques to reduce the temptation to overeat.

If it appears that Mrs. Jones is being overly critical of herself, it would be helpful to identify the negative automatic thoughts that are intensifying her feelings of disappointment and discouragement, and identify potential cognitive distortions (e.g., should statements, fortune-teller error, mental filter, discounting the positive). It is important to note that negative automatic thoughts are often based on some past truth. For example, an individual who has regained weight following every previous diet attempt would understandably predict that any future weight loss attempt will have the same outcome. Thought records are not meant to dismiss this past evidence, but rather to examine both the evidence supporting and not supporting the negative automatic thought, and to use cognitive restructuring to generate a more neutral or benign thought that leads to more adaptive behaviours.

In Mrs. Jones' case, some of the evidence supporting the thought, "I am never going to reach my goal weight" might include her occasional maladaptive eating behaviours and poor food choices and her recent weight plateau. Some of the evidence challenging the thought might include losing 70 pounds in 8 months, the overall improvement in her eating behaviours, and her regular exercise routine. An example of a balanced countering statement could include: "Even though I have not lost as much weight as I had originally expected, I have lost a significant amount of weight and have made improvements in many areas of my life including my eating habits, health, and fitness". To this end, it could also be beneficial to discuss some of the concrete improvements beyond her weight (e.g., increased strength and physical endurance, reduced joint pain, remission of diabetes). The balanced countering statements are intended to reduce the intensity of negative emotions (e.g., disappointment, discouragement) that could potentially lead to self-sabotaging behaviours and increase the likelihood that the client will persist with weight loss efforts.

18.7 Summary and Take Home Messages

- CBT is a short-term, psychosocial intervention that is based on the premise that thoughts (cognitions), emotions, and behaviours are all interconnected.
- CBT is a skills-based intervention that focuses on identifying and altering maladaptive cognitions and behaviours that perpetuate the cycle of maladaptive eating patterns.
- CBT is an effective treatment for severe obesity in non-surgical populations and results in improvements in eating-related and general psychopathology.
- CBT is effective in reducing binge eating in individuals with obesity and binge eating disorder.
- Research examining the efficacy of CBT in surgical populations is still in its infancy although preliminary results are promising.

References

1. Beck JS. Cognitive behaviour therapy: basics and beyond. 2nd ed. New York: Guilford; 2011.
2. Malik S, Mitchell JE, Engel S, Crosby R, Wonderlich S. Psychopathology in bariatric surgery candidates: a review of studies using structured diagnostic interviews. Compr Psychiatry. 2014;55(2):248–99.
3. Mitchell JE, Selzer F, Kalarchian MA, Devlin MJ, Strain GW, Elder KA, et al. Psychopathology before surgery in the longitudinal assessment of bariatric surgery-3 (LABS-3) psychosocial study. Surg Obes Relat Dis. 2012;8(5):533–41.
4. Mühlhans B, Horbach T, de Zwaan M. Psychiatric disorders in bariatric surgery candidates: a review of the literature and results of a German prebariatric surgery sample. Gen Hosp Psychiatry. 2009;31:414–21.
5. Taylor VH, McIntyre RS, Remington G, Levitan RD, Stonehocker B, Sharma A. Beyond pharmacotherapy: understanding the links between obesity and chronic mental illness. Can J Psychiatry. 2012;57(1):5–12.
6. Kalarchian MA, Wilson GT, Brolin RE, Bradley L. Binge eating in bariatric surgery patients. Int J Eat Disord. 1998;23(1):89–92.
7. Saunders R, Johnson L, Teschner J. Prevalence of eating disorders among bariatric surgery patients. Eat Disord. 1998;6(4):309–17.
8. Gariepy G, Nitka D, Schmitz N. The association between obesity and anxiety disorders in the population. Int J Obes (Lond). 2010;34(3):407–19.
9. Luppino FS, de Wit LM, Bouvy PF, Stijnen T, Cuijpers P, Pinninx BWJH, et al. Overweight, obesity, and depression: a systematic review and meta-analysis of longitudinal studies. Arch Gen Psychiatry. 2010;67(3):220–9.
10. Whiteside U, Chen E, Neighbors C, Hunter D, Lo T, Larimer M. Difficulties regulating emotions: do binge eaters have fewer strategies to modulate and tolerate negative affect? Eat Behav. 2007;8(2):162–9.
11. National Institute for Health and Care Excellence. Depression in adults: recognition and management. NICE clinical guideline 90. 2009. http://www.nice.org.uk/guidance/cg90
12. National Institute for Health and Care Excellence. Eating disorders in over 8s: management. NICE clinical guideline 9. 2004. http://www.nice.org.uk/guidance/cg9
13. Fairburn C. Overcoming binge eating. 2nd ed. New York: Guilford; 2013.
14. Apple RF, Lock J, Peebles R. Preparing for weight loss surgery: therapist guide. New York: Oxford University Press; 2006.
15. Cooper Z, Fairburn CG, Hawker DM. Cognitive behavioural treatment of obesity. New York: Guilford; 2004.
16. Laliberte M, McCabe RE, Taylor V. The cognitive behavioural workbook for weight management. Oakland: New Harbinger; 2009.
17. National Institute for Health and Care Excellence. Obesity: identification, assessment, and management. NICE clinical guideline 189. 2014. http://www.nice.org.uk/guidance/cg189
18. Cassin SE, Sockalingham S, Wnuk S, Strimas R, Royal S, Hawa R, et al. Cognitive behavioural therapy for bariatric surgery patients: preliminary evidence for feasibility, acceptability, and effectiveness. Cogn Behav Pract. 2013;20(4):529–43.
19. McManus F, Waller G. A functional analysis of binge eating. Clin Psychol Rev. 1995;15(8):845–63.
20. Schulte EM, Grilo CM, Gearhardt AN. Shared and unique mechanisms underlying binge eating disorder and addictive disorders. Clin Psychol Rev. 2016;44:125–39.
21. Burns DD. The feeling good handbook: revised edition. New York: Penguin; 1999.
22. Greenberger D, Padesky CA. Mind over mood. New York: Guilford; 1995.
23. Marchesini G, Natale S, Chierici S, Manini R, Besteghi L, Di Domizio S, et al. Effects of cognitive-behavioural therapy on health-related quality of life in

obese subjects with and without binge eating disorder. Int J Obes Relat Metab Disord. 2002;26(9):1261–7.
24. Stahre L, Hällström T. A short-term cognitive group treatment program gives substantial weight reduction up to 18 months from the end of treatment: a randomized controlled trial. Eat Weight Disord. 2005;10(1):51–8.
25. Munsch S, Biedert E, Keller U. Evaluation of a lifestyle change programme for the treatment of obesity in general practice. Swiss Med Wkly. 2003;133(9-10):148–54.
26. Sbrocco T, Nedegaard R, Stone J, Lewis E. Behavioural choice treatment promotes continuing weight loss: preliminary results of a cognitive-behavioural decision-based treatment for obesity. J Consult Clin Psychol. 1999;67:260–6.
27. Nauta H, Hospers H, Kok G, Jansen A. A comparison between a cognitive and a behavioural treatment for obese binge eaters and obese non-binge eaters. Behav Ther. 2000;31(3):441–61.
28. Nauta G, Hospers H, Jansen A. One-year follow-up effects of two obesity treatment on psychological well-being and weight. Br J Health Psychol. 2001;6(3):271–84.
29. Painot D, Jotterand S, Kammer A, Fossati M, Golay A. Simultaneous nutritional cognitive—behavioural therapy in obese patients. Patient Educ Couns. 2001;42(1):47–52.
30. Dennis K, Pane K, Adams B, Qi BB. The impact of a shipboard weight control program. Obes Res. 1999;7(1):60–7.
31. Werrij MQ, Jansen A, Mulkens S, Elgersma HJ, Ament AJHA, Hospers HJ. Adding cognitive therapy to dietetic treatment is associated with less relapse in obesity. J Psychosom Res. 2009;67(4):315–24.
32. de Zwaan M. Binge eating disorder and obesity. Int J Obes Relat Metab Disord. 2001;25(1):51–5.
33. Spitzer RL, Devlin M, Walsh BT, Hasin D, Wing R, Marcus M, et al. Binge eating disorder: a multisite field trial of the diagnostic criteria. Int J Eat Disord. 1992;11(3):191–203.
34. Spitzer RL, Yanovski S, Wadden T, Wing R, Marcus M, Stunkard AJ, et al. Binge eating disorder: its further validation in a multisite study. Int J Eat Disord. 1993;13(2):137–53.
35. Telch CF, Stice E. Psychiatric comorbidity in women with binge eating disorder: prevalence rates from a non-treatment seeking sample. J Consult Clin Psychol. 1998;66(5):768–76.
36. Marchesini G, Solaroli E, Baraldi L, Natale S, Migliorini S, Visani E, et al. Health-related quality of life in obesity: the role of eating behaviour. Diabetes Nutr Metab. 2000;13(3):156–64.
37. Brownley KA, Berkman ND, Sedway JA, Lohr KN, Bulik CM. Binge eating disorder treatment: a systematic review of randomized controlled trials. Int J Eat Disord. 2007;40:337–48.
38. Duchesne M, Appolinario JC, Range BP, Freitas S, Papelbaum M, Coutinho W. Evidence of cognitive-behavioural therapy in the treatment of obese patients with binge eating disorder. Rev Psiquiatr Rio Gd Sul. 2007;29(1):80–92.
39. Iacovino JM, Gredysa DM, Altman M, Wilfley DE. Psychological treatment for binge eating disorder. Curr Psychiatry Rep. 2012;14(4):432–46.
40. Agras WS, Telch CF, Arnow B, Eldredge K, Detzer MJ, Henderson J, et al. Does interpersonal therapy help patients with binge eating disorder who fail to respond to cognitive-behavioural therapy? J Consult Clin Psychol. 1995;63(3):356–60.
41. Munsch S, Biedert E, Meyer A, Michael T, Schlup B, Tuch A, et al. A randomized comparison of cognitive behavioural therapy and behavioural weight loss treatment for overweight individuals with binge eating disorder. Int J Eat Disord. 2007;40(2):102–13.
42. Grilo CM, Masheb RM. A randomized controlled comparison of guided self-help cognitive behavioural therapy and behavioural weight loss for binge eating disorder. Behav Res Ther. 2005;43:1509–25.
43. Grilo CM, Masheb RM, Gueorguieva R, Wilson GT, White MA. Cognitive-behavioural therapy, behavioural weight loss, and sequential treatment for obese patients with binge eating disorder. J Consult Clin Psychol. 2011;79(5):675–85.
44. Wilson GT, Wilfley DE, Agras WS, Bryson SW. Psychological treatments of binge eating disorder. Arch Gen Psychiatry. 2010;67(1):94–101.
45. Wilson GT, Grilo CM, Vitousek KM. Psychological treatments of eating disorders. Am Psychol. 2007;62(3):199–216.
46. Hilbert A, Bishop ME, Stein RI, Tanofsky-Kraff M, Swenson AK, Welch RR, Wilfley DE. Long-term efficacy of psychological treatment for binge eating disorder. Br J Psychiatry. 2012;200(3):232–7.
47. Ricca V, Mannucci E, Mezzani B, Moretti S, Di Bernardo M, Bertelli M, et al. Fluoxetine and fluvoxamine combined with individual cognitive-behaviour therapy in binge eating disorder: a one-year follow-up study. Psychother Psychosom. 2001;70(6):298–306.
48. Eldredge KL, Steward Agras W, Arnow B, Telch CF, Bell S, Castonguay L, et al. The effects of extending cognitive-behavioural therapy for binge eating disorder among initial treatment nonresponders. Int J Eat Disord. 1997;21(4):347–52.
49. Agras WS, Telch CF, Arnow B, Eldredge K, Wilfley DE, Raeburn SD, et al. Weight loss, cognitive-behavioural and desipramine treatments in binge eating disorder: an addictive design. Behav Ther. 1994;25(2):209–38.
50. Wilfley DE, Welch RR, Stein RI, Spurrell EB, Cohen LR, Saelens BE, et al. A randomized comparison of group cognitive-behavioural therapy and group interpersonal psychotherapy for the treatment of overweight individuals with binge-eating disorder. Arch Gen Psychiatry. 2002;59(8):713–21.
51. Grilo CM, Masheb RM, Wilson GT. Efficacy of cognitive behavioural therapy and fluoxetine for the treatment of binge eating disorder: a randomized

double-blind placebo-controlled comparison. Biol Psychiatry. 2005;57(1):301–9.
52. Agras WS, Telch CF, Arnow B, Eldredge K, Marnell M. One-year follow-up of cognitive-behavioural therapy for obese individuals with binge eating disorder. J Consult Clin Psychol. 1997;65(2):343–7.
53. Devlin MJ, Goldfein JA, Petkova E, Jiang H, Raizman PS, Wolk S, et al. Cognitive behavioural therapy and fluoxetine as adjuncts to group behavioural therapy for binge eating disorder. Obes Res. 2005;13(6):1077–88.
54. Fossati M, Amati F, Painot D, Reiner M, Haenni C, Golay A. Cognitive-behavioural therapy with simultaneous nutritional and physical activity education in obese patients with binge eating disorder. Eat Weight Disord. 2004;9(2):134–8.
55. Coucoulas AP, Christian NJ, Belle SH, Berk PD, Flum DR, Garcia L, et al. Weight change and health outcomes at 3 years after surgery among individuals with severe obesity. JAMA. 2013;310:2416–25.
56. Shah M, Simha V, Garg A. Review: long term impact of bariatric surgery on body weight, comorbidities, and nutritional status. J Clin Endocrinol Metab. 2006;91:4223–31.
57. Wolnerhanssen BK, Peters T, Kern B, Schotzau A, Ackermann C, von Flue M, Peterli R. Predictors of outcome in treatment of morbid obesity by laparoscopic adjustable gastric banding: results of a prospective study of 380 patients. Surg Obes Relat Dis. 2008;4(4):500–6.
58. Kalarchian MA, Wilson GT, Brolin RE, Bradley E. Effects of bariatric surgery on binge eating and related psychopathology. Eat Weight Disord. 1999;4(1):1–5.
59. Sallet PC, Sallet JA, Dixon JB, Collis E, Pisani CE, Levy A, et al. Eating behaviour as a prognostic factor for weight loss after gastric bypass. Obes Surg. 2007;17(4):445–51.
60. Abiles V, Rodriguez-Ruis S, Abiles J, Obispo A, Gandara N, Luna V, et al. Effectiveness of cognitive-behavioural therapy in morbidity obese candidates for bariatric surgery with and without binge eating disorder. Nutr Hosp. 2013;28(5):1523–9.
61. Ashton K, Drerup M, Windover A, Heinberg L. Brief, four-session group CBT reduces binge eating behaviours among bariatric surgery candidates. Surg Obes Relat Dis. 2009;5(2):257–62.
62. Ashton K, Heinberg L, Windover A, Merrell J. Positive response to binge eating intervention enhances postoperative weight loss. Surg Obes Relat Dis. 2011;7(3):315–20.
63. Cassin SE, Sockalingam S, Du C, Wnuk S, Hawa R, Parikh S. A pilot randomized controlled trial of telephone-based cognitive behavioural therapy for preoperative bariatric surgery patients. Behav Res Ther. 2016;80:17–22.
64. Gade H, Hjelmesæth J, Rosenvinge JH, Friborg O. Effectiveness of a cognitive behavioural therapy for dysfunctional eating among patients admitted for bariatric surgery: a randomized controlled trial. J Obes. 2014;21:127936.
65. Gade H, Friborg O, Rosenvinge JH, Smastuen MC, Hjelmesæth J. The impact of a preoperative cognitive behavioural therapy (CBT) on dysfunctional eating behaviours, affective symptoms and body weight 1 year after bariatric surgery: a randomized controlled trial. Obes Surg. 2015;25(11):2112–9.
66. Leahey TM, Crowther JH, Irwin SR. A cognitive-behavioural mindfulness group therapy intervention for the treatment of binge eating in bariatric surgery patients. Cogn Behav Pract. 2008;15(4):364–75.
67. Kalarchian MA, Marcus MD, Courcoulas AP, Cheng Y, Levine MD. Preoperative lifestyle intervention in bariatric surgery: a randomized clinical trial. Surg Obes Relat Dis. 2016;12(1):180–7. doi:10.1016/j.soard.2015.05.004.
68. Lier HO, Biringer E, Stubhaug B, Tangen T. The impact of preoperative counseling on postoperative adherence in bariatric surgery patients: a randomized controlled trial. Patient Educ Couns. 2012;87(3):336–42.
69. Kalarchian MA, Marcus MD, Courcoulas AP, Cheng Y, Levine MD, Josbeno D. Optimizing long-term weight control after bariatric surgery: a pilot study. Surg Obes Relat Dis. 2012;8(6):710–6.
70. Kalarchian MA, Marcus MD. Psychosocial interventions pre and post bariatric surgery. Eur Eat Disord Rev. 2015;23(6):457–62.

Behavioural Interventions for Weight Management Among Patients with Schizophrenia

19

Markus Duncan, Karen Davison, Gary Remington, and Guy Faulkner

19.1 Behavioural Interventions for Weight Management Among Patients with Schizophrenia

This chapter will focus on behavioural interventions for patients with schizophrenia and obesity. Building on previous chapters focused on assessment of obesity, this chapter will use a case vignette to apply an approach to assessing and treating obesity in patients with schizophrenia. We will summarize the evidence for behavioural interventions for weight management among patients with schizophrenia and specific components of behavioural approaches will be discussed.

M. Duncan • G. Faulkner (✉)
School of Kinesiology, University of British Columbia, 2146 Health Sciences Mall, Room 4606, Vancouver, BC, Canada V6T 1Z3
e-mail: mark.duncan@alumni.ubc.ca; guy.faulkner@ubc.ca

K. Davison, Ph.D., M.Sc., B.A.Sc., R.D.
Faculty of Health and Faculty of Science and Horticulture, Kwantlen Polytechnic University, 12666 72nd Avenue, Surrey, BC, Canada V3W 2M8
e-mail: karen.davison@kpu.ca

G. Remington, M.D., Ph.D., F.R.C.P.C.
Schizophrenia Division, Centre for Addiction and Mental Health, 250 College Street, Toronto, ON, Canada M5T 1R8
e-mail: gary.remington@camh.ca

Case Vignette

Amanda is a 24-year-old female who first became ill at the age of 18. Up until then, she had been functioning well, doing reasonably well at school but much more interested in sports. As the illness unfolded, she became increasingly withdrawn, labile, and religiously preoccupied. At her parents' recommendation, she visited the family doctor who felt she might be depressed. Antidepressants were offered but she declined.

Her performance at school deteriorated with the change in behaviour, as did her involvement with friends and the athletic activities she was routinely so interested in. Things worsened and her behaviour became more erratic; for example, she began to believe she had special powers in terms of intellect and, in addition, had a special relationship with God. She believed God could predict the future and acknowledged hearing voices that encouraged these ideas. She also became paranoid, concerned that others envious of his special powers were plotting to harm her. A confrontation on the street with a stranger who she accused of this led to the police becoming involved, and she was admitted to hospital involuntarily.

(continued)

S. Sockalingam, R. Hawa (eds.), *Psychiatric Care in Severe Obesity*,
DOI 10.1007/978-3-319-42536-8_19

(continued)

It was in hospital that she was first diagnosed with psychosis. There was a positive family history, with several family members on her father's side diagnosed with schizophrenia. Substance abuse did not appear to be a factor. Amanda was started on one of the newer antipsychotics because of evidence that they have less risk of the motor side effects that were so prevalent with the older agents. However, as a class these newer antipsychotics have been associated with greater liability in terms of weight gain and associated metabolic difficulties. She was started on risperidone.

She was discharged after approximately 2 weeks, with the symptoms modestly improved. Regular follow-up visits were scheduled but she was non-adherent with treatment and required re-hospitalization. In this instance, she was switched to a long-acting injectable antipsychotic (fluphenazine) because she had not been adherent with her medications as an outpatient.

Once again, she was discharged from hospital and while improved over the next 6 months, she continued to experience symptoms that interfered with functioning. She did not feel she could return to school or work, and her interest in sports was not there. She spent much of the time at home and alone in her room.

Also with time, she became more accepting of the need for treatment. Because she was still manifesting psychotic symptoms, it was felt that she could be tried again on an oral medication and was started on another of the newer antipsychotics, olanzapine. Over the next 2 months, she showed progressive improvement and symptoms remitted entirely. Accompanying this was renewed interest in continuing school and returning to sports.

Unfortunately, while she responded very well to olanzapine, she also experienced one of its most common side effects—weight gain. She had gained approximately 2 kg since the onset of the illness prior to its initiation, but this was not associated with her previous medications and thought to reflect inactivity. On the olanzapine, though, her weight ballooned; within 18 months, she had gained 14 kg, and now with a BMI of 34. She was being followed regularly by her family doctor because of olanzapine's association with weight gain and metabolic side effects. Within this period of 18 months, lab reports indicated elevated fasting blood glucose levels as well as abnormal HbA1C levels; in addition, there was evidence of elevated cholesterol and triglycerides.

She did return to school and began to become more active once more, but she acknowledged she was not able to bring the same effort to either that she had before becoming ill. In terms of weight, she was able to see very modest changes with the amount of exercise she was involved with (e.g. walking 20 min 3–4 times weekly) but was unable to shed more than 1 kg. Because of the concerns related to her lab work, she was also started on metformin to address the abnormal glucose and a statin for the abnormal lipid profile. She subjectively reported having much more difficulty controlling her appetite than before being put on olanzapine.

Because of concerns regarding her physical health over the longer term, it was decided to taper and discontinue the olanzapine, replacing it with a newer antipsychotic that carried a lower liability for weight gain. Two such trials were undertaken, but in both cases the psychotic symptoms reappeared. Following discussions that involved her, the family doctor, and the psychiatrist, olanzapine was reinstated.

At present, she has returned to school and is doing well. Despite efforts to control her eating, her BMI hovers between 33 and 36. She remains on metformin and a statin. Because of the weight gain, it has been hard for her to re-engage in sports and, in fact, she now complains of joint pain that compromises her further. Socially, Amanda struggles and indicates this is related to her weight and increased self-consciousness.

19.2 Schizophrenia

Schizophrenia is a disabling and enduring form of serious mental illness. It is typically considered a disease related to brain abnormalities caused by a range of specific genetic and/or environmental factors [1]. The annual incidence of schizophrenia is approximately 15 per 100,000, and the risk of developing the illness over one's lifetime is 0.7 % [2]. The usual presentation in late adolescence/early adulthood places very high demands on individuals, their families, and society itself. In particular, the economic burden of schizophrenia has been estimated to range from 0.02 to 1.65 % of many high-income nations' gross domestic product [3]. The symptoms of schizophrenia can be divided into positive, negative, and cognitive symptoms [4]. Positive symptoms are those that appear to reflect an excess or distortion of normal functions and are manifested in symptoms such as delusions, hallucinations, and thought disorder. Negative symptoms are those that appear to reflect a reduction or loss of normal functions and reflect symptoms such as affective flattening, apathy, social withdrawal, and cognitive impairments. Cognitive symptoms can adversely affect functions such as attention, memory, and concentration.

Schizophrenia is a chronic and relapsing disorder with incomplete remission in most cases [4]. Antipsychotic medication is the primary treatment for schizophrenia. While such medication can help control the positive symptoms, they are less effective in alleviating negative symptoms and cognitive deficits [5, 6]. Unfortunately, it appears that the negative symptoms and cognitive deficits can substantially interfere with functional recovery [7]. Some researchers have also suggested that motivational deficits are the central link between negative symptoms and functional impairment in schizophrenia [8]—a particular challenge for developing and implementing behavioural interventions in this population.

For individuals with schizophrenia, there is a decreased life expectancy of approximately 20–25 years in comparison to the general population [9, 10]. Some data also suggest that this mortality gap is increasing [11]. This increased rate of mortality is reflected in higher rates of morbidity. Almost all disorders occur at higher than expected rates but the prevalence of cardiovascular disease and diabetes is markedly elevated [12].

Potential causes of this excess mortality and morbidity are varied but can be broadly categorized in terms of treatment (metabolic side-effects of atypical antipsychotic medication), greater engagement in unhealthy behaviours such as smoking, physical inactivity, and poor nutritional habits, and limited access to health care [13]. The clinical case of Amanda highlights one very common outcome associated with schizophrenia—increased weight gain and an increased risk of obesity. The impact of obesity on cardiovascular health of people with schizophrenia is double as compared to the general population [14]. Weight gain is largely mediated by antipsychotic medication based on evidence of patients with schizophrenia before the development of such medication or drug naïve patients (e.g. [15]). The antipsychotic Amanda is taking, olanzapine; has been associated with severe weight gain although all antipsychotics are associated with weight gain [16]. Similarly, the risk of metabolic syndrome is significantly higher with clozapine and olanzapine than other antipsychotics [17]. A recent meta-analysis demonstrated that clinically significant weight gain risk increased about twofold with antipsychotic use in first-episode patients [18]. Compared to placebo, mean weight gain was 3.22 kg and 1.4 points BMI in the short term, and 5.30 kg and 1.86 points BMI in the long term [18]. Recognition of the metabolic side effects of antipsychotic medication has rightly focused attention on addressing the physical health needs of individuals with schizophrenia. With significant weight gain or emerging metabolic effects, the risk and benefit of antipsychotic choice should be re-evaluated from both a psychiatric and a metabolic perspective, and at this stage, patients like Amanda should ideally be referred to a more structured and supervised behavioural intervention to manage weight gain [19].

19.3 Behavioural Interventions for Weight Management in Schizophrenia: What Does the Evidence Tell Us?

We performed a systematic search of MEDLINE and EMBASE for systematic reviews and meta-analyses concerning behavioural interventions for weight management. The search terms included combinations of terms by study type (e.g. systematic review), population (e.g. schizophrenia), intervention (e.g. non-pharmacological), and outcome (e.g. weight). To be included in this review of reviews, the reviews had to (1) use a systematic search strategy (e.g. systematic review and/or meta-analysis), (2) provide data on weight loss or management (e.g. prevention of weight gain), (3) include studies assessing non-pharmacological interventions to manage weight, and this data had to be interpreted separately from pharmacological evidence (e.g. sub-analysis of only behavioural studies; details of studies are presented individual), and (4) include studies where the sample was predominantly individuals with a serious mental illness (SMI) such as schizophrenia or taking antipsychotic medication. The search was restricted to the last five years (January 2011–April 2016).

Ten reviews were ultimately included (see Table 19.1; [20–29]). Across all reviews, 46 unique studies pertaining to behavioural interve ntions for weight management in SMI were included. With regard to interventions, three reviews [22, 26, 27] were focused on physical activity, another on diet advice [25], and the remaining six included any non-pharmacological, behavioural, or lifestyle intervention to change body weight [20, 21, 23, 24, 28, 29].

Results were mixed among the seven reviews that performed meta-analyses. Two found no significant difference between interventions and controls [22, 26], four found an effect in favour of interventions [20, 23, 27, 29], while one did not find any studies that met the inclusion criteria [25]. Both meta-analyses that found no effect for the intervention included interventions focused on physical activity. The only other meta-analysis to limit interventions solely to physical activity did find a positive effect in favour of physical activity, but included studies that were not limited to SMI [27]. These results indicate that exercise only interventions are unlikely to assist weight management. Rather multifaceted and comprehensive weight management programmes that aim to improve diet, increase physical activity, and provide counselling are likely to be more successful in improving weight management.

The reviews conducted by Bonfioli et al. [20], Caemmerer et al. [29], and Gierisch et al. [23] could be considered the most comprehensive due to their inclusion of any non-pharmacological intervention to target weight management. These reviews are also specific to people with SMI, rather than all mental illnesses, and each provide meta-analyses of randomized controlled trials providing high quality level of evidence. Caemmerer et al.'s [29] review meta-analysed 17 studies, the majority of which (nine) were described as cognitive behavioural therapy or a psychoeducational programme, and another four were described as a combination of nutrition and exercise. Treatment programmes lasted 8–72 weeks. The average treatment period was 19.6 weeks. Overall, the weighted mean difference across all trials was significant for weight (−3.12 kg, CI: −4.03 to −2.21, $p<0.001$) and BMI (−0.94 kg/m^2, CI: −1.45 to −0.43, $p<0.001$), indicating that small reductions in weight are feasible with non-pharmacological therapies and these changes can be accrued within an approximate 6-month treatment period. Furthermore, this review provides evidence that weight loss can be maintained. Five programmes had follow-up periods 8–52 weeks (mean 14.4 weeks) after the treatment ended. Significantly greater weight loss persisted in favour of the intervention group compared to control (−3.48 kg, CI: −6.37 to −0.58, $p=0.02$).

Caemmerer and colleagues [29] also performed several sub-analyses to identify moderating variables. Intervention trials to reduce weight gain among individuals taking antipsychotics were separated from prevention trials aiming to minimize weight gain after initiating antipsychotic medication. There was no significantly different effect for prevention (−3.23 kg, CI: −4.37 to −2.04, $p<0.001$) versus treatment interventions (−3.12 kg, CI: −4.39 to −2.21, $p<0.001$).

Table 19.1 Summary of reviews

Author, date	Type of review (K)	Sample description	Intervention variables	Outcome measures	Types of research design	Weight management findings	Comments
Bonfioli et al., 2012 [20]	SR and MA (13)	Adults 18–64, at least 50 % with SZ-like illness, bipolar disorder, or depression with psychotic features	Psychoeducational, cognitive-behavioural, nutritional or physical activity-based interventions, aimed at weight reduction or prevention of weight gain	BMI	RCT	Compared to controls, experimental groups showed a mean BMI reduction of –0.98 kg/m^2 (95 % CI: –1.31 to –0.65 kg/m^2). Equivalent to loss of 3.12 % of initial weight. Prevention studies with individual psychoeducational programmes that include diet and/or physical activity have the highest impact	
Cimo et al., 2012 [21]	SR (4) (One of these was a follow-up to previous study)	Type 2 diabetes and SZ/SZA	Must target a lifestyle factor associated with diabetes self-care, such as problem-solving skills, education classes, diet, or exercise	HbA1c, fasting blood glucose (FBG), BMI or weight lost (measured in pounds or kilograms)	Various	Only one study reported weight loss in an RCT Authors conclude diabetes education is effective when it incorporates diet and exercise components. Weight loss is possible	Low number of included studies, and inclusion of a variety of study designs makes it difficult to draw conclusions
Firth et al., 2015 [22]	SR (20) and MA (11)	Non-affective psychotic disorders (but including SZA) or first episode psychosis	Exercise	At least one quantitative measure of physical or mental health	Interventions (RCT, non-randomized controlled trial, case series/uncontrolled longitudinal) Only RCT for MA	Body weight/BMI studies in SR (K=9) and MA (K=4). Exercise did not significantly reduce BMI in meta-analysis: mean difference = –0.98 kg/m^2; 95 % CI –3.17 to 1.22 kg/m^2. Systematic review results of other studies were mixed	
Gierisch et al., 2014 [23]	SR (33) and MA (11) (10 Behavioural)	Adults with SMI	Patient-focused behavioral interventions/peer or family support intervention/ pharmacological treatments targeting weight control/glucose levels/lipid levels/overall CVD risk	Key outcomes were weight (kg), glycosylated haemoglobin A1c (HbA1c), total and low-density lipoprotein (LDL) cholesterol	RCT	Behavioural significantly reduced BMI in meta-analysis of behavioural interventions (K=10): mean difference = –3.14 kg/m^2; 95 % CI –4.33 to –1.96 No peer or family support studies; Insufficient strength of evidence for any intervention having effect on glucose control (glycosylated haemoglobin) or lipid control	Metformin (K=5, mean difference = –4.13 kg/m^2; 95 % CI –6.58 to –1.68) and anti-convulsant medication (K=4, mean difference = –5.11 kg/m^2; 95 % CI –9.48 to –0.74) also effective pharmacological interventions

(continued)

Table 19.1 (continued)

Author, date	Type of review (K)	Sample description	Intervention variables	Outcome measures	Types of research design	Weight management findings	Comments
Hjorth et al., 2014 [24]	SR (23)	>50 % SZ, SZA or schizophreniform disorder	Non-pharmacological interventions (diet, exercise, cognitive behavioural therapy, or combined) aimed at weight reduction/reducing physical illness compared to with standard care	Weight loss/ weight maintenance, other physical health outcomes	Interventions (Randomized and Non-randomized clinically controlled)	*Diet* ($K=4$) three studies demonstrated improved weight management; one study offering free fruits and vegetables did not show any health parameter change	Two diet interventions included walking, but were not considered "combinations"
						Exercise ($K=5$): four studies reported weight loss/better weight management with exercise, one did not report weight outcomes but reported improved cardiovascular fitness	One pedometer and motivational interviewing, one fitness training and nutritional advice
						Cognitive/Behavioural-Therapy ($K=3$): two studies showed significant better weight management; one not significant at study end, but significant at 6-month follow-up	
						Combined ($K=11$): improved weight control in ten studies (two of these reported improved metabolic profile), remaining study demonstrated reduction in metabolic syndrome (weight not reported in review)	
Pearsall et al., 2016 [25]	SR and MA (0)	Any age, schizophrenia, or other types of schizophrenia-like psychosis	dietary advice, with the aim of changing and improving dietary intake; only diet, no exercise/ supplements	Nutritional intake; BMI/ weight	RCT	No studies eligible for inclusion	Cochrane Review

Pearsall et al., 2014 [26]	SR and MA (8)—Body weight/BMI in SR (4) and MA (4)	Adults with schizophrenia, schizoaffective disorders, or bipolar-affective disorder	Promote exercise or physical activity	Any outcome (not specified in methods, post hoc analysis)	RCT	MA showed no difference in BMI ($K=4$) or weight ($K=2$) between standard care and exercise at end of trials. Change in BMI/weight not in MA, but SR reported one study showed reduction in body weight greater in intervention than control, other study no significant difference. Change in BMI for only one study reported in SR, with no significant difference between intervention and control	MA appears to just evaluate final BMI and weight, not change. This does not account for initial differences between groups
Rosen-baum et al., 2014 [27]	SR and MA (39) (12 schizophrenia, 1 bipolar disorder, 1 first episode psychosis; 1 severe mental illness); (11 for anthropometric measures)	18 years of age or older, in whom a DSM or ICD diagnosis of mental illness was made. Dysthymia, "mild-depression", and eating disorders were excluded	Any form of physical activity	Various health outcomes, including BMI/Weight	RCT	Pooled anthropometric measures indicate effect in favour of exercise: SMD = 0.24; 95 % CI, 0.06–0.41; $p<0.05$; $I^2=0\%$	8 of 11 studies analysed in anthropometric MA described sample as SMI
Whitney et al., 2015 [28]	SR (17)	>50 % of participants treated with clozapine (all treated with antipsychotics)	Pharmacological and non-pharmacological weight management interventions	BMI/Weight	Various	*Non-Pharmacological* ($n=2$): Only one intervention study which found significant reduction in weight (–5.2 kg) and BMI with diet and exercise intervention versus control	
						Combination ($K=1$): Sibutramine + behavioural and nutritional counselling found no change in weight	
Caem-merer et al., 2012 [29]	SR and MA (17)	Implied: individuals with antipsychotic weight gain	Any non-pharmacological interventions to address antipsychotic associated weight	BMI/Weight	RCT	Interventions led to a significant reduction in weight (–3.12 kg; CI:–4.03, –2.21, $p<0.001$) and BMI (–0.94 kg/m^2; CI:–1.45, –0.43, $p<0.001$) compared with control groups	Prevention and intervention trial sub-analyses performed, similar to pooled results

Note: *K* Number of Studies, *SR* Systematic Review, *MA* Meta-analysis, *BMI* Body mass index, *SZ* Schizophrenia, *SZA* Schizoaffective Disorder, *SMI* Severe Mental Illness, *RCT* Randomized controlled trial, *CI* Confidence interval, *DSM* Diagnostic and Statistical Manual of Mental Disorders, *ICD* International Classification of Disease, *SMI* Severe Mental Illness

Additional sensitivity analyses found comparable results between interventions >3 months and <3 months, as well as group-based and individual treatments. Cognitive-behavioural interventions had a smaller effect size than nutrition and/or exercise programmes though both were significantly better than controls. Finally, weight and BMI were significantly improved only in outpatient trials but not in inpatient or mixed samples. Overall, these analyses indicate that both prevention and intervention trials are roughly equivalent in effect, weight loss can be achieved in under 3 months, and that both group-based and individual interventions are similarly effective.

Gierisch and colleagues' [23] review included ten behavioural interventions in their meta-analysis, all of which included either cognitive behavioural therapy or multiple lifestyle change factors. Pooled effects favoured behavioural interventions with a mean difference of −3.13 kg (CI: −4.21 to −2.05, $p<0.05$). This review also reported positive effects for metformin (mean difference=−4.13 kg CI: −6.58 to −1.68, $p<0.05$), and anticonvulsive medications topiramate and zonisamide (mean difference=−5.11 kg, CI: −9.48 to −0.74, $p<0.05$). Bonfioli et al. [20] identified 17 studies in their systematic review, of which four were excluded from meta-analysis due to missing information. The remaining 13 studies all included elements of cognitive behavioural therapy or psychoeducation as opposed to diet or exercise alone. Overall, the findings were very similar to Caemmerer et al.'s [29] review, which found a weighted mean difference in BMI of −0.98 kg/m^2 (CI: −1.31 to −0.65 kg/m^2, $p<0.05$), compared to control. In contrast to the findings reported by Caemmerer and colleagues [29], the sub-analyses reported by Bonfioli et al. [20] found that weight gain prevention studies were slightly more effective than treatment interventions, and group interventions were less effective than individual interventions. These differences in the results of sub-analyses reflect different inclusion criteria of the two reviews.

Taken together these three meta-analyses provide consistent evidence that lifestyle interventions that include diet and physical activity are feasible and are effective in reducing weight by approximately 3 kg or a BMI reduction of 0.9–1 kg/m^2. Weight loss can also be maintained. However, the optimal duration and intensity (e.g. number of counselling sessions) of intervention is still unclear. At the least, meta-analyses suggest that optimal interventions should consider both diet and physical activity and include psychological/behavioural components. A more focused discussion is now provided concerning dietary and physical activity strategies that could be applied in the case of Amanda.

19.4 Intervening with Amanda

19.4.1 Nutrition

Nutrition interventions, as part of programmes that include regular physical activity and quality sleep, are an important component of healthy weight management. The dietary patterns of people with schizophrenia or those at high risk for psychosis are typically high in energy mainly contributed from excess fat (particularly saturated fat) and low in fruits, vegetables, and dietary fibre [30–34]. These eating patterns contribute both to dietary energy excess and gut microbiome alterations [35], which lead to subsequent weight gain, risks of conditions such as heart disease, type 2 diabetes, osteoarthritis, and exacerbation of mental health symptoms.

The causes of overeating are multifactorial [36]. Genetics, which can affect metabolic rate and weight status, and physiologic factors (e.g. leptin, ghrelen, uncoupling proteins, beta-endorphins, neuropeptide Y, decreased blood glucose) can reduce satiety or increase hunger. Recurrent and frequent binge eating can cause significant weight gain, and food environments, which offer an abundance of good-tasting, cheap food, makes it difficult for susceptible individuals to avoid such overeating triggers. Night eating, where most food energy is consumed between 8 p.m. and 6 a.m., is another common contributor to overeating.

For those with schizophrenia, other condition-related determinants contribute to excess food intake. As in Amanda's case, psychiatric medications such as the second-generation antipsychotics, are associated with metabolic side effects of weight gain, dyslipidemia, insulin resistance, susceptibility to type 2 diabetes, and metabolic syndrome ([37–40]), which may be coupled by an a priori increased risk of obesity that has been reported in schizophrenia [41, 42]. Structural factors such as the built environment that controls food availability and social barriers such as negative discrimination and stigma can also contribute to the etiology of overeating and excess weight. Individual factors such as a history of trauma, memory or cognitive impairment, food-related hallucinations or delusions, comorbid eating disturbances, poor condition self-management skills, proneness to food fads and use of natural health products, concurrent substance use, social avoidance, symptoms of depression, anxiety, and poor sleep, and determinants of health such as low socioeconomic status, and food insecurity can create barriers to health services access and behavioural interventions [43–48].

Figure 19.1 outlines an algorithm that may be used in the assessment and management of weight and nutrition for individuals such as Amanda. Her initial assessment would include examining health status, nutrition-related biochemical measures and genomic markers where feasible, medication and natural health product use, food intake and eating behaviours, anthropometric measurements (e.g. height, weight, waist and hip circumferences), and

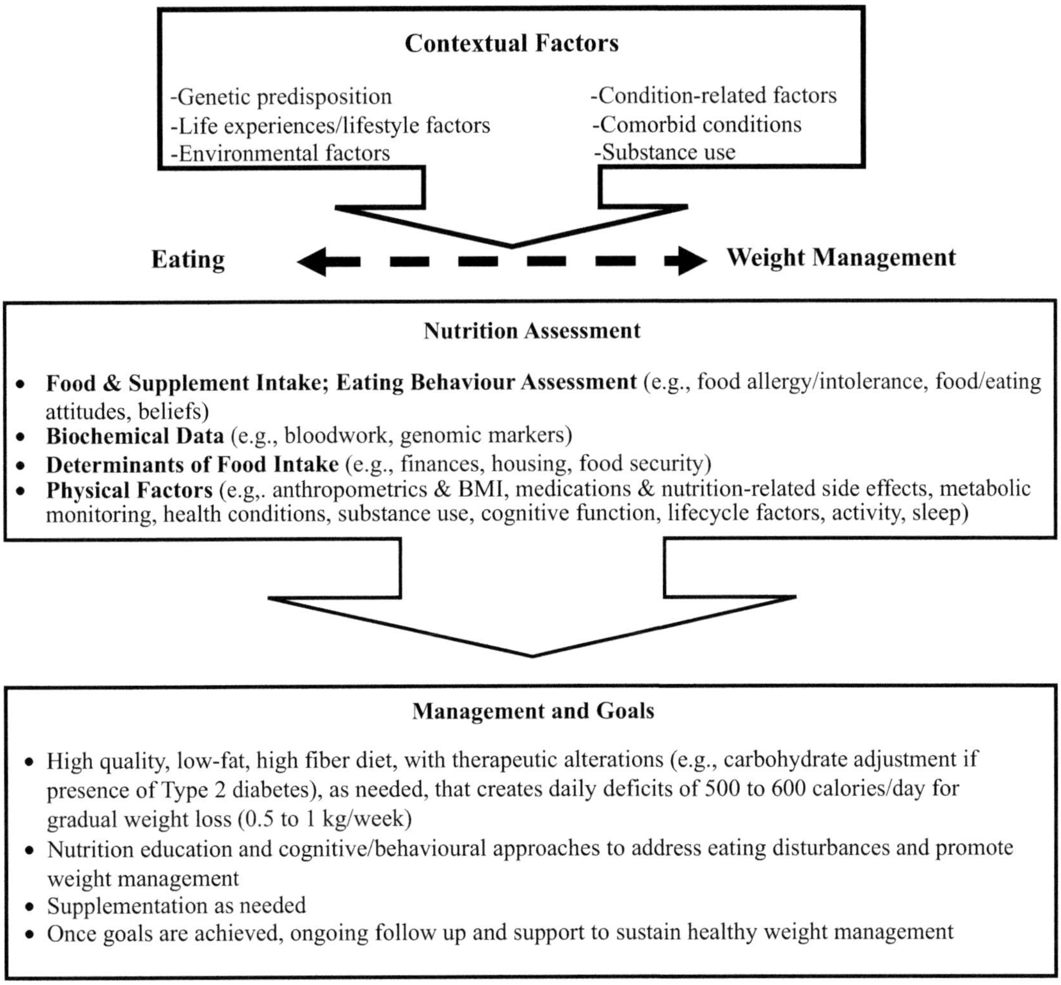

Fig. 19.1 Assessment and Weight Management Algorithm

health determinants such as income, food security, and living situation. Subsequently, an individualized lifestyle intervention would be negotiated where the nutrition component would focus on reducing energy intake in the range of 500–600 cal/day and applying cognitive and behavioural techniques aimed at dietary restructuring. The recommended macronutrient composition would emphasize high complex carbohydrates with moderate fat and protein levels where total energy is distributed as 20–30 % fat, 55–60 % carbohydrates, and 15–20 % protein to help reduce weight and control LDL-cholesterol, blood triglycerides, and blood glucose levels [49, 50], even in the context of antipsychotic medication use [45, 51]. The minimum caloric level for women such as Amanda is 1000 cal/day; for men no less than 1200 kcal/day should be consumed to ensure all nutrient requirements are being met. If the individual's food intake is not balanced and varied, then fibre and micronutrients such as zinc, calcium, iron, and vitamin B_{12} may be lacking and supplementation may be required. Furthermore, should the person be pregnant or lactating, or have significant eating disturbances these lower calorie diets should be avoided. In designing a weight management plan for Amanda, a personalized non-complex approach is needed that incorporates three core strategies:

1. *Determining readiness for change and setting realistic goals*: Discussions about weight should be non-judgemental and explore the individual's readiness for change [52]. If the individual has concerns about their weight, then goals should be set that are specific, reasonable, measurable, and promote gradual weight loss of 0.5–1 kg/week.
2. *Consuming less food energy*: Nutrition education would focus on learning appropriate serving sizes, facilitating lowered energy intake by consuming less added and hidden fats, switching to low- and non-caloric beverages, and emphasizing consumption of vegetables and fruits to provide important micronutrients and promote satiety.
3. *Incorporate appropriate eating behaviour modifications*: Exemplars of these include eating at set regular times in one location to avoid mindless eating, keeping a log of what is eaten, when, and why to identify social or emotional cues of overeating, saving high-calorie snacks foods for occasional special treats, avoiding purchases of problem foods, serving food portions on smaller dishes, and chewing foods slowly and stopping when feeling full.

As is the case with Amanda, several condition specific factors should be considered in the management of weight. While for some the structure of a diet plan may be helpful, therapeutic interventions may be needed alone or as adjunct to a diet plan to help correct eating disturbances and manage weight. Although a number of strategies may be used, evidence is currently lacking about their utility in mental health populations. For those who do not connect with hunger or satiety cues, mindful and intuitive eating counselling can help promote awareness of bodily sensations, self-care, and valuing health more than appearance [53, 54]. Motivational interviewing can also be used as a tool in weight management to help the individual resolve ambivalence about eating behaviour change and build intrinsic motivation [55]. Cognitive behaviour therapy (CBT) is a core strategy that can be used to address binge eating and improve body image [56]. Dialectical behaviour therapy is a form of CBT often used in more complex cases that can facilitate learning and skills development such as emotion regulation and distress intolerance that improve abilities to manage negative affect adaptively [57]. Should cognitive-behavioural and dialectical behaviour therapies not be effective, an alternative is acceptance and commitment therapy that can help the person work toward valued goals and life directions [58]. For individuals with cognitive impairments, cognitive adaptive training (CAT) may be used to help overcome challenges such as initiating and sustaining task behaviour (e.g. preparing meals). Exemplars of CAT environmental supports include separating foods into bins labelled by day of the week, using checklists, lists outlining steps for food preparation, and electronic auditory prompts, as well as practicing shopping at grocery stores using a food list [59]. While mobile electronic devices are popular tools to facilitate and maintain weight loss among overweight and obese populations, evidence on their sustained benefit and utility in mental health populations is currently lacking [60].

19.4.2 Physical Activity

Physical inactivity is itself a major cause of morbidity and mortality, and merits the same level of concern as other cardiovascular disease risk factors like smoking (e.g. [61]). Studies consistently highlight that individuals with schizophrenia are less active than the general population [62, 63]. This is reflected in the demonstration of significantly lower cardiorespiratory fitness among individuals with schizophrenia in comparison to the general population (e.g. [64]). Given the compelling evidence that regular physical activity is an effective preventative strategy against premature mortality, cardiovascular disease, stroke, hypertension, colon cancer, breast cancer, and type 2 diabetes for the general population [65], promoting physical activity is important irrespective of weight loss.

We have adapted a form of physical activity counselling that is designed to increase physical activity by addressing an individual's needs, motivation, and barriers to activity [66]. Physical activity counselling draws from numerous theories of behaviour change including social cognitive theory and the transtheoretical model (TTM) [67, 68]. Social cognitive theory states that behaviour is influenced and influences both environmental and personal factors. Environmental factors include group structures, equipment, or various facilities. Personal factors include cognitions such as self-efficacy, mood, and attitudes. Together, these three determinants influence one another and form what is known as triadic reciprocal causation [67]. The TTM allows a clinician to assess whether an individual is ready to change a particular behaviour. Depending on their readiness to change, clients are placed into one of six stages: precontemplation (not considering changing behaviour), contemplation (intending to change behaviour in the next 6 months), preparation (intending to change behaviour in next 30 days), action (actively engaged in behaviour change for 6 months), maintenance (actively engaged in behaviour change for more than 6 months), and termination (actively engaged in behaviour change for more than 5 years). This then directs attention to those individuals who are contemplating or preparing to increase their physical activity. The TTM also provides stage specific strategies that strengthen a client's self-efficacy and highlight the positive, rather than the negative, attributes of increasing physical activity. Self-efficacy has been shown to be an important mediator of physical activity behaviour change in people with schizophrenia [69].

The intervention was conducted over 2 months and included four 60 min weekly individual sessions that could be replicated:

Session one: Build rapport and gather knowledge. This first session provided an opportunity to assess current levels of physical activity and explore commitment to increasing physical activity. As a starting point, physical activity was assessed using the International Physical Activity Questionnaire (IPAQ; [70]). The IPAQ has previously been validated as a measure of physical activity behaviour for adults with schizophrenia [71]. Throughout the first session, various techniques were used to assess readiness to change. First, past, present, and future interests and physical activity were explored. Given Amanda's prior interest in sport and exercise there is an excellent basis for establishing rapport. Additionally, confidence and importance scales were used to assess how confident each participant was about becoming more physically active and how important physical activity was to him or her [72, 73]. A similar approach could be taken in assessing interest in modifying dietary behaviour and a decision taken to focus on one or both behaviours. The first session provided a better understanding of why physical activity may or may not be important to the participant and what potential barriers existed. In addition to the confidence and importance scales, the participants completed a decisional balance exercise [72, 73]. This exercise helped participants explore and overcome their ambivalence to behaviour change by attempting to establish a discrepancy between the advantages and disadvantages of changing their behaviour.

Session two: Goal setting. The second session helped participants develop an action plan to become more physically active by setting specific goals and strategies. Participants were guided by two sets of questions. First, participants had to establish a particular physical activity goal, identify its importance, create a series of steps to help them follow through with their goal, and be provided with a list of available support structures both in- and outside the hospital or home. Second, participants were asked to identify how to handle potential barriers and seek out individuals who may render assistance. Throughout this session, participants were asked about their goals, their goals' perceived importance, and also how to overcome potential barriers. These questions were intended to increase the level, strength, and specificity of not only exercise self-efficacy, but also barrier self-efficacy through verbal persuasion [67].

Walking is recommended as an initial form of physical activity given its low cost, relative ease for most people in engaging in, and safety. Pedometers are useful tools for monitoring steps accrued through walking. Typically, we have asked participants to wear a pedometer for a week to get a baseline of their steps before then gradually increasing walking to 3000 steps/day above baseline. This is typically ramped such that individuals increase their steps by 1000 over baseline for 2 weeks, and then 2000 steps above baseline for a further 2 weeks, before increasing and maintaining their steps by 3000 over their initial baseline. This is approximately equivalent to 30 min of daily physical activity for the average person [74].

Sessions three and four: Evaluate, revise, inform. During sessions three and four, the action plan was reviewed and adjusted, if necessary. Participants were encouraged to discuss their set goals and any anticipated and unanticipated barriers they may have encountered during the previous week. Throughout these sessions, participants were reminded about their individual personal strengths and support systems, asked to brainstorm ideas of how to overcome difficult barriers, and provided with additional information about various resources to help them achieve their physical activity goals.

In the single case experimental study, this approach was found to be a feasible and acceptable intervention to help improve the psychological mediators associated with physical activity [66]. Two participants moved from the preparation stage to the action stage while one participant moved from contemplation to the preparation stage. One participant did not shift from the preparation stage throughout the study. Importantly, self-efficacy improved for all participants throughout the intervention. While promising, further development and longitudinal evaluation of such a counselling approach is required. It does provide a structure for consultation with clients in attempting to develop the self-regulatory skills needed to maintain physical activity participation. More structured exercise interventions with ongoing support may be necessary for some individuals with schizophrenia [75]. Exercise interventions in supervised or group settings, can be feasible and effective interventions for schizophrenia [22]. A recent meta-analysis of exercise intervention studies in this population recommended clinicians implement supervised group exercise programmes of at least 30 min/day, 3 times per week for at least 12 weeks [76]. However, the need for such intensive support has clear implications for the sustainability of such interventions. Such specialized interventions may also not be readily accessible for many individuals with schizophrenia. A focus on modifying habitual physical activity might be more feasible.

19.5 Summary

The case of Amanda is unfortunately the norm in the clinical management of schizophrenia. The prevalence of obesity and metabolic syndrome is significantly elevated compared to the general population. Behavioural interventions for weight gain in schizophrenia are feasible although weight loss appears to be modest. Given this modest weight loss, the first strategy in preventing or alleviating weight gain is to appraise metabolic risk when prescribing antipsychotic medication although priority remains on achieving good control of the mental illness [19]. Ideally, the clinical management of Amanda would be interdisciplinary where team members would include physicians, registered dieticians, psychologists, kinesiologists, and social workers working collaboratively to manage the various factors that contribute to her weight status.

National weight loss guidelines suggest that a daily calorie deficit of 500–600 kcal through combined diet and moderate intensity activity is required for weight loss in overweight and obese adults [77]. The American College of Sports Medicine (ACSM) Position Stand on activity for weight loss proposes a weekly duration for moderate intensity physical activity of up to 250–300 min [78]. The feasibility of such a goal for most individuals with schizophrenia remains to be tested. The most effective dose of physical activity is likely one that individuals enjoy. The benefits of increased physical activity, independent of weight loss, should be emphasized. A range of physical activity modes and intensities should also be recommended based on the participant's prior experiences, preferences and goals.

Dietary interventions that promote healthy weight management should be based on a comprehensive assessment of nutritional status and personalized approaches that incorporate appropriate diet plans, nutrition education, and eating behaviour modifications. For those with eating disturbances and significant impairments, therapeutic interventions such as mindful and intuitive eating counselling, motivational interviewing, cognitive behaviour therapy, dialectical behaviour therapy, and cognitive adaptive training may also be used to help manage overeating and excess weight. Any dietary interventions must have buy-in of the individual and be offered in a tailored and non-complex way. However, given the limited resources allocated to nutrition and physical activity support for individuals like Amanda within mental health services, the implementation of these ideal weight management interventions is challenging. Similar to service models for diabetes, individuals who are initially diagnosed with schizophrenia would likely benefit from referral to an interdisciplinary healthcare team who can provide education and guidance with chronic condition self-management skills to prevent and ameliorate overeating, physical inactivity, and excess weight.

However, it is important to acknowledge that behavioural interventions may not be appropriate for many individuals with schizophrenia due to significant impairment in functioning and insight. Intervention also needs to be directed toward how the environment, in which many people with schizophrenia inhabit (e.g. psychiatric facilities; community care homes), can be modified to promote physical activity and reduce energy intake [79]. Such settings may facilitate increased energy intake (e.g. overeating, easy access to high-calorie snacks and beverages, and skipping breakfast) and reduce opportunities for energy expenditure (e.g. not having access to staircases; availability of screen time). For example, the modified buffet service form of food delivery (food is plated in the dining area by food service staff based on patient choice) was associated with overeating in one institution. In an uncontrolled natural experiment, we examined the impact of introducing an individualized tray service that allowed for control over portion size [80]. There was a significant reduction in body weight compared with pre-intervention measures at 3 and 6 months. At 6 months, 74 % of the 53 patients lost weight with 14 (26 %) losing more than 7 % body weight. As a group, mean BMI dropped 1 point over 6 months, from 29.8 to 28.8. This is comparable to the weighted mean differences reported in the meta-analyses of behavioural interventions (e.g. [23]). In complementing behavioural interventions, this study illustrates the potential effectiveness of environmental interventions in assisting population level approaches to weight management [80].

19.6 Take Home Messages

- Although priority should be given to achieving good control of the mental illness, the first strategy in preventing or alleviating weight gain or metabolic disturbance is to appraise metabolic risk when prescribing antipsychotic medication.

- Patients, family, and caregivers should be educated about metabolic risks and receive lifestyle advice regarding diet and physical activity. Baseline screening and a monitoring plan should be initiated on commencement of antipsychotic treatment.
- With significant weight gain or emerging metabolic effects, patients should be referred to a more structured and supervised lifestyle intervention where available.
- Intervention components should focus on reducing caloric intake (changing types of food consumed and reducing portion sizes) rather than complex dietary change, and support people in gradually increasing their levels of physical activity. However, the best physical activity dose is the one that can be sustained by an individual—some physical activity is better than none and more is better. Cognitive-behavioural strategies to facilitate changes in diet and physical activity that are tailored to this population need development.

References

1. Tandon R, Keshavan MS, Nasrallah HA. Schizophrenia, "Just the Facts": what we know in 2008. Part 1: overview. Schizophr Res. 2008;100:4–19. doi:10.1016/j.schres.2008.01.022.
2. Tandon R, Keshavan MS, Nasrallah HA. Schizophrenia, "just the facts" what we know in 2008. Part 2. Epidemiology and etiology. Schizophr Res. 2008;102:1–18. doi:10.1016/j.schres.2008.04.011.
3. Chong HY, Teoh SL, Wu DB, Kotirum S, Chiou CF, Chaiyakunapruk N. Global economic burden of schizophrenia: a systematic review. Neuropsychiatr Dis Treat. 2016;12:357–73. doi:10.2147/NDT.S96649.
4. Tandon R, Nasrallah HA, Keshavan MS. Schizophrenia, "just the facts" 4. Clinical features and conceptualization. Schizophr Res. 2009;110:1–23. doi:10.1016/j.schres.2009.03.005.
5. Tandon R, Belmaker RH, Gattaz WF, Lopez-Ibor Jr JJ, Okasha A, Singh B, et al. World Psychiatric Association Pharmacopsychiatry Section statement on comparative effectiveness of antipsychotics in the treatment of schizophrenia. Schizophr Res. 2008;100:20–38. doi:10.1016/j.schres.2007.11.033.
6. Harvey RC, James AC, Shields GE. A systematic review and network meta-analysis to assess the relative efficacy of antipsychotics for the treatment of positive and negative symptoms in early-onset schizophrenia. CNS Drugs. 2016;30:27–39. doi:10.1007/s40263-015-0308-1.
7. Remington G, Foussias G, Agid O. Progress in defining optimal treatment outcome in schizophrenia. CNS Drugs. 2010;24:9–20. doi:10.2165/11530250-000000000-00000.
8. Foussias G, Mann S, Zakzanis KK, van Reekum R, Remington G. Motivational deficits as the central link to functioning in schizophrenia: a pilot study. Schizophr Res. 2009;115:333–7. doi:10.1016/j.schres.2009.09.020.
9. Hennekens CH, Hennekens AR, Hollar D, Casey DE. Schizophrenia and increased risks of cardiovascular disease. Am Heart J. 2005;150:1115–21.
10. McGrath J, Saha S, Chant D, Welham J. Schizophrenia: a concise overview of incidence, prevalence, and mortality. Epidemiol Rev. 2008;30:67–76. doi:10.1093/epirev/mxn001.
11. Saha S, Chant D, McGrath J. A systematic review of mortality in schizophrenia: is the differential mortality gap worsening over time? Arch Gen Psychiatry. 2007;64:1123–31. doi:10.1001/archpsyc.64.10.1123.
12. Ventriglio A, Gentile A, Stella E, Bellomo A. Metabolic issues in patients affected by schizophrenia: clinical characteristics and medical management. Front Neurosci. 2015;9:297. doi:10.3389/fnins.2015.00297.
13. Casey DE, Hansen TE. Excessive mortality and morbidity associated with schizophrenia. In: Meyer JM, Nasrallah HA, editors. Medical illness and schizophrenia. 2nd ed. Washington, DC: American Psychiatric; 2009. p. 17–35.
14. Ratliff JC, Palmese LB, Reutenauer EL, Srihari VH, Tek C. Obese schizophrenia spectrum patients have significantly higher 10-year general cardiovascular risk and vascular ages than obese individuals without severe mental illness. Psychosomatics. 2013;54:67–73. doi:10.1016/j.psym.2012.03.001.
15. Padmavati R, McCreadie RG, Tirupati S. Low prevalence of obesity and metabolic syndrome in never-treated chronic schizophrenia. Schizophr Res. 2010;121:199–202. doi:10.1016/j.schres.2010.05.010.
16. Bak M, Fransen A, Janssen J, van Os J, Drukker M. Almost all antipsychotics result in weight gain: a meta-analysis. PLoS One. 2014;9:e94112. doi:10.1371/journal.pone.0094112.
17. Vancampfort D, Stubbs B, Mitchell AJ, De Hert M, Wampers M, Ward PB, et al. Risk of metabolic syndrome and its components in people with schizophrenia and related psychotic disorders, bipolar disorder and major depressive disorder: a systematic review and meta-analysis. World Psychiatry. 2015;14:339–47. doi:10.1002/wps.20252.
18. Tek C, Kucukgoncu S, Guloksuz S, Woods SW, Srihari VH, Annamalai A. Antipsychotic-induced weight gain in first-episode psychosis patients: a meta-analysis of differential effects of antipsychotic

medications. Early Interv Psychiatry. 2016;10:193–202. doi:10.1111/eip.12251.
19. Faulkner G, Cohn T, Remington G. Interventions to reduce weight gain in schizophrenia. Cochrane Database Syst Rev. 2007;24:CD005148. doi:10.1002/14651858.CD005148.pub2.
20. Bonfioli E, Berti L, Goss C, Muraro F, Burti L. Health promotion lifestyle interventions for weight management in psychosis: a systematic review and meta-analysis of randomised controlled trials. BMC Psychiatry. 2012;12:78. doi:10.1186/1471-244X-12-78.
21. Cimo A, Stergiopoulos E, Cheng C, Bonato S, Dewa CS. Effective lifestyle interventions to improve type II diabetes self-management for those with schizophrenia or schizoaffective disorder: a systematic review. BMC Psychiatry. 2012;12:24. doi:10.1186/1471-244X-12-24.
22. Firth J, Cotter J, Elliott R, French P, Yung AR. A systematic review and meta-analysis of exercise interventions in schizophrenia patients. Psychol Med. 2015;45:1343–61. doi:10.1017/S0033291714003110.
23. Gierisch JM, Nieuwsma JA, Bradford DW, Wilder CM, Mann-Wrobel MC, McBroom AJ, et al. Pharmacologic and behavioral interventions to improve cardiovascular risk factors in adults with serious mental illness: a systematic review and meta-analysis. J Clin Psychiatry. 2014;75:e424–40. doi:10.4088/JCP.13r08558.
24. Hjorth P, Davidsen AS, Kilian R, Skrubbeltrang C. A systematic review of controlled interventions to reduce overweight and obesity in people with schizophrenia. Acta Psychiatr Scand. 2014;130:279–89. doi:10.1111/acps.12245.
25. Pearsall R, Thyarappa Praveen K, Pelosi A, Geddes J. Dietary advice for people with schizophrenia. Cochrane Database Syst Rev. 2016;3:CD009547. doi:10.1002/14651858.CD009547.pub2.
26. Pearsall R, Smith DJ, Pelosi A, Geddes J. Exercise therapy in adults with serious mental illness: a systematic review and meta-analysis. BMC Psychiatry. 2014;14:117. doi:10.1186/1471244X-14-117.
27. Rosenbaum S, Tiedemann A, Sherrington C, Curtis J, Ward PB. Physical activity interventions for people with mental illness: a systematic review and meta-analysis. J Clin Psychiatry. 2014;75:964–74. doi:10.4088/JCP.13r08765.
28. Whitney Z, Procyshyn RM, Fredrikson DH, Barr AM. Treatment of clozapine-associated weight gain: a systematic review. Eur J Clin Pharmacol. 2015;71:389–401. doi:10.1007/s00228-0151807-1.
29. Caemmerer J, Correll CU, Maayan L. Acute and maintenance effects of non pharmacologic interventions for antipsychotic associated weight gain and metabolic abnormalities: a meta-analytic comparison of randomized controlled trials. Schizophr Res. 2012;140:159–68. doi:10.1016/j.schres.2012.03.017.
30. Brown S, Birtwistle J, Roe L, Thompson C. The unhealthy lifestyle of people with schizophrenia. Psychol Med. 1999;29:697–701. doi:10.1017/S0033291798008186.
31. Dipasquale S, Pariante CM, Dazzan P, Aguglia E, McGuire P, Mondelli V. The dietary pattern of patients with schizophrenia: a systematic review. J Psychiatr Res. 2013;47:197–207. doi:10.1016/j.jpsychires.2012.10.005.
32. Manzanares N, Monseny R, Ortega L, Montalvo I, Franch J, Gutiérrez-Zotes A, et al. Unhealthy lifestyle in early psychoses: the role of life stress and the hypothalamic-pituitary-adrenal axis. Psychoneuroendocrinology. 2014;39:1–10. doi:10.1016/j.psyneuen.2013.09.023.
33. McCreadie R, Scottish Schizophrenia Lifestyle Group. Diet, smoking, and cardiovascular risk in people with schizophrenia: descriptive study. Br J Psychiatry. 2003;183:534–9. doi:10.1192/03-162.
34. Nunes D, Eskinazi B, Camboim Rockett F, Delgado VB, Schweigert Perry ID. Nutritional status, food intake and cardiovascular disease risk in individuals with schizophrenia in southern Brazil: a case-control study. Rev Psiquiatr Salud Ment. 2014;7:72–9. doi:10.1016/j.rpsm.2013.07.001.
35. Ng M, Fleming T, Robinson M, Thomson B, Graetz N, Margono C, et al. Global, regional, and national prevalence of overweight and obesity in children and adults during 1980–2013: a systematic analysis for the Global Burden of Disease Study 2013. Lancet. 2014;384:766–81. doi:10.1016/S0140-6736(14)60460-8.
36. Zhang Y, Ren J. Epigenetics and obesity cardiomyopathy: from pathophysiology to prevention and management. Pharmacol Ther. 2016;161:52–66. doi:10.1016/j.pharmthera.2016.03.005.
37. Graham KA, Perkins DO, Edwards LJ, Barrier RC Jr, Lieberman JA, Harp JB. Effect of olanzapine on body composition and energy expenditure in adults with first-episode psychosis. Am J Psychiatry. 2005;162:118–23. http://dx.doi.org/10.1176/appi.ajp.162.1.118
38. McEvoy JP, Meyer JM, Goff DC, Nasrallah HA, Davis SM, Sullivan L, et al. Prevalence of the metabolic syndrome in patients with schizophrenia: baseline results from the Clinical Antipsychotic Trials of Intervention Effectiveness (CATIE) schizophrenia trial and comparison with national estimates from NHANES III. Schizophr Res. 2005;80:19–32.
39. Newcomer JW. Second-generation (atypical) antipsychotics and metabolic effects: a comprehensive literature review. CNS Drugs. 2005;19:1–93.
40. Sharpe JK, Stedman TJ, Byrne NM, Hills AP. Low-fat oxidation may be a factor in obesity among men with schizophrenia. Acta Psychiatr Scand. 2009;119:451–6. doi:10.1111/j.1600-0447.2008.01342.x.
41. Spelman LM, Walsh PI, Sharifi N, Collins PB, Thakore JH. Impaired glucose tolerance in first-episode drug-naive patients with schizophrenia. Diabet Med. 2007;24:481–5. http://dx.doi.org/10.1176/appi.ajp.160.2.284
42. van Nimwegen LJM, Storosum JG, Blumer RME, Allick G, Venema HW, de Haan L, et al. Hepatic insulin resistance in antipsychotic naive schizophrenic patients: stable isotope studies of glucose metabolism. J Clin Endocrinol Metab. 2008;93:575–7. http://dx.doi.org/10.1210/jc.2007-1167#sthash.D3vQiUHW.dpuf

43. Agerbo E, Byrne M, Eaton WW, Mortensen PB. Marital and labor market status in the long run in schizophrenia. Arch Gen Psychiatry. 2004;61:28–33.
44. Bou Khalil R, Hachem D, Richa S. Eating disorders and schizophrenia in male patients: a review. Eat Weight Disord. 2011;16:e150–6. doi:10.1007/BF03325126.
45. Daumit GL, Dickerson FB, Wang NY, Dalcin A, Jerome GJ, Anderson CA, et al. A behavioral weight-loss intervention in persons with serious mental illness. N Engl J Med. 2013;368:1594–602. doi:10.1056/NEJMoa1214530.
46. Elsey J, Coates A, Lacadie CM, McCrory EJ, Sinha R, Mayes LC, et al. Childhood trauma and neural responses to personalized stress, favorite-food and neutral-relaxing cues in adolescents. Neuropsychopharmacology. 2015;40:1580–9. doi:10.1038/npp.2015.6.
47. Garrett M. Psychosis, trauma, and ordinary mental life. Am J Psychother. 2016;70:35–62.
48. Owen MJ, Sawa A, Mortensen PB. Schizophrenia. Lancet. 2016;388(10039):86–97. doi:10.1016/S0140-6736(15)01121-6.
49. Foreyt JP, Salas-Salvado J, Caballero B, Bulló M, Gifford KD, Bautista I, et al. Weight-reducing diets: are there any differences? Nutr Rev. 2009;67:S99–101. doi:10.1111/j.1753-4887.2009.00169.x.
50. Freedman MR, King J, Kennedy E. Popular diets: a scientific review. Obes Res. 2001;9:1S–40.
51. Green CA, Yarborough BJ, Leo MC, Yarborough MT, Stumbo SP, Janoff SL, et al. The STRIDE weight loss and lifestyle intervention for individuals taking antipsychotic medications: a randomized trial. Am J Psychiatry. 2015;172:71–81. doi:10.1176/appi.ajp.2014.14020173.
52. Campos C. Tips for communicating with overweight and obese patients. J Fam Pract. 2014;63:S11–4.
53. Bays JC. Mindful eating: a guide to rediscovering a healthy and joyful relationship with food. Boston: Shambhala; 2009.
54. Godfrey KM, Gallo LC, Afari N. Mindfulness-based interventions for binge eating: a systematic review and meta-analysis. J Behav Med. 2015;38:348–62. doi:10.1007/s10865-014-9610-5.
55. Methapatara W, Srisurapanont M. Pedometer walking plus motivational interviewing program for Thai schizophrenic patients with obesity or overweight: a 12-week, randomized, controlled trial. Psychiatry Clin Neurosci. 2011;65:374–80.doi:10.1111/j.1440-1819.2011.02225.x.
56. Jones S, Barrowclough C, Allott R, Day C, Earnshaw P, Wilson I. Integrated motivational interviewing and cognitive-behavioural therapy for bipolar disorder with comorbid substance use. Clin Psychol Psychother. 2011;18:426–37. doi:10.1002/cpp.783.
57. Klein AS, Skinner JB, Hawley KM. Targeting binge eating through components of dialectical behavior therapy: preliminary outcomes for individually supported diary card self-monitoring versus group-based DBT. Psychotherapy. 2013;50:543–52. doi:10.1037/a0033130.
58. Juarascio AS, Forman EM, Herbert JD. Acceptance and commitment therapy versus cognitive therapy for the treatment of comorbid eating pathology. Behav Modif. 2010;34:175–90. doi:10.1177/0145445510363472.
59. Draper ML, Stutes DS, Maples NJ, Velligan DI. Cognitive adaptation training for outpatients with schizophrenia. J Clin Psychol. 2009;65:842–53. doi:10.1002/jclp.20612.
60. Khokhar B, Jones J, Ronksley PE, Armstrong MJ, Caird J, Rabi D. Effectiveness of mobile electronic devices in weight loss among overweight and obese populations: a systematic review and meta-analysis. BMC Obes. 2014;1:22. doi:10.1186/s40608-014-0022-4.
61. Wei M, Kampert JB, Barlow CE, Nichaman MZ, Gibbons LW, Paffenbarger Jr RS, et al. Relationship between low cardiorespiratory fitness and mortality in normal weight, overweight and obese men. JAMA. 1999;282:1547–53. doi:10.1001/jama.282.16.1547.
62. Daumit GL, Goldberg RW, Anthony C, Dickerson F, Brown CH, Kreyenbuhl J, et al. Physical activity patterns in adults with severe mental illness. J Nerv Ment Dis. 2005;193:641–6. doi:10.1097/01.nmd.0000180737.85895.60.
63. Lindamer LA, McKibbin C, Norman GJ, Jordan L, Harrison K, Abeyesinhe S, et al. Assessment of physical activity in middle-aged and older adults with schizophrenia. Schizophr Res. 2008;104:294–301. doi:10.1016/j.schres.2008.04.040.
64. Vancampfort D, Stubbs B, Sienaert P, Wyckaert S, De Hert M, Soundy A, et al. A comparison of physical fitness in patients with bipolar disorder, schizophrenia and healthy controls. Disabil Rehabil. 2016;1–5. doi:10.3109/09638288.2015.1114037 [Epub ahead of print].
65. Warburton DER, Charlesworth S, Ivey A, Nettlefold L, Bredin SSD. A systematic review of the evidence for Canada's Physical Activity Guidelines for Adults. Int J Behav Nutr Phys Act. 2010;7:39. doi:10.1186/1479-5868-7-39.
66. Gorczynski P, Faulkner G, Cohn T, Remington G. Examining the efficacy and feasibility of exercise counseling in individuals with schizophrenia: a single-case experimental study. Ment Health Phys Act. 2014;7:191–7. doi:10.1016/j.mhpa.2014.04.002.
67. Bandura A. Social foundations of thought and action. Englewood Cliffs: Prentice-Hall; 1986.
68. Prochaska JO, DiClimente CC. Toward a comprehensive model of change. In: Miller WR, Heather N, editors. Treating addictive behavior: processes of change. New York: Plenum; 1986. p. 3–27.
69. Faulkner G, Gorczynski P. Evidence of impact of physical activity on schizophrenia. In: Clow A, Edmunds S, editors. Physical activity and mental health: theory and practical applications. Champaign: Human Kinetics; 2014. p. 215–35.
70. Craig CL, Marshall AL, Sjöström M, Baumanm AE, Booth ML, Ainsworth BE, et al. International physical activity questionnaire: 12-country reliability and validity. Med Sci Sports Exerc. 2003;35:1381–95. doi:10.1249/01.MSS.0000078924.61453.FB.
71. Faulkner G, Cohn T, Remington G. Validation of a physical assessment tool for individuals with schizo-

phrenia. Schizophr Res. 2006;82:225–31. doi:10.1016/j.schres.2005.10.020.

72. Carey KB, Leontieva L, Dimmock J, Maisto SA, Batki SL. Adapting motivational interventions for comorbid schizophrenia and alcohol use disorders. Clin Psychol. 2007;14:39–57.doi:10.1111/j.1468-2850.2007.00061.x.
73. Miller WR, Rollnick S. Motivational interviewing: preparing people for change. 2nd ed. New York: Guilford; 2002.
74. Tudor-Locke C. Steps to better cardiovascular health: how many steps does it take to achieve good health and how confident are we in this number? Curr Cardiovasc Risk Rep. 2010;4:271–6. doi:10.1007/s12170-010-0109-5.
75. Hodgson MH, McCulloch HP, Fox KR. The experiences of people with severe and enduring mental illness engaged in a physical activity programme integrated into the mental health service. Ment Health Phys Act. 2011;4:23–9. doi:10.1016/j.mhpa.2011.01.002.
76. Dauwan M, Begemann MJ, Heringa SM, Sommer IE. Exercise improves clinical symptoms, quality of life, global functioning, and depression in schizophrenia: a systematic review and meta-analysis. Schizophr Bull. 2016;42:588–99. doi:10.1093/schbul/sbv164.
77. Mabire L. Physical activity guidelines for weight loss: global and national perspectives. Br J Sports Med. 2016. doi:10.1136/bjsports-2015-095863 [Epub ahead of print].
78. Donnelly JE, Blair SN, Jakicic JM, Manore MM, Rankin JW, Smith BK, et al. Appropriate physical activity intervention strategies for weight loss and prevention of weight regain for adults. Med Sci Sports Exerc. 2009;41:459–71. doi:10.1249/MSS.0b013e3181949333.
79. Faulkner G, Gorczynski P, Cohn T. Dissecting the obesogenic nature of psychiatric settings. Psychiatr Serv. 2009;60:538–41.
80. Cohn T, Grant S, Faulkner GE. Schizophrenia and obesity: addressing obesogenic environments in mental health settings. Schizophr Res. 2010;121:277–8. doi:10.1016/j.schres.2010.05.024.

20 Young Adulthood and Obesity Management: Developmental Issues and Transition of Care

Marlene Taube-Schiff and Shira Yufe

20.1 Introduction

In this chapter, we provide the reader with an overview of issues facing young obese adults from both a developmental and social perspective. We then review transitions of care, as individuals with chronic health issues that reach adulthood are often faced with several difficulties in making the leap from paediatric care to the adult healthcare system. Transition guidelines and their effectiveness are described to allow the reader to begin to understand key elements. Finally, we provide the reader with the journey of "Sally" as she transferred her care from a paediatric centre in Toronto to an adult bariatric surgery centre. In doing so, we illustrate the program that was developed at the Toronto Western Hospital and data from the patient narrative to illustrate the impact of this type of a program. We hope this case study will bring to life for the reader the type of program components to consider creating as a model of care for young adult bariatric patients undergoing a transition of obesity management treatment.

M. Taube-Schiff, Ph.D., C. Psych. (✉)
Department of Psychiatry, Sunnybrook Health Sciences Centre, 2075 Bayview Avenue, Toronto, ON, Canada M4N 3M5

Department of Psychiatry, University of Toronto, 250 College Street, Toronto, ON, Canada M5T 1R8
e-mail: marlene.taubeschiff@sunnybrook.ca

S. Yufe, B.A.
Department of Psychology, York University, 4700 Keele Street, Behavioral Science Building, Toronto, ON, Canada M3J 1P3
e-mail: syufe@yorku.ca

Case Vignette

Sally is 16-and-a-half years old when she initially begins her obesity management treatment at a paediatric centre of care. Within this model of care, she received extensive counselling and support from her interdisciplinary team (nurses, dietitians, psychologists, psychiatrists, and social workers) as well as individual and family therapy services. Her parents felt very involved in this treatment and were constantly attending appointments with her and supervising her dietary and lifestyle changes. She received a sleeve gastrectomy when she was 17 years old, still under the care of the paediatric treatment centre. This procedure was chosen for her (i.e. as opposed to the Roux-en-Y) as there are less nutritional supplements to adhere to, and her team thought this was a better option, given her age. Sally, with extensive support from others, has done well since having this

(continued)

S. Sockalingam, R. Hawa (eds.), *Psychiatric Care in Severe Obesity*,
DOI 10.1007/978-3-319-42536-8_20

(continued)

procedure 1 year ago. She has lost 60 lbs and has made a number of changes in terms of her eating habits and has started an exercise program with her mother. However, her family feels that her weight loss could potentially be enhanced by now undergoing a Roux-en-Y procedure. Her mother speaks with the paediatric team and while they do support this revision surgery, they recommend that she seek this treatment at an adult centre, given she is now 18 years old. Both Sally and her parents are disappointed with this news and feel at a loss for where treatment can now be received. The paediatric team is not connected to any specific adult obesity treatment program. The team recommends that Sally speak with her family doctor and get a referral to an adult bariatric surgery centre. Sally's family decides to pursue this route.

Sally's family is also concerned with school-related difficulties that Sally has been experiencing. She is struggling academically and feels socially isolated. On a few occasions, she has been called offensive names in the hallway by her peers. Sally attributes her low marks to bullying. Sally's parents are concerned that Sally is undergoing so many transitions in her life; developmentally and now in the context of needing to switch healthcare systems.

Six months following discharge from the paediatric centre, Sally receives a call directly from the adult treatment centre and feels unprepared because her mother always spoke with staff and booked appointments for her. She writes down where she needs to go and with whom she needs to meet with but feels overwhelmed by the differences in hospital approaches. Sally debates whether she wants to meet a team of strangers and manage appointments by herself. She feels confused and uncertain with respect to how she can continue with her obesity management treatment.

20.2 Young Adulthood and Obesity: Developmental Issues

The physical and psychiatric issues associated with childhood obesity are often maintained into adulthood and may worsen over time [1, 2]. Severe obesity is commonly treated with bariatric surgery, and research supports the safety and effectiveness for bariatric surgery for adolescents and young adults [3, 4]. When medical treatment begins during childhood or adolescence and continues into adulthood, medical professionals are often concerned with the transition from a paediatric obesity management centre to an adult facility or hospital, where the environments and level of care are different.

Most of what we know about surrounding developmental issues with obesity is from research with adolescents. Studies are done with this population far more than with young adults. Often times, the research will include 18 year olds, but the age range from 18 to 25 is, unfortunately, understudied. We will discuss what we know both from the adolescent and young adult obesity literature concerning key developmental issues.

Apart from the known risk factors for developing childhood and adolescent obesity, such as low socioeconomic status, family history of obesity, and maltreatment [5, 6], growing up with obesity also poses significant risks to the individual's mental health. High rates of psychopathology are common, such as depressive and anxiety disorders [7, 8], as well as attention-deficit hyperactivity disorder [9]. We will focus on some specific psychosocial issues unique to the developmental trajectories of adolescents and young adults with obesity, such as school performance, early onset puberty, body image, and weight victimization.

20.2.1 School and Work Difficulties

Many challenges may develop in the school environment. A number of studies show lower academic achievement in children and adolescents with obesity [10, 11]. Arithmetic and spelling have been shown to be significantly lower in students aged 14 to 20 years old with obesity as compared to age-matched non-obese students. Cognitive functions are also affected, such as working memory, attention, psychomotor efficiency, and mental flexibility [12]. However, the relationship between obesity and lower academic achievement may be more complex, given that one study found that students in middle school, community college, and university across the USA received significantly lower grades in these educational institutions, yet surprisingly showed no statistically significant differences in nationally standardized vocabulary and mathematics tests [13]. Clinicians and researchers speculate that the reason for the observed lower academic achievement is due to discrimination (direct or indirect) by their teachers and peers. Thus, less attentional resources, stereotypes, and lowered expectations for students with obesity may contribute to the underlying mechanisms of their poor performance [13, 14].

Disruptive behavior has also been found to be problematic within the school environment. Chronic obesity is associated with oppositional defiant disorder in both boys and girls [15] as well as more general behavioural issues, such as poor self-control, acting out behaviours (i.e., arguing), and internalizing behaviours such as loneliness [16]. Obesity is also a risk factor for high school dropout; this finding has been found to be particularly true for white adolescents who develop obesity in adolescence [17]. One study found that females who were overweight or obese between adolescence and adulthood fared worse in terms of educational achievements and economic stability [18]. Moreover, Class III obesity (BMI>40) and diabetes are associated with a higher likelihood of worker illness absenteeism [19]. Jung and Chang (2015) found that obesity is associated with increased mental health sick days [20], and they hypothesize that a substantial growth in weight stigma and weight-related discrimination in recent years have led to increased mental distress in individuals with obesity. Lastly, a high percentage of workers with obesity face challenges in employment settings, such as weight-based discrimination in job evaluations and hiring decisions, as well as wage penalties [21].

20.2.2 Weight-Based Bullying and Discrimination

Weight-based bullying and stigmatizing attitudes towards adolescents with obesity is highly common and is associated with poor health outcomes [21, 22]. The consequences of such experiences include social marginalization, difficulty forming and maintaining peer relationships, and heightened symptoms of existing co-morbid psychopathology such as depression and anxiety [23]. Adolescents with obesity are more likely to be bullied by their peers than their average-weight counterparts [24] with teasing, social exclusion (e.g. ignoring, avoiding), and physical harassment [25]. Weight stigmatization experiences may decrease motivation and self-efficacy to engage in physical activity and increase sedentary behaviours [23, 26]. Sedentary behaviours cultivated in childhood contribute to a "never-ending spiral" of obesity and health consequences, leading to an increase or maintenance of obesity [27]. Importantly, it is unclear whether severe obesity precedes these issues or whether psychosocial issues contribute to severe obesity in adolescents [28]. For instance, the presence of a psychiatric disorder and school difficulties is associated with a higher BMI [5]. Although some issues remain to be clarified in the literature, there is no doubt that weight stigmatization has significant lasting impacts on health and interpersonal relationships.

20.2.3 Body Image and Early Onset Puberty

Adolescents and adults with obesity are at risk for poor health-related quality of life (HRQOL) [29, 30]. This means they may have a lower capacity for physical activity, poor self-esteem, and body dissatisfaction, to name just a few difficulties. Disturbances of body image have a particularly strong association with predicting poor HRQOL

[29]. New research points to an additional challenge for adolescents with obesity, which is—early onset puberty. During puberty, the adolescent body undergoes changes in terms of location and quantity of body fat, insulin sensitivity, and physical fitness capabilities [31]. Evidence shows that adolescents with obesity can enter puberty and achieve later stages of puberty earlier than non-obese controls [31]. This tends to be the case more so for girls than boys [31, 32]. These findings require more conclusive research in order to clarify the factors which promote early onset puberty, as well as to determine the relationship of early onset puberty and difficulties with body image.

Having reviewed the myriad of developmental issues facing adolescents (for a summary, please see Table 20.1), we hope that the reader has been given a sense of the challenges that youth with obesity face – given their age and co-morbid obesity-related issues. The additional burden of seeking treatment for obesity management and transitioning between paediatric and adult healthcare centres is another typical and problematic developmental challenge that this age group often faces.

Table 20.1 Summary of developmental issues among adolescents and young adults with obesity

Developmental issues	Examples
School difficulties	– Lower academic achievement
	– Diminished cognitive functions
	– Disruptive behaviour
	– School dropout
Work difficulties	– Decreased economic stability
	– Worker illness absenteeism (physical and mental health related)
Weight-based bullying discrimination	– Stigmatizing attitudes (e.g. stereotypes, teasing, marginalization)
	– Compromised peer relationships
Body image	– Poor self-esteem
	– Body dissatisfaction
	– Early onset puberty

20.3 Young Adulthood and Transitions of Care: What Do We Know?

Transition of care has been defined by the Society of Adolescent Medicine as "the purposeful, planned movement of adolescents and young adults with chronic physical and medical conditions from child-centred to adult-centred health systems" [33]. Transitional care research has been conducted within a variety of chronic illnesses, including cerebral palsy, diabetes, transplantation, cardiac care, and oncology [34–38]. A number of challenges have been well-documented when individuals turn 18- years- old and transfer their care from a paediatric to an adult healthcare centre. These often include non-compliance with life-saving medication regimens [39]; loss to follow-up; and increased hospitalizations post transfer of care [40–43]. Illness-specific difficulties have also been documented in the literature. For example, in terms of renal transplant patients, it has been documented that young adults are four times more likely to lose their organ grafts due to lack of medication adherence as compared to any other age group [44], suggesting that outcomes are the worst for this particular age group [45].

Developmental issues are often suspect of underlying many of these poor medical outcomes. The adolescent/young adult brain is still in a stage of development, particularly the frontal lobe [46]. The frontal lobes have been found to be responsible for executive functioning, including planning and reasoning skills. The interested reader is referred to Colver and Longwell (2015) for a review of adolescent brain development. Within the context of healthcare, an individual would require these frontal lobe functions for: making and attending appointments, taking one's medication, and, possibly, engaging in healthy lifestyle modifications (e.g., healthy dietary changes and routine blood tests). Therefore, without these abilities fully acquired, one can imagine that carrying out the above tasks independently might be difficult and result in poor healthcare compliance. Due to these developmental issues, young adults who have experienced the transition from a paediatric to adult bariatric surgery centre may desire (and benefit from) ongoing and age appropriate parental and healthcare provider support [47].

We can also learn about transition of care issues by turning to the "emerging adulthood" literature. Arnett [48] has written extensively on the idea of "emerging adulthood". This is proposed to be a stage of life in which individuals aged 18–25 are believed to be "in-between" being an adolescent and being an adult. In fact, when individuals within this age group were asked whether they believe themselves to be adults they answered that in some ways they do feel like adults, but, in other ways they do not [49]. During this stage of life, individuals have not yet decided on where they belong in terms of many cultural expectations and identity, such as romance, vocation, and life outlooks. Many potential future directions remain possible, and the opportunity to explore life in an independent manner is often greater during this period of one's life compared to other phases within one's development [48]. A recent study examined experiences of young adult bariatric surgery patients who transitioned their care from a paediatric centre to an adult surgical centre [47]. Participants interviewed in this study reported that they felt they had not yet figured out "who they are" and that it would be beneficial for adult healthcare providers to be more sensitive to these issues. They expressed a desire for adult healthcare providers to be more sensitive to their unique needs (as young adults). In addition to their healthcare being in a time of transition, they themselves actually felt that they were in a time of transition and that their identity was still forming. Consistent with this was a desire to be allowed to be "irresponsible" and concern that it might be difficult to adhere to post-surgical guidelines given this lingering desire to not be as accountable as an adult would be [47].

Several guidelines have been established for transition of care within the context of chronic medical illness and disease. These guidelines have been published in the form of consensus statements and committee guidelines for medical issues, such as organ transplantation, diabetes care, and special care needs. Recommendations often include (1) transfer information being provided during adolescence and if that is not possible then at least 1 year prior to transfer [44, 50]; (2) a transition "champion" (often referred to as a coordinator) should be in place to ensure transition services are organized and coordinated [35, 44, 51]; (3) older adolescents should begin to take on management of their health prior to transfer and parents can aid in this transition [35, 44, 50]; (4) transition clinics should be implemented which often involve the adult healthcare professionals meeting with the older adolescent patient prior to transfer of care along with members from the paediatric team [35, 44]; (5) provision of information to parents and older adolescents concerning different environments within the paediatric versus adult healthcare system [50]; and, finally (6) prior to the transfer process it has been recommended that the paediatric team send along an assessment of transfer readiness in addition to any important medical and psychosocial information (i.e. medical concerns; psychiatric issues; current medications) concerning the patient [35, 44, 50, 52]. Please see Table 20.2 for a summary of these recommendations.

Although many guidelines exist to guide the process of transfer of care between the paediatric and adult healthcare systems, fewer studies have focused on changes in patient outcomes as a result of these initiatives. A recent study found that transition clinic attendance improved renal function for kidney transplant patients in addition to overall adherence 1 year following the transfer of care [36]. Cadario and colleagues [53] implemented a number of transition initiatives for adolescents with Type I diabetes and results were

Table 20.2 Quick check: summary of transition guidelines

Transition care guidelines and recommendations	References
Begin transition process in paediatric centres (e.g. deliver patient education)	[44, 50]
Transition champion	[35, 44, 51]
Self-management of healthcare by adolescent	[35, 44, 50]
Transition clinics	[35, 44]
Education regarding different cultures in paediatric care versus adult care	[35, 44, 50]
Transfer readiness information sent to adult healthcare centre	[35, 44, 50, 52]

favourable. Patients were found to have enhanced glycemic control; improved adherence to appointments; and enhanced service satisfaction as well as earlier attendance to appointments within the adult healthcare system. Services that were implemented included coordinator of transition services; information summary was transferred from the paediatric system to the adult healthcare team; transition clinics; and the involvement of a paediatrician in the first appointment that occurred on the adult side [53]. Also, McDonagh and others [51] found that when transition initiatives were implemented (including templates for individualized transition plans that were based on developmental stages of adolescence as well as a project coordinator and resources for both youth and parents), patients with juvenile idiopathic arthritis had improved patient knowledge as well as the ability to self-manage health-related behaviours. Furthermore, health-related quality of life improved [51]. Therefore, these three studies provide encouraging evidence that implementation of transition services can be beneficial for adolescents prior to their transfer to adult healthcare.

Some researchers have sought to gain a sense of the transition experience and transition initiatives that have been implemented within programs through self-report measures and qualitative research design. For example, Fernandes and colleagues [54] recently surveyed a sample of youth (ages 16–25 years old) that had a variety of childhood onset chronic diseases (including cancer, Type I diabetes, congenital heart disease, and solid organ transplant) as well as their parents. Overall, most patients and parents felt they received adequate education and information regarding the transition of care process. However, participants felt that they did not receive satisfactory education regarding reproductive issues (including birth control and childbearing issues), recreational substance use, as well as future vocational issues in terms of the impact of the ongoing chronic medical condition. In terms of barriers to transfer of care, patients and parents reflected on the emotional bond they have towards the paediatric centre as well as a perceived lack of adult specialty care providers [54]. Within transplant transition of care, McCurdy and colleagues [55] found patients spoke about differences between the paediatric and adult hospital, often citing the former as "more fun" and "nicer". Participants also remarked that the actual transfer of care was an important event and constituted a significant change; often one that was met with emotions such as disappointment, shock, and sadness [55].

Recently, an international Delphi study examined the key elements important for successful transfer from paediatric to adult healthcare systems [56]. A key element was the importance of having effective communication between the paediatric and adult healthcare centre. This corroborates well with the existing guidelines and patient narratives of transition and transfer of care issues. Overall, consensus statements, guidelines, and the voice of the patient shed light on important elements to incorporate within any type of transition program to allow for a seamless transfer of care from paediatric to adult healthcare for a variety of chronic medical conditions. We will now turn to a discussion on transition issues within the context of obesity and bariatric surgery specifically.

20.4 Young Adulthood and Bariatric Surgery: An Example of a Seamless Transition of Care Program

The literature does not provide a great deal of insight with respect to transition of care for young adult bariatric surgery candidates. A recent paper by Shrewsbury and colleagues [57] highlighted the fact that little work has been done to establish guidelines or models of care for transitions in obesity management. In fact, they stated that "there is no obvious transition pathway" from paediatric obesity treatment to adult care (p. 478). Therefore, clinicians and researchers in this area have only been able to turn to the established guidelines and models of care, as described above for other areas of chronic illness and disease. The Toronto Western Hospital Bariatric Surgery Program (TWH-BSP) set out to create a model of transition of care for patients transferring from a paediatric obesity management facility to their adult bariatric surgery program. The team at TWH-BSP researched the impact of this transition care model on young adult transfer patients. We will describe this model of care (below) and our research findings in the hopes of aiding other healthcare clinicians building a transition pathway for this specific population. Let's return to our patient Sally to illustrate the transition process she would have undergone with the model of care that has been created by our group.

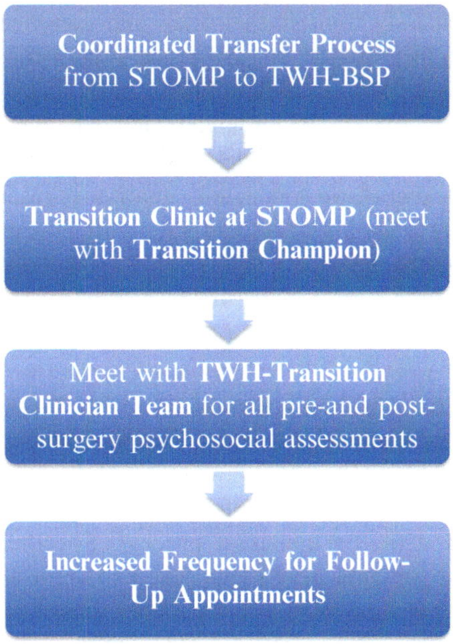

Diagram 20.1 Flow of patients from STOMP to TWH-BSP (*Transition initiatives in bold*)

In 2012, TWH-BSP partnered with the Sick Kids Obesity Management Program (STOMP) to create transition initiatives and a clear transition pathway for patients that transferred their care from the Hospital for Sick Children to the Toronto Western Hospital. Please refer to Diagram 20.1 for an illustration of the pathway created for patients transferring their care from STOMP to the TWH-BSP. In order for Sally to begin her treatment at the TWH-BSP, she would have been referred through the Ontario Bariatric Network (OBN). When an individual is seeking surgical weight loss, they must be referred to either STOMP or the OBN; the latter is a centralized provincial registry. Our team worked closely with the OBN to ensure that patients arriving from our partner paediatric program seamlessly transferred their care into our program. Prior to this transfer, the adult care transition champion (from TWH-BSP) would have been contacted by the transition champion at the paediatric centre (from STOMP) to come and meet with Sally. As we know from the literature described above, transition clinics often ease the transfer process and allow for individuals to become more comfortable with the healthcare professionals that will be involved in their care. During this transition clinic, Sally would not only meet with the TWH-BSP's transition champion but would also receive a transition resource booklet. This booklet was developed in partnership by both teams and provides our young adults with information regarding what they should expect during the transfer of care, along with the different types of support that can be accessed through the TWH-BSP and their community. Once Sally begins her treatment at the TWH-BSP, she will then undergo her preoperative assessment process with a team of clinicians that have been designated to follow young adult transfers along their surgical and post-operative trajectories. There is one transition clinician from every discipline in the team (psychology/psychiatry; social work; nursing; and dietetics). This allows for consistency of care, which likely allows the transfer patient to be less overwhelmed by the different culture within the adult system and allows them to feel a sense of safety within an environment that is much larger and busier than the paediatric centre. Once Sally has undergone bariatric surgery, she will also receive more frequent follow-up appointments during her routine post-operative care. After the first year of surgery, most patients only receive care on an annual basis. Due to the known challenges with adherence and compliance in this age group, we implemented semi-annual appointments with the designated transition clinicians to ensure that patients feel engaged within the program and that any non-compliance issues will be picked up on fairly quickly. When creating and implementing this program, our hope was that it would allow patients such as Sally to easily and seamlessly transfer their care and continue on with the bariatric surgical process, be it for surgery or post-operative follow-up care.

In order to better understand whether this transition of care model was advantageous for our patients, we conducted a qualitative research study to identify: (1) themes regarding the experience of our young adults (18–24 years old) as they transferred their care from a paediatric to an adult care hospital; (2) transition challenges that young adults experienced upon transfer; and (3) how developmental issues for this population impacted their transition of care experience [47]. Results suggested that there were both negative and positive experiences associated with the transition process. Specifically, some patients would have liked to learn about the transition process even sooner than they did and hoped for a process that was even more explicit than our team had delivered. Participants also cited a desire for more parental involvement and hoped that adult healthcare providers would be more compassionate towards young adults given the fact that they are not "quite adults" and are still learning about who they are. In this regard, patients spoke about themselves as being emerging adults and the impact this has on self-management, such as having a desire to be irresponsible and needing some understanding in that regard. On the positive side, many participants valued having a transition champion that could guide them through the process [47]. We believe these findings are important to consider when it comes to encouraging regular follow-up appointments (i.e. consider asking about parental involvement) and adherence to lifestyle issues (i.e. vitamin use and proper nutrition). Overall, our findings and the experience of our patients fit well with the literature that has been reviewed from chronic healthcare. As discussed, the developmental stage of emerging adulthood also impacted the transition process for our patients. Gaining insight from patients who are undergoing this process can allow for transition programs and healthcare bridging to meet the needs of our patients on an ongoing basis.

20.5 Summary

Given that more research is now supporting the safety and effectiveness of bariatric surgery for adolescents, it is paramount for adult bariatric centres to understand the unique developmental and psychosocial issues and challenges that must be addressed when treating young adult bariatric surgery patients. Ensuring that medical teams have the knowledge and education regarding these unique issues, such as weight victimization and school-related difficulties, is an important first step. Furthermore, ensuring the development of transition initiatives within their centres is also an extremely important issue. While there might not be resources available to implement all of the strategies discussed within this chapter, we would encourage healthcare professionals to regard these initiatives as a menu of options and choose a few that would best fit their particular healthcare team. It is clear from the literature reviewed that emerging adults are aware of their differences and hope that their healthcare teams will be able to offer some sensitivity towards their ongoing development. Furthermore, the involvement of parents, in a respectful way, might be very beneficial for some young adults. We hope the description of Sally and her process from the paediatric to adult bariatric centre helps to illustrate to the reader a potential model of care that can be designed to ensure a seamless transfer of services and enhanced quality of care for young adult bariatric patients.

Take Home Messages

- Young adults (i.e. 18 to 25 years old) are in a unique stage of life developmentally; not quite adults yet and not quite adolescents.
- Young adults with obesity struggle with a variety of developmental issues, obesity-related stigma, and weight victimization.
- Research from chronic health illness and disease has established that this age group tends to fare less well in terms of health-related outcomes as compared to their adult counterparts.
- Young adults seeking obesity management in an adult centre might have to deal with an

extra burden of transition of care if treatment has begun within a paediatric centre.

- Transition of care is considered to be a process that occurs when paediatric patients begin the process of graduating from a paediatric centre and gradually transferring their care to the adult healthcare system.
- Guidelines have been created to enhance healthcare professionals' understanding of transition and transfer of care, such as having transition clinics and a transition coordinator ensuring seamless care is delivered.
- Research has found a positive impact from the use of these different types of transition initiatives.
- Healthcare providers working in obesity management and bariatric surgery centres must consider the value and importance of ensuring some of these transition guidelines are adhered to when treating this unique age group within their centre; this will allow for best practice and possibly enhanced long-term medical outcomes.

Appendix: Transition Checklist: Points to Consider When Young Adults Transfer to Adult Bariatric Surgical Centres

- Transition clinics to welcome young adult to adult healthcare system
- Transition champion to coordinate services and ensure seamless transfer of care
- Designated transition clinicians to allow for familiarity and consistency with healthcare team (more similar to paediatric centres)
- Increased follow-up (ensure difficulties caught sooner and adherence to lifestyle changes are being managed)
- Adult healthcare providers are open to familial involvement when it is welcomed by the young adult
- Adult healthcare providers consider development age and stage (young adults are emerging adults; neither adolescents nor fully formed adults)

References

1. Hilty DM, Parish MB, Callahan E. The effectiveness of telemental health: a 2013 review. Telemed J E Health. 2013;19(6):444–54.
2. Whitaker RC, Wright JA, Pepe MS, Seidel KD, Dietz WH. Predicting obesity in young adulthood from childhood and parental obesity. N Engl J Med. 1997;337(13):869–73.
3. DuCoin C, Moon RC, Mulatre M, Teixeira AF, Jawad MA. Safety and effectiveness of Roux-en-Y gastric bypass in patients between the ages of 17 and 19. Obes Surg. 2015;25(3):464–9.
4. Inge TH, Courcoulas AP, Jenkins TM, Michalsky MP, Helmrath MA, Brandt ML, et al. Weight loss and health status 3 years after bariatric surgery in adolescents. N Engl J Med. 2016;374(2):113–23.
5. Gonzalez A, Boyle MH, Kyu HH, Georgiades K, Duncan L, MacMillan HL. Childhood and family influences on depression, chronic physical conditions, and their comorbidity: findings from the Ontario Child Health Study. J Psychiatr Res. 2012;46(11):1475–82.
6. Wells NM, Evans GW, Beavis A, Ong AD. Early childhood poverty, cumulative risk exposure, and body mass index trajectories through young adulthood. Am J Public Health. 2010;100(12):2507–12.
7. Hillstrom KA, Graves JK. A review of depression and quality of life outcomes in adolescents post bariatric surgery. J Child Adolesc Psychiatr Nurs. 2015;28(1):50–9.
8. Jarvholm K, Olbers T, Marcus C, Marild S, Gronowitz E, Friberg P, et al. Short-term psychological outcomes in severely obese adolescents after bariatric surgery. Obesity (Silver Spring). 2012;20(2):318–23.
9. Kim J, Mutyala B, Agiovlasitis S, Fernhall B. Health behaviors and obesity among US children with attention deficit hyperactivity disorder by gender and medication use. Prev Med. 2011;52(3-4):218–22.
10. Booth JN, Tomporowski PD, Boyle JM, Ness AR, Joinson C, Leary SD, et al. Obesity impairs academic attainment in adolescence: findings from ALSPAC, a UK cohort. Int J Obes (Lond). 2014;38(10):1335–42.
11. Black N, Johnston DW, Peeters A. Childhood obesity and cognitive achievement. Health Econ. 2015;24(9):1082–100.
12. Yau PL, Kang EH, Javier DC, Convit A. Preliminary evidence of cognitive and brain abnormalities in uncomplicated adolescent obesity. Obesity (Silver Spring). 2014;22(8):1865–71.
13. MacCann C, Roberts RD. Just as smart but not as successful: obese students obtain lower school grades but equivalent test scores to nonobese students. Int J Obes (Lond). 2013;37(1):40–6.
14. Falkner NH, Neumark-Sztainer D, Story M, Jeffery RW, Beuhring T, Resnick MD. Social, educational, and psychological correlates of weight status in adolescents. Obes Res. 2001;9(1):32–42.
15. Mustillo S, Worthman C, Erkanli A, Keeler G, Angold A, Costello EJ. Obesity and psychiatric disorder:

developmental trajectories. Pediatrics. 2003;111(4 Pt 1):851–9.

16. Judge S, Jahns L. Association of overweight with academic performance and social and behavioral problems: an update from the early childhood longitudinal study. J Sch Health. 2007;77(10):672–8.
17. Lanza HI, Huang DY. Is obesity associated with school dropout? Key developmental and ethnic differences. J Sch Health. 2015;85(10):663–70.
18. Chung AE, Skinner AC, Maslow GR, Halpern CT, Perrin EM. Sex differences in adult outcomes by changes in weight status from adolescence to adulthood: results from Add Health. Acad Pediatr. 2014;14(5):448–55.
19. Howard JT, Potter LB. An assessment of the relationships between overweight, obesity, related chronic health conditions and worker absenteeism. Obes Res Clin Pract. 2014;8(1):e1–15.
20. Jung H, Chang C. Is obesity related to deteriorating mental health of the U.S. working-age population? J Behav Med. 2015;38(1):81–90.
21. Puhl R, Suh Y. Health consequences of weight stigma: implications for obesity prevention and treatment. Curr Obes Rep. 2015;4(2):182–90.
22. Browne NT. Weight bias, stigmatization, and bullying of obese youth. Bariatr Nurs Surg Patient Care. 2012;7(3):107–15.
23. Yufe SJ, Taube-Schiff M, Fergus KD, Sockalingam S. Weight-based bullying and compromised peer relationships in young adult bariatric patients. J Health Psychol. 2016. http://hpq.sagepub.com/content/early/2016/01/27/1359105315622559.abstract
24. Fox CL, Farrow CV. Global and physical self-esteem and body dissatisfaction as mediators of the relationship between weight status and being a victim of bullying. J Adolesc. 2009;32(5):1287–301.
25. Puhl RM, Luedicke J, Heuer C. Weight-based victimization toward overweight adolescents: observations and reactions of peers. J Sch Health. 2011;81(11):696–703.
26. Pearl RL, Dovidio JF, Puhl RM, Brownell KD. Exposure to weight-stigmatizing media: effects on exercise intentions, motivation, and behavior. J Health Commun. 2015;20(9):1004–13.
27. Williams EP, Mesidor M, Winters K, Dubbert PM, Wyatt SB. Overweight and obesity: prevalence, consequences, and causes of a growing public health problem. Curr Obes Rep. 2015;4(3):363–70.
28. Kelly AS, Barlow SE, Rao G, Inge TH, Hayman LL, Steinberger J, et al. Severe obesity in children and adolescents: identification, associated health risks, and treatment approaches: a scientific statement from the American Heart Association. Circulation. 2013;128(15):1689–712.
29. Kolodziejczyk JK, Gutzmer K, Wright SM, Arredondo EM, Hill L, Patrick K, et al. Influence of specific individual and environmental variables on the relationship between body mass index and health-related quality of life in overweight and obese adolescents. Qual Life Res. 2015;24(1):251–61.
30. Herranz Barbero A, Lopez de Mesa MR, Azcona San Julian C. [Influence of overweight on the health-related quality of life in adolescents]. An Pediatr (Barc). 2015;82(3):131–8.
31. Alberga AS, Sigal RJ, Goldfield G, Prud'homme D, Kenny GP. Overweight and obese teenagers: why is adolescence a critical period? Pediatr Obes. 2012;7(4):261–73.
32. Crocker MK, Stern EA, Sedaka NM, Shomaker LB, Brady SM, Ali AH, et al. Sexual dimorphisms in the associations of BMI and body fat with indices of pubertal development in girls and boys. J Clin Endocrinol Metab. 2014;99(8):E1519–29.
33. Blum RW, Garell D, Hodgman CH, Jorissen TW, Okinow NA, Orr DP, et al. Transition from child-centered to adult health-care systems for adolescents with chronic conditions. A position paper of the Society for Adolescent Medicine. J Adolesc Health. 1993;14(7):570–6.
34. Lariviere-Bastien D, Bell E, Majnemer A, Shevell M, Racine E. Perspectives of young adults with cerebral palsy on transitioning from pediatric to adult healthcare systems. Semin Pediatr Neurol. 2013;20(2):154–9.
35. Saidi A, Kovacs AH. Developing a transition program from pediatric- to adult-focused cardiology care: practical considerations. Congenit Heart Dis. 2009;4(4):204–15.
36. McQuillan RF, Toulany A, Kaufman M, Schiff JR. Benefits of a transfer clinic in adolescent and young adult kidney transplant patients. Can J Kidney Health Dis. 2015;2:45.
37. Garvey KC, Beste MG, Luff D, Atakov-Castillo A, Wolpert HA, Ritholz MD. Experiences of health care transition voiced by young adults with type 1 diabetes: a qualitative study. Adolesc Health Med Ther. 2014;5:191–8.
38. Rosenberg-Yunger ZR, Klassen AF, Amin L, Granek L, D'Agostino NM, Boydell KM, et al. Barriers and facilitators of transition from pediatric to adult long-term follow-up care in childhood cancer survivors. J Adolesc Young Adult Oncol. 2013;2(3):104–11.
39. Rianthavorn P, Ettenger RB. Medication non-adherence in the adolescent renal transplant recipient: a clinician's viewpoint. Pediatr Transplant. 2005;9(3):398–407.
40. Pyatak EA, Sequeira PA, Whittemore R, Vigen CP, Peters AL, Weigensberg MJ. Challenges contributing to disrupted transition from paediatric to adult diabetes care in young adults with type 1 diabetes. Diabet Med. 2014;31(12):1615–24.
41. Nakhla M, Daneman D, To T, Paradis G, Guttmann A. Transition to adult care for youths with diabetes mellitus: findings from a Universal Health Care System. Pediatrics. 2009;124(6):e1134–41.
42. Pacaud D, Yale JF, Stephure D, Trussel R, Davies HD. Problems in transition from pediatric care to adult care for individuals with diabetes. Can J Diabetes. 2005;29:13–8.

43. Van Walleghem N, Macdonald CA, Dean HJ. Evaluation of a systems navigator model for transition from pediatric to adult care for young adults with type 1 diabetes. Diabetes Care. 2008;31(8): 1529–30.
44. Bell LE, Bartosh SM, Davis CL, Dobbels F, Al-Uzri A, Lotstein D, et al. Adolescent transition to adult care in solid organ transplantation: a consensus conference report. Am J Transplant. 2008;8(11):2230–42.
45. Magee JC, Bucuvalas JC, Farmer DG, Harmon WE, Hulbert-Shearon TE, Mendeloff EN. Pediatric transplantation. Am J Transplant. 2004;4 Suppl 9:54–71.
46. Colver A, Longwell S. New understanding of adolescent brain development: relevance to transitional healthcare for young people with long term conditions. Arch Dis Child. 2013;98(11):902–7.
47. Taube-Schiff M, Yufe S, Dettmer E, D'Agostino N, Sockalingam S. Bridging the gap: patient experiences following transfer of care from a pediatric obesity management program to an adult bariatric surgery program. Bariatr Surg Pract Patient Care. 2016;11(2):67–72.
48. Arnett JJ. Emerging adulthood. A theory of development from the late teens through the twenties. Am Psychol. 2000;55(5):469–80.
49. Arnett JJ. Conceptions of the transition to adulthood among emerging adults in American ethnic groups. New Dir Child Adolesc Dev. 2003;100:63–75.
50. Peters A, Laffel L. Diabetes care for emerging adults: recommendations for transition from pediatric to adult diabetes care systems: a position statement of the American Diabetes Association, with representation by the American College of Osteopathic Family Physicians, the American Academy of Pediatrics, the American Association of Clinical Endocrinologists, the American Osteopathic Association, the Centres for Disease Control and Prevention, Children with Diabetes, The Endocrine Society, the International Society for Pediatric and Adolescent Diabetes, Juvenile Diabetes Research Foundation International, the National Diabetes Education Program, and the Pediatric Endocrine Society (formerly Lawson Wilkins Pediatric Endocrine Society). Diabetes Care. 2011;34(11):2477–85.
51. McDonagh JE, Southwood TR, Shaw KL. The impact of a coordinated transitional care programme on adolescents with juvenile idiopathic arthritis. Rheumatology (Oxford). 2007;46(1):161–8.
52. American Academy of Pediatrics, American Academy of Family Physicians, American College of Physicians-American Society of Internal Medicine. A consensus statement on health care transitions for young adults with special health care needs. Pediatrics. 2002;110(6 Pt 2):1304–6.
53. Cadario F, Prodam F, Bellone S, Trada M, Binotti M, Trada M, et al. Transition process of patients with type 1 diabetes (T1DM) from paediatric to the adult health care service: a hospital-based approach. Clin Endocrinol (Oxf). 2009;71(3):346–50.
54. Fernandes SM, O'Sullivan-Oliveira J, Landzberg MJ, Khairy P, Melvin P, Sawicki GS, et al. Transition and transfer of adolescents and young adults with pediatric onset chronic disease: the patient and parent perspective. J Pediatr Rehabil Med. 2014;7(1):43–51.
55. McCurdy C, DiCenso A, Boblin S, Ludwin D, Bryant-Lukosius D, Bosompra K. There to here: young adult patients' perceptions of the process of transition from pediatric to adult transplant care. Prog Transplant. 2006;16(4):309–16.
56. Suris JC, Akre C. Key elements for, and indicators of, a successful transition: an international Delphi study. J Adolesc Health. 2015;56(6):612–8.
57. Shrewsbury VA, Baur LA, Nguyen B, Steinbeck KS. Transition to adult care in adolescent obesity: a systematic review and why it is a neglected topic. Int J Obes (Lond). 2014;38(4):475–9.

21 Technology to Promote Obesity Self-Management

Melvyn W.B. Zhang and Roger C.M. Ho

21.1 Objectives and Topics to be Covered

The objective of this chapter is to explore how bariatric care has been influenced and transformed by technological innovations. A clinical vignette will be used to highlight the potential benefits of such innovations for bariatric patient care. The role of technology in general self-management and the influence of health technology in bariatric care will be discussed. This will be followed by an overview of the potential role of technology in bariatric care and its accompanying benefits. The authors will then provide an overview of the potential limitations of bariatric applications that are currently made available on the respective application stores. Taking into consideration these limitations, examples of evidence-based technological interventions for bariatric care will be illustrated and further discussed.

M.W.B. Zhang, M.B.B.S., D.C.P., M.R.C.Psych. (✉)
Biomedical Institute for Global Health Research & Technology (BIGHEART), National University of Singapore, Md6 14 Medical Drive, #14-01, Singapore 117599, Singapore
e-mail: ciezwm@nus.edu.sg

R.C.M. Ho, M.B.B.S(H.K)., D.P.M(Ire)., M.R.C.Psych(U.K)., F.R.C.P.C.
Department of Psychological Medicine, National University of Singapore, Level 9, NUHS Tower Block, 1E Kent Ridge Road, Singapore 119228, Singapore
e-mail: pcmrhcm@nus.edu.sg

Case Vignette

Carla was a 30-year-old female who has been referred by her family physician for bariatric surgery. She stays around 40 miles from the bariatric surgery center. When she was assessed initially, her body mass index was 38. She also has had other obesity-related medical complications. Upon assessment by the psychiatrist, she was diagnosed with binge eating disorder, along with depressive disorder. It was recommended that she undergo sessions with the psychologist prior to proceeding for surgery. However, she cited that it was not possible for her to attend the sessions as she is the sole breadwinner at home and she needs to be working full time. She is also having much trouble with traveling to the bariatric center as she does not drive. She wanted to know whether there were viable alternatives to which she could still partake in the program prior to her undergoing the necessary bariatric surgery.

21.2 Role of Technology in General Self-Management

Over the past decade, technology has transformed and has revolutionized conventional healthcare. The introduction of the iPhone by Apple in 2007

S. Sockalingam, R. Hawa (eds.), *Psychiatric Care in Severe Obesity*, DOI 10.1007/978-3-319-42536-8_21

was pivotal as it led subsequently to the launch of applications store, to further enhance the capabilities of smartphone devices, which at that point in time, already enabled mobile computing and has made healthcare more accessible on the go [1]. A recent survey done [2] showed the massive increment in the number of applications that are downloaded off the application stores. Psychiatry has tapped onto the recent advances in technology and used it to help transform existing care models. For example, patients with schizophrenia could now make use of their smartphone application to complete a self-report questionnaire on their current psychotic symptoms [3]. This has enabled psychiatrists to recognize potential stressors that might lead to their patients having a relapse of their underlying condition. In addition, others have made use of smartphones and wearable sensors to help in identifying changes in mood symptoms [4]. Routine pen and paper questionnaires are now integrated into an application, and patients could use these validated questionnaires to help themselves self-monitor their own conditions [5]. Apart from the utilization of smartphone technologies in symptoms monitoring and self-management, studies have found smartphone technologies to be a viable tool to help augment face-to-face therapy sessions for patients who are diagnosed with substance disorder. The rapid advances in technologies have enabled smartphones to be used as safety tools for patients who are diagnosed with dementia as well [6]. Smartphone applications could detect the precise location of elderly demented patients and send immediate alerts and notifications to their caregivers if the sensors detect a change in the preset parameters, indicating that the demented patient might have wandered out of his or her own home [6]. The above illustration has only covered some of the evidence-based innovations that are currently available for patients with mental health-related disorders. There are many other applications in the application store that might be of use for psychiatric patients, but have not been extensively peer reviewed or are in the midst of being peer reviewed.

21.3 Influence of Health Technology in Bariatric Clinical Care

Given the rapid advances in technology and how pervasive its influence has been, bariatric care has been transformed by technological innovations and advances as well. There have been previous reviews looking into the currently available bariatric- and obesity-related applications on the respective application stores. Katie et al. [7] and Daniel et al. [8] have previously done a comprehensive search through the application store in 2013 for bariatric-related applications. They have identified applications that were useful for educating patients more about their condition. They have also identified applications that were useful for patients, as these applications enabled patients to connect with others on a support forum. Hence, there are indeed a wide variety of bariatric-related applications on the application stores.

21.4 Role of Technology in Bariatric Care

There are indeed numerous benefits of having bariatric applications for patient care. Prior studies have shown that there is an association between the success rates of bariatric surgery and psychological factors. Studies have highlighted that obesity is very often associated with other psychiatric disorders, such as that of anxiety disorder and depressive disorder, as well as binge eating disorder. Some review studies have shown that the presence of depressive disorder and binge eating disorder would result in poor maintenance of the gains made by bariatric surgery. Given these associations, various bariatric programs have recognized the need for individuals to be involved in psychological therapy. Cognitive behavioral therapy has been found to be useful for bariatric patients. Prior studies have demonstrated the initial feasibility of implementation of a telephone-based bariatric cognitive behavioral therapy program in Toronto [9]. With the current advances in technology, web-based and smartphone innovations could potentially be used to reach out to individuals who might have issues coming for their regular therapy program. Web-based and smartphone-based cognitive behavioral therapy could be used as a stand-alone therapy, or they could also be used as an adjunctive therapy to help individuals better manage their weight conditions and their psychiatric conditions in between the routine sessions.

Apart from the potential utilization of web and smartphone technologies to cater to the psychosocial care needs of patients, web and smartphone technologies could also help patients to self-manage their own condition. It is believed that this would give them more ownership and more motivation in their recovery process. In addition, the information contained within the applications would help to better educate patients about their preexisting conditions, as well as their loved ones and caregivers. The fact that they have better knowledge about their condition is crucial as it would help them progress towards recovery. In addition, bariatric applications could be used as tool kits to prevent patients from relapse into their preexisting habits, thus negating the gains they have made in consultation with the multidisciplinary team. At times, pertinent information could be stored on their downloaded applications, and these logs would be useful for members of the multidisciplinary team who are seeing them to review. This helps the multidisciplinary team to have better insights into the patient's condition during the time he/she was out of consult.

21.5 Understanding Potential Limitations of Bariatric Applications

21.5.1 Gaps in Knowledge and Limitations of Current Applications

Despite the numerous advantages, there are some limitations with regard to the applications currently made available on the application store. What seemed to be particularly concerning is the lack of the evaluation of these applications that are made available on the current application stores as was highlighted by Katie et al. [7] and Daniel et al. [8]. They have underlined that most of the applications has been developed by developers, with medical professionals not being involved. Hence, they have raised concerns with regard to the current evidence base of the applications currently available in the app store.

21.5.2 Critical Appraisal and Evaluation of Information Quality of Bariatric Applications

Zhang et al. [10] in their recent paper have conducted an analysis of the information quality of bariatric surgery smartphone applications using the Silberg scale. Based on their evaluation of 39 applications that they have identified from the individual application stores, they have found that most of the current applications have not provided references and have not fully disclosed the sponsorship of the application. More importantly, most of the current applications have not specified when they were last updated. These factors are essential, as they would have an implication on the evidence base of the application.

The Silberg scale assesses the information quality of a smartphone application across four domains. These include that of authorship, attribution, disclosure, and currency. For authorship, it is essential to determine whether authors are credited, whether the affiliations of the authors are recorded, and whether the credentials of the authors are provided. For attribution, the scale looks into whether information sources are given and whether appropriate references are provided for. For disclosure, the scale takes into account whether the ownership of the application and sponsorship have been disclosed. For currency, it looks at whether the application has been modified in the previous month and whether the application has included a creation or a last-modification date. The scale rates the information quality of an application out of a cumulative total of 9 points. While there may be new scales that have been developed to rate smartphone applications, the above-mentioned scale has been utilized widely in the assessment of other psychiatric information available online.

In summary, a critical appraisal of applications enables healthcare professionals to understand how best to conceptualize new applications to overcome the existing limitations.

21.5.3 Privacy and Confidentiality Issues

In addition to the above, there are always concerns about the storage of patient's sensitive data and concerns pertaining to privacy and confidentiality, especially so when the data are stored on today's cloud-based servers. It is also essential for patients themselves to recognize that the information available within the application are not specific for their own condition and that the applications are no replacement for an evaluation by the multidisciplinary team that they are in touch with. Patients should be cognizant of this and seek consults with their regular health providers if they have any new symptoms. In addition, it is highly possible that certain innovative technologies developed are not made equally available to all patients. Some of the limiting factors might include the compatibility between the technologies and the existing phones that patients might have, and some disadvantaged patients might also not have access to the technology as they do not have a smartphone.

21.6 Examples of Technology for Bariatric Care

Taking these limitations into account, the authors would try to demonstrate how web-based and smartphone-based innovations could be applied for bariatric care and in particular for the management of obesity. The authors would comment how these technologies could be applied for the case described in the clinical vignette.

21.6.1 Bariatric Intervention Application

Psychosocial factors could be both a precipitating factor leading an individual towards obesity and a perpetuating factor that is responsible for the maintenance of obesity. Hence, over the years, various bariatric surgery programs have started to recognize the need to integrate psychological programs into the existing bariatric program structure. Psychological programs could help equip individuals with skills that could help them deal with binge eating, as well as correct maladaptive cognitive schemas about eating that might negate the health benefits resulting from bariatric surgery. Cognitive behavioral therapy has been increasingly recognized to be helpful for bariatric patients, and it has been gradually integrated into various bariatric programs. However, one of the major limitations with the implementation of such programs has to do with the existence of geographical barriers. Very often, psychosocial programs require individuals to engage with a mental health provider on a regular basis. The existence of geographical barriers may prevent certain individuals from accessing their mental health specialist and hence limit the effectiveness of these psychosocial interventions. Hence, telephone-based CBT was conceptualized and implemented in response to this treatment need. Previous studies have demonstrated that individuals are as satisfied with telephone-based CBT as with face-to-face CBT sessions [9]. With the recent advances in information technology, psychosocial programs are now not only limited to delivery via the telephone. Previous studies have compared live therapy against self-help therapy and Internet-based therapy and have demonstrated that there are slightly superior long-term effects of online as compared to conventional face-to-face sessions.

A literature search conducted to date of the online published literature also showed that there has been a paucity of research into the utilization of web-based technologies and smartphone technologies to deliver psychosocial care for bariatric patients. Tapping onto the latest developments in web-based and smartphone technologies, a bariatric online portal was created. The online psychosocial program comprises six modules, which includes that of a general introduction to CBT and the cognitive behavior model of overeating; how to use food records to normalize eating; identification of pleasurable alternatives to overeating; identification of problem-solving high-risk eating situations; challenging counterproductive thoughts; and preparing for bariatric surgery as well as an additional module of how best to keep on track following surgery. Figure 21.1 illustrates the web-based portal that the authors have conceptualized and implemented previously.

Figure 21.2 illustrates the smartphone version of the online web-based cognitive behavioral portal. The smartphone version includes not only the six core modules of the cognitive behavioral therapy programs but has also included other innovative features. The smartphone application includes a weekly weigh tracker as well as a daily mood tracker for patients to monitor their weight and mood accordingly. In addition, the smartphone application also features a unique visual pill tracker to help patients monitor their vitamin supplementations that they might be prescribed. It also includes a contact resource for patients. Based on the analysis of the initial data, it showed that patients were receptive towards such a modality of intervention. In particular, participants who stayed more than 40 miles from a bariatric center are particularly receptive towards such an intervention.

21.6.2 Bariatric Aftercare Application

Based on the previous reviews, most of the current obesity or weight management applications on the app stores are limited to the following: patient education, patient discussion forums, and weight management using hypnosis. There seemed to be a paucity of smartphone innovations and applications that could help individuals self-manage their weight issues. In contrast, conditions such as cystic fibrosis have applications that

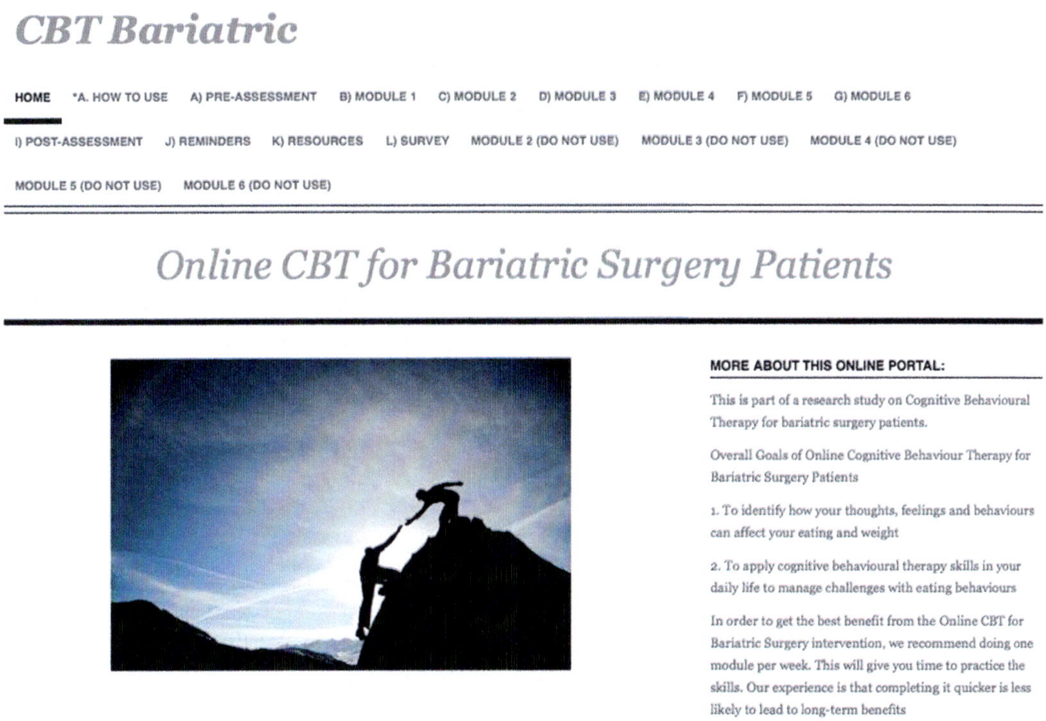
CBT Bariatric
HOME
*A. HOW TO USE
A) PRE-ASSESSMENT
B) MODULE 1
C) MODULE 2
D) MODULE 3
E) MODULE 4
F) MODULE 5
G) MODULE 6
I) POST-ASSESSMENT
J) REMINDERS
K) RESOURCES
L) SURVEY
MODULE 2 (DO NOT USE)
MODULE 3 (DO NOT USE)
MODULE 4 (DO NOT USE)
MODULE 5 (DO NOT USE)
MODULE 6 (DO NOT USE)
Online CBT for Bariatric Surgery Patients
MORE ABOUT THIS ONLINE PORTAL:
This is part of a research study on Cognitive Behavioural Therapy for bariatric surgery patients.
Overall Goals of Online Cognitive Behaviour Therapy for Bariatric Surgery Patients
1. To identify how your thoughts, feelings and behaviours can affect your eating and weight
2. To apply cognitive behavioural therapy skills in your daily life to manage challenges with eating behaviours
In order to get the best benefit from the Online CBT for Bariatric Surgery intervention, we recommend doing one module per week. This will give you time to practice the skills. Our experience is that completing it quicker is less likely to lead to long-term benefits

Fig. 21.1 Web-based interface

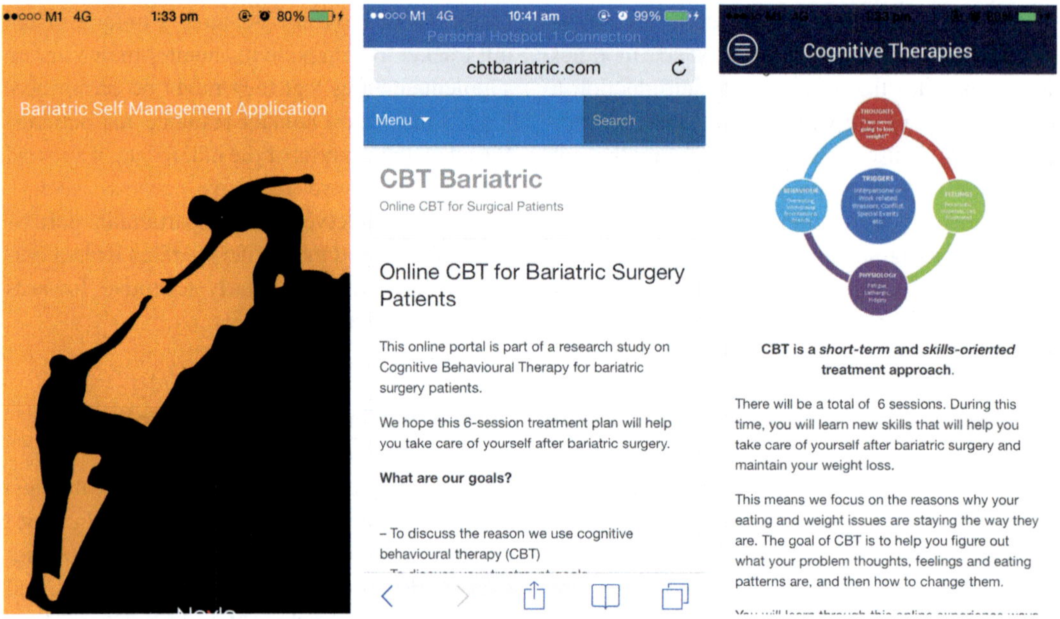

Fig. 21.2 Smart-phone interface

helped individuals self-manage their own conditions [11]. Conditions such as pain disorders also have smartphone applications that allow individuals to manage and monitor their own pain [12].

Taking into consideration previous literature, the team at TWH-BSP conceptualized and developed an aftercare application. The conceptualized application contains information about the various appointments, as well as information about routine blood works and vitamin supplementation. A user perspective survey was conducted after implementation and showed that the vast majority of patients felt that the information components of the application were useful, especially so with regard to the aspect of the application that provides information about each appointment. The vast majority of the participants also felt that the ability of the application to help them in rescheduling their appointment was also significantly helpful. Of importance, the introduction of the smartphone application has helped to change users' perceptions and confidence about their ability to manage their own condition. After the implementation of the smartphone application, 25 % of the sample group reported being extremely confident about managing their own condition, as compared to 17 % prior [13].

Case Vignette Discussion

As mentioned, Carla is a 30-year-old female with severe obesity who has been referred for bariatric surgery. She has comorbid psychiatric conditions, and hence she has been recommended to see the team psychologist prior to undergoing surgery. The web-based and smartphone CBT module might be applicable in her case, as she lives far from the hospital and cannot miss additional days from work. It could be used as a replacement for in-person CBT or as an adjunct to the existing sessions that she could be attending at her town.

The bariatric aftercare self-management application would also be helpful for her to monitor her progress after the surgery. She would be provided with updated information about what to expect at each of the appointments, as well as the required labo-

(continued)

(continued)

ratory investigations that would have to be done at specific time points post-surgery. In addition, she would also be able to find out more about her required vitamin supplementations after surgery and the potential changes in her psychiatric medications.

The physical activity tracker application would help her to track her daily physical activity levels and enable her to keep a log of her daily activities. In addition, it would also help her to trend her weight loss over time.

21.7 Summary and Take Home Messages

With the rapid advances in technology, bariatric care, like other specialties, has been massively transformed by technological innovations. There are a multitude of bariatric-related applications in the smartphone stores currently. Prior research has highlighted the limitations of these smartphone innovations, in that most of them are lacking in evidence base. A recent analysis of the information quality of bariatric smartphone applications has also reinforced this viewpoint. It is the objective of this chapter to illustrate to healthcare professionals how advances in technology could be implemented successfully in promoting obesity self-management. In addition, the authors also wish to highlight how evidence-based approaches could be incorporated into bariatric applications could be incorporated into bariatric applications to better support patients and their providers in severe obesity care.

Take Home Messages

(a) Given the rapid advances in technology and how pervasive its influence has been, bariatric care has been transformed by technological innovations and advances as well.

(b) There are indeed numerous benefits of having bariatric applications for patient care, including increasing access to psychosocial supports during severe obesity care.

(c) There are some limitations with regard to the applications currently made available on the application stores. Data suggests that there has been a lack of evaluation data related to these applications.

(d) There are indeed numerous benefits of having bariatric applications for patient care. Web-based and smartphone-based cognitive behavioral therapy could be used as a standalone therapy, or they could also be used as an adjunctive therapy to help individuals better manage their weight conditions and their psychiatric conditions in between the routine sessions. Web and smartphone technologies could also help patients to self-manage their own condition.

References

1. Abu SMM, Illhoi Y, Lincoln S. A systematic review of healthcare applications for smartphones. BMC Med Inform Decis Mak. 2012;12:67.
2. Karl FBP, Heather W, Kim W. Smartphone and medical related App use among medical students and junior doctors in the United Kingdom (UK): a regional survey. BMC Med Inform Decis Mak. 2012;12:121.
3. Palmier-Claus JE, et al. The feasibility and validity of ambulatory self-report of psychotic symptoms using a smartphone software application. BMC Psychiatry. 2012;12:172.
4. Grunerbl A, et al. Smart-phone based recognition of states and state changes in bipolar disorder patients. IEEE J Biomed Health Inform. 2015;19(1):140–8.
5. Palmier-Claus JE, et al. Integrating mobile-phone based assessment for psychosis into people's everyday lives and clinical care: a qualitative study. BMC Psychiatry. 2013;13:34.
6. Sposaro F, Danielson J, Tyson G. iWander: an android application for dementia patients. Conf Proc IEEE Eng Med Biol Soc. 2010;2010:3875–8.
7. Katie C, Richard RWB, Bruce T, Andrew DB. Smartphone applications (Apps) for the bariatric surgeon. Obes Surg. 2013;2013(23):1669–72.
8. Daniel JS, John AJ, Noah H, Justin M. Obesity surgery smartphone apps: a review. Obes Surg. 2014;2014(24):32–6.
9. Sockalingam S, Cassin S, Chan D, Parikh SV. A pilot randomized controlled trial of telephone-based cognitive behavioral therapy for preoperative bariatric surgery patients. Surg Obes Relat Dis. 2015;1(6):S53–4.
10. Zhang MW, Ho RC, Hawa R, Sockalingam S. Analysis of the information quality of bariatric surgery smart-

phone applications using the Silberg scale. Obes Surg. 2016;26(1):163–8.
11. Hillard ME, Hahn R, Ridge AK, Eakin MN, Riekert KA. User preferences and design recommendations for an mHealth app to promote cystic fibrosis self-management. JMIR Mhealth Uhealth. 2014;2(4):e44.
12. Stinson JN, Lallo C, Harris L, Isaac L, Campbell F, Brown S, Ruskin D, Gordon M, Pink LR, Buckley N, Henry JL, White M, Karim A. iCanCope with Pain™: user-centred design of a web- and mobile based self-management program for youth with chronic pain based on identified health care needs. Pain Res Manag. 2014;19(5):257–65.
13. Zhang MW, Ho RC, Hawa R, Sockalingam S. Pilot implementation and user preferences of a Bariatric After-care application. Technol Health Care. 2015;23(6):729–36. doi:10.3233/THC-151025.

Part V

Psychopharmacological Considerations in Severe Obesity and Bariatric Surgery Care

Choosing Psychiatric Medications for Patients with Severe Obesity and Pharmacological Treatments for Severe Obesity in Patients with Psychiatric Disorders: A Case Study

22

Giovanni Amodeo, Mehala Subramaniapillai, Rodrigo B. Mansur, and Roger S. McIntyre

Case Vignette

David is a 38-year-old Caucasian male. He is married, with two children. He visits the Mood Disorders Clinic for a comprehensive second opinion, as requested by his current psychiatrist. He denies any perinatal problems or developmental delays. He is the second oldest son of three children and describes having close, affectionate relationships with both parents. His father was a lawyer and his mother was a homemaker. His childhood is described as happy and supportive. He had several close friends, enjoyed playing football and working on cars. He describes himself as an excellent student. He was very motivated in high school and his academic performance was good. After graduating from high school, he received his master's degree in law with exceptional grades. According to the patient, he had been "happily high" most of his life, which has helped him to be very successful at work and to accomplish many things in his life.

However, he also reports experiencing seasonal, episodic periods of sadness, irritability, and some loss of self-esteem, slight decrease in concentration, occasional fatigue, and mild anhedonia. These symptoms tend to occur in the fall and winter if he remains in a cold, dark climate and it tends to disappear in spring and summer.

Until the age of 24, the patient had been treated by his primary care physician for intermittent symptoms of depression, with citalopram, mirtazapine, paroxetine, sertraline, and bupropion at different times. He reports to have discontinued all the medications above after a few weeks, due to excessive irritability. However, the onset of more severe symptoms started approximately at age 25. He reports that he had an epiphany while he was a passenger on a train. At that

(continued)

G. Amodeo, M.D.
Department of Psychiatry, Department of Molecular Medicine and Development, University of Siena School of Medicine, Viale Bracci, 1, Via XXIV Maggio, 23, Tuscany, Siena 53100, Italy
e-mail: giovanniamodeo86@gmail.com

M. Subramaniapillai, H.B.Sc., M.Sc. (✉)
R.B. Mansur, M.D. • R.S. McIntyre, M.D., F.R.C.P.C.
Mood Disorders Psychopharmacology Unit, University Health Network, 399 Bathurst Street, MP 9-325, Toronto, ON, Canada M5T 2S8
e-mail: m.subram@mail.utoronto.ca; Rodrigo.Mansur@uhn.ca; roger.mcintyre@uhn.ca

S. Sockalingam, R. Hawa (eds.), *Psychiatric Care in Severe Obesity*,
DOI 10.1007/978-3-319-42536-8_22

(continued)

time, he had a vision of St. Peter and he believed he was "called to serve in a mission." He became religiously preoccupied, with grandiose thinking and behavior.

During that time, his wife describes observing continued symptoms of marked irritability, sharp responses when engaged in conversation and general self-absorption. Over time, his symptoms continued to escalate with marked grandiose thinking, impulsive and excessive spending, decreased sleep, and increased contact with individuals via telephone and e-mails at all hours of the day and night on six computers that he had recently bought. He also experienced difficulty focusing and psychomotor agitation.

The patient realized at this point that he was experiencing difficulties and agreed to speak with a psychiatrist who made a diagnosis of bipolar disorder with psychotic features and started him on divalproex (Divalproate) 500 mg twice a day and olanzapine 10 mg a day. After 1 week, the serum valproic acid level was 37 ug/mL and the dose was titrated up to 1500 mg/day. Since his symptoms did not resolve completely, his olanzapine dose was then raised to 20 mg/day and valproate was titrated to his current dose of 2000 mg/day. His most recent valproic acid level was 59 ug/mL.

His symptoms gradually improved and olanzapine was gradually discontinued after approximately 6 months of remission, primarily due to significant weight gain (i.e., more than 40 lb). The patient continued to feel relatively well for a few months. However, the following spring, he suffered from the change in daylight hours and temperature and started to experience irritability, reduced sleep, flight of ideas, and rapid speech. His appetite was reduced while the level of interest and energy in a number of activities were all reported as extremely high. He also started thinking that he was about to be called to serve on a special mission on behalf of God.

His psychiatrist proposed to restart olanzapine, but the patient and his family asked for a second opinion, owing to his reluctance to gain more weight. The patient is presently obese. He is a 6-foot-tall man (183 cm) and weighs 230 lbs (104 kg), with a body mass index (BMI) of 31.05 kg/m^2. Active medical problems include dyslipidemia, coronary artery disease, and hypothyroidism, all responding relatively well to his current medication regimen, which includes atorvastatin 10 mg 1 tablet a day, nitroglycerin 0.4 mg sublingual tablet every 5 min, if needed, and l-thyroxine 75 mcg/day. He is also taking divalproex 1000 mg twice a day.

At the present visit, he denies drug/alcohol abuse. He denies suicidal/homicidal ideation, plan, intent, or attempt. He describes his mood as irritable with periods of happiness and sadness. Throughout the evaluation, his mood appears elevated with an excessive range of affect. Rate of speech is rapid at times and difficult to interrupt. Content of speech is focused on his disorder, but he also reports having visions and hearing voices and talks about a special mission that he has to perform, which indicates the presence of mood congruent psychotic symptoms. Patient was recently seen for a neurological evaluation, MRI without contrast and proton MR spectroscopy, with no sign or major neurological/organic disorder.

He is oriented in all spheres and shows an above average intellectual functioning. He recognizes his mood/emotional dysregulation has had a negative impact on his life and in his relationships with others but is not completely insightful into his present condition. However, he seems invested in seeking treatment that will maximize stabilization.

Based on the clinical interview, collaborative information from his wife and the review of previous records, our primary diagnosis is bipolar I disorder, most recent episode, mania, with psychotic features.

22.1 Introduction

David has a history of bipolar disorder with psychotic features. He has been treated with success in the past, using a combination of olanzapine and divalproex. However, the discontinuation of olanzapine, primarily due to weight gain and dyslipidemia, has led to a recurrence of manic and psychotic symptoms. With a new course of olanzapine, David would likely achieve a rapid remission. However, a longer term course of olanzapine treatment would contribute to further weight gain and dyslipidemia or, at least, complicate his efforts to lose weight and improve these conditions.

Patients with psychiatric disorders are at high risk of gaining weight and developing metabolic illnesses for several reasons, including unhealthy eating, low energy expenditure, and sedentary lifestyle and lack of physical exercise, as well as intrinsic factors of these diseases, such as genetic factors. For instance, the absence of an allele variant of the 5-HT2C receptor gene in a Chinese cohort predicted a weight gain of greater than 7 % of total body weight with chlorpromazine, fluphenazine, risperidone, clozapine, and sulpiride [1]. Undoubtedly, however, one of the major drivers for weight gain in patients with psychiatric conditions is their pharmacologic treatment.

Hence, patients with mood and psychotic disorders, including patients with bipolar disorder like David, are at a high risk for medical comorbidities in general and metabolic diseases in particular. Not only do metabolic comorbidities add to risk for cardiovascular disease, but they also associate with greater mental disorder severity [2–4], morbidity, mortality, and disability [4, 5].

For these reasons, the risk of metabolic illness has become one of the major determinants of treatment choice. In fact, the growing knowledge about the devastating impact of metabolic illness, as well as the increasing attention to physical health in patients with psychiatric diseases, has prompted a change in prescribers' attitude and behavior in cases like David's. Indeed, accumulating evidence shows that rates of obesity also increase in response to treatment. Therefore, this is another reason why psychiatrists must consider metabolic concerns when considering pharmacologic therapy.

Herein, we evaluate a range of possible psychiatric medications for a patient like David and discuss the specific risks and benefits of each medication with particular consideration given to the risk of causing metabolic illnesses in general, and weight gain and obesity in particular. Specifically a range of anticonvulsants (valproate, carbamazepine), lithium and antipsychotics (olanzapine, clozapine, risperidone, quetiapine, ziprasidone, asenapine, lurasidone, and aripiprazole) will be discussed. Furthermore, we aim to describe the most promising anti-obesity agents (orlistat, lorcaserin, combined treatment of phentermine and topiramate, combined treatment of bupropion and naltrexone and liraglutide) and their application in mental health settings. An overall view of the psychotropic medications is presented in Tables 22.1 and 22.2.

22.2 Anticonvulsants

Anticonvulsants have well-established effectiveness for acute and maintenance phases of bipolar disorder. They are called "anticonvulsants" because they are used to treat patients with epilepsy and include medications such as valproate, carbamazepine, and lamotrigine. Their mechanism of action is not fully understood. Their main mechanism is thought to be the blockage of voltage-gated sodium channels, which would affect glutamatergic signaling. However, it is very likely that their pharmacological profile is more complex and involves other monoamine pathways, enzymes complexes (GSK-3B), and gene transcriptions (such as BDNF).

22.2.1 Valproate

Valproate may cause significant weight gain, which may be due to increased appetite and food intake, reduced energy expenditure or slower metabolism. One particular study of interest found that a group of subjects with epilepsy treated with valproate who gained weight also manifested a reduced metabolic rate, rather than an increased intake of calories [6]. A review of weight gain in patients with epilepsy showed that

Table 22.1 Psychotropic medications and their involvement in weight gain/obesity and metabolic risk

Psychotropic drugs and their respective metabolic effects		
Psychotropic drug	Weight gain/ obesity and metabolic risk	References
Valproate	↑ weight, appetite, food intake	[6, 7, 9, 10]
	↓ energy expenditure, metabolic rate	
Lithium	↑ weight, energy consumption, appetite, edema	[16, 18, 21, 59]
	↑ risk of dyslipidemia and diabetes	
Carbamazepine	Mild effect on weight gain	[7, 12, 13]
	↑ cholesterol and triglycerides	
Olanzapine	↑ weight	[21, 30]
	↑ risk of dyslipidemia and diabetes	
Clozapine	↑ weight	[27, 32]
	↑ risk of dyslipidemia and diabetes	
Risperidone	Low risk of weight gain, dyslipidemia, or diabetes	[21, 35]
	↑ prolactin	
Quetiapine	Low risk of weight gain, dyslipidemia, or diabetes	[36]
Ziprasidone	↓ weight	[37, 38]
	↑ glucose or glycosylated hemoglobin	
	↓ cholesterol and triglycerides	
Asenapine	↓ weight	[40]
Aripiprazole	Low risk of weight gain, dyslipidemia, or diabetes	[21, 44]

up to 71 % of patients treated with valproate gained weight (*M*=22 kg, ranging from 8 to 49 kg) [7]. Furthermore, a recent study of patients who gained weight during valproate therapy also presented with significantly higher serum leptin concentrations. This may be indicative of leptin resistance and thus a reduced sensitivity of hypothalamic receptors to leptin action. This may produce a dysfunction in the sense of satiety and food intake control—more in women than in men [8]. The frequency of carbohydrate craving was 25.8 % higher in women and 14.3 % in men. In a study by Pylvänen and colleagues [9, 10], 51 patients receiving monotherapy with valproate and 45 healthy controls were evaluated, after an overnight fast, for differences in fasting plasma glucose and serum insulin, as well as in proinsulin and C-peptide, which are precursor molecules to insulin, synthesized in the beta cells of the pancreas. Patients receiving valproate showed fasting hyperinsulinemia although the fasting serum proinsulin and C-peptide levels were not higher in patients compared to control subjects, indicating that valproate did not increase insulin secretion, but may have altered insulin metabolism in the liver. In addition, proinsulin/insulin and C-peptide/insulin ratios results were lower in patients compared to controls. Moreover, valproate also is associated with increased androgen levels, which along with weight gain and hyperinsulinemia, is a feature of polycystic ovary syndrome (PCOS) [11].

Finally, valproate-treated patients had lower fasting plasma glucose concentrations than the control subjects. These changes were seen regardless of concomitant weight gain, suggesting that weight gain may be induced by increased insulin concentrations and not vice versa. In another study [9, 10], the same authors observed an association of valproate therapy with increased circulating insulin concentrations relative to body mass index. The participant sample in this trial was composed of lean and obese outpatients treated with valproate and a control group, which also included lean and obese subjects. The results suggest that the high insulin levels are not a consequence of obesity, as the rate of hyperinsulinemia

Table 22.2 Anti-obesity agents and their implications in psychiatric settings

Anti-obesity medication and their respective psychotropic effects			
Anti-obesity agent	Mechanism of action	Psychotropic side effects or pharmacological interaction	References
Orlistat	Reversible inhibitor of gastrointestinal lipases	Mild anxiety No pharmacological interaction with antidepressants and antipsychotics	[47]
Lorcaserin	Selective 5-HT 2C receptor agonist	Use of lorcaserin associated with SSRI, TCA, I-MAO, triptans, or other serotonin medications may potentiate the risk of Serotonin Syndrome, via CYP450 2D6 inhibition.	[50]
		Possible Psychiatric Side Effects: • Depressive behavior • Cognitive deficits • Suicidal thoughts and ideation • Mood changes • Hallucinations and delusions	Lorcaserin—Belviq prescribing information, accessed on April 24, 2016
Phentermine/topiramate	TAAR1 agonist/multiaction (ion channel, GABA inhibitor, glutamatergic agonist)	Possible Psychiatric Side Effects: • Depressive behavior • Anxiety/agitation • Cognitive deficits • Sleep disorder • Suicidal thoughts and ideation Co-administration with TCAs may increase the risk of cardiovascular events (e.g., hypertension, arrhythmia, tachycardia)	[53]
Naltrexone/bupropion	Selective opioid receptor (μ)/nicotinic acetylcholine receptor antagonist and reuptake inhibitor and releasing agent of NE	Bipolar disorder: higher risk of switching to mania or developing mixed features Schizophrenia: higher risk of developing agitation, hallucinations, and delusions May exacerbate existing anxiety Increased risk of depression and suicide thoughts	[54]
Liraglutide	GLP-1 receptor agonist	Mood changes Increased depressive behavior and symptoms Increased risk of suicide	[58]

SSRI Selective Serotonin Re-uptake Inhibitor, *TCA* Tricyclic Antidepressant, *I-MAO* Inhibitor of Monoamino Oxidase, *TAAR1* Trace Amino-Associated Receptor 1, *GABA* Gamma Amino Butyric Acid, *NE* Norepinephrine, *GLP-1* Glucagon-like peptide-1

was higher in patients treated with valproate than control subjects, and also higher in lean and obese patients treated with valproate than in lean and obese control subjects.

Although valproate is likely contributing to David's obesity, due to David's current unstable clinical situation, this may not be the best time to switch mood stabilizers. A change to a new mood stabilizer, with a reduced propensity for weight gain would be best considered as an adjunct treatment first, followed by a completed switching during the maintenance treatment phase.

22.2.2 Carbamazepine

Considering David's diagnosis of bipolar I disorder, carbamazepine (CBZ) could be another pharmacological choice. Indeed, the majority of the published studies report a relatively low rate and magnitude of weight gain in patients treated with CBZ. Specifically, in a review, weight gain has been reported in 2.5–14 % of patients with epilepsy who were treated with CBZ [7] and a 6-month study by Ketter and colleagues [12] suggested that weight gain in patients with bipolar disorder is minimal during long-term treatment with CBZ. In fact, this study reported a mean weight gain of 0.7 %. However, treatment with CBZ may affect blood-cholesterol concentrations. CBZ's effects on lipid metabolism were observed in a prospective study of adults with normal lipid indexes [13]. Significant increases in total cholesterol (by 13 +/− 15 %; $p = 0.02$), apolipoprotein B (apoB)-containing lipoproteins (very-low-density lipoprotein [VLDL], intermediate-density lipoprotein [IDL], and low-density lipoprotein [LDL]) and increased levels of triglycerides were noted, with no increase in high-density lipoprotein (HDL). According to the authors, this could be due to changes in the conversion cascade of IDL particles, possibly as an indirect effect related to a thyroid hormone decrease.

Carbamazepine would have a lower risk of obesity. However, co-administration of valproate and CBZ is not recommended due to their pharmacodynamic interactions, as CBZ usually decreases valproate levels, and valproate may alter CBZ levels in unpredictable ways. Furthermore, valproate may prolong the elimination half-life of CBZ [14]. However, a possible change to carbamazepine may be considered in the future and we may opt to increase his dosage of valproate in the meantime as David's latest blood concentration of valproate was 59 ug/mL at 2000 mg/day.

22.3 Lithium

Similar to valproate, lithium is a first-line treatment for bipolar disorder [15], but it has been similarly associated with weight gain, which is observed in 30–65 % of patients [16–18]. There is evidence that this weight gain could be due to a direct effect on carbohydrate [19] and fat metabolism [20] or due to lithium-induced hypothyroidism and consequential increased appetite and thirst [21].

David is already taking another mood stabilizer (valproate) and furthermore, the patient has a history of hypothyroidism and obesity. Co-administration of valproate and lithium would be a rationale option, but we prefer to increase valproate dosage (last valproate blood concentration 59 ug/mL) and keep lithium as a second choice compound at this stage of the illness.

22.4 Antipsychotics

Returning to David's case, we believe that his current symptoms and history suggest starting an antipsychotic. In fact, current available data suggest that combining a second-generation antipsychotic with an anticonvulsant or lithium is an efficacious treatment option for acute mania [22]. Atypical, second-generation antipsychotics are usually preferred to first-generation antipsychotics in patients with mood disorder because they are more efficacious in depressive symptoms and also have a lower risk of exprapyramidal symptoms (EPS; e.g., dystonia, akathisia, parkinsonism, tardive dyskinesia) [23], and decreased risk of worsening depressive symptoms [24]. Indeed, patients with bipolar disorder are even more susceptible to EPS than those with schizophrenia [25, 26]. Atypical antipsychotics, as a class, are very frequently prescribed to persons with bipolar disorder. However, a major limitation is that they have also been strongly implicated with weight gain, dyslipidemia, and diabetes mellitus. For instance, some atypical antipsychotics have a high affinity for serotonin 5-HT2C receptor and histaminergic receptor with an antagonist effect (linked to increased food intake) which may play a synergistic role in weight gain [27]. The most promising atypical antipsychotics are discussed below.

22.4.1 Olanzapine

Weight gain has been reported in virtually all published studies of this medication [21]. In particular, in a 4-week, randomized, double-blind, parallel study with a sample of 115 bipolar patients, Tohen and colleagues [28] described a weight gain of 2.11 kg (SD = 2.83 kg), and in a 6-month, double-blind study with 113 bipolor I patients, Sanger and colleagues [29] described a weight gain of 6.64 kg (SD = 8.51 kg).

Dyslipidemia has been well documented as one of the most common side effects. For instance, the association between olanzapine and hyperlipidemia was evaluated in a sample of 18,309 individuals with schizophrenia, with a finding that olanzapine use was associated with a nearly fivefold increase in the odds for developing hyperlipidemia, compared with no antipsychotic exposure (odds ratio [OR] = 4.65; 95 % CI: 2.44–8.85; $p<0.01$) as well as a greater than threefold increase compared with those receiving conventional agents (OR = 3.36; 95 % CI: 1.77–6.39; $p<0.01$) [30]. Moreover, several studies, including prospective trials, retrospective studies and single case reports, have increasingly implicated olanzapine as causing or exacerbating type 2 diabetes [21]. Indeed, Koller and Doraiswamy [31] documented 237 cases of olanzapine-associated hyperglycemia, where most cases (73 %) occurred within 6 months of therapy initiation, and 188 patients developed a new-onset of diabetes. Glucose levels were greater than 1000 mg/dL in 41 patients and 78 % of patients improved following medication discontinuation or dose reduction. Hyperglycemia recurred in 80 % of cases that were recruited for new course of olanzapine.

Although David's manic symptoms have been historically managed well with olanzapine, it would be worth trying a medication with a lower metabolic risk.

22.4.2 Clozapine

Clozapine has an even greater propensity than olanzapine toward weight gain, diabetes, and hypertriglyceridemia [27, 32]. A 3-year, large, non-randomized, observational study evaluating 10,972 schizophrenic patients showed that clozapine ($n=188$) induced body weight gain, ranging from 3.3 to 6.6 kg [33]. This evidence is supported by a review covering 16 clinical trials ($n=798$) with early onset of schizophrenia that also highlights relevant weight gain due to the treatment with clozapine with an incidence of 20–64 %. Clozapine may contribute to the development of metabolic abnormalities, in particular hypertriglyceridemia (8–22 %) and diabetes (6 %) [34].

Clozapine is not approved for use in any phase of bipolar disorder although it has been used in treatment-resistant bipolar patients. Therefore, this is not an evidence-based treatment option for David.

22.4.3 Risperidone

Although the risk of weight gain, diabetes, and dyslipidemia is lower with risperidone than with olanzapine, this compound is associated with a significant risk of hyperprolactinemia. For instance, in a randomized controlled trial [35], 90.5 % of subjects who received risperidone showed an increase in serum prolactin levels above the upper limit of the reference range (2–29 ng/mL). Only a few case reports and studies have suggested risperidone as an agent that increases the risk for diabetes and many schizophrenia trials suggest that risperidone does not have a high risk for hyperlipidemia or increase the incidence of diabetes [21].

Risperidone would represent an acceptable option for David's manic symptomathology, but the risk for hyperprolactinemia is high and thus avoiding a further endocrinological worsening is warranted.

22.4.4 Quetiapine

Quetiapine, compared to olanzapine and clozapine, has a lower propensity toward weight gain, but a higher one compared to risperidone. In a study by Brecher and colleagues [36], 352 patients were treated with quetiapine for 52 weeks. Overall, 37 % of patients gained 7 % or more of their baseline body weight. Interestingly, the rate of weight gain was inversely related to baseline body mass index. The mean weight gain at study end was 3.19 kg. In patients treated with <200 mg/day of quetiapine, mean weight gain was 1.54 kg, compared with 4.08 kg for 200–399 mg/day, 1.89 kg for 400–599 mg/day, and 3.57 kg for > or = 600 mg/day; median weight gain was 0.95 kg, 3.40 kg, 2.00 kg, and 3.34 kg, respectively. Of note, most weight gain (>60 %) occurred within the first 12 weeks of quetiapine treatment, with modest changes after 6 months. In a large study for patients with psychosis, quetiapine and risperidone patients had estimated odds of receiving treatment for type 2 diabetes that were no different than those of subjects who were never treated with antipsychotics or who were treated with conventional antipsychotics. However, other studies have suggested that quetiapine may share with other dibenzodiazepine-derived atypical antipsychotics, primarily olanzapine and clozapine, with a propensity to increase serum triglycerides levels [21].

Given that David is in a phase of his disease also characterized by delusional thoughts, we would like to choose a drug with timely action on these psychotic symptoms, but the pharmacological profile of quetiapine gives a high affinity to dopamine receptors only at high doses (600–800 mg/day), and this would require a longer time of titration than other atypical antipsychotics. For these reasons above, we decided not to introduce quetiapine.

22.4.5 Ziprasidone

Ziprasidone treatment is associated with low metabolic risks and analysis of laboratory data from the short-term studies showed that the incidence of abnormal elevations in random glucose measurements was the same as placebo (8 %). In the Clinical Antipsychotic Trials of Intervention Effectiveness (CATIE) study [37], patients with schizophrenia treated with ziprasidone ($n = 185$) lost a median of 0.91 kg, with no significant change in serum glucose or glycosylated hemoglobin levels. Also, a reduction in total cholesterol and triglycerides (possibly due to the discontinuation of previous medications) was observed. Other switch studies with ziprasidone showed a reduction in body weight and other metabolic effects [38].

Ziprasidone could be a viable option for David. However, we decided to not prescribe ziprasidone medication at this point because of its risk of QTc interval prolongation, an electrocardiographic abnormality which increases the risk of irregular heart rhythm and "torsades de pointes." Although the clinical relevance of this risk for ziprasidone has been recently questioned [39], we preferred to avoid this medication as a first choice drug because of David's preexisting coronary artery disease and the risk of ischemia-induced arrhythmia.

22.4.6 Asenapine

Asenapine has shown a relatively low weight gain liability. A recent meta-analysis [40] showed that asenapine produces significantly less weight gain than many other antipsychotics. For instance, the standard mean difference (SMD) in weight gained in those on placebo versus asenapine was 0.23 (95 % CI: 0.07–0.39) which was significantly superior compared to risperidone (SMD = 0.42; 95 % CI: 0.33–0.50), quetiapine (SMD = 0.43; 95 % CI: 0.34–0.53), clozapine (SMD = 0.65;

95 % CI: 0.31–0.99), and olanzapine (SMD = 0.74; 95 % CI: 0.67–0.81). Aripiprazole (SMD = 0.17; 95 % CI: 0.05–0.28) and ziprasidone (SMD = 0.10; 95 % CI: –0.02 to 0.22) also demonstrated a reduced weight gain.

We decided not to prescribe asenapine, owing to the fact that the patient has a history of emetophobia (fear of vomiting) and refused to take a sublingual medication that could give dysgeusia.

22.4.7 Lurasidone

Evidence about lurasidone-induced weight gain/obesity is not unique. In a meta-analysis by De Hert and colleagues [41], treatment with lurasidone was found not to induce statistically significant weight gain in patients with schizophrenia and bipolar disorder (six trials, $n = 1793$). However, short-term trials (five trials, $n = 999$) demonstrated a significant weight gain >7 % from baseline among patients treated with lurasidone compared to patients in the placebo group [42]. In a long-term, open-label extension trial in patients with schizophrenia or schizoaffective disorder, percentages of weight gain and weight loss differed considerably depending on the pre-switch agent. Significant weight loss (+/– 7 % from baseline) was more often seen than significant weight gain [43].

Lurasidone may be a possible option to treat David. However lurasidone is not well studied for the treatment of mania, as previous use has largely focused on the treatment of bipolar depression. Since there is little direct evidence, we will not be prescribing lurasidone at the present moment. It may be reconsidered in the future if David does not respond to other medication or if more evidence comes to light regarding its effectiveness for mania.

22.4.8 Aripiprazole

Aripiprazole has been associated with a relatively low risk of weight gain, dyslipidemia, and diabetes [44]. No difference in mean weight change between aripiprazole (0 kg) and placebo (–0.2 kg) were seen in four trials that were 3 weeks in duration [21]. In a randomized, double-blind, 26-week, placebo-controlled, maintenance study of aripiprazole treated patients with bipolar I disorder, the mean weight gain was 0.5 kg (SD = 0.8 kg), with a weight gain of 7 % or greater occurring in 13 % of patients. The difference between aripiprazole and placebo groups was not statistically significant. Also, no significant difference was seen between aripiprazole and placebo for median fasting glucose and cholesterol levels [45].

We decided to prescribe aripiprazole. The medication is started at 15 mg daily, as an adjunct to the ongoing valproate, which is increased to a dose of 2500 mg/day (previous blood level, at 2000 mg/day: 59 ug/mL). We have also instructed the patient to take lorazepam 1 mg in the morning and 2 mg at bedtime to alleviate anxiety and irritability.

The patient's symptoms significantly improve over time and lorazepam is gradually tapered off in the following weeks, up to complete discontinuation at week 5. Valproate is kept at 2500 mg/day (blood level 84 ug/mL) for 2 months and then decreased back to 2000 mg/day. Once remission is achieved, we will attempt a gradual switch from valproate to carbamazepine (CBZ), which is successfully completed over a period of 4 weeks. Given the pharmacokinetic interaction with CBZ (CYP3A4 inducer), aripiprazole dose is escalated to 30 mg/day. Additional treatment recommendations include the addition of psychotherapy to address psychosocial/psychoeducational issues. Also, we discussed the risks of impaired judgment during manic episodes and the risk that he will experience new manic episodes in the future. We have also advised him to consider safeguarding his assets to prevent future irreparable financial damage during manic episodes.

22.5 Metabolic Illness Monitoring and Treatment

David's metabolic illness is monitored in the following months. Indeed, we recommend that all individuals with psychiatric disorders be assessed at baseline for personal and family history of dyslipidemia, cardiovascular disease, and hyperglycemia. Baseline assessments should include waist circumference, weight, blood pressure, lipid panel, blood glucose, and thyroid function. Body weight, waist circumference, fasting serum lipids, glucose, and TSH should then be monitored at regularly scheduled intervals thereafter [44].

After consulting with his cardiologist, David is also invited to participate in a healthy lifestyle intervention, which includes psychoeducation, dietary consults, and motivational-behavioral interventions to avoid a sedentary lifestyle. The patient's metabolic condition gradually improves and his body weight decreases from 104 to 85 kg.

For patients who do not improve with an appropriate choice of psychiatric medications and education, dietary and exercise programs, consideration should be given to an appropriate pharmacological treatment of their metabolic illness with medications such as orlistat, lorcaserin, combination of phentermine and topiramate, combination of naltrexone and bupropion, or liraglutide.

22.5.1 Orlistat

Orlistat is a reversible inhibitor of gastrointestinal lipases indicated for obesity management including weight loss and weight maintenance when used in conjunction with a reduced-calorie diet. Orlistat is also indicated to reduce the risk for weight regain after prior weight loss [46]. The medication inhibits gastrointestinal lipases, thus lowering the absorption of dietary fat. However, orlistat may also decrease absorption of fat-soluble vitamins (A, D, E, and K) and certain concomitantly administered drugs in some individuals. Patients taking the drug should take a daily vitamin pill at bedtime to maximize absorption of the vitamins. Hilger and colleagues [47] monitored plasma levels of several psychotropic agents in eight psychiatric patients receiving orlistat to determine the potential influence of this medication on the bioavailability of these drugs. No clinically relevant changes in plasma concentrations of haloperidol, clozapine, clomipramine, desipramine, or carbamazepine were found over an 8-week period in orlistat recipients. Nonetheless, plasma level monitoring is recommended whenever possible. Orlistat was tested in obese or overweight adults with schizophrenia, with no concomitant hypocaloric diet or behavioral interventions. The medication caused moderate weight loss only in men. However, some subgroups showed favorable changes in several metabolic parameters. Prolonged (32 weeks) orlistat treatment yielded no additional benefits as compared to short (16 weeks) treatment [48]. Golay and colleagues [49] tested orlistat for the efficacy in obese patients with binge eating disorder and found that at 24 weeks, the mean weight loss from baseline for orlistat-treated patients was significantly greater than for patients receiving placebo (−7.4 % vs. −2.3 %; $p=0.01$). The most common side effects of orlistat include oily spotting, flatus with discharge, fecal urgency, fatty/oily stool, oily evacuation, increased defecation and fecal incontinence [46].

22.5.2 Lorcaserin

Lorcaserin is a selective serotonin 2C receptor agonist able to reduce appetite and food intake. Different from other serotonergic medications that had been previously used for weight loss, such as fenfluramine, this medication is a selective serotonin 2c receptor agonist and is less likely to cause cardiac valve disease. Lorcaserin is contraindicated in patients with renal failure. Concomitant use of lorcaserin with agents that possess or enhance serotonergic activity, such as selective serotonin reuptake inhibitors (SSRIs), selective serotonin-norepinephrine reuptake inhibitors (SNRIs), monoamine oxidase inhibitors (MAOIs), and tricyclic antidepressants (TCAs), 5-HT1 receptor agonists (triptans), may potentiate the risk of serotonin syndrome, which is a rare but serious and potentially fatal condition thought to result from hyperstimulation of brainstem 5-HT1A and 2A receptors. Although lorcaserin is primarily a serotonin 2C receptor agonist, the safety of concomitant use with other serotonergic agents has not been established.

Lorcaserin inhibits CYP450 2D6, thus increasing the plasma concentrations of drugs that are primarily metabolized by this enzyme complex, including many antidepressants (e.g., SSRIs, TCAs, trazodone). Lorcaserin is prescribed as a 10-mg tablet twice daily [50]. In one large randomized, double-blind placebo-controlled, parallel trial including 4008 obese patients, approximately half of the patients who took the drug for 12 months lost at least 5 % of their weight [51]. The most common side effects of lorcaserin are headache, dizziness, fatigue, nausea, dry mouth, and constipation.

22.5.3 Combined Treatment: Phentermine and Topiramate

A combination of phentermine (a sympathomimetic amine which acts as an appetite suppressant and stimulant) and extended-release topiramate (an anticonvulsant and antimigraine medication with the ability to induce weigh loss) was approved by the US Food and Drug Administration (FDA) in 2012. Approval was denied by European regulatory authorities, which cited potential risk to the heart and blood vessels, psychiatric side effects, and cognitive side effects in explaining their decision [52]. Among other issues, there were concerns about the long-term psychiatric effects (depression and anxiety were reported in studies) and cognitive effects (related to the topiramate component of the medication). In clinical trials, phentermine/topiramate was associated with modest yet statistically significant weight loss when compared with placebo [53]. Of note, the weight loss was associated with improvements in weight-related comorbidities such as improved glycemia, decreased blood pressure, and improved cholesterol. In clinical trials, the most common adverse events which occurred at a rate ≥5 % and ≥1.5 times placebo included paraesthesia, dizziness, dysgeusia, insomnia, constipation, and dry mouth. In the United States, the drug label contains warnings for increased heart rate, suicidal behavior and ideation, glaucoma, mood and sleep disorders, creatine elevation, and metabolic acidosis. Some of these warnings are based on historical observations in epilepsy patients taking topiramate. Because of the stimulant component, patients should not use this medication if they have uncontrolled high blood pressure or heart disease. Also, the medication may cause anxiety, agitation, and insomnia. Patients treated with this medication should be monitored for the emergence or worsening of depression, suicidal thoughts or behavior, and/or any unusual changes in mood or behavior. In fact, antiepileptic drugs (AEDs), including topiramate, a component of this medication, increase the risk of suicidal thoughts or behavior in patients taking these drugs for any indication. Because of a risk of fetal malformations, women of childbearing age should have a monthly pregnancy test while taking phentermine-topiramate [53].

22.5.4 Combined Treatment: Bupropion and Naltrexone

A combination of bupropion (an antidepressant and smoking cessation medication) and naltrexone (a medication for alcohol and opioid dependence) was approved by the FDA in September 2014 [54]. Both drugs have individually shown evidence of effectiveness in weight loss, and the combination is intended to have a synergistic effect [55]. Bupropion is a nicotinic acetylcholine receptor antagonist and a reuptake inhibitor and releasing agent of norepinephrine. Bupropion activates pro-opiomelanocortin (POMC) neurons in the hypothalamus, resulting in loss of appetite and increased energy output. Of interest, the POMC is regulated by endogenous opioids via opioid-mediated negative feedback. Naltrexone is instead a pure opioid antagonist, further augmenting bupropion's activation of the POMC [56]. The combination of bupropion and naltrexone has an effect on the reward pathway that results in reduced food craving [57]. Most common adverse events (greater than or equal to 5 %) include nausea, constipation, headache, vomiting, dizziness, insomnia, dry mouth, and diarrhea. The medication is contraindicated in subjects with uncontrolled hypertension, seizure disorders, anorexia nervosa or bulimia, subjects undergoing abrupt discontinuation of alcohol, benzodiazepines, barbiturates, and anticonvulsant drugs, subjects using other products containing bupropion, chronic opioid use, during or within 14 days of taking monoamine oxidase inhibitors (MAOI), and pregnant women. Most common adverse reactions (greater than or equal to 5 %): include nausea, constipation, headache, vomiting, dizziness, insomnia, dry mouth, and diarrhea [54]. The presence of an antidepressant (bupropion) indicates the need for caution in patients with mental illness. For instance, patients with bipolar disorder may switch to mania or develop mixed features, patients with schizophrenia may develop agitation, and patients with anxiety may develop an exacerbation of their symptoms. The risk of suicide may be also increased.

22.5.5 Liraglutide

Liraglutide is a compound that was previously approved for type 2 diabetes and has been recently approved as an anti-obesity agent in a higher dose, for patients with or without diabetes. Liraglutide is a glucagon-like peptide-1 (GLP-1) receptor agonist, which helps control blood sugar and also promotes weight loss and maintenance. A higher dose is used to treat obesity than to treat diabetes alone. In fact, the dose to treat obesity is 3.0 mg, in contrast to 1.2 mg or 1.8 mg for diabetes. The medication is available only as a once-daily injection. Most common adverse reactions, reported in greater than or equal to 5 % are: nausea, hypoglycemia, diarrhea, constipation, vomiting, headache, decreased appetite, dyspepsia, fatigue, dizziness, abdominal pain, and increased lipase. The efficacy and safety of liraglutide in patients with psychiatric conditions is yet to be demonstrated. Liraglutide was studied in three clinical trials of obese and overweight participants. However, patients who had a history of major depressive disorder or suicide attempt were excluded from these studies. In these clinical trials, 6 (0.2 %) of 3384 liraglutide- treated patients and none of the 1941 placebo-treated patients reported suicidal ideation; one of these liraglutide-treated patients attempted suicide. Liraglutide is contraindicated during pregnancy because it may cause fetal harm. This medication has a boxed warning stating that thyroid C-cell tumors have been seen in rodents but that the risk in humans is not known. However, liraglutide should not be used in patients with a personal or family history of medullary thyroid carcinoma (MTC) or in patients with multiple endocrine neoplasia syndrome type 2 [58].

22.6 Conclusions

Patients with psychiatric disorders are at a high risk for obesity and metabolic illnesses, and the treatments for their mental illness may significantly increase such a risk, leading to even greater mortality, morbidity, and disability. Therefore, new paradigms for the management of psychiatric disorders are required. It is paramount that health care professionals be aware that, when exposed to psychotropic medications, many patients gain significant weight and/or develop dyslipidemia, hyperglicemia, thyroid dysfunction, hyperprolactinemia, or other endocrine/metabolic conditions. Whenever possible, the development of weight gain and other metabolic illnesses should be *prevented* or minimized by choosing agents with a lower metabolic risk, both for acute and long-term treatments, as reported above in our clinical case.

Centrally, anti-obesity drugs modulate several neurochemical pathways involved in mood, cognition, sleep, anxiety, and suicidal ideation. Surprisingly, clinical studies explaining their effect on different mental illnesses are scarce. However, mental illness is often an exclusion criterion for the treatment of severe obesity with anti-obesity agents, and this may explain the lack of studies on this specific focus.

Educational and behavioral programs for healthier lifestyle, weight management or loss should be incorporated into a personalized treatment plan, and obesity should be considered a direct target for clinical intervention, rather than an indicator for lipid-modifying drug treatments.

Clearly, mental health professionals need to play an active role in patients' weight-maintenance and, when needed, weight loss efforts. A team working toward a patient's healthy weight, with at least a psychiatrist, psychotherapist, internist, dietician, and endocrinologist, is required.

22.7 Summary and Take Home Messages

- Psychiatric disorders and the subsequent use of psychotropic medications can both independently and in combination increase the risk of weight gain/obesity and the development of a metabolic diseases.
- Adequate assessment of psychiatric patients at baseline (medical history, metabolic risk factors, comorbidities, clinical history of relatives, body weight, waist circumference, BMI, lipid and glycemic evaluations) is necessary to detect risk factors for weight gain/obesity.
- Weight gain and subsequent obesity can be managed by choosing psychotropic medications with lower metabolic implications in patients with genetic, lifestyle, and environmental risk factors.
- It is necessary for health care providers to educate psychiatric patients and their caregivers about making healthy lifestyle choices (i.e., diet, exercise, and smoking cessation) in order to manage weight.
- When psychiatric patients require an anti-obesity agent, the costs and benefits of each medication should be considered, including the mechanism of action, the neurochemical pathways involved, as well as pharmacological interactions to avoid relapses and/or new psychiatric symptoms.

References

1. Reynolds GP, Zhang ZJ, Zhang XB. Association of antipsychotic drug-induced weight gain with a 5-HT2C receptor gene polymorphism. Lancet. 2002;359:2086–7.
2. Fagiolini A, Frank E, Scott JA, et al. Metabolic syndrome in bipolar disorder: findings from the Bipolar Disorder Center for Pennsylvanians. Bipolar Disord. 2005;7:424–30.
3. Fagiolini A, Kupfer DJ, Houck PR, et al. Obesity as a correlate of outcome in patients with bipolar I disorder. Am J Psychiatry. 2003;160:112–7.
4. Fagiolini A, Kupfer DJ, Rucci P, et al. Suicide attempts and ideation in patients with bipolar I disorder. J Clin Psychiatry. 2004;65:509–14.
5. Kupfer DJ. The increasing medical burden in bipolar disorder. JAMA. 2005;293:2528–30.
6. Gidal BE, Anderson GD, Spencer NW, et al. Valproate-associated weight gain: potential relation to energy expenditure and metabolism in patients with epilepsy. J Epilepsy. 1996;9:234–41.
7. Jallon P, Picard F. Bodyweight gain and anticonvulsants: a comparative review. Drug Saf. 2001;24:969–78.
8. Kwon O, Kim KW, Kim MS. Leptin signalling pathways in hypothalamic neurons. Cell Mol Life Sci. 2016;73(7):1457–77. Epub 19 Jan 2016.
9. Pylvänen V, Pakarinen A, Knip M, et al. Characterization of insulin secretion in valproate-treated patients with epilepsy. Epilepsia. 2006;47:1460–4.
10. Pylvänen V, Pakarinen A, Knip M, et al. Insulin-related metabolic changes during treatment with valproate in patients with epilepsy. Epilepsy Behav. 2006;8:643–8.
11. McIntyre RS, Mancini DA, McCann S, Srinivasan J, Kennedy SM. Valproate, bipolar disorder and polycystic ovarian syndrome. Bipolar Disord. 2003;5(1):28–35.
12. Ketter TA, Kalali AH, Weisler RH, et al. A 6-month, multicenter, open-label evaluation of beaded extended-release carbamazepine capsule monotherapy in bipolar disorder patients with manic or mixed episodes. J Clin Psychiatry. 2004;65:668–73.
13. Brämswig S, Kerksiek A, Sudhop T. Carbamazepine increases atherogenic lipoproteins: mechanism of action in male adults. Am J Physiol Heart Circ Physiol. 2002;282:H704–16.
14. Kondo T, Otani K, Hirano T, et al. The effects of phenytoin and carbamazepine on serum concentrations of mono-unsaturated metabolites of valproic acid. Br J Clin Pharmacol. 1990;29:116–9.
15. Goodwin FK. Rationale for long-term treatment of bipolar disorder and evidence for long-term lithium treatment. J Clin Psychiatry. 2002;63 Suppl 10:5–12.
16. Aronne LJ, Segal KR. Weight gain in the treatment of mood disorders. J Clin Psychiatry. 2003;64 Suppl 8:22–9.
17. Baptista T, Teneud L, Contreras Q, et al. Lithium and body weight gain. Pharmacopsychiatry. 1995;28:35–44.
18. Chengappa KN, Chalasani L, Brar JS, et al. Changes in body weight and body mass index among psychiatric patients receiving lithium, valproate, or topiramate: an open-label, nonrandomized chart review. Clin Ther. 2002;24:1576–84.
19. Mellerup ET, Grondlund Thompson H, Bjorum N, et al. Lithium, weight gain and serum insulin in

manic-depressive patients. Acta Psychiatr Scand. 1972;48:332–6.
20. Birnbaumer L, Pohl SL, Rodbell M. Adenyl cyclase in fat cells. 1. Properties and the effects of adrenocorticotropin and fluoride. J Biol Chem. 1969;244: 3468–76.
21. Fagiolini A, Chengappa KN. Weight gain and metabolic issues of medicines used for bipolar disorder. Curr Psychiatry Rep. 2007;9(6):521–8.
22. Scherk H, Pajonk FG, Leucht S. Second-generation antipsychotic agents in the treatment of acute mania: a systematic review and meta-analysis of randomized controlled trials. Arch Gen Psychiatry. 2007;64(4): 442–55.
23. Correll CU, Leucht D, Kane JM. Lower risk for tardive dyskinesia associated with second-generation antipsychotics: a systematic review of 1-year studies. Am J Psychiatry. 2004;161:414–25.
24. Esparon J, Kolloori J, Naylor GJ, McHarg AM, Smith AH, Hopwood SE. Comparison of the prophylactic action of flupenthixol with placebo in lithium treated manic-depressive patients. Br J Psychiatry. 1986;148: 723–5.
25. Cavazzoni PA, Berg PH, Kryzhanovskaya LA, Briggs SD, Roddy TE, Tohen M, Kane JM. Comparison of treatment-emergent extrapyramidal symptoms in patients with bipolar mania or schizophrenia during olanzapine clinical trials. J Clin Psychiatry. 2006;67: 107–13.
26. Mukherjee S, Rosen AM, Caracci G, Shukla S. Persistent tardive dyskinesia in bipolar patients. Arch Gen Psychiatry. 1986;43:342–6.
27. Masand PS. Relative weight gain among antipsychotics. J Clin Psychiatry. 2001;60:706–8.
28. Tohen M, Jacobs TG, Grundy SL, et al. Efficacy of olanzapine in acute bipolar mania: a double-blind, placebo-controlled study. The Olanzipine HGGW Study Group. Arch Gen Psychiatry. 2000;57:841–9.
29. Sanger TM, Grundy SL, Gibson PJ, Namjoshi MA, Greaney MG, Tohen MF. Long-term olanzapine therapy in the treatment of bipolar I disorder: an open-label continuation phase study. J Clin Psychiatry. 2001;62:273–81.
30. Koro CE, Fedder DO, L'Italien GJ, et al. An assessment of the independent effects of olanzapine and risperidone exposure on the risk of hyperlipidemia in schizophrenic patients. Arch Gen Psychiatry. 2002;59:1021–6.
31. Koller EA, Doraiswamy PM. Olanzapine-associated diabetes mellitus. Pharmacotherapy. 2002;22:841–52.
32. Melkersson KI, Dahl ML. Relationship between levels of insulin or triglycerides and serum concentrations of the atypical antipsychotics clozapine and olanzapine in patients on treatment with therapeutic doses. Psychopharmacology (Berl). 2003;170:157–66.
33. Bushe CJ, Slooff CJ, Haddad PM, Karagianis JL. Weight change from 3-year observational data: findings from the worldwide schizophrenia outpatient health outcomes database. J Clin Psychiatry. 2012;73(6):e749–55.
34. Schneider C, Corrigall R, Hayes D, et al. Systematic review of the efficacy and tolerability of Clozapine in the treatment of youth with early onset schizophrenia. Eur Psychiatry. 2014;29(1):1–10.
35. Potkin SG, Saha AR, Kukawa MJ, et al. Aripiprazole, an antipsychotic with a novel mechanism of action, and risperidone vs placebo in patients with schizophrenia and schizoaffective disorder. Arch Gen Psychiatry. 2003;60:681–90.
36. Brecher M, Leong RW, Stening G, Osterling-Koskinen L, Jones AM. Quetiapine and long-term weight change: a comprehensive data review of patients with schizophrenia. J Clin Psychiatry. 2007;68(4):597–603.
37. Lieberman JA, Stroup ST, McEvoy JP, et al. Effectiveness of antipsychotic drugs in patients with chronic schizophrenia. N Engl J Med. 2005;353:1209–23.
38. Weiden PJ, Simpson GM, Potkin SG, et al. Effectiveness of switching to ziprasidone for stable but symptomatic outpatients with schizophrenia. J Clin Psychiatry. 2003;64:580–8.
39. Strom BL, Eng SM, Faich G, Reynolds RF, D'Agostino RB, Ruskin J, Kane JM. Comparative mortality associated with ziprasidone and olanzapine in real-world use among 18,154 patients with schizophrenia: the Ziprasidone Observational Study of Cardiac Outcomes (ZODIAC). Am J Psychiatry. 2011;168(2):193–201.
40. Leucht S, Cipriani A, Spineli L, Mavridis D, Orey D, Richter F, Samara M, Barbui C, Engel RR, Geddes JR, Kissling W, Stapf MP, Lässig B, Salanti G, Davis JM. Comparative efficacy and tolerability of 15 antipsychotic drugs in schizophrenia: a multiple-treatments meta-analysis. Lancet. 2013;382(9896):951–62.
41. De Hert M, Yu W, Detraux J, et al. Body weight and metabolic adverse effects of asenapine, iloperidone, lurasidone and paliperidone in the treatment of schizophrenia and bipolar disorder: a systematic review and exploratory meta-analysis. CNS Drugs. 2012;26(9):733–59.
42. Spielmans GI, Berman MI, Linardatos E, et al. Adjunctive atypical antipsychotic treatment for major depressive disorder: a meta-analysis of depression, quality of life, and safety outcomes. PLoS Med. 2013;10(3):e1001403.
43. Citrome L, Weiden PJ, McEvoy JP, et al. Effectiveness of lurasidone in schizophrenia or schizoaffective patients switched from other antipsychotics: a 6-month, open-label, extension study. CNS Spectr. 2013;19:1–10.
44. American Diabetes Association, American Psychiatric Association, American Association of Clinical Endocrinologists, North American Association for the Study of Obesity. Consensus development conference on antipsychotic drugs and obesity and diabetes. Diabetes Care. 2004;27:596–601.
45. Keck Jr PE, Calabrese JR, McQuade RD, et al. A placebo-controlled 26-week trial of aripiprazole in recently manic patients with bipolar I disorder. J Clin Psychiatry. 2006;67:626–37.

46. Orlistat—FDA Xenical prescribing information. http://www.gene.com/download/pdf/xenical_prescribing.pdf. Accessed 24 Apr 2016.
47. Hilger E, Quiner S, Ginzel I, Walter H, Saria L, Barnas C. The effect of orlistat on plasma levels of psychotropic drugs in patients with long-term psychopharmacotherapy. J Clin Psychopharmacol. 2002;22(1):68–70.
48. Tchoukhine E, Takala P, Hakko H, Raidma M, Putkonen H, Räsänen P, Terevnikov V, Stenberg JH, Eronen M, Joffe G. Orlistat in clozapine- or olanzapine-treated patients with overweight or obesity: a 16-week open-label extension phase and both phases of a randomized controlled trial. J Clin Psychiatry. 2011;72(3):326–30.
49. Golay A, Laurent-Jaccard A, Habicht F, Gachoud JP, Chabloz M, Kammer A, Schutz Y. Effect of orlistat in obese patients with binge eating disorder. Obes Res. 2005;13(10):1701–8.
50. Chan EW, He Y, Chui CS, Wong AY, Lau WC, Wong IC. Efficacy and safety of lorcaserin in obese adults: a meta-analysis of 1-year randomized controlled trials (RCTs) and narrative review on short-term RCTs. Obes Rev. 2013;14(5):383–92.
51. Fidler MC, Sanchez M, Raether B, et al. A one-year randomized trial of lorcaserin for weight loss in obese and overweight adults: the BLOSSOM trial. J Clin Endocrinol Metab. 2011;96(10):3067–77.
52. European Medicines Agency. Refusal of the marketing authorisation for Qsiva (phentermine/topiramate). http://www.ema.europa.eu/docs/en_GB/document_library/Summary_of_opinion_-_Initial_authorisation/human/002350/WC500139215.pdf. Accessed 24 Apr 2016.
53. Phentermine and topiramate extended-release—QSYMIA FDA prescribing information. https://qsymia.com/pdf/prescribing-information.pdf. Accessed 24 Apr 2016.
54. Naltrexone-Buproprion—Contrave FDA prescribing information. http://general.takedapharm.com/content/file.aspx?filetypecode=CONTRAVEPI&cacheRandomizer=53f72244-55c9-405a-845d-07e7526280f0. Accessed 24 April 2016.
55. Sinnayah P, Wallingford N, Evans A, Crowley MA. Bupropion and naltrexone interact synergistically to decrease food intake in mice. Obesity. 2007;15(9):A179.
56. Greenway F, Whitehouse MJ, Guttadauria M, Anderson J. Rational design of a combination medication for the treatment of obesity. Obesity. 2007;17:30–9.
57. Apovian C, Aronne L, Rubino L, Still C. A randomized, phase 3 trial of naltrexone SR/bupropion SR on weight and obesity-related risk factors (COR-II). Obesity. 2013;21:935–43.
58. Liraglutide—Saxenda prescribing information. http://www.novo-pi.com/saxenda.pdf. Accessed 24 Apr 2016.
59. Vestergaard P, Amdisen A, Schou M. Clinically significant side effects of lithium treatment. A survey of 237 patients in long-term treatment. Acta Psychiatr Scand. 1980;62:193–200.

Psychopharmacology in Bariatric Surgery Patients

23

Kathleen S. Bingham and Richard Yanofsky

23.1 Introduction

Bariatric surgery patients have a high degree of psychiatric comorbidity, with the prevalence of any DSM-IV defined Axis I disorder approaching 40 % [1]. Antidepressant medications are the most commonly used psychotropic medication in this population by far: 35 % of patients in a large, multisite cohort ($n = 2146$) were found to be taking at least one antidepressant medication on a daily basis [2]. However, bariatric surgery is projected to become more widespread and accessible in the coming years, and therefore more likely to include persons with severe mood and psychotic disorders [3]. This factor, coupled with the expanding indication list for various psychotropic medication classes (particularly second-generation antipsychotics), means that clinicians working in the bariatric surgery field must be familiar with a variety of psychopharmacological management issues in this population.

In the following chapter, we describe pharmacological alterations associated with bariatric surgery, and suggest management strategies to address clinically relevant issues. We begin with an illustrative case of a bariatric surgery candidate who is taking several psychiatric medications. Next, we briefly review the pharmacokinetic steps, and discuss the impact of bariatric surgery on each of these steps, paying particular attention to medication absorption. We will then discuss various medication formulation options before moving on to the bulk of the chapter: a review of the effect of bariatric surgery on the major classes of psychiatric medications and management suggestions for each.

Case Vignette

Ms. P is a 42-year-old woman presenting to the bariatric surgery clinic for consideration of gastric bypass surgery. She is seen by the psychiatrist in consultation. Ms. P's BMI is 37 kg/m^2 and she has several obesity-related medical conditions, including hypertension, dyslipidemia, and gastroesophageal reflux disease. Her psychiatric history is notable for bipolar II disorder, with onset in her early 20s and three previous hypomanic episodes (ages 22, 28, and 35). She has had multiple previous depressive episodes, the

(continued)

K.S. Bingham
University Health Network,
399 Bathurst Street, Toronto, ON, Canada M5T 2S8
e-mail: Kathleen.bingham@mail.utorono.ca

R. Yanofsky (✉)
Toronto Western Hospital Bariatric Surgery Program,
University Health Network, Toronto, ON, Canada

Department of Psychiatry, University of Toronto,
Toronto, ON, Canada
e-mail: richard.yanofsky@uhn.ca

S. Sockalingam, R. Hawa (eds.), *Psychiatric Care in Severe Obesity*,
DOI 10.1007/978-3-319-42536-8_23

(continued)

most recent being 2 years ago, and two previous suicide attempts (ages 25 and 40), both resulting in psychiatric hospitalizations. Ms. P was also diagnosed with panic disorder at age 18, but these symptoms have been well controlled by paroxetine since that time. Overall, her mood has been stable since the initiation of her current medication regimen 2 years ago. Her medications include lithium 1200 mg once daily at bedtime (typical serum level 0.7), quetiapine XR 300 mg once daily at bedtime, paroxetine 20 mg once daily, lorazepam 1 mg once daily at bedtime as needed, atorvastatin 20 mg once daily at bedtime, and amlodipine 5 mg once daily.

Questions for the psychiatrist to consider:

- How will gastric bypass impact Ms. P's medication absorption?
- Should any of the medications be adjusted preoperatively?
- Are there any early signs of decreased medication absorption for which the psychiatrist should monitor?
- How will gastric bypass surgery impact lithium serum levels?
- How frequently should lithium levels be monitored in the perioperative period?

23.2 Pharmacokinetic Changes Following Bariatric Surgery

Bariatric surgery procedures all involve some element of restriction of the capacity of the digestive system, reduction of the digestive system's ability to absorb nutrients (via intestinal diversion), or a combination of both restrictive and malabsorptive elements. Examples of each category of procedure include the following: gastric banding and gastric sleeve (predominantly restrictive), biliopancreatic diversion and jejunoileal bypass (predominantly malabsorptive), and gastric bypass (mixed restrictive/malabsorptive).

Gastric bypass, specifically roux-en-Y gastric bypass (RYGB), and sleeve gastrectomy are the two most commonly performed bariatric surgery procedures in the United States as of the time of writing [3]. All bariatric surgery procedures can theoretically impact drug absorption since they all change gastrointestinal (GI) function to some degree. However, despite the emerging popularity of the gastric sleeve procedure in recent years [3], the literature regarding psychopharmacology after bariatric surgery is primarily focused on RYGB. This emphasis is likely due to RYGB's historical predominance, combined with its potential to significantly impact drug absorption via its potent effect on GI structure and function. Therefore, this chapter will largely refer to RYGB patients, but management strategies for RYGB may be generally applied to all bariatric surgery patients.

The pharmacology branch of pharmacokinetics refers to the effect of the body on an externally administered substance. It is generally understood to encompass the following steps: (1) absorption of the substance into the blood circulation; (2) distribution of the substance throughout the body tissues and fluids; (3) the body's metabolism of the substance into modified (usually more readily excreted) products, typically via enzymatic systems in the liver; and (4) excretion, whereby the substance is removed from the body [4]. The impact of bariatric surgery on the various pharmacokinetic steps is discussed below.

23.2.1 Absorption

Although bariatric surgery can theoretically impact all of the pharmacokinetic steps outlined above, its primary effects are on drug absorption. Numerous studies involving various procedures and medications have demonstrated evidence of reduced drug absorption post-bariatric surgery [5]. In a systematic review, Padwal et al. (2010) describe the steps involved in drug absorption and the theoretical impact that bariatric surgery has on these steps [5]. Firstly, in order for a drug to be absorbed into systemic circulation, it has to disintegrate and dissolve in the stomach, actions that can be affected by changes in gastric pH and gastric mixing following restrictive bariatric surgeries. Next, the drug has to be emptied out of the stomach and into the small intestine, a process that is also often altered after surgeries involving gastric restriction, and which impacts the rate of drug absorption. Most drug absorption occurs in the small intestine, where substances are exposed to the intestinal mucosa and transported across the epithelium, via passive diffusion or active transport, into the portal circulation. Thus, diversionary bariatric procedures (e.g., RYGB, jejunoileal bypass, biliopancreatic diversion) have the potential to profoundly impact drug absorption since they reduce functional gastrointestinal length significantly. Procedures that bypass the proximal small intestine can affect lipophilic drugs in particular, since these medications may require bile acid mixing in the small intestine to increase solubility. Lipophilic drugs are also often dependent upon enterohepatic recirculation to enhance absorption, a phenomenon that is limited by bypass of the proximal intestine. Furthermore, some drugs undergo metabolism within the intestinal wall, a factor that influences absorption and, along with drug efflux, may vary across the length of the intestine under normal circumstances. Therefore, it is theoretically possible that different types of malabsorptive procedures involving different portions of the intestine may produce variable changes in drug absorption, though this effect has not been studied. Figure 23.1 outlines the steps involved in oral drug absorption and the differential impact of various types of bariatric surgery procedures on these steps.

23.2.2 Distribution

Drug distribution, the process by which drugs enter the body's interstitial and intracellular fluids, can be influenced by any physiological factor

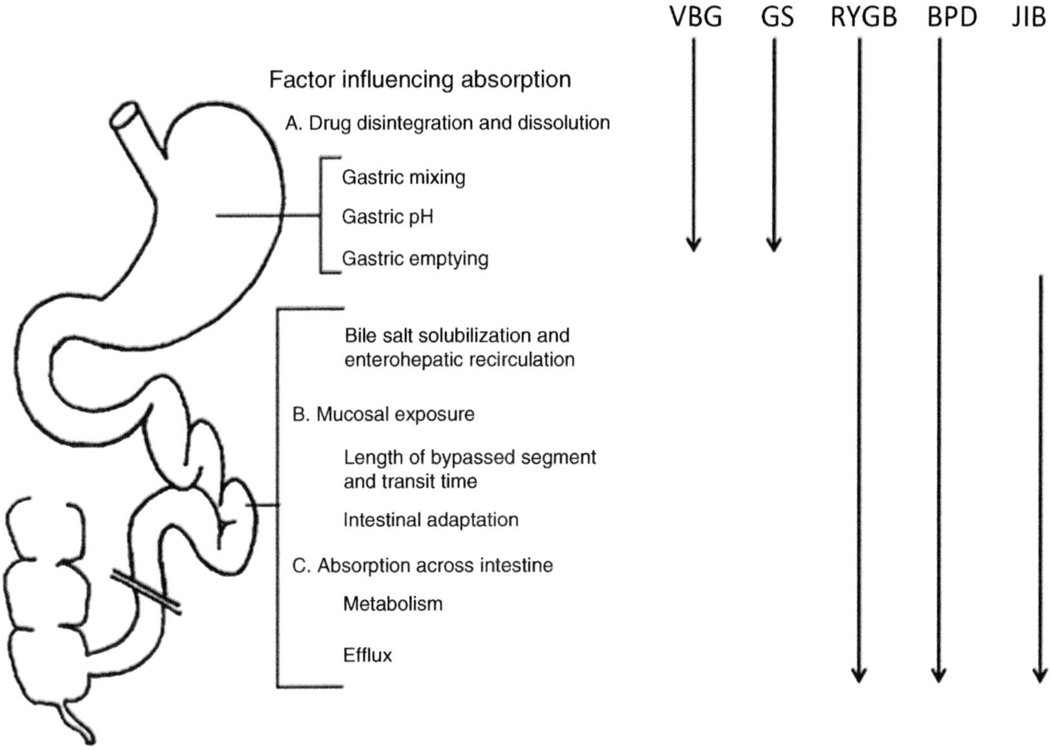

Fig. 23.1 Summary of the theoretical effect of various bariatric procedures on factors influencing drug absorption. The factors influencing drug absorption are shown in the *center*. For each factor, the major site gastrointestinal site involved is indicated on the *left*. The major types of bariatric surgery are listed on the *right*. The *arrows* summarize the potential spectrum of influence for each type of bariatric procedure. *VBG* vertical banded gastroplasty, *GS* gastric sleeve, *RYGB* Roux-en-Y gastric bypass, *BPD* biliopancreatic diversion, *JIB* jejunoileal bypass. Figure modified, with permission, from Padwal et al., 2010 [5]

that affects vascular volume, plasma protein binding, tissue volume, or tissue binding [6]. Several obesity-related physiologic changes, such as increased blood volume [7] and increased cardiac output [8], can influence drug distribution, and higher total body weight generally increases drug distribution [6]. Furthermore, obesity and weight loss result in altered blood concentrations of drug-binding proteins, such as lipoproteins, alpha acid glycoprotein, and (less commonly) albumin, thus changing a drug's plasma protein binding, and therefore its distribution [9]. Generally, lipid-soluble drugs have higher volumes of distribution (a measure that is correlated with the amount of a drug stored in body tissue vs. plasma), and are therefore more likely to be influenced by obesity and substantial changes in body weight than are water-soluble drugs [6]. The clinical effect of changes in drug distribution with significant weight loss (such as the type of weight loss seen after bariatric surgery) depends on the properties of the individual medication, but could include issues such as increased adverse effects and toxicity.

23.2.3 Metabolism and Excretion

Metabolism and excretion are the steps whereby drugs are processed and cleared from the body. The majority of drug metabolism occurs in the liver, primarily via phase I (modification; includes the actions of the cytochrome P450 system) and/or phase II (conjugation) reactions [4]. Drugs are then excreted via the urine, bile, feces, and other bodily fluids. Although theoretical, changes in hepatic function associated with significant weight loss, along with improvement in common obesity-associated conditions such as nonalcoholic fatty liver disease, may impact drug metabolism and excretion [3]. The clinical effect of these changes would hypothetically be an improvement in drug metabolism, and therefore the emergence of adverse effects associated with a patient's typical dose. Obesity and weight loss can also be associated with changes in renal drug clearance [6], a factor that would also affect the levels of renally excreted medications.

23.2.4 Summary

Bariatric surgery has the potential to affect all pharmacokinetic steps, though drug absorption is the parameter that has been most studied and is hypothetically most likely to be impacted, given that many procedures are malabsorptive by nature, and all involve substantial changes to the anatomy and function of the gastrointestinal system. However, pharmacokinetic changes post-bariatric surgery may be difficult to predict given the complex interplay of medication, patient, and surgical factors. More definitive and systematic research in this area is needed in order to fully understand the scope of the issue.

23.3 Medication Formulations

Because we recommend the use of various medication formulations in the management of bariatric surgery patients, in this section we describe the formulations discussed in the text and the particulars of their use in this population. Specifically, we refer to controlled release, orodispersible and liquid formulations. Readers should note that the availability of various medication formulations differs internationally.

In the context of oral medications, "controlled release," and its various synonyms, such as "extended" and "sustained" release, refers to capsules and tablets that are modified using technology to alter the rate or timing of drug delivery. This mechanism is in contrast to conventional pills and tablets, which release the drug immediately upon oral administration (i.e., "immediate release" formulations) [10]. Pharmaceutical companies have developed a number of mechanisms to achieve controlled release, e.g., enteric coating, the use of coated beads/granules within a capsule, and the use of outer semipermeable membranes. Controlled release medications are designed to achieve a therapeutic objective, such as reduced side effect burden, or to enhance patient adherence by minimizing the need for divided dosing. However, any medication formulation that prolongs drug disintegration and dissolution has the potential to impede absorption following bariatric surgery [5]. Therefore, although data regarding the use of controlled release medications after bariatric surgery is very limited, clinicians commonly convert these medications to their immediate release formulations prior to surgery [3]. We currently suggest this strategy based on expert clinical recommendation [5, 6]. Not all controlled release medications come in an immediate release formulation. If switching formulations is not an option, we recommend consulting with pharmacy colleagues regarding other potential modifications to controlled release medications that may improve dissolution and disintegration (e.g., opening and sprinkling capsules, crushing tablets). If controlled release medications cannot be modified, a clinical decision must be made to switch to a different medication or to continue the same medication with close monitoring after bariatric surgery.

Medication tablets may also be modified by drug manufacturers so that they are orodispersible, or orally disintegrating. Such tablets disintegrate and, at least partially, dissolve in the mouth. One benefit of this formulation is that tablets can be taken without water, and it overcomes issues such as dysphagia and trouble swallowing pills. However, it must be noted that not all orally disintegrating tablets are absorbed via the oral mucosa (a characteristic that would clearly benefit bariatric surgery patients). Depending on the particular pharmacological properties of the drug, some medications travel to the gastrointestinal system after disintegration and dissolution in the mouth, whereby they are absorbed across the small intestine like conventional oral tablets. Therefore, while orally disintegrating tablets that are absorbed in the GI system may still optimize absorption by enhancing disintegration and dissolution (often altered in the bariatric surgery gastrointestinal environment), many still require a functioning GI system to enter systemic circulation. We suggest that clinicians consult pharmacy colleagues or check product monographs when uncertain about the route of absorption of orally disintegrating tablets.

Lastly, a number of psychiatric medications are available in liquid formulations. Again, this formulation may enhance absorption in bariatric surgery patients, since liquid medications do not have to be disintegrated and dissolved in the GI tract the way pills do. Liquid formulations are therefore an option for patients exhibiting signs of reduced medication absorption while taking solid pills.

23.4 Antidepressants

23.4.1 Evidence

Like most oral medications, antidepressants are maximally absorbed in the small intestine and therefore have the potential to be significantly impacted by malabsorptive bariatric procedures. In addition, they are lipophilic and generally highly protein bound, meaning that they are hypothetically vulnerable to the changes in volume of distribution and concentration of drug-binding proteins that accompany rapid weight loss [6, 11].

Although the literature is far from robust, antidepressants are the best-studied psychotropic medication in the bariatric population. At the time of writing, there have been four small pharmacokinetic studies evaluating the effect of RYGB on antidepressant levels [12–15]. Two cross-sectional studies compared the area under the plasma concentration time curve (AUC; a measure of the medication's bioavailability) between patients who were 1-year post-RYGB and age-, sex-, and body mass index-matched control subjects who had not undergone bariatric surgery [14, 15]. In one study, all participants ($n=5$ RYGB subjects and five controls) were given a single dose of sertraline 100 mg [15], and in the other study, participants ($n=10$ subjects per group) were given a single dose of duloxetine 60 mg [14]. Serial plasma medication levels were collected following medication administration in both studies. For both sertraline and duloxetine, the post-RYGB group demonstrated a significantly and substantially lower mean AUC compared to the nonsurgical control group, suggesting lower bioavailability of these medications 1 year post-RYGB surgery. However, since this data is from a cross-sectional study in a nonclinical sample, it does not provide evidence as to the effect of bariatric surgery on antidepressant bioavailability in patients taking the medication on a daily basis over time.

In a case series following 12 RYGB patients taking venlafaxine ($n=5$), citalopram ($n=2$), duloxetine ($n=1$), escitalopram ($n=2$), and sertraline ($n=2$), Hamad et al. (2012) evaluated AUC at preoperative baseline, and 1, 6, and 12 months post-surgery [13]. Eight of the 12 patients experienced a significant drop in AUC at the 1-month time point (range 36–80 %), though this decrease was only significant for the sample as a whole and the SSRI group. AUC returned to baseline (or increased) for the majority of patients by 6 months, although three patients did not return to their baseline levels by 1 year. The authors postulated that the improved bioavailability at 6 months was due to the adaptive increase in the absorptive component of the intestinal mucosa that occurs postoperatively. From a clinical perspective, four patients experienced a relapse of their depression postoperatively, and improvement in their symptoms correlated with a return to baseline antidepressant bioavailability. Data from a case series involving four RYGB patients supported the evidence of decreased escitalopram absorption post-RYGB initially identified by Hamad et al. (2012): escitalopram plasma concentrations decreased by 4–71 % compared to baseline 2 weeks post-surgery and by a further 16–19 % by 6 weeks in this study [12].

All pharmacokinetic studies on antidepressant use in bariatric surgery patients have involved SSRIs and SNRIs. Thus, there is almost no evidence regarding the effect of bariatric surgery on patients taking other classes of antidepressant medication. An in vitro study comparing drug dissolution between a simulated RYGB GI tract and a control environment found that amitriptyline dissolved significantly less in the RYGB vs. the control model, and that immediate release bupropion dissolved more [16]. Of interest, fluoxetine, paroxetine, and sertraline were found to dissolve significantly less in the RYGB model and citalopram and venlafaxine were found to dissolve equally in both models. Although one cannot extrapolate as to the real world, clinical impact of these in vitro findings, they demonstrate the potential inter-drug variability of pharmacokinetic changes post-bariatric surgery.

Overall, although sample sizes have been small, all studies in this area have demonstrated evidence of reduced antidepressant bioavailability post-RYGB. Therefore, clinicians working with bariatric surgery patients taking antidepressants must be alert for signs and symptoms of reduced antidepressant absorption. Management strategies are discussed in the section below.

23.4.2 Management

Since we are unable to predict which patients are at highest risk of experiencing the clinical effects of reduced antidepressant absorption postoperatively, we do not recommend routinely increasing antidepressant doses preoperatively. Rather, all bariatric surgery patients on antidepressant medication should be monitored postoperatively for changes in mental status, and patients should be counseled to self-monitor for mental status changes [13]. A potential early symptom of reduced antidepressant bioavailability is the antidepressant discontinuation syndrome: the cluster of neurological, emotional, and somatic phenomena associated with abrupt antidepressant discontinuation or dose reduction [17]. Common symptoms would typically appear in the first few days postoperatively, and include dizziness, vertiginous sensations, gait incoordination, nausea, headache, fatigue, insomnia, anxiety, and irritability [17]. Discontinuation symptoms must be differentiated from relapse of the primary psychiatric disorder, which would typically happen over a period of months [18]. Bingham et al. (2014) report on a case of severe antidepressant discontinuation syndrome post-RYGB, and describe the management strategies that were helpful for this patient, namely increasing and dividing the medication dose [19].

Management strategies for patients demonstrating evidence of reduced antidepressant absorption (e.g., discontinuation symptoms or worsening psychiatric symptoms) include increasing the medication dose, dividing the dose (smaller amounts dissolve, and are therefore absorbed, more easily), crushing pills if feasible, and switching to a liquid or orally disintegrating formulation if available. These strategies may be implemented in a stepwise manner, depending on the clinical situation and patient preference.

As discussed in the section above (*Medication Formulations*), any controlled release antidepressant medication should be switched to its immediate release formulation prior to surgery. If an immediate release formulation is not available, some controlled release tablets may be crushed and some capsules may be opened and sprinkled, but, as previously mentioned, we suggest consulting with pharmacy colleagues prior to making these recommendations. Depending on the clinical situation, some patients on controlled release antidepressants may benefit from switching preoperatively to another type of antidepressant with an available immediate release or liquid formulation.

Of note, Hamad et al. found that antidepressant bioavailability normalized or increased for some patients in their small sample by 6 months post-surgery [13]. For this reason, clinicians and patients should be aware of the potential emergence of antidepressant adverse effects starting several months postoperatively, particularly in patients whose antidepressant doses were increased from baseline in the postoperative period to address signs of reduced absorption.

We suggest using rating scales to systematically monitor symptoms in perioperative patients with a history of anxiety or depression. This strategy provides longitudinal data and allows for early identification of symptom recurrence. The Patient Health Questionnaire-9 (PHQ-9) [20] is an example of such a rating scale, and has been validated as a depression-screening tool in the bariatric population [21].

In terms of laboratory monitoring, while most antidepressants do not have established therapeutic ranges, some of the tricyclic antidepressants do, and these may be used for monitoring drug levels. We suggest obtaining baseline preoperative levels as well as levels at regular intervals over the first year postoperatively, after which point patients may return to routine monitoring, provided they are stable.

Given the potential for persistent absorption changes for at least 6–12 months postoperatively [13], along with the potentially latent effects of reduced medication absorption, patients on antidepressant medication require enhanced monitoring for complications of pharmacokinetic changes, including antidepressant discontinuation syndrome, worsening of their primary psychiatric disorder, and antidepressant adverse effects, over the course of at least the first postoperative year.

23.5 Mood Stabilizers

The literature addressing mood stabilizers in bariatric surgery patients is limited to a small number of case reports. However, given the comorbidity between obesity and mood disorders [22], in conjunction with the increasing accessibility of bariatric surgery, this is a topic that deserves attention.

23.5.1 Lithium

Due to its narrow therapeutic index, lithium is the mood stabilizer that presents the greatest management challenge in the perioperative period. In terms of pharmacokinetics, lithium is readily and completely absorbed in the small intestine. It is hydrophilic and nonprotein bound, is not metabolized, and is almost completely renally excreted. These characteristics mean that it is particularly vulnerable to fluid shifts, a significant concern in the postoperative period. Serum levels between 0.6 and 1.2 mmol/L are considered therapeutic for bipolar disorder treatment, and levels above 1.5 mmol/L are toxic. Lithium dissolution was shown to be higher in an in vitro RYGB model [16], and there are several case reports describing lithium toxicity following RYGB [23–25].

Although toxicity is the immediate concern for patients on lithium undergoing bariatric surgery, subtherapeutic levels can also have devastating consequences for patients with severe mood disorders. Given the unpredictability of absorption and other pharmacokinetic changes associated with bariatric surgery and significant weight loss, clinicians should be prepared to manage both subtherapeutic and elevated lithium levels. Furthermore, not only can lithium levels be affected following bariatric surgery, they can be altered in the preoperative phase, where many patients are prescribed a liquid diet in order to lose weight and reduce the risk of surgical complications. Liquid meal replacement may alter patients' usual fluid and salt intake, which, in turn, may impact lithium levels.

For these reasons, bariatric surgery patients on lithium require particularly close monitoring throughout the perioperative period. Patients and health care providers should be carefully educated about adequate fluid intake and symptoms of lithium toxicity, and patients should be advised to seek medical attention at the first sign of any of these symptoms, or if they are not tolerating oral intake. Conversely, if a patient is experiencing subtherapeutic lithium levels in the postoperative period, physicians may try the management strategies suggested for reduced antidepressant absorption, such as increasing and dividing the doses or switching to lithium citrate syrup (available in some regions). Considering the complexities associated with caring for bariatric surgery patients on lithium, the psychiatrists at the Toronto Western Hospital Bariatric Surgery Psychosocial program created a protocol to guide management (see Table 23.1). The protocol provides suggestions for fluid intake, frequency of lithium monitoring, and additional education for clinicians managing bariatric surgery patients on lithium.

23.5.2 Valproic Acid and Other Anticonvulsants

Valproic acid (VPA) is rapidly and completely absorbed in the GI tract, though absorption can be delayed if taken with food [28]. It is highly protein bound, mainly to albumin. It comes in various forms, including as VPA, itself, the salt

Table 23.1 Perioperative bariatric surgery lithium protocol

Bariatric surgery perioperative phase	Recommendations
Presurgery: while taking liquid meal replacement[a]	• Weekly lithium levels
	• Educate patient to drink 2.5–3 L per day (includes liquid meal replacement)
	• Consider lithium dose decrease if lithium levels *approach* 1.2 mmol/L or increase by >25 % from baseline
	• Hold and reassess dose if signs of lithium toxicity
	• Monitor depressive or manic symptoms (consider using standardized scales[b])
Post-surgery: 0–6 weeks post-surgery	• Weekly lithium levels as fluid intake will increase gradually over initial months post-surgery[c]
	• Ask about food intolerance and vomiting as it can impact fluid intake
	• Consider lithium dose decrease if lithium levels *approach* 1.2 mmol/L or increase by >25 % from baseline
	• Hold and reassess dose if signs of lithium toxicity
	• Monitor depressive or manic symptoms (consider standardized scales)
Post-surgery: >6 weeks post-surgery	• Monitor lithium levels q2weeks *until 6 months post-surgery* and then proceed to monthly lithium levels until 1 year post-surgery
	• Ask about food intolerance and vomiting as it can impact fluid intake
	• *After 1 year post-surgery*, resume routine lithium monitoring

Note: Lithium levels should be trough levels

[a]Duration of meal replacement is based upon presurgery weight

[b]Standardized rating scales include the Hamilton Depression Rating Scale [26] or Patient Health Questionnaire-9 [20] for depression and the Young Mania Rating Scale for mania [27]

[c]Gradual increase from ~1–1.5 L/day to 2–2.5 L/day first few months post-surgery

of VPA (sodium valproate), the amide of VPA (valpromide; available in Europe), and a compound of both VPA and sodium valproate in a 1:1 ratio (divalproex sodium). There are also a number of possible VPA formulations, including immediate and delayed release capsules, controlled release tablets, suppositories, intravenous and oral solutions, and syrup [28].

Two case reports describe the use of intravenous valproate following gastric bypass surgery [29, 30]. One involves a patient with schizoaffective disorder who, in the first week post-surgery, developed severe manic symptoms that did not respond to clozapine (his usual medication), but were controlled when intravenous valproate was added (later switched to oral divalproex with adequate serum levels) [29]. The second describes a patient with bipolar II disorder who was unable to take anything by mouth for a prolonged period after gastric bypass due to surgical complications [30]. After her mood became unstable, her medical team initiated intravenous valproate with good effect.

Toxicity from VPA is less of a concern in the postoperative period than it is with lithium, given VPA's wider therapeutic range (50–125 μg/mL), but there are some particular issues to bear in mind with respect to postoperative VPA monitoring. Although the free (biologically active) and protein-bound VPA fractions are typically in stable ratios in the blood, the free VPA fraction can increase disproportionately with medical conditions associated with low protein levels (such as rapid weight loss) [28]. This imbalance would not be reflected in routine VPA laboratory assays, which represent both protein-bound and free VPA. Thus, there is a theoretical possibility that routine VPA blood levels may underestimate the concentration of the biologically active, free VPA level in bariatric surgery patients. This phenomenon is unlikely to be a concern for most patients, since VPA is primarily bound to albumin, the concentration of which is not as impacted by rapid weight loss as other proteins (e.g., alpha-1-acid glycoprotein) [6, 28]. Nevertheless, clinicians should keep this possibility in mind for patients experiencing increased VPA side effects or toxicity despite apparently appropriate serum levels.

The Toronto Western Hospital Bariatric Surgery Psychosocial program has also developed a protocol for bariatric surgery patients on VPA (see Table 23.2). The protocol includes guidelines regarding VPA dosing and monitoring in the perioperative period. As with other medications, VPA extended release or enteric-coated preparations should be switched to immediate release formulations. VPA is available in liquid form, and this formulation should be considered for patients who have difficulty tolerating solid forms and/or who demonstrate evidence (by blood levels or clinically) of reduced absorption, not responsive to increased and divided doses. Lastly, given the potential underestimation of free VPA levels, we also suggest monitoring platelets and liver enzymes so that clinicians can intervene at the earliest signs of thrombocytopenia or hepatotoxicity (rare, but established adverse effects of VPA).

The bariatric surgery literature addressing other anticonvulsants used in psychiatric care is extremely limited. Though not a psychiatric case, Koutsavlis et al. (2015) reported on a patient with a history of epilepsy, maintained on carbamazepine, who developed life-threatening agranulocytosis and febrile neutropenia 4 weeks post-gastric sleeve surgery [31]. Carbamazepine levels were found to be elevated at 15.9 mg/L (therapeutic range 4–12 mg/L). Given that agranulocytosis is a well-established side effect of carbamazepine, the authors postulated that a change in carbamazepine pharmacokinetics post-bariatric surgery (e.g., increased hepatic metabolism or another weight loss-associated phenomenon) induced carbamazepine toxicity. In this case, the patient stabilized with reduction in carbamazepine dose. In another case from the epilepsy literature, Pournaras et al. (2011) reported on a patient who developed a relapse of his seizure disorder after experiencing reduced phenobarbitone and phenytoin levels post-RYGB, but was subsequently started on lamotrigine and achieved therapeutic levels of this medication [32].

One cannot make conclusions from two cases, but these reports further demonstrate the significant variability in pharmacokinetic changes among patients and medications post-bariatric

Table 23.2 Perioperative bariatric surgery VPA protocol

Bariatric surgery perioperative phase	Recommendations
Presurgery	*Dosing*
	• Switch extended release formulations to immediate release preparations of equivalent dosing
	Monitoring • Baseline valproic acid level[a]
	• Baseline liver enzymes and liver function tests
	• Baseline CBC with platelets
Post-surgery: 0–6 months post-surgery	*Dosing*
	• Should ideally take valproic acid on an empty stomach, if tolerated
	• Suggest using TID (rather than BID) dosing until serum levels are stable and patient is tolerating po intake, unless there is significant difficulty with adherence that requires a simplified regimen
	Monitoring
	• Obtain valproic acid levels q4 weeks and 1 week after changes to dosage or formulation
	• Consider dose decrease if valproic acid levels approach 700 micromol/L and/or if patient develops new adverse effects
	• Hold and reassess dose if symptoms of toxicity develop
	• Obtain liver enzymes and liver function tests q4 weeks
	• If signs of hepatotoxicity develop, hold and reassess
	• Obtain CBC at the 12-week mark and repeat monthly if platelet level is lower than baseline. Obtain CBC for any signs of thrombocytopenia
	• Monitor depressive and/or manic symptoms and suicidality (consider using standardized rating scales[b])
	• If patient experiences breakthrough mood symptoms, consider increasing the valproic acid dose and/or switching to a liquid formulation
	• If the valproic acid levels are lower than baseline and patient is symptomatic, or at risk of becoming symptomatic (e.g., highly recurrent illness), consider increasing the dose and/or switching to a liquid formulation
Post-surgery: >6 months post-surgery	*Dosing*
	• Consider consolidating dosing to BID if appropriate/not already done
	Monitoring
	• Continue to monitor valproic acid levels q4 weeks if there are ongoing fluctuations
	• Continue to monitor liver enzymes and liver function tests q4 weeks if there are ongoing fluctuations
	• Continue to monitor CBC q4 weeks if there are ongoing platelet fluctuations

[a]All levels should be trough levels

[b]Standardized rating scales include the Hamilton Depression Rating Scale [26] or Patient Health Questionnaire-9 [20] for depression and the Young Mania Rating Scale [27] for mania

surgery. Thus, we suggest that clinicians follow the same general rules for all mood-stabilizing medications: change all controlled release and enteric-coated medications to immediate release formulations whenever possible; obtain preoperative baseline blood levels; monitor patients closely in the perioperative period for medication adverse effects (considering both clinical symptoms and laboratory indices); and, for patients with signs of decreased medication absorption (again, based on both clinical presentation and medication blood levels), increase and divide doses and consider switching to a liquid formulation if available.

23.6 Antipsychotics

The 1990s saw a major shift in the landscape of antipsychotic use, with the widespread introduction of the second-generation ("atypical") antipsychotics. The second-generation antipsychotics were marketed as more effective and better tolerated than the first-generation ("typical") antipsychotics, though these assertions are controversial [33, 34]. Regardless, the use of second-generation antipsychotic medications has more than doubled since the 1990s [35]. Second-generation antipsychotics are now prescribed to a much larger and more diverse clinical population than first-generation agents ever have been, not only for FDA-approved indications, such as schizophrenia, bipolar disorder, and major depression, but for off-label use in a broad variety of conditions, including anxiety disorders, eating disorders, insomnia, and developmental disorders [35]. While a discussion about the clinical indications for second-generation antipsychotics is outside the scope of this text, their wide-ranging use means that bariatric clinicians must be familiar with them. Furthermore, the potentially severe weight gain associated with antipsychotics [36] may be a factor in some patients' decisions to pursue bariatric surgery.

Like antidepressants, antipsychotics are lipophilic and highly protein bound, meaning that they, too, are vulnerable to pharmacokinetic changes associated with bariatric surgery and weight loss [6, 37]. Unfortunately, data concerning the use of antipsychotics in bariatric surgery patients are limited to several small case reports ($n = 1$–5). General principles for prescription and monitoring of antipsychotics will be discussed here, with special attention paid to those agents that are more frequently clinically encountered, have more available data, or have known pharmacokinetic properties particularly likely to be affected by bariatric surgery procedures. Of note, in addition to conventional pills, many antipsychotics are available in orally disintegrating, liquid and intramuscular formulations, all of which may be used to optimize absorption following bariatric surgery. The available formulations, as well as the metabolic effects of the antipsychotic medications described here, are outlined in Table 23.3.

23.6.1 First-Generation Antipsychotics

Despite the increased popularity of second-generation antipsychotics, first-generation antipsychotics remain an important treatment option for many patients, particularly those with primary psychotic disorders [33]. First-generation antipsychotics have very little literature to guide their use in bariatric surgery patients. Fuller et al. (1986) described the case of a patient with schizophrenia maintained on haloperidol who exhibited similar haloperidol levels post-bariatric surgery to those generally reported in the literature [38], suggesting that, at least in this patient, absorption was not significantly affected. There are no studies reporting on the use of other typical antipsychotics. Despite the paucity of evidence in this area to guide clinical management, one benefit of many typical antipsychotics in the bariatric surgery population is their availability in long-acting injectable (LAI) formulations. Thus, for patients demonstrating evidence of reduced absorption (i.e., worsening or recurrence of symptoms), clinicians may have the option of switching to the LAI formulation, particularly for patients who do not respond to an increase in dose, or who are unable to tolerate oral medication (either due to complications of surgery or exacerbation of their underlying psychiatric illness). Close monitoring of patients on antipsychotic medications, especially in the early (i.e., <6 months) postsurgical period, should be performed as a matter of course.

23.6.2 Risperidone, Olanzapine, and Aripiprazole

Risperidone's use in the bariatric surgery population has been reported in both its immediate release tablet and LAI formulations. Hamoui et al. (2004) described a case–control study of

Table 23.3 Antipsychotic characteristics pertinent to the bariatric surgery population

	Metabolic adverse effects[a]			Immediate release tablet	Extended release tablet	Orally disintegrating tablet	Oral liquid	Immediate release injectable	Long-acting injectable
	Weight gain	Diabetes risk	Dyslipidemia risk						
Haloperidol	Low/neutral	Low	Low	X	–	–	X	X	X
Risperidone	Mod	Low	Low	X	–	X	X	–	X
Paliperidone	Mod	Low	Low	–	X[b]	–	–	–	X
Olanzapine	High	High	High	X	–	X	–	X	X
Quetiapine	Mod	Mod	Mod	X	X	–	–	–	–
Aripiprazole	Low	Low	Low	X	–	–	–	–	X
Ziprasidone	Low/neutral	Low	Low	X	–	–	X[c]	X	–
Lurasidone[d]	Low/neutral	Low	Low	X	–	–	–	–	–
Asenapine	Low	Low	Low	–	–	X[e]	–	–	–
Clozapine	High	High	High	X	–	X	X	–	–

[a]Data compiled from De Hert et al., 2012 [55]; Klemp et al., 2011 [56]; Leucht et al., 2013 [57]; and American Diabetes Association, 2004 [58]
[b]There is no commercially available immediate release formulation of paliperidone
[c]Oral suspension ziprasidone does not obviate the requirement of intake with >500 kcal meal
[d]Limited long-term data
[e]Asenapine is only available in sublingual formulation

five patients with schizophrenia on antipsychotics, four of whom were taking risperidone [39]. One of these two patients suffered a decompensation that required stabilization with intravenous haloperidol and lorazepam. In a 2011 case report, Brietzke and Lafer described the utility of risperidone post-bariatric surgery in a patient with bipolar II disorder who was unable to tolerate oral medications, and whose psychiatric condition was stabilized on LAI risperidone [40]. Risperidone is also available in orally disintegrating and liquid formulations.

Though there are no reported cases for the use of olanzapine or aripiprazole in the bariatric surgery population, we have chosen to include these medications here because of their relative popularity [35] and the wide variety of available formulations (see Table 23.3). These alternate formulations provide clinicians with several options in the event that they suspect decreased absorption is contributing to psychiatric decompensation in postoperative patients. Given the limited literature in the area, as well as the variability in pharmacokinetic changes post-bariatric surgery among individual patients and medications, we do not, however, suggest that antipsychotics are routinely switched to liquid or LAI formulations preoperatively.

23.6.3 Quetiapine

Quetiapine is a frequently encountered low-potency (and sedating) atypical antipsychotic. It is prescribed for a wide variety of conditions [35], and doses often differ dramatically depending on the intended target of treatment (e.g., 25–150 mg for insomnia, 150–300 mg for depression, and 400–800 mg for mania or psychosis). The only data regarding the use of quetiapine in bariatric surgery patients comes from Hamoui et al.'s 2004 case–control series of five patients with schizophrenia, one of whom was prescribed quetiapine 400 mg [39]. This patient received a duodenal switch operation and did not experience relapse postoperatively, though he was also taking risperidone 2 mg, and the length of follow-up was not explicitly stated.

Bariatric clinicians must review prescription information carefully for patients taking quetiapine. The extended release formulation is frequently encountered in clinical practice, and, as discussed previously, should be converted to the immediate release formulation preoperatively. Furthermore, for individuals taking higher doses of quetiapine (i.e., ≥300 mg daily), we advise dividing of the dose, if tolerated, in order to optimize absorption.

23.6.4 Paliperidone

Paliperidone is the primary active metabolite of risperidone. There are no published reports on the use of paliperidone in bariatric surgery patients as of the time of writing. Clinicians assessing a preoperative patient stabilized on paliperidone must be cautious, since oral paliperidone is only available as an extended release tablet, increasing the risk for reduced absorption in the postoperative period. Several options exist for patients taking paliperidone, depending on history, clinical judgment, and patient preference. Patients could be maintained on paliperidone at their usual dose and monitored carefully for signs of decompensation postoperatively. If they experience decompensation, they could then have their paliperidone dose increased, switch to the equivalent dose of risperidone (available in multiple formulations) or switch to the LAI paliperidone formulation. Some patients and clinicians may wish to switch to either risperidone or LAI paliperidone preoperatively, for instance if patients are known to be at high risk of relapse or have experienced very severe illness. If switching medications preoperatively, patients should demonstrate a period of stability on the new medication prior to undergoing bariatric surgery.

23.6.5 Ziprasidone

We discuss ziprasidone separately because of the requirement that it be taken with a specified amount of food, an additional challenge in bariatric surgery patients. Hamoui et al. (2004) described one patient taking ziprasidone 240 mg daily in their case–control study [39]. The authors did not discuss the significant caloric intake (>500 kcal) known to be critical for adequate absorption of ziprasidone [41]. This patient underwent a duodenal switch operation (a procedure associated with significant malabsorption), and was not reported to experience any postoperative psychiatric decompensation, though length of follow-up was not clear.

Bariatric surgery patients taking ziprasidone are at risk of reduced absorption because of inconsistent (and low) caloric intake in the perioperative period. Gandelman et al. described absorption rates 60–90 % lower with 250 kcal meals than with 500 kcal meals [41]. This issue is potentially troublesome because ziprasidone absorption in the absence of sufficient caloric intake cannot be improved by increasing the prescribed dose [42]. Furthermore, according to the manufacturer's product monograph, the oral suspension formulation of ziprasidone requires co-ingestion with meals, and likely does not obviate absorption limitations below 500 kcal [43]. Most bariatric surgery programs require patients to exclusively consume meal replacement formula for several weeks prior to surgery. These meal replacements are usually approximately 225 kcal taken 4 times a day. In the postoperative period, patients are expected to eat between 300 and 500 kcal total per day, gradually increasing to 1000–1500 kcal of daily intake by 1 year. Compounded with the altered transit time associated with most bariatric surgeries, prolonged restricted caloric intake in bariatric surgery patients creates a context of highly unstable ziprasidone absorption. Therefore, clinicians assessing bariatric surgery patients who are taking this medication in the preoperative period, as well as clinicians treating postoperative patients on ziprasidone who are experiencing evidence of reduced medication absorption, must carefully consider the risk/benefit ratio of the patient remaining on this medication vs. switching to another medication that does not depend on food intake for optimal absorption.

23.6.6 Lurasidone

There are no reports on the use of lurasidone in bariatric surgery patients. Like ziprasidone, lurasidone is known to require co-ingestion with food for optimal absorption. Unlike ziprasidone, however, absorption is maximally achieved with a food intake of 350 kcal [44]. Lurasidone absorption on an empty stomach appears better than with ziprasidone (reduced by 50 % compared with 60–90 %) and may be improved by increasing the dose (personal correspondence with Sunovion, 2015). Thus, for patients eating meals that are less than 350 kcal in the perioperative period, one management option is to increase the lurasidone dose until meals are at least 350 kcal. Unfortunately, there is no literature to guide the amount that doses should be increased, so clinicians must rely on their judgment and consultation with pharmacy colleagues. Bariatric clinicians should also work closely with patients and their treating psychiatrists to discuss the risks and alternatives to this plan (e.g., a preoperative switch to another medication). Patients should be monitored carefully for both medication side effects and signs of relapse during the postoperative period.

23.6.7 Asenapine

Asenapine is only available in an immediate release sublingual formulation and is primarily absorbed in the oral mucosa [45]. There is one case report in the literature describing a patient who had previously undergone RYGB, with diagnoses of depression, anxiety, personality disorders, and pica, who responded well to a switch from ziprasidone to asenapine a number of years after her RYGB procedure [46]. While it is impossible to ascertain whether the improved absorption of asenapine vs. ziprasidone was the factor that led to clinical improvement in this case, the benefit of asenapine in the bariatric surgery population, as noted by the authors, is that it bypasses the GI tract. Therefore, depending on the clinical history, this medication may be a good option for bariatric patients requiring the use of antipsychotic medication, provided they are able to follow the manufacturer's recommendations to place the tablet under the tongue and allow it to dissolve completely, then to avoid eating or drinking for 10 min thereafter [47].

23.6.8 Clozapine

Unfortunately, like most antipsychotics, there are no studies addressing the use of clozapine in bariatric surgery patients. Clozapine is considered the "gold standard" in schizophrenia treatment [48], but it also has a severe side effect profile, and, in North America, requires registration under a central monitoring network and regular blood work for its continued prescription. Given the complexities associated with its use, it is typically reserved for treatment refractory patients with schizophrenia, and is less commonly prescribed than other antipsychotics, particularly in North America [48]. However, we include it here because there are several management strategies that can reduce the potential for serious adverse effects in perioperative patients taking clozapine.

Discussion about the full range clozapine-induced side effects is outside of the scope of this text, but there are several adverse effects that are of particular concern in the bariatric surgery population. One such adverse effect is constipation, which is common and potentially severe in patients on clozapine [49]. There are numerous case reports of intestinal obstruction, bowel perforation, and toxic megacolon associated with constipation from clozapine use [50]. Given the exacerbating effects of bariatric surgery on constipation [51], patients on clozapine should be monitored systematically and closely for this side effect, and constipation should be treated promptly, in consultation with primary care providers and other specialists as indicated.

The most infamous complication of clozapine use, and the primary reason its prescription requires regular blood work, is agranulocytosis. (Other significant clozapine adverse effects include myocarditis and seizures.) Agranulocytosis is a dangerously low white blood cell count that can lead to severe infection and death. The manufacturer recommends that blood work to screen for agranulocytosis is performed weekly for the first 6 months of clozapine prescription, every 2 weeks from 6 to 12 months, and then monthly thereafter, provided the hematological profile is stable [52]. If at any point an individual stops taking clozapine for ≥48 h, monitoring must increase for a duration of 6 weeks, and the product monograph suggests that it is re-titrated from a starting dose [52].

Patients taking clozapine who are undergoing bariatric surgery should be monitored very closely, especially in the acute postoperative period, for worsening psychotic symptoms and medication adverse effects associated with pharmacokinetic changes. Reference ranges for clozapine blood levels exist and, while not clearly correlated to therapeutic response or toxicity [53], may be used to establish patients' preoperative baseline level and monitor for changes in bioavailability postoperatively. For long-term clozapine patients who are receiving hematological laboratory monitoring monthly, clinicians may wish to consider more frequent monitoring in the postoperative period (e.g., every 1–2 weeks) to ensure that any serious adverse events associated with increased clozapine levels are identified early. General prescribing principles to counteract suspected decreased clozapine absorption, described elsewhere in this chapter, apply equally to clozapine use. There is no parenteral formulation of clozapine available, though there is an oral suspension and an orally disintegrating tablet available in some regions, and these may improve absorption.

Although we would primarily expect to see pharmacokinetic clozapine changes in the postoperative period, preoperative bariatric surgery patients who quit smoking in anticipation of surgery (often required in order to reduce postoperative complications) are also at risk. Clozapine is metabolized by the cytochrome P450 enzyme 1A2, which is induced by components of cigarette smoke. Therefore, clinicians should be aware that clozapine patients who quit smoking may experience worsening side effects, and may require a decrease in their regular dose [54].

Given the complexities associated with clozapine use, the management of bariatric surgery patients taking this medication requires close collaboration among the bariatric surgery team, the treating mental health team, primary care providers, and pharmacy colleagues.

23.7 Other Psychiatric Medications

There is no clinical literature addressing the effect of bariatric surgery on other classes of psychiatric medications (e.g., stimulants, anxiolytics/hypnotics). In an in vitro RYGB model, clonazepam was found to dissolve significantly less than in the control condition, whereas diazepam, lorazepam, trazodone, zolpidem, and buspirone dissolved equally in both models [16]. Methylphenidate was also found to dissolve equally between models [16]. However, as discussed previously in this chapter, while it is interesting to note the differences in dissolution (and, therefore, potentially absorption) among medications, one cannot draw conclusions about their pharmacokinetic changes post-bariatric surgery in real-life patients, where many more variables come into play.

We suggest generally following the same management guidelines described above and summarized below for patients on any psychiatric medication: close monitoring in the perioperative period, switching controlled release to immediate release formulations when possible, and increasing and dividing medication doses, along with possibly crushing pills or changing to more readily dissolvable formulations, when there is evidence of decreased absorption.

With respect to the stimulants and sedative/hypnotics mentioned above, there are several specific issues to consider. First, many stimulant medications come in controlled release formulations, though fortunately most also come in corresponding immediate release versions. Second, several sedative/hypnotic medications come in liquid formulations and orally dispersible sublingual formulations, a number of which are absorbed (at least partially) in the oral mucosa, thereby bypassing the GI tract and optimizing absorption post-bariatric surgery. Sublingual lorazepam and zolpidem tartrate oral spray (available in some regions) are examples of two medications that are absorbed via this route. As previously mentioned, however, not all orally disintegrating tablets are actually absorbed through the oral mucosa, so if clinicians are uncertain they should consult the product monograph or with pharmacy colleagues.

23.8 Summary of Perioperative Medication Management Recommendations

The following table outlines management suggestions that can be applied generally to all bariatric surgery patients on psychotropic medications. Note that since there is limited evidence in the literature from which to draw, these suggestions are based on expert consensus [3, 5, 6, 13, 19]. See Table 23.4.

Case Vignette

Returning to the case of Ms. P, we will now discuss management strategies for each of her psychiatric medications. From a clinical perspective, it is important to note that Ms. P is a patient who has achieved stability on her current medication regimen after experiencing severe depressive episodes as part of her bipolar disorder, including suicide attempts and hospitalizations. Thus, it is important for her medications to remain as consistent as possible. Her mood should be monitored carefully in the perioperative period, and clinicians should consider using formal rating scales. We discuss each medication sequentially below.

1. Lithium: A baseline level should be obtained prior to starting the liquid diet portion of the bariatric surgery process. Ms. P should be carefully educated about adequate fluid consumption and about the symptoms of lithium toxicity. She should be advised to seek medical attention if she develops any of these symptoms and/or if she is not tolerating oral intake postoperatively. Lithium levels should be monitored frequently in the perioperative period (see Table 23.2 for protocol with suggested monitoring frequency). If lithium levels approach 1.2 mmol/L or increase by >25 % from baseline, consider a dose reduction. Lithium should be held if symptoms of

(continued)

(continued)

toxicity develop or if levels are in the toxic range, and started at a lower dose when levels normalize. If levels are >25 % lower than baseline (particularly after two or more readings) and/or if symptoms of mood instability develop, there are several strategies that can be used to optimize absorption. These include increasing and dividing the dose and considering the use of lithium citrate syrup if available. Ms. P should continue on the enhanced monitoring protocol for at least the first year postoperatively. She may return to routine monitoring thereafter, provided her lithium levels are stable.

2. Quetiapine XR: This medication should be switched to its immediate release formulation prior to surgery. The dose may be increased postoperatively and divided (if tolerated) if Ms. P develops signs of reduced quetiapine absorption (e.g., insomnia, mood instability despite adequate lithium levels).
3. Paroxetine: Ms. P should be educated about the antidepressant discontinuation syndrome, particularly since SSRIs with short half-lives, such as paroxetine, are known to be most associated with discontinuation symptoms [59]. These symptoms are outlined in detail in the Discontinuation Emergent Signs and Symptoms Checklist [17], and would be expected to develop within the first week postoperatively. If Ms. P develops signs of reduced antidepressant absorption (discontinuation symptoms in the immediate postoperative period and/or a recurrence of panic attacks within the first postoperative year), then the paroxetine dose may be increased and divided. In the unlikely event that clinical signs of decreased paroxetine absorption continue despite these steps, clinicians might consider switching Ms. P to an antidepressant with an available liquid formulation. These adjustments would have to be done with caution in Ms. P's case, given her diagnosis of bipolar disorder, and provided that her lithium levels are therapeutic.
4. Lorazepam: Consider using the sublingual form of lorazepam if feasible, since this formulation is absorbed via the oral mucosa, negating the effect of reduced absorption in the post-RYGB gastrointestinal environment. Otherwise, if there are signs of decreased absorption in the postoperative period, the dose may be increased, or Ms. P could be switched to the liquid formulation of lorazepam (available in some regions), or to another benzodiazepine with an available liquid formulation.

Table 23.4 General recommendations for management of psychiatric medication in the perioperative period

Bariatric surgery perioperative phase	Recommendations	
	Monitoring strategies	Interventions
Preoperative	– Educate patients about adverse effects and signs of medication malabsorption that should be monitored postoperatively	– Switch controlled release medications to immediate release formulations
	– Consider whether medication pharmacokinetics will be affected by the use of a liquid meal replacement	– If controlled formulations are not available, consult with pharmacy colleagues about other options (e.g., crushing tablets, opening and sprinkling capsules)
	– Perform baseline medication blood levels if indicated	
	– Perform baseline symptom assessment using a formal rating scale specific to patient's psychiatric disorder	

(continued)

Table 23.4 (continued)

Bariatric surgery perioperative phase	Recommendations	
	Monitoring strategies	Interventions
Acute postoperative (0–6 weeks)	– Close monitoring for signs of medication adverse effects and signs of medication malabsorption (e.g., discontinuation symptoms, worsening of psychiatric symptoms; continue using clinical rating scales)	– If patient exhibits signs of medication malabsorption, consider the following suggestions:
	– Regular medication blood levels if indicated	1. Increase and divide the dose; consider crushing pills if feasible
	– Regular screening blood work for medication adverse effects if indicated	2. Switch to a more readily dissolvable formulation (e.g., orally dispersible tablets or liquid)
		3. Switch to an alternate medication with a more readily dissolvable formulation
		– If patient exhibits signs of medication toxicity: Reduce dose or hold medication and restart at lower dose, depending on severity of adverse effect
Later postoperative (>6 weeks)	– Continue regular clinical and laboratory monitoring, though frequency can be reduced if symptoms and laboratory indices remain stable	– May consider returning to presurgical medication dosing regimen and medication formulation after 1 year, depending on patient preference and clinical history
	– Monitor for an increase in medication adverse effects, particularly if the patient's dose was previously increased to optimize absorption in the acute postoperative period	

23.9 Conclusions

Bariatric surgery is an important and effective treatment option for patients with severe obesity. Candidates are known to have high rates of affective disorders, and experts anticipate that increasing numbers of patients with severe and persistent mental illnesses will seek bariatric surgery in the coming years [3]. Therefore, bariatric surgery clinicians must be comfortable managing a variety of psychiatric medications in the perioperative period.

Bariatric surgery (particularly malabsorptive procedures) has the potential to significantly impact medication absorption. When patients demonstrate signs of malabsorption, there are a number of dosing and medication formulation strategies that clinicians can employ to combat this problem. For patients taking more complex medication regimens, and when clinicians are unsure as to the availability of specific medication formulations, pharmacy colleagues can be an invaluable resource.

Although medication malabsorption is the primary concern following bariatric surgery, other pharmacokinetic steps are likely affected as well (particularly with rapid weight loss). Thus, clinicians must also be aware of the possibility of increased medication bioavailability postoperatively, and associated adverse effects.

Since postoperative pharmacokinetic changes can be unpredictable and vary among patients, medications, and types of surgery, bariatric clinicians' best tools are thorough patient education and careful and systematic monitoring in the perioperative period. Monitoring should always include inquiry into clinical symptoms of altered medication levels, and laboratory measurements (in both the pre- and postoperative periods) when indicated. We advocate the use of systematized protocols for higher risk medications (such as those described above for lithium and VPA) and clinical rating scales to monitor for psychiatric symptom worsening for all patients in the perioperative period. These strategies increase the likelihood that problems will be identified and addressed early.

The majority of research concerning pharmacokinetic changes in psychiatric medications following bariatric surgery has been conducted on patients who underwent RYGB and those taking antidepressants. Further research is needed involving other procedures (particularly the gastric sleeve, given its growing popularity [3]) and additional medication classes, so that clinicians have a strong evidence base to guide clinical practice.

Acknowledgement The authors wish to thank Sassha Orser RPh., ACPR for her assistance in preparing this chapter.

References

1. Kalarchian MA, Marcus MD, Levine MD, Courcoulas AP, Pilkonis PA, Ringham RM, et al. Psychiatric disorders among bariatric surgery candidates: relationship to obesity and functional health status. Am J Psychiatry. 2007;164:328–34. doi:10.1176/ajp.2007.164.2.328. Quiz 374.
2. Mitchell JE, King WC, Chen J-Y, Devlin MJ, Flum D, Garcia L, et al. Course of depressive symptoms and treatment in the longitudinal assessment of bariatric surgery (LABS-2) study. Obesity (Silver Spring). 2014;22:1799–806. doi:10.1002/oby.20738.
3. Roerig JL, Steffen K. Psychopharmacology and bariatric surgery. Eur Eat Disord Rev. 2015;23:463–9. doi:10.1002/erv.2396.
4. Katzung B. Basic and clinical pharmacology. 10th ed. New York: McGraw-Hill; 2007.
5. Padwal R, Brocks D, Sharma AM. A systematic review of drug absorption following bariatric surgery and its theoretical implications. Obes Rev. 2010;11:41–50. doi:10.1111/j.1467-789X.2009.00614.x.
6. Macgregor AM, Boggs L. Drug distribution in obesity and following bariatric surgery: a literature review. Obes Surg. 1996;6:17–27. doi:10.1381/096089296765557222.
7. Alexander JK. Obesity and cardiac performance. Am J Cardiol. 1964;14:860–5.
8. de Divitiis O, Fazio S, Petitto M, Maddalena G, Contaldo F, Mancini M. Obesity and cardiac function. Circulation. 1981;64:477–82.
9. Blouin RA, Kolpek JH, Mann HJ. Influence of obesity on drug disposition. Clin Pharm. 1987;6:706–14.
10. Shargel L, Wu-Pong S, Yu A. Applied biopharmaceutics & pharmacokinetics. 6th ed. New York: McGraw-Hill Education; 2012.
11. Yska JP, van der Linde S, Tapper VV, Apers JA, Emous M, Totté ER, et al. Influence of bariatric surgery on the use and pharmacokinetics of some major drug classes. Obes Surg. 2013;23:819–25. doi:10.1007/s11695-013-0882-6.
12. Marzinke MA, Petrides AK, Steele K, Schweitzer MA, Magnuson TH, Reinblatt SP, et al. Decreased escitalopram concentrations post-Roux-en-Y gastric bypass surgery. Ther Drug Monit. 2015;37:408–12. doi:10.1097/FTD.0000000000000146.
13. Hamad GG, Helsel JC, Perel JM, Kozak GM, McShea MC, Hughes C, et al. The effect of gastric bypass on the pharmacokinetics of serotonin reuptake inhibitors. Am J Psychiatry. 2012;169:256–63. doi:10.1176/appi.ajp.2011.11050719.
14. Roerig JL, Steffen KJ, Zimmerman C, Mitchell JE, Crosby RD, Cao L. A comparison of duloxetine plasma levels in postbariatric surgery patients versus matched nonsurgical control subjects. J Clin Psychopharmacol. 2013;33:479–84. doi:10.1097/JCP.0b013e3182905ffb.
15. Roerig JL, Steffen K, Zimmerman C, Mitchell JE, Crosby RD, Cao L. Preliminary comparison of sertraline levels in postbariatric surgery patients versus matched nonsurgical cohort. Surg Obes Relat Dis. 2012;8:62–6. doi:10.1016/j.soard.2010.12.003.
16. Seaman JS, Bowers SP, Dixon P, Schindler L. Dissolution of common psychiatric medications in a Roux-en-Y gastric bypass model. Psychosomatics. 2005;46:250–3. doi:10.1176/appi.psy.46.3.250.
17. Rosenbaum JF, Fava M, Hoog SL, Ascroft RC, Krebs WB. Selective serotonin reuptake inhibitor discontinuation syndrome: a randomized clinical trial. Biol Psychiatry. 1998;44:77–87.
18. Black K, Shea C, Dursun S, Kutcher S. Selective serotonin reuptake inhibitor discontinuation syndrome: proposed diagnostic criteria. J Psychiatry Neurosci. 2000;25:255–61.
19. Bingham K, Hawa R, Sockalingam S. SSRI discontinuation syndrome following bariatric surgery: a case report and focused literature review. Psychosomatics. 2014;55:692–7. doi:10.1016/j.psym.2014.07.003.
20. Spitzer RL, Kroenke K, Williams JB. Validation and utility of a self-report version of PRIME-MD: the PHQ primary care study. Primary Care Evaluation of Mental Disorders. Patient Health Questionnaire. JAMA. 1999;282:1737–44.
21. Cassin S, Sockalingam S, Hawa R, Wnuk S, Royal S, Taube-Schiff M, et al. Psychometric properties of the Patient Health Questionnaire (PHQ-9) as a depression screening tool for bariatric surgery candidates.

Psychosomatics. 2013;54:352–8. doi:10.1016/j.psym.2012.08.010.
22. McIntyre RS, Konarski JZ, Wilkins K, Soczynska JK, Kennedy SH. Obesity in bipolar disorder and major depressive disorder: results from a national community health survey on mental health and well-being. Can J Psychiatry. 2006;51:274–80.
23. Walsh K, Volling J. Lithium toxicity following Roux-en-Y gastric bypass. Bariatr Surg Pract Patient Care. 2014;9:77–80.
24. Nykiel J, Carino G, Levinson A. Lithium toxicity in the context of recent gastric bypass surgery. Case Vignettes Clin Care II Respir Crit Care Med Abstr Issue. 2014;189:A6203.
25. Tripp AC. Lithium toxicity after Roux-en-Y gastric bypass surgery. J Clin Psychopharmacol. 2011;31: 261–2. doi:10.1097/JCP.0b013e318210b203.
26. Hamilton M. A rating scale for depression. J Neurol Neurosurg Psychiatry. 1960;23:56–62.
27. Young RC, Biggs JT, Ziegler VE, Meyer DA. A rating scale for mania: reliability, validity and sensitivity. Br J Psychiatry. 1978;133:429–35.
28. Keck PE, McElroy SL. Clinical pharmacodynamics and pharmacokinetics of antimanic and mood-stabilizing medications. J Clin Psychiatry. 2002;63 Suppl 4:3–11.
29. Kaltsounis J, De Leon OA. Intravenous valproate treatment of severe manic symptoms after gastric bypass surgery: a case report. Psychosomatics. 2000;41:454–6. doi:10.1176/appi.psy.41.5.454.
30. Semion K, Dorsey J, Bourgeois J. Intravenous valproate use in bipolar II disorder after gastric bypass surgery. J Neuropsychiatry Clin Neurosci. 2005;17:427–9. doi:10.1176/jnp.17.3.427-a.
31. Koutsavlis I, Muayed L. Dose-dependent carbamazepine-induced agranulocytosis following bariatric surgery (Sleeve Gastrectomy): a possible mechanism. Bariatr Surg Pract Patient Care. 2014;10:130–4.
32. Pournaras DJ, Footitt D, Mahon D, Welbourn R. Reduced phenytoin levels in an epileptic patient following Roux-En-Y gastric bypass for obesity. Obes Surg. 2011;21:684–5. doi:10.1007/s11695-010-0107-1.
33. Jones PB, Barnes TRE, Davies L, Dunn G, Lloyd H, Hayhurst KP, et al. Randomized controlled trial of the effect on Quality of Life of second- vs first-generation antipsychotic drugs in schizophrenia: Cost Utility of the Latest Antipsychotic Drugs in Schizophrenia Study (CUtLASS 1). Arch Gen Psychiatry. 2006;63:1079–87. doi:10.1001/archpsyc.63.10.1079.
34. Lieberman JA, Stroup TS, McEvoy JP, Swartz MS, Rosenheck RA, Perkins DO, et al. Effectiveness of antipsychotic drugs in patients with chronic schizophrenia. N Engl J Med. 2005;353:1209–23. doi:10.1056/NEJMoa051688.
35. Maher AR, Maglione M, Bagley S, Suttorp M, Hu J-H, Ewing B, et al. Efficacy and comparative effectiveness of atypical antipsychotic medications for off-label uses in adults: a systematic review and meta-analysis. JAMA. 2011;306:1359–69. doi:10.1001/jama.2011.1360.
36. Allison DB, Mentore JL, Heo M, Chandler LP, Cappelleri JC, Infante MC, et al. Antipsychotic-induced weight gain: a comprehensive research synthesis. Am J Psychiatry. 1999;156:1686–96. doi:10.1176/ajp.156.11.1686.
37. Javaid JI. Clinical pharmacokinetics of antipsychotics. J Clin Pharmacol. 1994;34:286–95.
38. Fuller AK, Tingle D, DeVane CL, Scott JA, Stewart RB. Haloperidol pharmacokinetics following gastric bypass surgery. J Clin Psychopharmacol. 1986; 6:376–8.
39. Hamoui N, Kingsbury S, Anthone GJ, Crookes PF. Surgical treatment of morbid obesity in schizophrenic patients. Obes Surg. 2004;14:349–52. doi:10.1381/096089204322917873.
40. Brietzke E, Lafer B. Long-acting injectable risperidone in a bipolar patient submitted to bariatric surgery and intolerant to conventional mood stabilizers. Psychiatry Clin Neurosci. 2011;65:205. doi:10.1111/j.1440-1819.2010.02175.x.
41. Gandelman K, Alderman JA, Glue P, Lombardo I, LaBadie RR, Versavel M, et al. The impact of calories and fat content of meals on oral ziprasidone absorption: a randomized, open-label, crossover trial. J Clin Psychiatry. 2009;70:58–62.
42. Citrome L. Using oral ziprasidone effectively: the food effect and dose-response. Adv Ther. 2009;26: 739–48. doi:10.1007/s12325-009-0055-0.
43. Zeldox product monograph. 2014.
44. Preskorn S, Ereshefsky L, Chiu Y-Y, Poola N, Loebel A. Effect of food on the pharmacokinetics of lurasidone: results of two randomized, open-label, crossover studies. Hum Psychopharmacol. 2013;28: 495–505. doi:10.1002/hup.2338.
45. Bartlett JA, van der Voort Maarschalk K. Understanding the oral mucosal absorption and resulting clinical pharmacokinetics of asenapine. AAPS PharmSciTech. 2012;13:1110–5. doi:10.1208/s12249-012-9839-7.
46. Tabaac BJ, Tabaac V. Pica patient, status post gastric bypass, improves with change in medication regimen. Ther Adv Psychopharmacol. 2015;5:38–42. doi:10.1177/2045125314561221.
47. Saphris prescribing information. 2015.
48. Meltzer HY. Clozapine: balancing safety with superior antipsychotic efficacy. Clin Schizophr Relat Psychoses. 2012;6:134–44. doi:10.3371/CSRP.6.3.5.
49. Young CR, Bowers MB, Mazure CM. Management of the adverse effects of clozapine. Schizophr Bull. 1998;24:381–90.
50. Palmer SE, McLean RM, Ellis PM, Harrison-Woolrych M. Life-threatening clozapine-induced gastrointestinal hypomotility: an analysis of 102 cases. J Clin Psychiatry. 2008;69:759–68.
51. Afshar S, Kelly SB, Seymour K, Woodcock S, Werner A-D, Mathers JC. The effects of bariatric procedures on bowel habit. Obes Surg. 2016;26:2348–2354. doi:10.1007/s11695-016-2100-9.
52. Clozaril product monograph. 2015.
53. Stark A, Scott J. A review of the use of clozapine levels to guide treatment and determine cause of death.

Aust N Z J Psychiatry. 2012;46:816–25. doi:10.1177/0004867412438871.
54. Zhou S-F, Yang L-P, Zhou Z-W, Liu Y-H, Chan E. Insights into the substrate specificity, inhibitors, regulation, and polymorphisms and the clinical impact of human cytochrome P450 1A2. AAPS J. 2009;11:481–94. doi:10.1208/s12248-009-9127-y.
55. De Hert M, Yu W, Detraux J, Sweers K, van Winkel R, Correll CU. Body weight and metabolic adverse effects of asenapine, iloperidone, lurasidone and paliperidone in the treatment of schizophrenia and bipolar disorder: a systematic review and exploratory meta-analysis. CNS Drugs. 2012;26:733–59. doi:10.2165/11634500-000000000-00000.
56. Klemp M, Tvete IF, Skomedal T, Gaasemyr J, Natvig B, Aursnes I. A review and Bayesian meta-analysis of clinical efficacy and adverse effects of 4 atypical neuroleptic drugs compared with haloperidol and placebo. J Clin Psychopharmacol. 2011;31:698–704. doi:10.1097/JCP.0b013e31823657d9.
57. Leucht S, Cipriani A, Spineli L, Mavridis D, Orey D, Richter F, et al. Comparative efficacy and tolerability of 15 antipsychotic drugs in schizophrenia: a multiple-treatments meta-analysis. Lancet. 2013;382:951–62. doi:10.1016/S0140-6736(13)60733-3.
58. American Diabetes Association, American Psychiatric Association, American Association of Clinical Endocrinologists, North American Association for the Study of Obesity. Consensus development conference on antipsychotic drugs and obesity and diabetes. Diabetes Care. 2004;27:596–601.
59. Clerc GE, Ruimy P, Verdeau-Pallès J. A double-blind comparison of venlafaxine and fluoxetine in patients hospitalized for major depression and melancholia. The Venlafaxine French Inpatient Study Group. Int Clin Psychopharmacol. 1994;9:139–43.

Part VI

Putting It All Together: An Integrative Synthesis

Integrated Case Summary

24

Raed Hawa and Sanjeev Sockalingam

24.1 Introduction

Previous chapters in this book have focused on understanding predisposing factors of severe obesity, assessment approaches to psychiatric issues in severe obesity, potential treatments for severe obesity, and the evidence for pharmacological and non-pharmacological treatments in severe obesity management. This chapter will use an integrated case to revisit key concepts and recommendations from previous chapters in this book. Salient components to case formulation, assessment, and management will be highlighted. Using this illustrative case example, the chapter will review evidence-informed treatment interventions and their role in patient care.

R. Hawa (✉)
Toronto Western Hospital Bariatric Surgery Program, University Health Network, 399 Bathurst Street, Toronto, ON, Canada M5T 2S8

Department of Psychiatry, University of Toronto, Toronto, ON, Canada
e-mail: Raed.Hawa@uhn.ca

S. Sockalingam
Toronto Western Hospital Bariatric Surgery Program, Centre for Mental Health, University Health Network, 200 Elizabeth Street, Toronto, ON, Canada M5G 2C4

Department of Psychiatry, University of Toronto, Toronto, ON, Canada
e-mail: sanjeev.sockalingam@uhn.ca

24.2 An Integrated Approach to Psychiatric Care in Severe Obesity

Given the prevalence of psychiatric comorbidity in individuals with severe obesity, there is no doubt that obesity care must include an understanding, awareness, and approach to psychiatric conditions. Using the multiple lenses from past chapters, we will use the following case to untangle the psychiatric complexity in severe obesity care.

Case Vignette: Ms. A

Ms. A is a 45-year-old woman who was referred by her primary care physician to a weight management centre for an evaluation of her obesity and recommendations for treatment options. The center has a team of obesity specialists, including an internist, a nurse practitioner, a registered dietician, and a psychologist, who perform a comprehensive initial evaluation and make recommendations for obesity treatment. Ms. A presented to the weight center team reluctant to consider weight-loss sur-

(continued)

S. Sockalingam, R. Hawa (eds.), *Psychiatric Care in Severe Obesity*,
DOI 10.1007/978-3-319-42536-8_24

(continued)
gery due to fear regarding surgery and surgical complications.

Ms. A has type 2 diabetes, hypertension, hyperlipidemia, depression, and obstructive sleep apnea. Her medications include insulin, metformin, atorvastatin, paroxetine, and amlodipine. She is not using her CPAP machine. Her morning blood glucose levels are 100–130 mg/dL, her haemoglobin A_{1c} (A1C) level is 6.1 % (within normal limits), her triglyceride level is 190 mg/dL, and serum insulin is 19 mIU/mL. Her blood pressure is 140/90 mm Hg. Her BMI is 44.8 kg/m^2.

Ms. A developed obesity as a child and reports having gained weight since then. Her family history is positive for obesity; both of her parents are also obese. She describes her childhood as "difficult" where her family moved a lot to accommodate her father's job. She endorses difficulties in having long-term relationships and difficulty with intimacy.

Ms. A has participated in both commercial and medical weight-loss programmes but has regained any weight lost within months of discontinuing the programmes. She has seen an RD for weight loss in the past and has also participated in a group weight-loss programme in which she lost some weight but regained it all. She has tried many self-directed diets, but has had no significant or sustained weight loss.

Ms. A does not eat breakfast as "I am too busy". She reports eating in restaurants 4–5 times a week. Her alcohol intake consists of only an occasional glass of wine except on weekends when she would drink half a bottle of wine. She reports binge eating about once a month and says it is precipitated by stress.

Ms. A has been feeling more depressed due to increased stress at work related to conflict with her manager. She lives alone and spends little time cooking or grocery shopping. She prefers ordering in and eating at restaurants.

Ms. A says she is concerned about her health and wants to get her life back under control. Her primary care physician has been encouraging her to explore weight-loss surgery; she is worried about surgery as an option for weight loss.

How could her failed weight loss attempts impact her self-efficacy in this context and how does the team approach this during treatment?

Ms. A has experienced several "failed" weight-loss attempts and she may be ambivalent about a surgical treatment to her obesity due to her past experiences of ineffective weight loss through various interventions. It will be important for the registered dietician on the team to review Ms. A's past weight-loss attempts at her initial intake. During this assessment with the dietician on the team weaving in education on the differences between "fad diets" as highlighted in the chapter by Warwick and Gougeon, may help identify clarify assumptions and address weight-loss knowledge gaps.

Throughout this process, an empathic and validating approach can be helpful in establishing a therapeutic alliance. Consideration of Ms. A's attachment style and adapting the team approach to best engage her long term is key. For example, if she had an avoidant attachment style, it would be beneficial to provide her with opportunities for autonomy and arrange her follow-up around a team member with whom she has a stronger therapeutic alliance. Supportive interventions offered by telephone or through online platforms could be used to optimize the "relational distance" and comfort in the context of her avoidant attachment style.

How does the team address Ms. A's concern and ambivalence about weight-loss surgery?

Ms. A's ambivalence about surgery could be related to concerns about surgical complications; however, further exploration of her fears is needed. As discussed previously, bariatric surgery may result in several complications but these complications need to be discussed in the context of the efficacy and health benefits of bariatric surgery procedures. Further education, attending support groups on bariatric surgery and speaking with the surgical team members may assist in addressing fears and providing Ms. A with the necessary information to make an informed decision about surgery. Moreover, integrated approaches should also involve the primary care team who often work with patients longitudinally. Given the potential knowledge gaps in primary care regarding bariatric surgery [1], education and resources should be developed to equip primary care teams with the knowledge to educate patients on potential surgical risks and benefits. Working in collaboration with Ms. A, it may be helpful to identify supports in her life and to engage these professional supports in the bariatric surgery education process.

How should Ms. A's relationship difficulties and supports be addressed as part of her obesity management?

It is clear from Ms. A's history that there have been difficulties in her childhood including potential adversity. She is also able to reflect on her challenges with long-term intimacy and relationships, which could be a starting point for exploring the role of relationships on her obesity management. As summarized earlier in the chapter by Maunder, Hunter, and Le, there is a high prevalence of childhood trauma in patients with obesity, and it would be important to also ask Ms. A about past traumatic events and their potential impact on her weight trajectory.

In addition to trauma, her current social support system is essential to her assessment and treatment plan formulation. It is important to revisit the notion of matching social support with patient need. In Wallwork and Tremblay's chapter, the concept of social supports providing emotional or affective, information and instrumental assistance is important to delineate based on the patient's need. For Ms. A, there appears to be an absence of emotional or affective support, and this may be an area for the psychologist and dietician to explore in the context of their assessments. While social supports may encourage behavioural changes suggested by the interprofessional weight management team, Wallwork and Tremblay also identify the potential for being sources of stress. An inventory of existing supports, such as friends or family members, who may be sabotaging her weight management efforts is critical and can inform problem-solving around these difficult social interactions. There may also be a role for peer supports and support groups to supplement Ms. A's treatment with the weight management center.

What is the relationship between Ms. A's increased depressive symptoms and their effect on weight gain?

As noted in previous chapters, obesity has an established bidirectional relationship with depression and more generally, mood disorders [2, 3]. Further, shared neuropsychological deficits between obesity (and other metabolic disorders) and depression reinforce this association [4]. A careful history of the temporal onset of depressive symptoms and the course of Ms. A's obesity over her lifetime can elucidate potential associations between these two conditions. Additional variables, for example, education status, body image concerns, and binge eating, may also mediate this relationship between depression and obesity and warrant further clinical assessment during Ms. A's follow-up care.

In assessing Ms. A's decline in mood, consideration of atypical depression and symptoms of overeating should also be part of the assessment. Secondary symptoms of overeating and binge eating could be a result of her active depressive symptoms, and with appropriate treatment of her depression she may regain control over eating patterns and behaviours. Moreover, if Ms. A is contemplating bariatric surgery, as outlined in the chapter by Gondek, poorly controlled major depressive disorder would be a concern and reason to delay bariatric surgery at this time given the potential impact active depression could have on post-operative weight-loss and psychiatric sequalae post-surgery. Therefore, early intervention in terms of depression management is imperative to supporting Ms. A's weight loss.

What is the relationship between Ms. A's stress at work and its effect of her emotional eating?

As highlighted in the eating disorders chapter (see Chap. 10), further assessment of behavioural, cognitive, and affective components of eating disorders is a first step. Research described in previous chapters has shown the relationship between emotional distress and the inability to regulate this affective distress as a predictor of emotional and binge eating [5, 6]. It should be clarified if Ms. A has used eating to regulate her emotions throughout her life. In addition, it would be important to explore Ms. A's coping strategies in response to stress. She could benefit from assessment of her support network and potential opportunities to strengthen her supports and to expand her support network.

If her stress is persistent, cognitive behavioural therapy or mindfulness-based approach may improve Ms. A's affective regulation in the context of her problem eating. Components of cognitive behavioural therapy [7] and mindfulness-based eating awareness therapy (MB-EAT) [8] are outlined in previous chapters and the weight management programme psychologist could begin to introduce components of CBT and MB-EAT into individual treatment sessions. For example, the introduction of mindfulness may begin with "raisin exercise" and later proceed to integration of food diaries and thought records to make the link between thoughts, feelings, and eating behaviours.

How are Ms. A's antidepressant medications affecting her weight and how can this be addressed?

In McIntyre and Syeda's chapter, the propensity for some medications to increase weight gain is summarized. Ms. A is currently treated with paroxetine and based on studies; this medication could be impacting her weight gain [9]. Therefore, it is important to further assess the impact of this medication while considering the potential benefit. The following strategies could assist with determining whether switching from paroxetine is beneficial:

- ***What was her weight history after starting paroxetine and how did her weight change in the time following her antidepressant initiation?*** Mapping her weight and inquiring about other potential factors that could have contributed to weight changes can be helpful. As described earlier in Chap. 14 (Gougeon and Warwick chapter), it is important to use an empathic and non-judgemental approach to weight inquiry to build rapport during treatment.
- ***Are there any additional comorbidities that warrant treatment at this time?*** If so, there may be a possibility to consider parsimonious pharmacological alternatives that may address her depression and any additional co-occurring conditions. If other psychiatric comorbidities such as binge eating disorder are complicating her depression treatment, additional pharmacological and psychological interventions summarized in Chap. 10 (Wnuk, Van Exan, Hawa) should be considered.

What was her response to paroxetine and if relevant, what was her response to previous pharmacological trials?

Ms. A could have had failed trials with other antidepressants and perhaps paroxetine was the only agent that provided remission of her depressive symptoms. If alternatives with minimal weight gain potential, for example, bupropion, are suitable amidst Ms. A's presentation and comorbidities, a switch in her antidepressant may be indicated. If paroxetine was the only agent to stabilize a severe and difficult to treat depression course, the risk and benefit would have to be discussed with Ms. A in terms of continuing with this medication and additional weight-loss interventions, such as psychotherapy, would have to be examined. If Ms. A decides with the team to proceed with a malabsorptive bariatric surgery procedure then the potential pharmacokinetic changes post-surgery as outlined by Bingham and Yanofsky's chapter should be discussed.

What effects do Ms. A.'s obstructive sleep apnea and her non-adherence to apnea treatment have on her psychological well-being and weight management?

Lee and Hawa outline some of the options that are available to help Ms. A with treatment for her sleep apnea beyond CPAP as well explore the potential links between apnea, sleep disruption, and obesity and diabetes. It is imperative to explore the barriers to her apnea treatment as well identify the enablers to increase her adherence to treatment. Educating Ms. A about the medical consequences of untreated sleep apnea in terms of increased cardiovascular and neurological events and the potential of improving or clearing her apnea post weight loss might help engage the patient in coming up with options for treatment and increase the chances of success in following up with the treatment.

How can Ms. A's care be organized to provide an integrated care approach to her severe obesity and psychiatric management?

Within the weight management center, Ms. A would ideally be seen by a team member who could conduct the intake assessment and initial screening. The use of depression questionnaires, such as Patient Health Questionnaire-9 (PHQ9), with screening cut-offs established in bariatric patient populations can assist with case identification [10]. Eating disorder measures as highlighted in the eating disorder chapter could also be used to provide a baseline for eating psychopathology and to inform stepped care interventions. Identification of depressive symptoms and related eating psychopathology could activate algorithms for Ms. A's depression treatment involving medications with reduced metabolic risks and based on guideline concordant care [3]. With respect to Ms. A's eating psychopathology, the assessment of her eating disorder symptoms with clinical and self-report measures could assist in identifying her treatment need. Following this initial assessment, Ms. A would receive a stepped care approach to psychosocial care based on the severity of her symptoms:

Example of a stepped care approach to eating problems in severe obesity

Severity of eating problems	Non-pharmacological intervention	Pharmacological intervention
1	Psycho-education	–
	Nutrition group session	
	Peer Support Groups	
2	Online CBT	Psychologist/ Psychiatrist Assessment for Comorbidities
	Nutrition counselling	
3	In-person CBT or telephone-CBT	Pharmacological treatment for Binge Eating*
	MB-EAT Group	

CBT cognitive behavioural therapy, *MB-EAT* mindfulness-based eating awareness therapy

While this proposed model may provide benefit, Ms. A's care should generally include an interprofessional team-based approach consisting of a range of team members with expertise in treating physical and mental health in the context of obesity.

24.3 Summary and Future Directions

The above case is an example of the biopsychosocial approach to severe obesity management when psychiatric comorbidity is present. We know that psychiatric comorbidity and general psychosocial burden is the rule rather than the exception. This book emphasizes the need for an integrated understanding of patients' physical and mental health issues in order to effectively develop a multifaceted treatment plan that can be personalized to patients. We were deliberate in grounding this book in patients' experience and the two courageous stories early in this book exemplify the challenges and opportunities to support patient resiliency in the context of severe obesity.

It is clear that there is a growing evidence base for the pathoetiology of the relationship between obesity and mental illness. Moreover, this association is linked to several biological, psychological, and environmental mechanisms that must be considered when assessing patients with severe obesity and comorbid mental health conditions. It is evident from the research that further studies are needed to clearly elucidate risk factors and causal mechanisms linking mental health and obesity. Additional research on the impact on the relationship between bariatric surgery and mental health is needed to more accurately identify risk factors for psychiatric sequalae post-surgery, such as eating disorders and de novo addictive disorders. Longitudinal studies are needed to examine long-term psychiatric trends and opportunities for psychosocial intervention.

Furthermore, we have summarized a range of pharmacological and psychological treatments for mental health and addictions in the context of severe obesity that can be personalized to patients in clinical practice. The next wave of research will need to expand on these initial studies with more rigorous clinical trials and examination of predictors of treatment response. Improving access to these evidence-based treatments will also need to incorporate novel technology in order to address the burden of obesity more broadly.

Lastly, the previous chapters have underscored the centrality of an interprofessional approach to psychosocial care in severe obesity. While there is an emergence of integrated care models and an established evidence base for these integrated care programmes, specific research in non-surgical and surgical settings are needed to clearly study and articulate an evidence based model for severe obesity care. As more treatment interventions are shown to have effect, it will be important to examine stepped care approaches that match patients' mental and physical health needs.

The role of psychiatric care in severe obesity management is no longer debatable. Mental health professionals and general practitioners need to be equipped with skills in nutrition counselling, knowledge about obesity-related medical comorbidities, and obesity treatment options to effectively care for their patients given the strong association between mental health and obesity. If severe obesity management is going to succeed, thoughtful integration of psychosocial assessment and care is needed. Through this comprehensive review of the current state of psychiatric care in severe obesity, we hope clinicians are better equipped to better address the challenges so clearly articulated by our patients.

References

1. Auspitz M, Cleghorn MC, Azin A, Sockalingam S, Quereshy FA, Okrainec A, et al. Knowledge and perception of bariatric surgery among primary care physicians: a survey of family doctors in Ontario. Obes Surg. 2016;26(9):2022–8.
2. Preiss K, Brennan L, Clarke D. A systematic review of variables associated with the relationship between obesity and depression. Obes Rev. 2013;14(11):906–18.
3. McIntyre RS, Alsuwaidan M, Goldstein BI, Taylor VH, Schaffer A, Beaulieu S, et al. The Canadian Network for Mood and Anxiety Treatments (CANMAT) task force recommendations for the management of patients with mood disorders and comorbid metabolic disorders. Ann Clin Psychiatry. 2012;24(1):69–81.
4. Mansur RB, Brietzke E, McIntyre RS. Is there a "metabolic-mood syndrome"? A review of the relationship between obesity and mood disorders. Neurosci Biobehav Rev. 2015;52:89–104.
5. Shakory S, Van Exan J, Mills JS, Sockalingam S, Keating L, Taube-Schiff M. Binge eating in bariatric surgery candidates: the role of insecure attachment and emotion regulation. Appetite. 2015;91:69–75.
6. Taube-Schiff M, Van Exan J, Tanaka R, Wnuk S, Hawa R, Sockalingam S. Attachment style and emotional eating in bariatric surgery candidates: the mediating role of difficulties in emotion regulation. Eat Behav. 2015;18:36–40.
7. Cassin SE, Sockalingam S, Wnuk S, Strimas R, Royal S, Hawa R, et al. Cognitive behavioral therapy for bariatric surgery patients: preliminary evidence for feasibility, acceptability, and effectiveness. Cogn Behav Pract. 2013;20(4):529–43.
8. Kristeller JL, Wolever RQ. Mindfulness-based eating awareness training for treating binge eating disorder: the conceptual foundation. Eat Disord. 2011;19(1):49–61.
9. Dent R, Blackmore A, Peterson J, Habib R, Kay GP, Gervais A, et al. Changes in body weight and psychotropic drugs: a systematic synthesis of the literature. PLoS One. 2012;7(6):e36889.
10. Cassin S, Sockalingam S, Hawa R, Wnuk S, Royal S, Taube-Schiff M, et al. Psychometric properties of the Patient Health Questionnaire (PHQ-9) as a depression screening tool for bariatric surgery candidates. Psychosomatics. 2013;54(4):352–8.

Appendix: Sample Bariatric Surgery Clinical Assessment Measures

Toronto **B**ariatric **I**nterprofessional **P**sychosocial
Assessment of **S**uitability **S**cale (BIPASS™)

Sockalingam S, Hawa R 2015 ©

P Patient's Name: ______________________________

Assessors: ______________________________

EXCLUSION CRITERIA

- ☐ **Smoking** ______________________
- ☐ **Active substance use disorder or problem substance use** ______________________
- ☐ **Uncontrolled/severe active psychiatric illness** ______________________
- ☐ **Impaired cognitive functioning** ______________________

SUMMARY OF BIPASS™ SCORING

Section	Question	Score
A. Patient's Readiness Level	#1	
	#2	
	#3	
	#4	
	Section Total	**/ 18**
B. Social Support System	#5	
	#6	
	Section Total	**/ 12**
C. Psychiatric Illness	#7	
	#8	
	#9	
	#10	
	#11	
	Section Total	**/ 30**
D. General Assessment Features	#12	
	#13	
	#14	
	Section Total	**/ 15**
BIPASS TOTAL SCORE	____ **/ 75**	

S. Sockalingam, R. Hawa (eds.), *Psychiatric Care in Severe Obesity*,
DOI 10.1007/978-3-319-42536-8

Toronto **B**ariatric **I**nterprofessional **P**sychosocial **A**ssessment of **S**uitability **S**cale (BIPASS™)

Sockalingam S, Hawa R 2015 ©

Score Interpretation

☐ 0–16 **GREEN – Candidate for Surgery at this Time**

- Recommend for surgery; no reservations

☐ >16 **YELLOW – Candidate Requires Surgical Delay at this Time**

- Delay for surgery until concerns are satisfactorily addressed as per interprofessional team before reviewing patient for reconsideration.

☐ **RED - Meets Exclusion Criteria for Bariatric Surgery**

- Not suitable for bariatric surgery at this time; see exclusion criteria

STOPBang Questionnaire for Obstructive Sleep Apnea

Is it possible that you have … Obstructive Sleep Apnea (OSA)?

Please answer the following questions below to determine if you might be at risk by circling yes or no.

Yes	No	**Snoring?**
		Do you Snore Loudly (loud enough to be heard through closed doors or your bed partner elbows you for snoring at night)?
Yes	No	**Tired?**
		Do you often feel Tired, Fatigued, or Sleepy during the daytime (such as falling asleep during driving or talking to someone)?
Yes	No	**Observed?**
		Has anyone Observed you Stop Breathing or Choking/Gasping during your sleep?
Yes	No	**Pressure?**
		Do you have or are being treated for High Blood Pressure?
Yes	No	**Body Mass Index more than 35 kg/m²?**
Yes	No	**Age older than 50?**
Yes	No	**Neck size large? (Measured around Adams apple)**
		For male, is your shirt collar 17 in./43 cm or larger?
		For female, is your shirt collar 16 in./41 cm or larger?
		Or: Is your neck circumference >40 cm or 16 in.?
Yes	No	**Gender = Male?**

For General Population

OSA—Low Risk: Yes to 0–2 questions

OSA—Intermediate Risk: Yes to 3–4 questions

OSA—High Risk: Yes to 5–8 questions

or Yes to 2 or more of 4 STOP questions + male gender

or Yes to 2 or more of 4 STOP questions + BMI > 35 kg/m^2

or Yes to 2 or more of 4 STOP questions + neck circumference 17 in./43 cm in male or 16 in./41 cm in female

Modified from

Chung F et al. Anesthesiology 2008; 108: 812–821,

Chung F et al. Br J Anaesth 2012; 108: 768–775,

Chung F et al. J Clin Sleep Med Sept 2014.

Index

S. Sockalingam, R. Hawa (eds.), *Psychiatric Care in Severe Obesity*,
DOI 10.1007/978-3-319-42536-8

N

O

T

Printed by Printforce, the Netherlands